# Questions & Answers
*in*
# Medical Physiology

# Questions & Answers
*in*
# Medical Physiology

**Sabyasachi Sircar**
M.D., M.A.M.S.
Reader, Department of Physiology,
University College of Medical Sciences,
Delhi - 110095 (India)

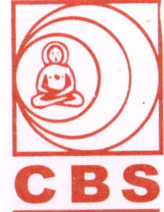

**CBS**

# CBS Publishers & Distributors Pvt. Ltd.
New Delhi • Bengaluru • Chennai • Kochi • Kolkata • Mumbai
Hyderabad • Nagpur • Patna • Pune • Vijayawada

ISBN: 81-239-1036-3

**First Edition: 2003**
Reprint: 2011, 2017

Published by **Satish Kumar Jain** and produced by **Varun Jain** for

**CBS Publishers & Distributors Pvt. Ltd.,**
4819/XI Prahlad Street, 24 Ansari Road, Daryaganj, New Delhi - 110002
delhi@cbspd.com, cbspubs@airtelmail.in • www.cbspd.com
Ph.: 23289259, 23266861, 23266867 • Fax: 011-23243014

*Corporate Office:* 204 FIE, Industrial Area, Patparganj, Delhi - 110 092
Ph: 49344934 • Fax: 011-49344935
E-mail: publishing@cbspd.com • publicity@cbspd.com

*Branches:*
- *Bengaluru:* 2975, 17th Cross, K.R. Road, Bansankari 2nd Stage,
  Bengaluru - 70 • Ph: +91-80-26771678/79 • Fax: +91-80-26771680
  E-mail: cbsbng@gmail.com, bangalore@cbspd.com
- *Chennai:* No. 7, Subbaraya Street, Shenoy Nagar, Chennai - 600030
  Ph: +91-44-26681266, 26680620 • Fax: +91-44-42032115
  E-mail: chennai@cbspd.com
- *Kochi:* Ashana House, 39/1904, A.M. Thomas Road, Valanjambalam,
  Ernakulum, Kochi • Ph: +91-484-4059061-65
  Fax: +91-484-4059065 • E-mail: cochin@cbspd.com
- *Kolkata:* 6-B, Ground Floor, Rameshwar Shaw Road, Kolkata - 700014
  Ph: +91-33-22891126/7/8 • E-mail: kolkata@cbspd.com
- *Mumbai:* 83-C, Dr. E. Moses Road, Worli, Mumbai - 400018
  Ph: +91-9833017933, 022-24902340/41 • E-mail: mumbai@cbspd.com

*Representatives:*

- Hyderabad: 0-9885175004
- Patna: 0-9334159340
- Vijayawada: 0-9000660880
- Nagpur: 0-9021734563
- Pune: 0-9623451994

*Printed at:*
Neekunj Print Process, Delhi (India)

# Apologia

Legend has it that when bandit *Ratnakar*, who later became saint *Valmiki*, was first asked to chant the name of Lord *Rama*, he failed to utter the word. In a clever move, *Brahma* asked him to chant the mantra *'mara'* meaning 'the dead'. As Ratnakar chanted *ma-ra-ma-ra*, he slowly succeeded in uttering '*Ra-ma-Ra-ma*' and went on to compose the *Ramayana*! There thus seems to exist a divine sanction for a morbid mantra when the malady is grave and the intent noble, not to mention the marvel that can be wrought when the teacher is ingenious.

Was it nature or nurture that made a bandit of *Ratnakar*? Nurture for sure, as his subsequent transformation confirmed. As for what makes our students scramble for an examination-oriented book of questions and answers, one has only to look at the syllabus, the time allotted, the overlaps and incongruities with complementary subjects, the quality of teaching and the nature of examinations.

A question-answer book is generally a forbidden word in the lexicon of teachers and its author is often accused of peddling a shortcut to success. However, it will continue to remain a favorite of students so long as the syllabus outline remains fuzzy and examination questions remain stereotype. Never an advocate of impromptu studies myself, I offer this book, an abridged textbook in the garb of a question-answer book, only as a tonic to the overburdened students, hoping that it would whet their appetite and encourage them to discover the joy of the wholesome intellectual diet offered by comprehensive textbooks.

**AUTHOR**

# Contents

## CARDIOVASCULAR SYSTEM

## RESPIRATORY SYSTEM

## EXCRETORY SYSTEM

## GASTROINTESTINAL SYSTEM

## METABOLISM AND NUTRITION

## ENDOCRINE SYSTEM

## REPRODUCTIVE SYSTEM

## CENTRAL NERVOUS SYSTEM

## SPECIAL SENSES

# *Principles of Physical Chemistry in Physiology*

## What is the Gibbs-Donnan equilibrium?

When two solutions of different strengths are separated by a permeable membrane, their concentration on both sides of the membrane equalizes due to diffusion of the solutes as well as the solvent. However, if there is an impermeable solute in one of the solutions, the concentration of the solutions do not equalize (Fig. 1.1). The final concentration of the solutions in such a situation is governed by the **Gibbs Donnan equilibrium**. One of the consequences of the Gibbs-Donnan equilibrium is that the *concentration of the solution with impermeable solutes remains higher even at equilibrium.*

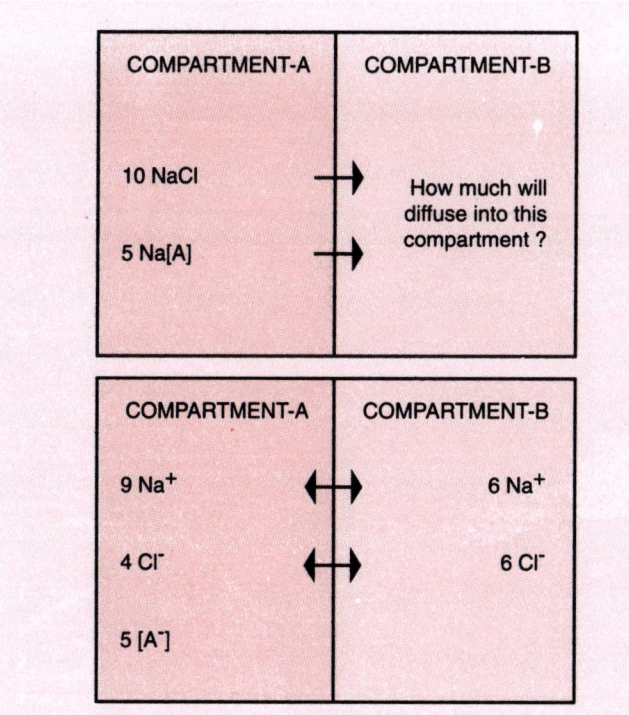

**Fig. 1.1**

Cells contain impermeable protein anions. Hence, its equilibrium with the extracellular fluid (ECF) is of the Gibbs-Donnan type. Thus, the intracellular fluid (ICF) always has a higher concentration of solutes than the ECF. This results in continuous osmosis of fluids into the cell, which threatens to burst the cell. To survive, the $Na^+$-$K^+$ pump in the cell membrane continuously pumps out excess cations.

## Define the terms osmoles, osmolarity and osmolality.

One mole of osmotically active particles is called one **osmole** (osm).

Thus, a molar solution of glucose contains 1 osmole, a molar solution of NaCl contains 2 osmoles (1 mole of $Na^+$ and 1 mole of $Cl^-$) while a molar solution of $CaCl_2$ contains 3 osmoles (1 mole of $Ca^{2+}$ and 2 moles of $Cl^-$).

The osmolar concentration of a solution (in osm/L) is called osmolarity. When expressed in osm/Kg of solution, it is called **osmolality**. Unlike **osmolality, osmolarity** is affected by temperature, which changes the volume of solution. Also, dissolution of solutes is associated with a slight rise in the volume of the solution. This increase is different for different solutes. Hence, when 1 mole of glucose is dissolved in 1 L of water, the osmolarity will be slightly less than 1 osm/L.

## Define tonicity.

When a membrane with unknown characteristics separates two solutions, osmosis may or may not occur between them. If no osmosis occurs, the two solutions are called **isotonic**. If osmosis occurs, then the solution that imbibes water is said to be **hypertonic** with respect to the other which is called **hypotonic**.

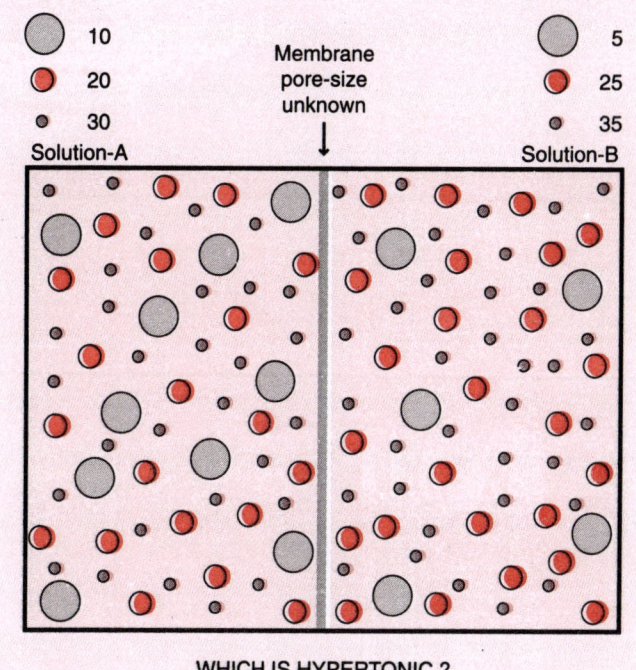

WHICH IS HYPERTONIC ?

**Fig. 1.2**

## Explain why two isoosmotic solutions are not necessarily isotonic.

Osmotic pressure depends on the total number of ions while tonicity depends on the total number of *permeable* ions. Two isoosmotic solutions have equal number of ions but not necessarily an equal number of *permeable* ions. In other words, toxicity depends on the membrane characteristics. In the example shown in Fig. 1.2, solution A will be hypotonic if the membrane is impermeable to all the molecules. Solution A will be hypertonic if the membrane is impermeable only to the largest molecules. The two solutions will be isotonic if the membrane is impermeable to the large and medium sized molecules.

## What is the osmolarity of 0.9% NaCl solution?

The osmolarity of 0.9% NaCl solution is approximately 300mOsm\L, as can be shown in the following calculations:

100 mL of 0.9% NaCl solution contains 0.9g of the NaCl.

∴ 1L of 0.9% NaCl solution contains 9g of NaCl.

The molecular weight of NaCl is 58.5.

∴ 58.5g of NaCl is equal to 1 mole of NaCl.

∴ 9g of NaCl is equal to $1/58.5 \times 9$ moles, i.e. 0.154 mole or 154 millimoles.

However, each mole of NaCl releases 2 osmoles: one osmole of $Na^+$ and one osmole of $Cl^-$. Thus, the osmolarity of 1 L of 0.9% NaCl solution is 308 mOsm ($154 \times 2$).

# The Cell & Intracellular Junctions

### Define a cell organelle.

An organelle is defined as a subcellular entity that is *membrane-limited* and can be *isolated by centrifugation* at high speeds. It includes the nucleus, mitochondria, endoplasmic reticulum, Golgi apparatus, peroxisome, lysosome and the plasma membrane. The *nucleolus, ribosomes and cytoskeleton proteins are not membrane-bound and therefore not organelles.*

### What is the function of the Golgi apparatus?

It is concerned with post-translational modification and packaging of secretory proteins into membranous vesicles.

### What are the functions of microsomes?

Microsome is another name for the **smooth endoplasmic reticulum** (ER). It is the *site of steroid synthesis* in steroid-secreting cells. Cells secreting steroid hormones like the testis and the ovaries are rich in smooth ER. It is also the *site of detoxification* of drugs and poisons in other cells, specially, liver cells. In skeletal and cardiac muscle, the smooth ER is called the **sarcoplasmic reticulum**. It stores $Ca^{2+}$ in high concentration and plays an important role in muscle contraction.

### What are the functions of peroxisomes?

Peroxisomes are *cellular storehouses of metabolic enzymes*. The peroxisome catalyzes a variety of anabolic and catabolic reactions. Peroxisomes in the liver detoxify alcohol and other harmful compounds.

### What are the functions of lysosomes?

A lysosome is a membranous bag containing **hydrolytic enzymes** that the cell uses to digest macromolecules. Lysosomes bud off from the Golgi apparatus. Some of the *granules of the granulocytic white blood cells* are lysosomes. Phagocytic vacuoles fuse with the lysosome, whose enzymes digest the phagocytosed matter. The lysosomes also engulf worn-out components of the cell in which they are located, forming *autophagic vacuoles*, and returns the digested products for reuse by the cell. When a cell dies, lysosomal enzymes cause **autolysis** of the remnants. Programmed cell destruction by lysosomal enzymes is often important in the process of development. For example, in the embryonic stage, the hands are webbed till lysosomes digest the tissues between the fingers. Small amounts of enzymes that leak out of lysosomes into the cytosol normally get inactivated due to the absence of acidic pH. However, large leakages cause tissue destruction. In gout, phagocytes ingest uric acid crystals and such ingestion triggers the extracellular release of lysosomal enzymes, which contribute to the inflammatory response in the joints.

### Compare and contrast microtubules and microfilaments.

**SIMILARITIES**

Both are made of protein subunits.

Both maintain the structure of the cell and also permit it to change shape and move.

Both are long polymers that move about by depolymerization at one end (the plus end) and polymerization at the other (the minus end).

Both serve as 'railroads' on which certain proteins called 'molecular motors' can 'walk'.

Both lend some amount of structural solidity to the cell.

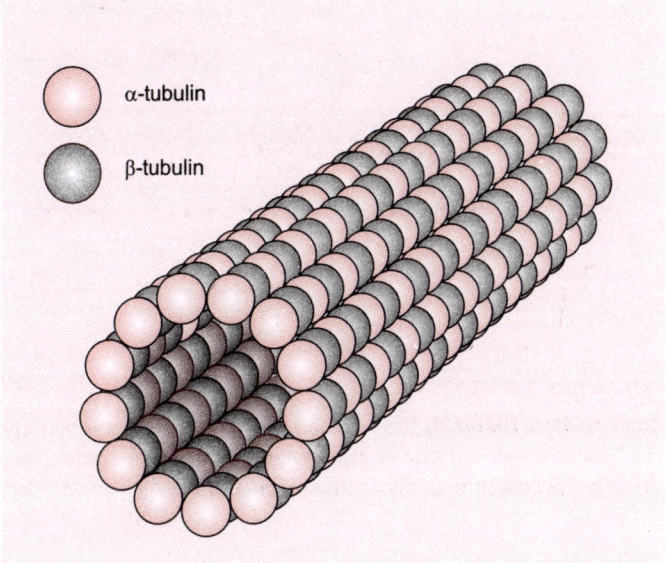

α-tubulin

β-tubulin

**Fig. 2.1**

**DIFFERENCES**

| Microtubules (Fig. 2.1) | Microfilaments (Fig. 2.2) |
| --- | --- |
| Tubular strucrures with a central lumen (~15nm in diameter). | Filamentous structures. |
| 20 nm in diameter. | 3-5 nm in diameter. |
| Made up of **α tubulin** and **β tubulin** subunits that form stacks of rings containing 13 subunits. | Made up of **G-actin** that are polymerized into two **F-actin** strands. The strands are coiled helically. |

| | |
|---|---|
| The 'molecular motors' are **kinesin** and **dynein.** | The 'molecular motor' is myosin. |
| Form the spindle, which moves the chromosomes in mitosis. | When a cell divides, it is pinched into two by a constricting band of microfilaments. |
| Transport secretory granules, vesicles, and mitochondria from one part of the cell to another. | Abundant at the *desmosomes* and *zonulae adherentes* (intercellular junctions). |
| | Abundant in *lamellipodia,* and in the core of intestinal microvilli. |
| | Microfilaments (actin) in skeletal muscle bring about contraction. |

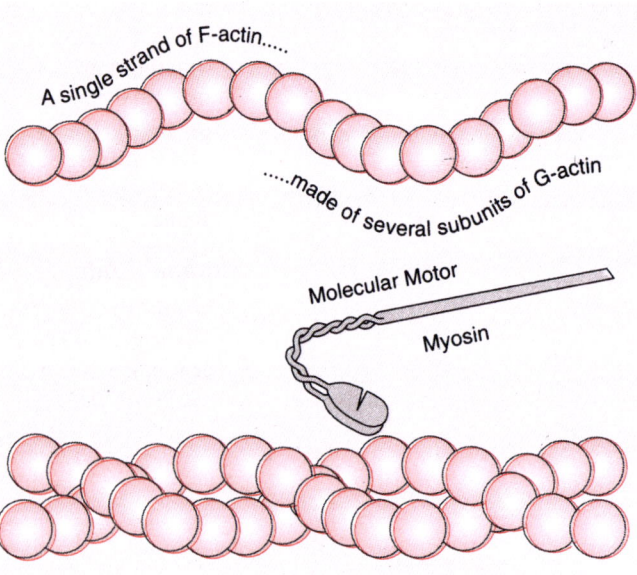

**Fig. 2.2**

### What are the other types of filaments found in the cell?

**Intermediate filaments** have a diameter (8 – 10 nm) that is between (i.e., intermediate to) that of microtubule and microfilament. They are more abundant than either microtubule or microfilament. They are made of **cytokeratin**. Unlike microtubule or microfilaments, these proteins are very stable and remain mostly polymerized. They serve as the 'bones' of the cell, giving structural strength to the cell. For example, the nucleus sits in a cage made of intermediate filaments. In axons, the intermediate filaments are called **neurofilaments**. They maintain the axonal diameter.

### What are the filamentous structures in the cell?

The filamentous structures include the centrioles, cilia and flagella. All are hollow cylindrical structures with microtubules running in their wall longitudinally.

### Name the different types of intercellular junction.

The different types of intercellular junctions (Fig. 2.3) are: (i) zona occludens (or tight junction), (ii) zona adherens, (iii) desmosome (or macula adherens) and (iv) gap junctions.

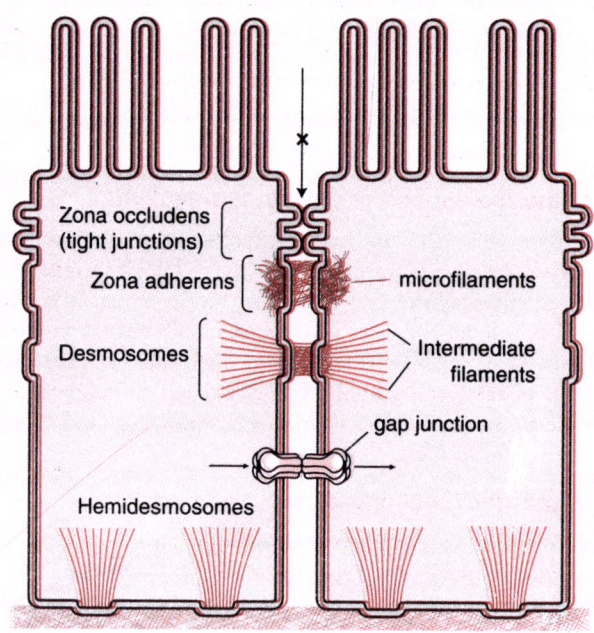

**Basal Membrane**

**Fig. 2.3**

# Composition & Structure of the Cell Membrane

## What are the constituents of cell membranes?

Membranes are complex structures composed of lipids, proteins, and carbohydrates. The major membrane lipids are **phospholipids**, **glycosphingolipids**, and **cholesterol**. Membrane phospholipids are broadly of two types: **phosphoglycerides**, which are relatively more abundant, and **sphingomyelins**, which is prominent in myelin sheath. Membrane glycosphingolipids include **cerebrosides** and **gangliosides**. Both are derivatives of sphingosine.

## Briefly describe the structure of the membrane.

Membrane lipids exist as **closed bilayers** in which the hydrophobic regions of the phospholipids are protected from the aqueous environment, while the hydrophilic regions are immersed in water. Membranes contain two types of proteins: integral proteins and peripheral proteins. **Integral proteins** are anchored to membrane through a direct interaction with the lipid bilayer. **Peripheral proteins** are weakly bound to the hydrophilic regions of specific integral proteins. They are located on both surfaces of the membrane.

## What are the functions of membrane proteins?

**Integral proteins** serve as: (i) *channels* that permit the passage of selected ions through the membrane; (ii) *carriers* (or transporters) that ferry substances across the membrane by binding to them; (iii) *pumps* that are carriers which can split ATP and use the energy derived for membrane transport of substrates; (iv) *receptors* (located on the outside) which bind to specific molecules and send a chemical signal to the cell interior, initiating intracellular reactions; (v) *enzymes*, catalyzing reactions at the membrane surfaces – both outer and inner. **Peripheral proteins**: (i) serve as *cell adhesion molecules* (CAM) that anchor cells to neighboring cells to the basal lamina; (ii) contribute to the *cytoskeleton* when present on the cytoplasmic side of the membrane.

## What are the factors affecting membrane fluidity?

The fluidity of a cellular membrane depends on the *lipid composition of the membrane*, the *density of integral proteins*, and the *temperature*. The presence of **cholesterol** in the membrane makes it possible for the cell membrane to *maintain its fluidity across a wide range of temperatures*.

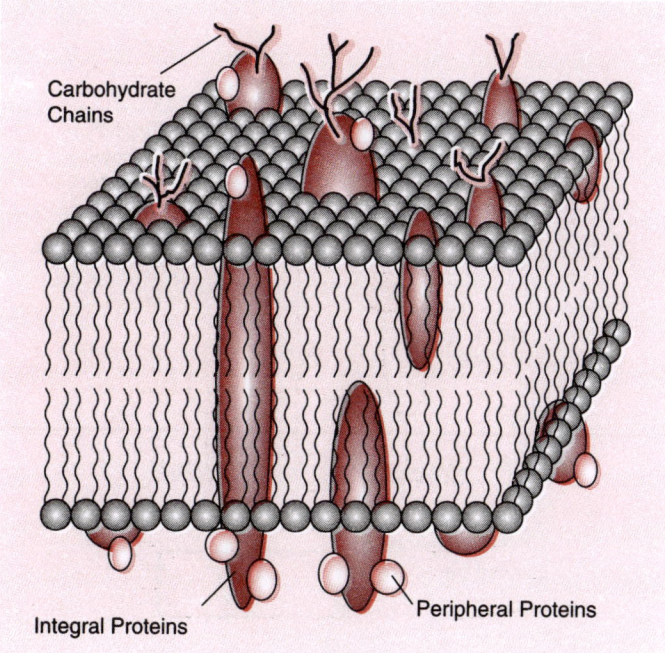

Carbohydrate Chains

Integral Proteins

Peripheral Proteins

**Fig. 3.1**

# Membrane Transport & Membrane Channels

**Compare and contrast simple diffusion and facilitated diffusion.**

**SIMILARITIES**

Neither of them involves energy expenditure and therefore, can occur only from a higher to a lower solute concentration.

Both are bidirectional, i.e., can occur in either direction depending on the concentration gradient.

**DIFFERENCES**

| Simple diffusion | Facilitated diffusion |
|---|---|
| The rate of simple diffusion is directly proportional to the concentration gradient across the membrane and the permeability of the membrane to the solute. | The rate of facilitated diffusion is governed by the kinetics of carrier-mediated transport and cannot exceed a certain maximum, called the *Vmax* (Fig. 4.1). However, at low concentration gradients, its rate is higher than in simple diffusion. |
| Examples of simple diffusion include diffusion of gases across the respiratory membrane and diffusion of solutes from blood to the cells through the interstitial spaces. | Examples of facilitated diffusion are: (i) the *cotransport* of $Na^+$ with sugars (glucose, galactose, fructose) and amino acids in renal tubular cells and intestinal mucosal cells, and (ii) the *counter-transport* of $Cl^-$—$HCO_3^-$ in renal tubular cells and gastric parietal cells. |

**Compare and contrast facilitated diffusion and primary active transport.**

**SIMILARITIES**

Both of them are carrier-mediated transport, the rate of which cannot exceed a certain maximum called the Vmax. The rate depends on three factors: (i) the concentration gradient across the membrane; (ii) the amount of carrier available (this is a key control step); and (iii) the rapidity of bonding and dissociation of the carrier with its substrate.

**DIFFERENCES**

| Facilitated diffusion | Primary active transport |
|---|---|
| It is bidirectional, i.e., can occur in either direction depending on the concentration gradient. | It is unidirectional: the direction of transport depends on the disposition of the carrier in the membrane. |
| It can never occur against a concentration gradient. | It can occur against a concentration gradient. It can build up a concentration gradient where there is none initially. |

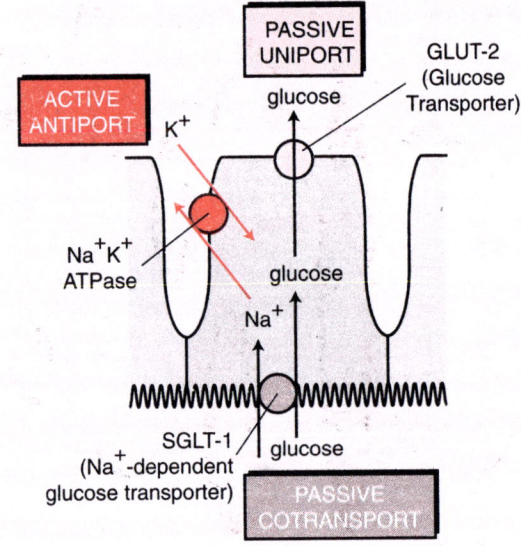

**Fig. 4.2**

**What is secondary active transport?**

Secondary active transport represents a combination of primary active transport and facilitated diffusion. The primary active transport builds up a concentration gradient, which in turn

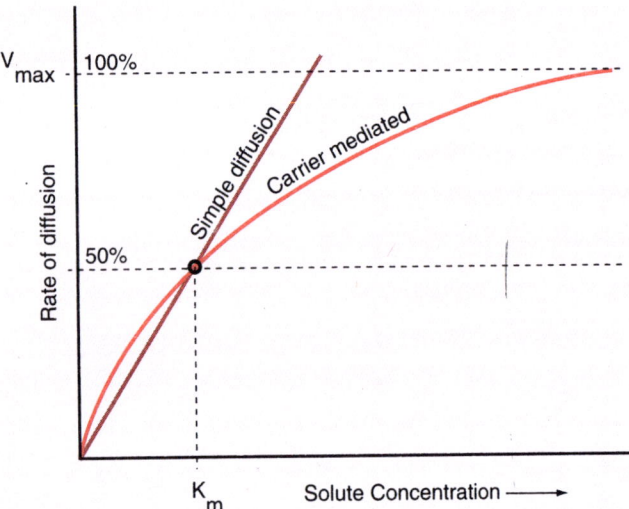

**Fig. 4.1**

provides energy for facilitated diffusion. It is exemplified by glucose transport across renal tubular cells or intestinal mucosal cells.

## What are the different types of membrane channels?

Depending on the factor(s) that produce their opening and closing (gating), ion channels are classified into four types: the **voltage-gated channels** that are gated by changes in membrane potential; the **ligand-gated channels** that are regulated by ligands, i.e., chemicals that bind to it; the **mechanically gated channels** that are ion channels whose pore responds to mechanical stimuli like stretch; and **resting channels** that are not gated at all.

## Briefly outline the ping-pong model of carrier-mediated transport.

The carriers for membrane transport are integral membrane proteins. In carrier-mediated transport, the *carriers do not move*

*through the thickness of the membrane*, carrying its substrate with it. Rather, a **ping-pong mechanism** is proposed. In this model, the carrier protein exists in two principal conformations: ping and pong. In the *pong state*, it is exposed to high concentrations of solute, and molecules of the solute bind to specific sites on the carrier protein. Transport occurs when the conformation changes to the *ping state*, exposing the carrier to a lower concentration of solute. In facilitated diffusion, the energy for the transition between the ping and pong states comes from the binding of the substrate to the carrier. In active transport, additional energy comes from the binding of ATP to the carrier.

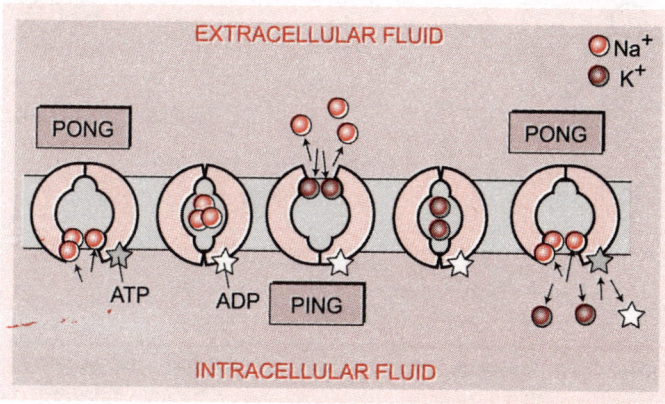

**Fig. 4.3**

# Mitosis, Meiosis & Apoptosis

### Define mitosis and name its stages.

Mitosis is a type of cell division in which each of the two daughter cells receives exactly the same number and the same kind of chromosomes contained in the parent cell. Mitosis occurs in five stages: **interphase**, **prophase**, **metaphase**, **anaphase** and **telophase**.

### What is mitotic chromosomal dysjunction and what are its consequences?

Non-separation of chromosomes (**chromosomal dysjunction**) results in abnormal mitosis. It usually occurs immediately after zygote formation and results in **mosaicism**. In mosaicism, the number of chromosomes is not the same in all the cells of the body. For example, nearly 50% of the body cell population may have a certain number of chromosomes while the remaining 50% may have a different number of chromosomes (*mosaic* = designs by inlaying small bits of colored stone, glass, tile, etc. in mortar). If half the cells in the body are 44 + XY and the remaining cells are 44 + XXY, the mosaicism is denoted symbolically as XY/XXY. Its mechanism is depicted diagrammatically in Fig. 5.1.

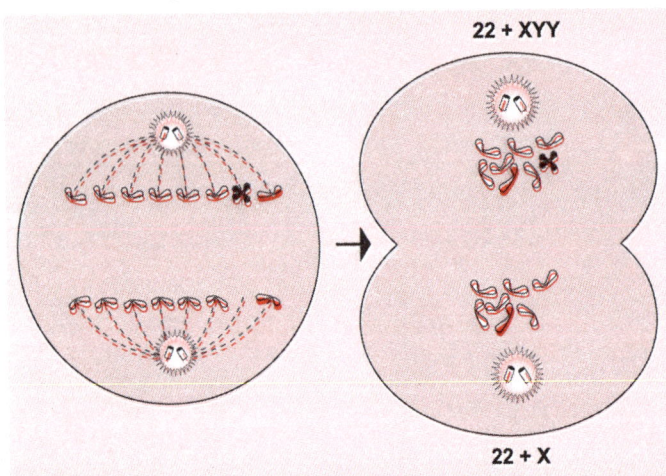

**Fig. 5.1**

### Define meiosis and name its stages.

Meiosis occurs during gamete formation (**spermatogenesis** and **oogenesis**). Like mitosis, it is preceded by the duplication of the chromosomes during interphase, but this duplication is followed by two successive cell divisions, **meiosis-I** and **meiosis-II**, both of which have the stages: interphase, prophase, metaphase, anaphase and telophase. *Meiosis-II is almost identical to mitosis.* The result is the formation of four haploid daughter cells.

### What is interkinesis?

The typical meiosis described above is seen only in the male. The

**primary spermatocyte** of the male forms two **secondary spermatocytes** (after meiosis-I) and finally four **spermatids** (after meiosis-II). Both stages of meiosis begin after puberty, and are completed within a few days. However, the prophase-I takes about 22 days – a disproportionately long time.

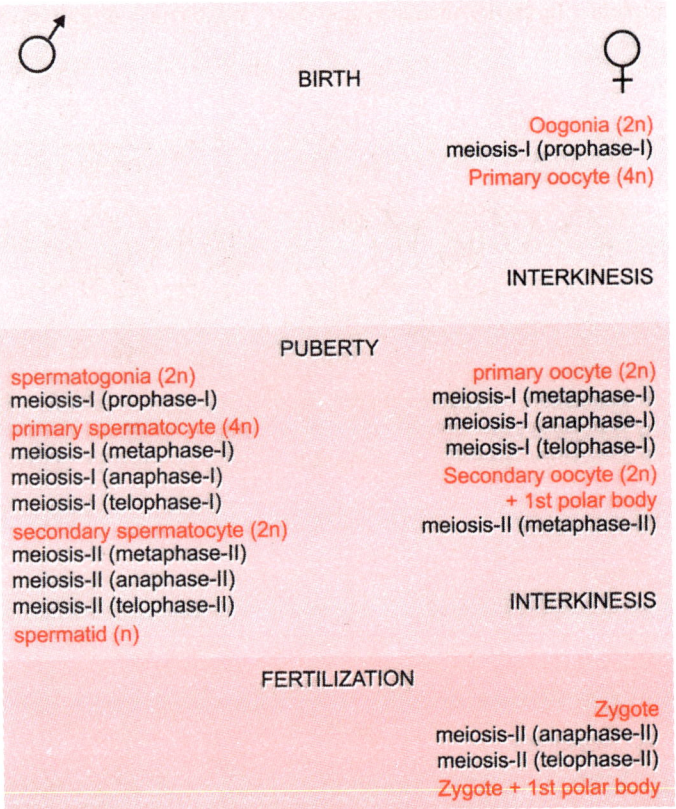

**Fig. 5.2**

In the female, however, there are long intervals (**interkinesis**) separating the different phases of meiosis, as shown in Fig. 5.2. Meiosis-I begins immediately after birth but gets arrested after prophase, only to resume after puberty. Meiosis-II also gets arrested in metaphase, only to be completed after fertilization. Moreover, in meiosis-I as well as in meiosis-II, the two daughter cells are not uniform in size: one gets most of the cytoplasm while the other gets little of it and is called the **polar body**. The polar bodies degenerate after sometime.

### What is meiotic chromosomal dysjunction?

Meiotic chromosomal dysjunction results in abnormal gametogenesis. In the classical form of **Klinefelter syndrome**, chromosomal dysjunction during meiosis results in formation of an abnormal ovum. When fertilized, the abnormal ovum results in a zygote with the chromosomal configuration of XXY. The mechanism through which the abnormal ovum is formed is depicted diagrammatically in Fig 5.3.

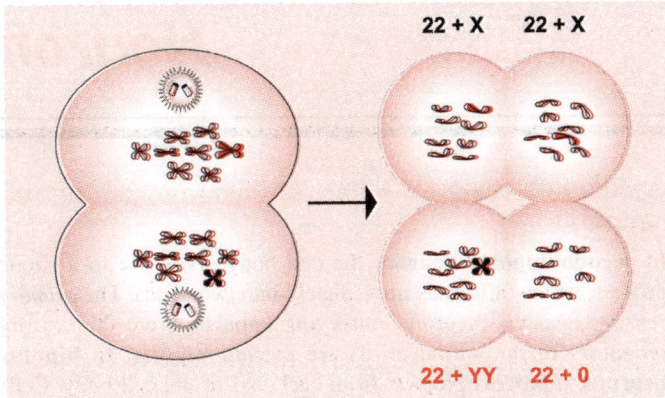

**Fig. 5.3**

## What is apoptosis? What are its phases?

Apoptosis is genetically programmed cell death that does not significantly affect neighboring cells and tissues. It is distinct from necrosis, which is an unregulated cell death destroying larger tissue areas. Apoptosis is responsible for: (i) death of intestinal mucosal cells as they reach the tip of the villus to be sloughed off; (ii) death of epidermal cells as they reach the surface; (iii) death of large number of neurons in the CNS that do not make appropriate synaptic contact with their target organs; (iv) death of clones of lymphocytes that are likely to react with 'self'; (v) removal of the webs between the fingers in fetal life; (vi) regression of one or the other of Wollfian duct and Mullerian duct systems in the course of sexual differentiation in the fetus; (vii) regression of incompletely developed Graafian follicles in ovary after ovulations; (viii) cyclic breakdown of the endometrium, leading to menstruation; (ix) lens protein 'crystalline' that is derived from the remnants of apoptotic cells.

The phases of apoptosis are induction, initiation, execution and disposal. The **induction phase** is the stage of gene activation. Several endogenous and exogenous stimuli activate the apoptotic genes through signal transduction. In the **initiation phase**, the activated gene initiates a proteolytic cascade involving a family of proteases named *caspases* (cysteine aspartase). In the **execution phase** completes the death program. The dying cell shrinks and loses its contact with neighboring cells. The cell DNA gets fragmented and the cytoplasm and chromatin condense. The nucleus and cytoplasm eventually fragment into multiple, small apoptotic bodies (*karyorrhexis*). The cytoplasmic blebs break away from the cell surface and eventually the entire cell breaks up (*karyolysis*). In the **disposal phase**, the cell remnants, called *apoptotic bodies*, are either phagocytosed, or are lost from the epithelial surfaces.

### Define a dendrite and an axon. How does conduction in a dendrite differ from that in an axon?

The axon is the single long process of the cell body. Dendrites are the multiple cell processes which branch extensively immediately after taking root from the soma. (It is wrong to define axon as the process carrying impulses *away from* the cell body. For example, the peripheral processes of the dorsal root ganglion are axons that carry impulses *towards* the cell body.) Axons conduct action potentials. *Dendrites usually do not produce action potentials:* they mostly conduct graded potentials.

### Compare and contrast peripheral and central myelination.

| SIMILARITY | |
|---|---|
| Both types of myelination are brought about by neuroglial cells that encircle the axon forming around it a thin sleeve (Fig. 6.1). | |

| DIFFERENCES | |
|---|---|
| Peripheral myelination occurs in the peripheral nervous system | Central myelination occurs in the central nervous system |
| The myelin sheath is produced by neuroglial cells called Schwann cells. | Myelination is made by a type of neuroglial cell called the oligodendrocyte. |
| A Schwann cell myelinates a single neuron. | An oligodendrocyte can myelinate 10 – 60 axons. |

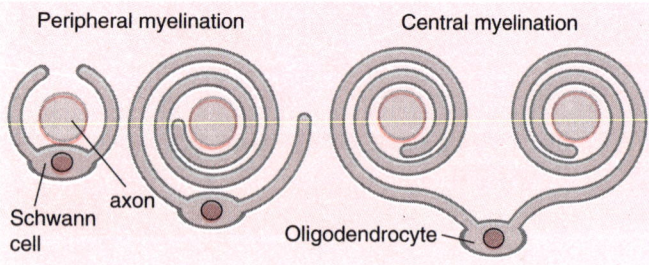

**Fig. 6.1**

### What are Golgi Type-I and Type-II neurons?

Large cells with long axons are called **Golgi type-I** neurons or **projection neurons**. They include the neurons forming peripheral nerves and long tracts of the brain and spinal cord. Small neurons with relatively short axon are called **Golgi type-II** neurons or **local circuit neurons**. They are usually small and especially numerous in the retina, cerebral cortex and cerebella cortex.

### What are pseudounipolar, bipolar and multipolar neurons?

In **pseudounipolar neuron**, the cell body gives rise to a single process, which bifurcates immediately into two axons. The *primary sensory neurons* (neurons conveying impulses from the sensory receptors to the spinal cord) are pseudounipolar. In **bipolar neurons**, a process projects from each end of the cell body. Cells of this type are found in the *vestibular* and *cochlear ganglia* and in the *nasal olfactory epithelium*. A **multipolar neuron** gives rise to numerous dendrites and usually a single axon. Most neurons in the brain are multipolar (Fig. 6.2).

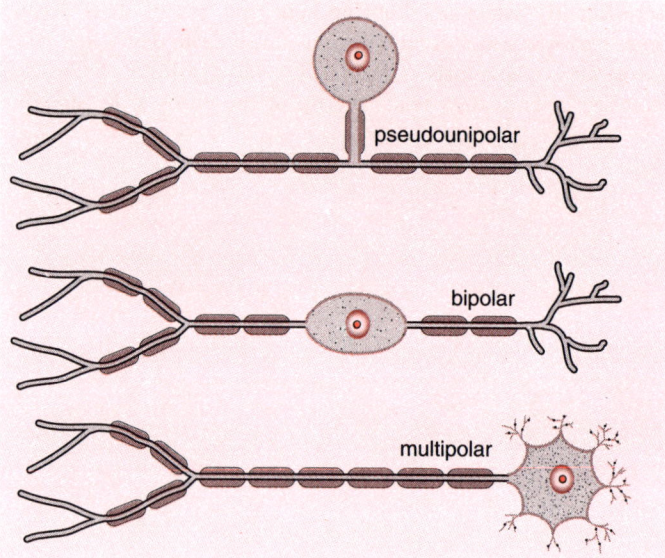

**Fig. 6.2**

### What are the 3 different types of synaptic vesicles?

There are 3 types of synaptic vesicles: (i) small, clear vesicles containing acetylcholine, glycine, GABA or glutamate; (ii) small, dense-core vesicles containing catecholamines; (iii) large, dense-core vesicles containing neuropeptides. In general, circular synaptic vesicles contain excitatory neurotransmitters while flat or elongated vesicles contain inhibitory neurotransmitters. Exceptions to the above rule include the neuropeptides and neurosecretory granules that are definitely produced in the cell body. In neurons that use biogenic amines as transmitters, large dense-cored vesicles can be seen in the cell body and traveling along the axon.

### Define a nucleus, a ganglion, a tract and a nerve.

An aggregation of neuronal cell bodies that is located inside the

CNS is called a **nucleus**. An aggregation of neuronal cell bodies that is located outside the CNS is called a **ganglion**. A compact bundle of axons located inside the CNS is called a **tract**. A compact bundle of axons located outside the CNS is called a **nerve**.

## Compare and contrast fast and slow axoplasmic transport.

### SIMILARITY

Both of them are concerned with transport of organelles and cell proteins between the cell body and the axon terminal.

### DIFFERENCES

| Fast axoplasmic transport | Slow axoplasmic transport |
| --- | --- |
| It has a velocity of 20 to 400 mm per day. | It occurs at 0.2—0.4 mm per day. |
| It may be anterograde or retrograde in direction. | It is always anterograde. |
| **Anterograde transport** moves membrane-bounded organelles like short tubules of reticulum, mitochondria, small vesicles, actin, myosin, and the clathrin used in recycling of synaptic vesicle membrane. **Retrograde transport** returns materials from the nerve terminals to the cell body for degradation or reuse. | It carries protein subunits of neurofilaments, tubulins of the microtubules, and soluble enzymes and also moves some cytosol with it. |
| It occurs along microtubules using molecular motors **dyenin** (for retrograde transport) or **kinesin** (for anterograde transport) | The cytoskeleton moves as a whole due to continual polymerization at the leading end and depolymerization at the trailing end. The axoplasmic matrix moves with the cytoskeleton. |

# Muscle & Neuromuscular Junction

## Briefly describe the structure of a skeletal muscle fiber.

Skeletal muscle fibers are cylindrical and multinucleate. They are 10 – 30 cm in length – long enough to justify the term 'fiber'. They are formed by fusion of several smaller cells into a *multinucleate syncitium*. Skeletal muscles are so named because they are *attached to bones* by tendons and move these bones and the loads borne by them. They are the only muscles *under voluntary control*.

Like all other cells, the striated muscle fiber also has a cell membrane (called *sarcolemma*), a smooth endoplasmic reticulum (called *sarcoplasmic reticulum*), cytoplasm (called sarcoplasm) and *cytoskeletal proteins* which are of 3 types: (i) **Contractile proteins**: *myosin* and *actin*. These two proteins interact to generate the contractile force in a muscle. (ii) **Regulatory proteins**: *tropomyosin* and *troponin*. Also called the '*relaxation proteins*', these regulate the interaction between actin and myosin (Fig. 7.1). (iii) **Anchoring proteins**: $\alpha$-*actinin, titin, nebulin* and *dystrophin*. These proteins anchor the cytoskeletal proteins to each other as well as to the sarcolemma and the extracellular matrix.

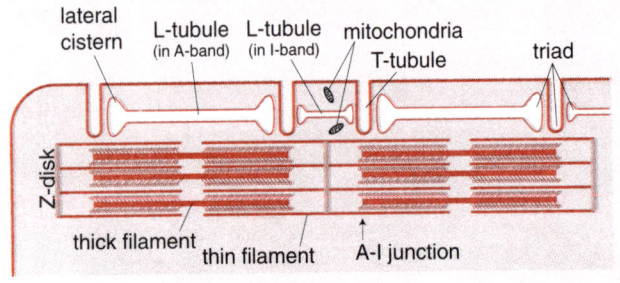

**Fig. 7.1**

The cytoskeletal proteins are disposed in a remarkably orderly configuration, which shows in gross morphology as striations, and on light microscopy as the **dark (A)** and **light (I)** bands. The **Z-line** is located in the middle of the I-band. The part of the muscle fiber that extends between two consecutive Z-lines is called a **sarcomere**, which is the *contractile unit of muscle* (Fig. 7.2).

## Describe the sarcoplasmic reticulum in a skeletal muscle.

In a muscle cell, parts of the sarcoplasmic reticulum run parallel to the length of the fiber (the longitudinal or **L-tubules**) while others are disposed radially, coursing from the surface towards the center of the fiber (the transverse or **T-tubules**). The transverse tubules are transverse invaginations of the sarcolemma into the cell. They typically occur *at the A-I junctions* in mammals (and at the Z disc in amphibians). Being extensions of the sarcolemma, the transverse tubules conduct the action potentials from the sarcolemma into

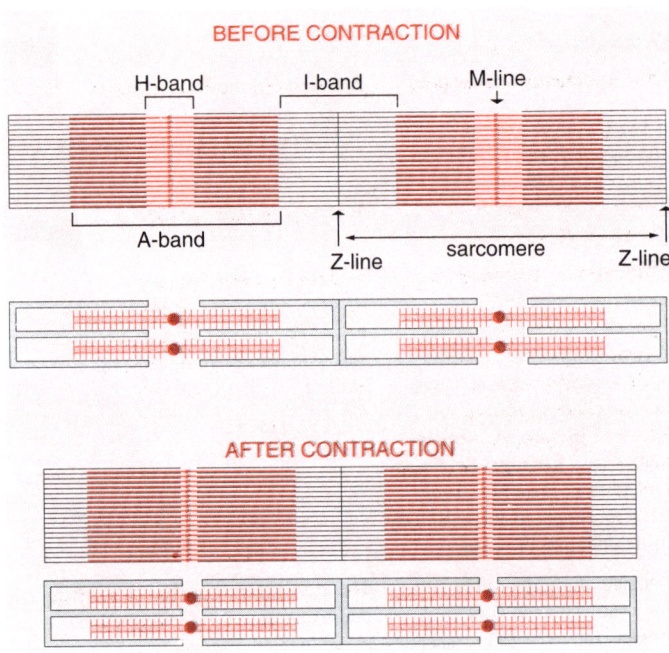

**Fig. 7.2**

the interior of the cell along its membranes. The longitudinal tubules are disposed longitudinally along the entire length of the A band. They end in dilated sacs called **lateral cisterns** (Fig. 7.1).

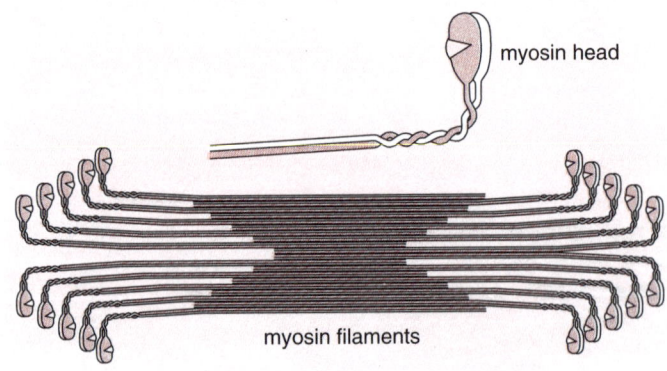

**Fig. 7.3**

## Describe the structure of the contractile filaments.

The **myosin filaments** (680 kDa) are thick and disposed longitudinally at the center of a sarcomere. It has a globular head and a fibrous tail. The fibrous tails are grouped into a bundle from which the globular heads called **myosin heads** project out (Fig. 7.3). The myosin heads have two special sites on them: (i) a site with ATPase activity (the myosin ATPase), and (ii) an actin-binding site.

The **actin filament** (F-actin) is a double helical filament. It is made of globular subunits called G-actin (43 kDa). In a sarcomere, actin filaments are attached at one end to the Z disc. During contraction, the actin filaments slide over myosin filament. This is made possible by the presence of active sites on the actin filament that bind to the myosin head.

**Tropomyosin** is a fibrous molecule that consists of 2 chains - α and β. It lies in the grove between the two filaments of actin. Each tropomyosin filament spans 7 G-actin subunits. It serves to cover and uncover the active sites of the actin molecules during muscle contraction and relaxation.

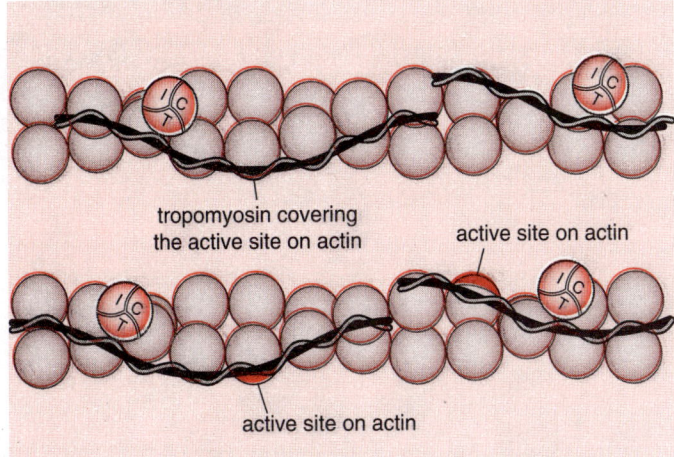

tropomyosin covering
the active site on actin

active site on actin

active site on actin

**Fig. 7.4**

**Troponin** is attached to tropomyosin. It has 3 subunits : (i) **Troponin-T** (TpT) binds to tropomyosin; (ii) **Troponin-C** (TpC) is a calcium-binding protein. Each molecule of TpC binds to 4 molecules of $Ca^{2+}$ ions; (iii) **Troponin-I** (TpI) prevents the interaction of the myosin heads with the active sites on actin when TpC is bound to $Ca^{2+}$. The inhibition occurs possibly due to the rolling of the tropomyosin molecule into a position that blocks the active sites (Fig. 7.4).

### Compare the structure of a smooth muscle fiber with that of a skeletal muscle fiber.

The sarcolemma show short invaginations into the cytoplasm called **caveoli**, which are analogous to the T-tubules in skeletal fibers (Fig. 7.5). There are several fusiform densities present in the cytoplasm (**cytoplasmic dense bodies**) and along the inner surface of the sarcolemma (**subsarcolemmal dense plaque**). The *ratio of actin and myosin* filaments is ~ 12:1 in smooth muscles compared to ~2:1 in skeletal muscles. The myosin filaments are biochemically different in skeletal and smooth muscles. In smooth muscles, the projecting heads of the myosin molecules, which form cross-bridges to the surrounding actin filaments are found along their entire length, whereas thick filaments of skeletal muscle have a bare central segment that is devoid of cross-bridges. The regulatory proteins tropomyosin and troponin that are present in skeletal muscle are absent in smooth muscle. Instead, smooth muscles contain **calmodulin**, which is analogous to troponin.

### Briefly describe the structure of a neuromuscular junction in skeletal muscle.

As the axon supplying a skeletal muscle fiber approaches its termination, it loses its myelin sheath. The axis cylinder then branches into a number of bulb-shaped endings called **terminal buttons**. The terminal buttons contain many small, synaptic vesicles containing acetylcholine (ACh). The terminal buttons come in close proximity with a thickened trough on the muscle membrane called the **motor end plate**, which bears receptors for ACh. The end plate is thrown into folds called the **junctional folds**. The 25 nm wide space between the terminal button and the motor end plate is called the **myoneural cleft**. The cleft is filled with the **basal lamina**, which contains the enzyme *acetylcholinesterase (AchE)*. The part of the terminal button membrane from which synaptic vesicles are released is called the **prejunctional membrane**. The part of the endplate membrane where the ACh receptors are located is called the **postjunctional membrane**.

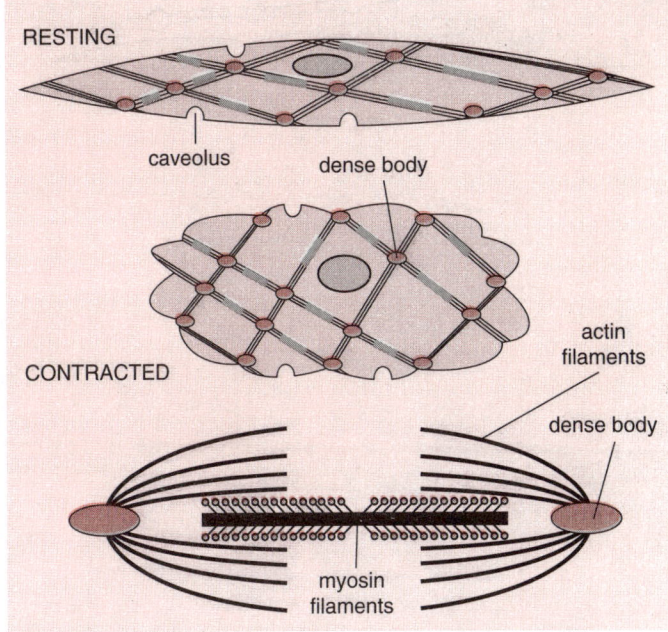

RESTING

caveolus

dense body

actin
filaments

CONTRACTED

dense body

myosin
filaments

**Fig. 7.5**

### What is meant by the term synapse enpassant?

Unlike the motor end plate of a skeletal muscle fiber, smooth muscles do not show any specialization at its site of contact with the axon. The axon innervating smooth muscle does not end at the site of innervation. Rather, it shows multiple swellings or varicosities along its course that liberate neurotransmitters. Each axon forms multiple junctions with muscle cells along its passage – the *synapse en passant* (Fig. 7.6). This is unlike in skeletal muscle where the neuron must branch to innervate multiple fibers.

### What are the transmitters released at the synapse enpassant?

The varicosities release either *acetylcholine* or *norepinephrine*. This is unlike the axonal ending in skeletal muscle, which releases only acetylcholine.

### What is the difference between contact junction and diffuse junction?

In multi-unit smooth muscles, the varicosities come in close contact with individual cells forming **contact junctions**. Here, the

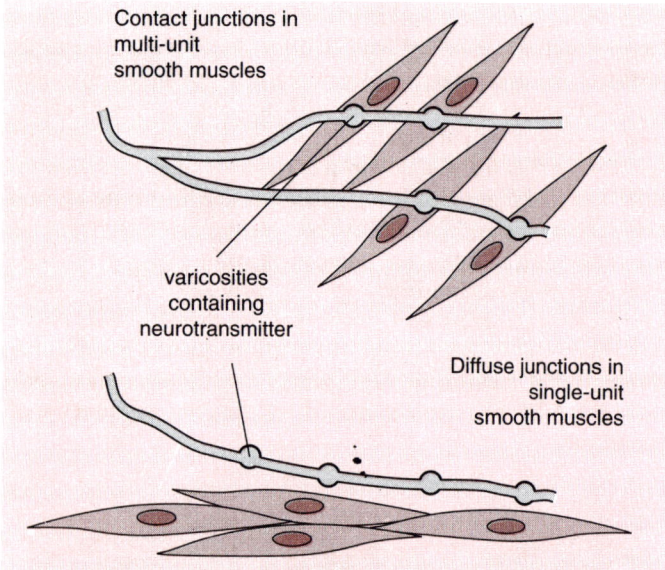

Contact junctions in
multi-unit
smooth muscles

varicosities
containing
neurotransmitter

Diffuse junctions in
single-unit
smooth muscles

**Fig. 7.6**

muscle membrane is separated from the varicosity by a gap of ~25 nm, the same as in a neuromuscular junction. Hence, the junctional delay (i.e., time taken for the impulse to travel from the neuron to the muscle membrane) is comparable to that in a neuromuscular junction of a skeletal muscle.

In single-unit smooth muscle, the varicosities do not come in close contact with any cell. Neurotransmitters from the varicosities diffuse away to reach all the muscle cells. This arrangement has been called a **diffuse junction**. The junction delay is considerably longer in diffuse junctions.

# Degeneration & Regeneration of Nerve & Muscle

## What are the salient changes associated with nerve degeneration?

When an axon is crushed or severed, it results in degeneration of the neuron both distal (anterograde) and proximal (retrograde) to the site of injury.

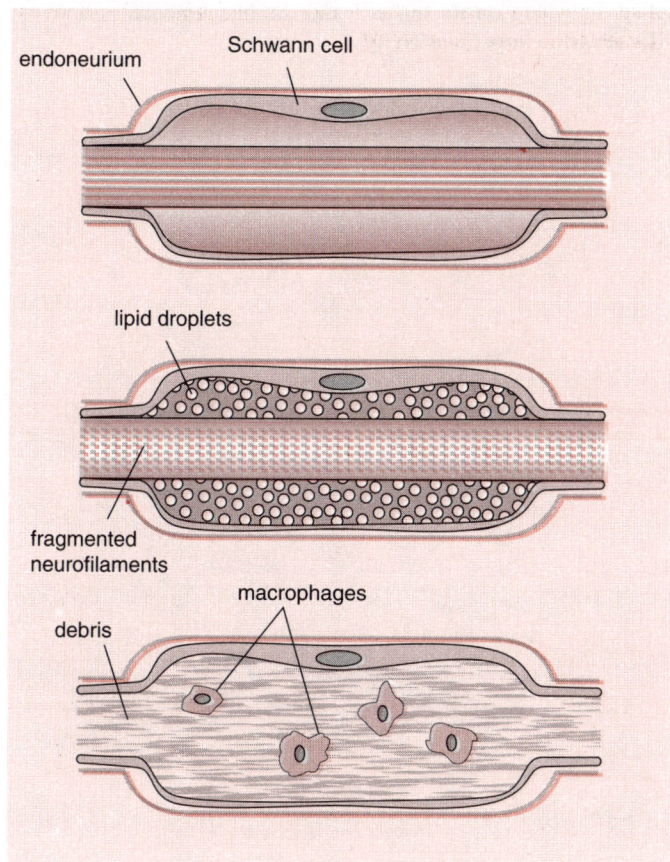

**Fig. 8.1**

*Anterograde degenerative changes* starts within 24 hours and is called **Wallerian degeneration**. The neurofilaments break up, and the axon breaks up into short lengths. *Within 10 days*, the myelin sheath breaks down into lipid droplets around the axon. *Within 30 days*, the myelin gets denatured chemically. *Within 3 months*, macrophages from the endoneurium invade the degenerating myelin sheath and axis cylinder and phagocytose the debris, leaving behind only the endoneurial tube (Fig. 8.1).

*Retrograde degenerative changes* affect the dendritic tree, the parent cell body and the part of the axon proximal to the lesion. Acute retrograde (**chromatolytic**) changes start after 24 hours

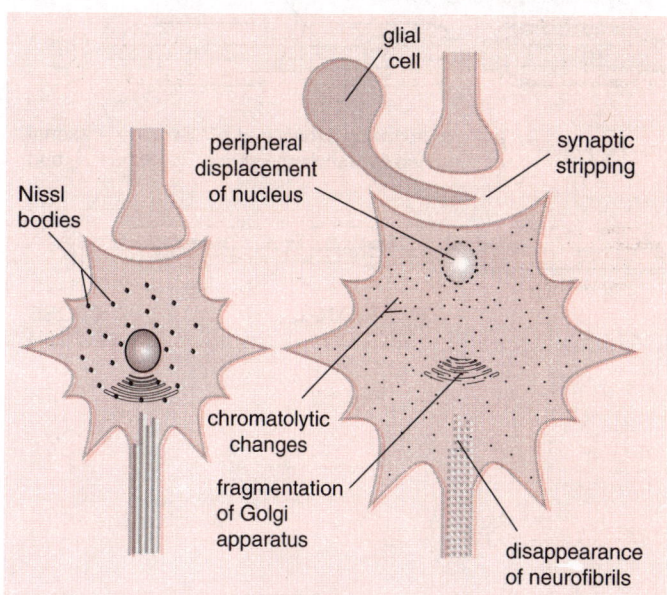

**Fig. 8.2**

and are characterized by the break up of the Nissl substance in the cell body (Fig. 8.2). Chronic retrograde atrophic response involves the atrophy of the nerve cell body with all its processes.

## What are the salient changes associated with nerve regeneration?

Nerve regeneration begins about 20 days after nerve section and is complete in 3 months. The Schwann cells at the site of injury multiply and grow at the rate of up to 1 mm per day, forming a solid cord of elongated cells (**band of Bungner**) within the endoneurial tube (Fig. 8.3). The plasmalemma of the Schwann cells and adjacent basal lamina separate creating an annular compartment between the Schwann cells and the endoneurium. Up to 100 axonal sprouts, each containing a neurofibril in it, grow out in all directions from the proximal axon. Some of them grow into the distal annular compartment. The daily rate of growth is up to 3—4 mm in the peripheral stump. Eventually all but one axonal sprout degenerate. The surviving fibril enlarges to fill the distal tube. The Schwann cells in the Band of Bungner form myelin sheath around the reinnervating axonal sprout. The sheath begins to develop in about 15 days and is completed in one year. The Nissl substance and Golgi apparatus gradually reappear. The cell regains its normal size and the nucleus returns to its central position.

## How are nerve injuries classified?

According to Seddon's classification, nerve injuries are of three types: (i) **neuropraxia**, which occurs due to minor nerve stretch

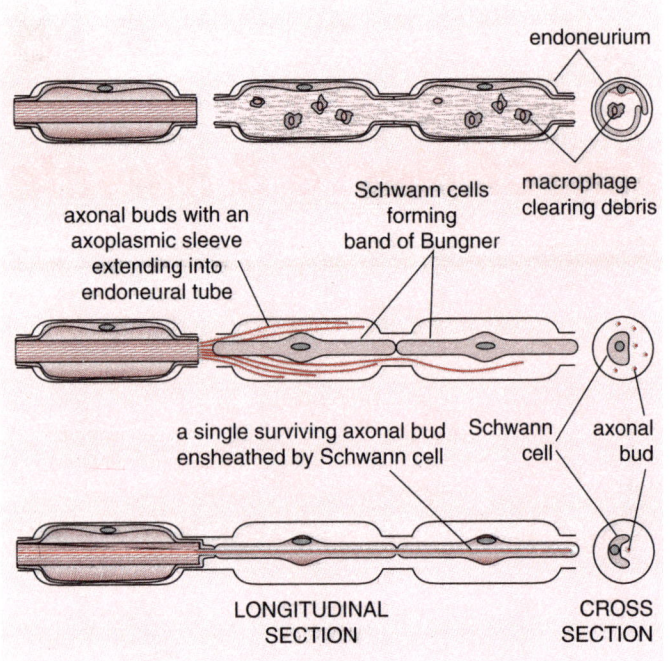

axonal buds with an
axoplasmic sleeve
extending into
endoneural tube

Schwann cells
forming
band of Bungner

macrophage
clearing debris

endoneurium

a single surviving axonal bud
ensheathed by Schwann cell

Schwann
cell

axonal
bud

LONGITUDINAL
SECTION

CROSS
SECTION

**Fig. 8.3**

or pressure causing ischemic injury to the nerve. It results in conduction block without causing any structural damage; (ii) **axonotemesis**, which occurs due to excessive stress injury to the nerve. It results in Wallerian degeneration. The basal lamina of Schwann cells and other sheaths are all intact, and (iii) **neurotemesis**, which as a result of penetrating injury to the nerve. All the sheaths are disrupted.

## What is denervation supersensitivity of muscle?

Each motor endplate contains about 50 million ACh receptors, which are highly concentrated near the mouths of the postjunctional folds. Few ACh receptors are located elsewhere on the muscle membrane (sarcolemma). Following section of a motor nerve, the ACh receptors (ACh-R) increase more than 10-fold in number and become dispersed over the entire surface of the sarcolemma. The muscle cell then becomes sensitive to ACh applied anywhere on its surface, and the phenomenon is known as **denervation supersensitivity**.

# Resting Membrane Potential

## What is the resting membrane potential?

The inner surface of the cell membrane is covered with a layer of anions while the outer surface is layered with cations. This makes the interior of the cell membrane negative with respect to its exterior. This potential difference is called the **resting membrane potential (RMP)**, which is especially marked in neurons and muscle cells. In a neuron, the RMP is about -70mV.

## How is the resting membrane potential (RMP) produced?

Whenever an ion diffuses across the membrane, it renders the membrane positive on one side and negative on the other. The polarity of this membrane potential depends on the direction of the diffusion and the charge carried by the ion. It also depends on the simultaneous diffusion of other ions. If an outward diffusion of cations is accompanied by an outward diffusion of equal amounts of anions or an inward diffusion of other cations, then no membrane potential will be produced. This rarely happens since all ions diffuse at different rates depending on their concentration gradients (Fig. 9.1). The resultant membrane potential is called the **resting membrane potential**. The ionic concentration gradients across the membrane (which drives the ionic diffusion) are created by the activity of the **Na⁺-K⁺ pump**. Hence, the pump is only indirectly involved in the production of the RMP, and the *inhibition of the pump does not immediately abolish the RMP*.

## How is the RMP calculated?

When a *single diffusible ion* is distributed asymmetrically across the membrane, its diffusion produces a diffusion potential, the magnitude of which can be calculated using the **Nernst equation.** This diffusion potential (Vm) produced by a single diffusible ion is called the **Nernst potential** of that ion.

$$Vm = \frac{61}{z} \log \frac{[C_o]}{[C_i]}$$

where $C_o$ and $C_i$ are the ionic concentration outside and inside the cell, and 'z' is the valence of the ion.

When *several diffusible ions* are distributed asymmetrically across a membrane, *each ion tries to drive the membrane potential towards its own Nernst potential*. The resultant diffusion potential (Vm) is called the **equilibrium potential of the membrane**. It is given by the **Goldman equation**

$$Vm = 61 \log \frac{P_K[K^+_o] + P_{Na}[Na^+_o] + P_{Cl}[Cl^-_i]}{P_K[K^+_i] + P_{Na}[Na^+_i] + P_{Cl}[Cl^-_o]}$$

where $P_K$, $P_{Na}$ and $P_{Cl}$ are the conductances (permeability) of K⁺, Na⁺ and Cl⁻ respectively.

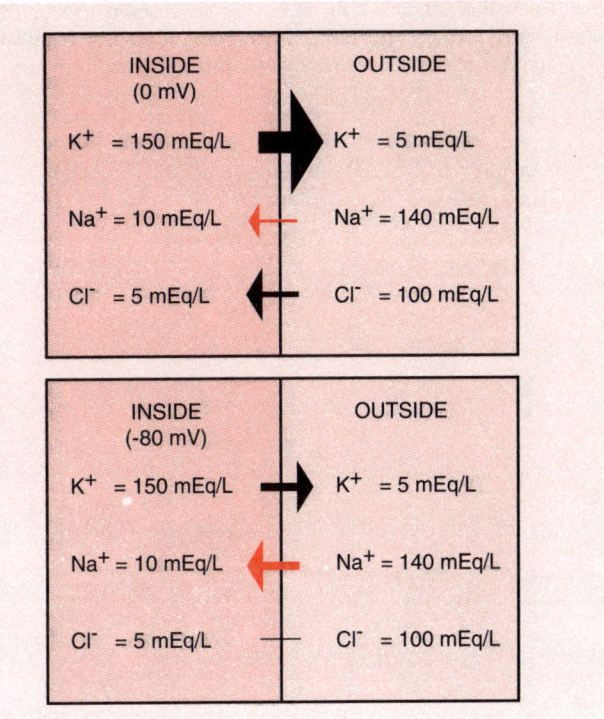

Fig. 9.1

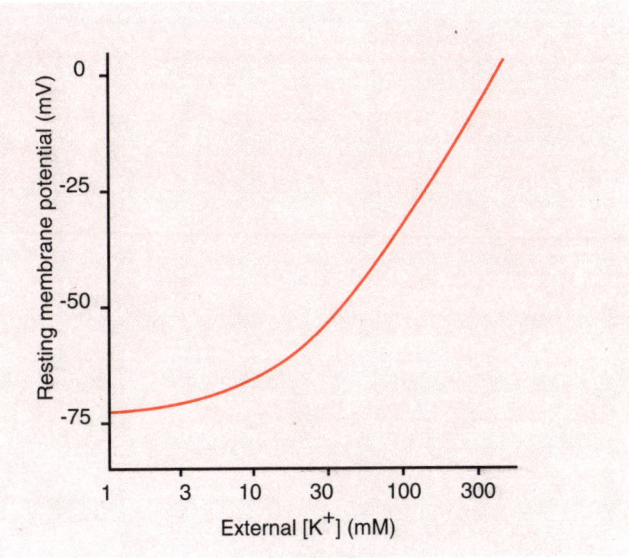

Fig. 9.2

## How does a change in ionic permeability affect the membrane potential?

When the permeability of the membrane to an ion increases, the membrane potential moves towards the Nernst potential of the same ion.

*Example:*

Suppose the membrane potential is –70mV, the equilibrium potential of Na$^+$ (E$_{Na}$) is +60mV and the equilibrium potential of K$^+$ (E$_K$) is –90mV. If the membrane permeability to Na$^+$ increases, the membrane potential will change from –70mV towards (but not up to) +60mV. In other words, the membrane will depolarize. If the membrane permeability to K$^+$ increases, the membrane potential will change from –70mV towards (but not up to) –90mV. In other words, the membrane will hyperpolarize.

## What is the effect of addition of KCl in the bathing fluid?

Addition of KCl (say, 5mEq/dl) to the bathing fluid of an excitable tissue will depolarize the membrane (Fig. 9.2).

# Membrane Excitation & Action Potential

## Describe the phases of action potential.

The action potential which is recorded using an intracellular electrode has 5 phases: (i) **Catelectrotonic potential.** Also called the pre-potential or the 'foot' of the action potential, this is a slow drift of the membrane potential towards –55 mV which is called the *threshold potential* or the *firing level*. (ii) **Depolarization.** The potential shoots up to +40 mV in less than a millisecond. The depolarization occurs only if the stimulus raises the membrane potential above ~ -55mV. The minimum strength of stimulus that can trigger an action potential is called a *threshold stimulus*. (iii) **Repolarization.** The potential drops to near resting levels, i.e. approximately – 40 mV. This phase also lasts less than a millisecond. (iv) **After-depolarization.** The rate of repolarization slows down and gradually reaches the resting potential of –70 mV. This slow phase of repolarization is called 'after-depolarization'. It lasts about 2 milliseconds. (v) **Hyperpolarization.** The intracellular negativity overshoots the normal resting value (which is –70mV) to reach a more negative value (about -75mV). It lasts for nearly 40 milliseconds before slowly returning to the normal resting potential of –70 mV (Fig. 10.1).

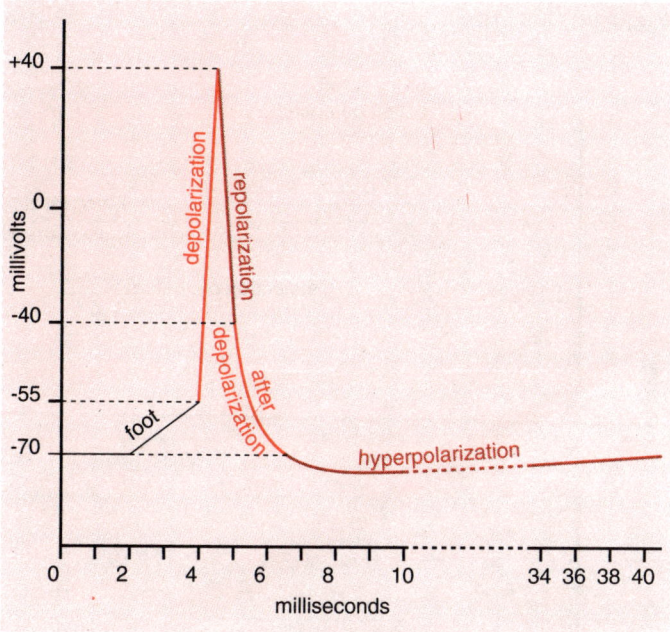

**Fig. 10.1**

## What is meant by the spike potential?

The depolarization and repolarization phases of the action potential together comprise the **spike potential** which serves as the actual neuronal signal. Although the total duration of the action potential is ~ 40 ms, the spike lasts only about 1ms.

## Describe the changes in membrane excitability during action potential.

The membrane is **refractory** (i.e. not responsive) to a second stimulus during most of the spike. From the spike onset till repolarization is about one-third complete, the membrane is **absolutely refractory** i.e. no stimulus howsoever strong can elicit a response. Thereafter, till the onset of after-depolarization, the membrane is **relatively refractory** i.e. a sufficiently high stimulus can elicit a response. During after-depolarization, the membrane is **hyperexcitable**. Having just come out of the refractory period, the membrane is fully excitable. Also, the membrane is closer to the firing level, which makes it hyperexcitable. During hyperpolarization, the membrane excitability is low but slowly returns to normal (Fig. 10.2).

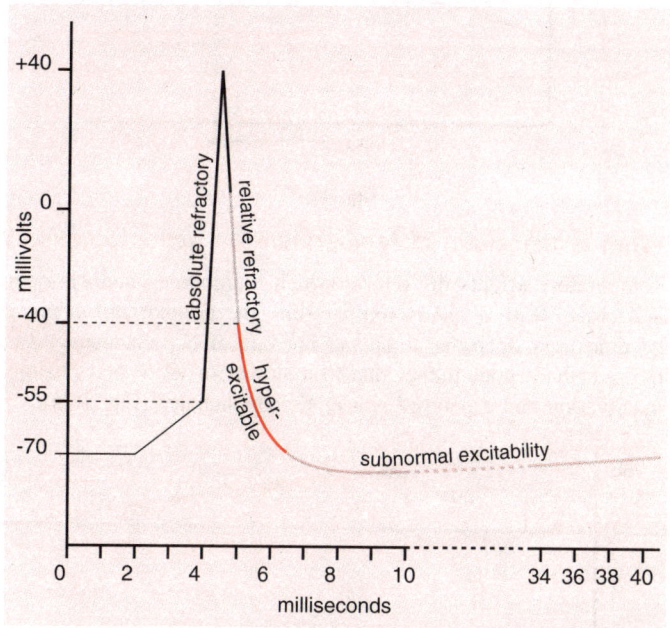

**Fig. 10.2**

## What is effective refractory period?

The **effective refractory period** (**ERP**) includes the absolute refractory period and the early part of the relative refractory period. At the end of ERP, the membrane is able to conduct physiologically produced action potentials. If the membrane is in the relative refractory period, the actions potentials are conducted slowly.

## Why is meant by the term all-or none law in relation to an action potential?

Each spike has a fixed amplitude of about 110 mV (–70 to +40mV). Subthreshold stimuli cannot trigger spikes. Conversely, all suprathreshold stimuli will trigger a full-fledged spike of 110mV. In other words, the magnitude of spike does not increase in a graded manner with the stimulus strength: it is either 110 mV (**all**) or 0 mV (**none**).

## Briefly explain the ionic basis of action potential.

Depolarization occurs due to a large increase in $Na^+$ permeability. Repolarization occurs due to a rise in $K^+$ permeability. Another cause of repolarization is **$Na^+$ channel inactivation**. Inactivation (closure) of $Na^+$ channels results in a fall in $Na^+$ permeability (Fig. 10.3).

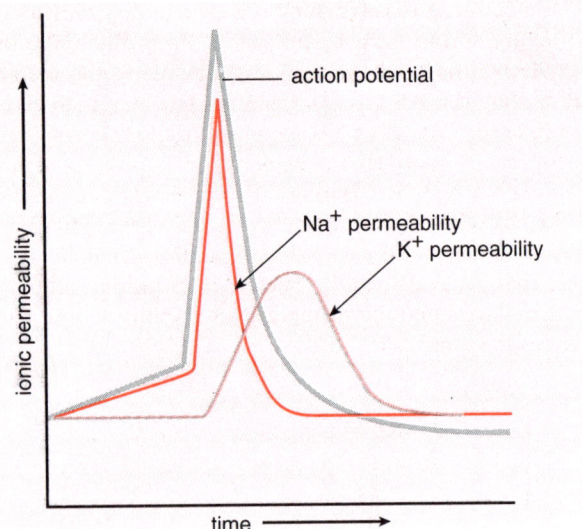

**Fig. 10.3**

## What is the effect of temperature on action potential?

Temperature affects the rate at which membrane channels open and close. With a fall in temperature, the depolarization phase becomes less steep due to slower opening of $Na^+$ channels. Also, the overshoot goes higher due to a slower onset of $Na^+$ channel inactivation and a delayed rise in $K^+$ conductance (Fig. 10.4).

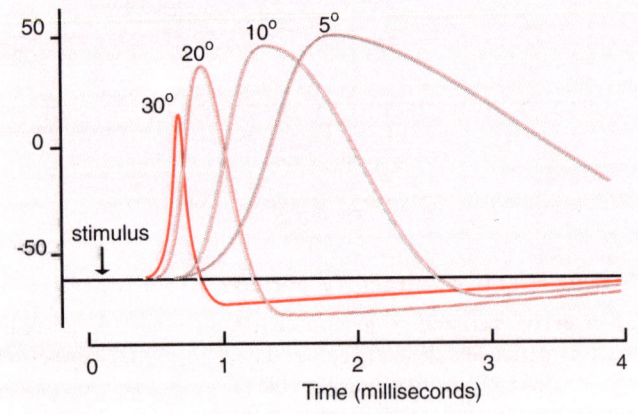

**Fig. 10.4**

## What is membrane accommodation? What is its mechanism?

When a catelectrotonic potential depolarizes the membrane rapidly to the firing level, an action potential is triggered off. However, when the catelectrotonic potential is made to depolarize the membrane slowly to the firing level, the action potential often fails to get triggered. This phenomenon is called **membrane accommodation** and is due to *$Na^+$ channel inactivation*.

When the membrane depolarizes, both $Na^+$ and $K^+$ channels open up. However, if the depolarization occurs very slowly, more and more $Na^+$ channels open up, only to get inactivated quickly. The $K^+$ channels remain open and tend to restore the membrane potential. By the time the potential touches the firing level, most of the $Na^+$ channels have got inactivated while the $K^+$ channels remain open. Therefore, the explosive depolarization fails to occur. If however the membrane depolarizes rapidly to the firing level, a large number of $Na^+$ channels open all at once. Before they get inactivated, they are able to trigger off the action potential by overcoming the effect of $K^+$ channels.

## What are catelectrotonic and anelectrotonic potentials?

When a cathode is brought near the external surface of the membrane, the internal surface of the membrane becomes positive in relation to the exterior. This depolarization induced by the cathode is called **catelectrotonic potential**. Similarly, an anode induces a hyperpolarizing **anelectrotonic potential**. Both types of *electrotonic potentials fade away as soon as the electrode is taken away from the membrane*. However, in case of the catelectrotonic potential, if the depolarization touches the firing level, a full-fledged action potential is triggered (Fig. 10.5).

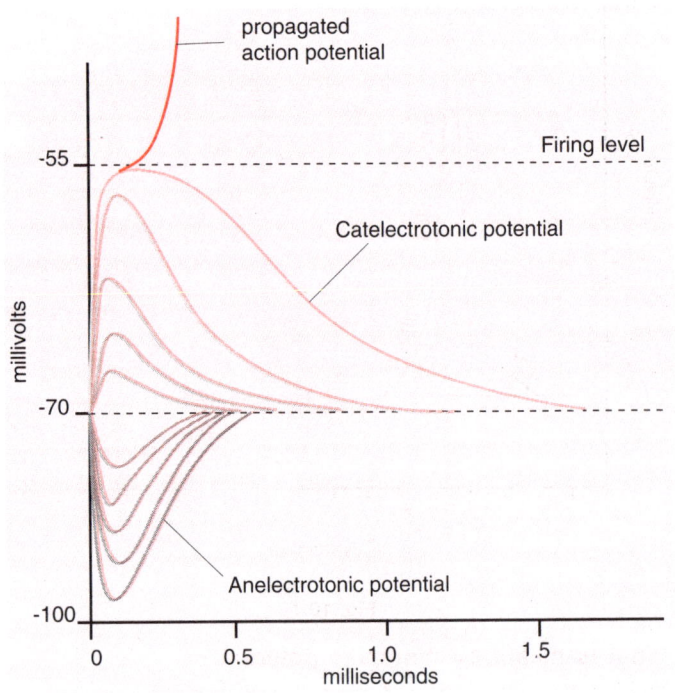

**Fig. 10.5**

## What are the differences between graded potentials and action potential?

| Graded potential | Action potential |
| --- | --- |
| Amplitude proportionate to stimulus strength and can get summated | Amplitude constant for all supra-threshold stimuli and cannot be summated |
| Can be a depolarization or hyperpolarization | Always a depolarization |
| Conduction is associated with reduction in amplitude | Conducted without reduction in amplitude |
| Can be generated spontaneously or in response to physical or chemical stimuli | Generated only in response to membrane depolarization |
| Examples are receptor potential and end plate potential. | Examples are the different types of action potentials recordable in skeletal, smooth (single-unit) and cardiac muscle fibers as well as neurons. |

## Describe the strength-duration curve and the indices derived from it.

The ease with which a membrane can be stimulated depends on two factors: the strength of a stimulus and the duration for which the stimulus is applied. As the strength of stimulus increases, the time required to excite the membrane decreases and *vice versa*. Any index of membrane excitability must therefore take into account both the above factors. Three such indices of membrane excitability are rheobase, utilization time and chronaxie. **Rheobase** is the theoretical minimum *current* of electrical stimulus which when applied for an *infinite length of time* will excite the membrane. **Utilization time** is the time taken by a stimulus of rheobase strength to excite the membrane. **Chronaxie** is the *time* required

to stimulate the membrane using *double the rheobase strength* of stimulus (Fig. 10.6).

Chronaxie is a practical index of membrane excitability. Its value ranges from 0.02 ms in the largest peripheral neurons (Aa) to a

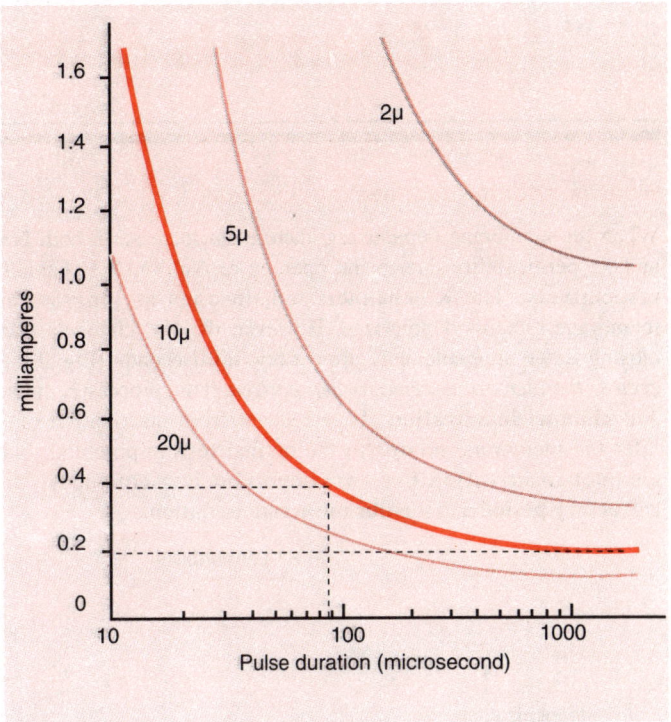

**Fig. 10.6**

maximum of 1.5 ms in the smallest C-fibers. A low chronaxie means greater membrane excitability. Serial measurements of chronaxie provide useful information regarding the progress of nerve healing following injury and surgical repair.

# Ion Channels & their Role in Action Potential

## What is sodium channel inactivation?

When the membrane depolarizes, there is an increase in both Na⁺ and K⁺ permeability due to the opening of Na⁺ and K⁺ channels respectively. The K⁺ channels remain open as long as the membrane remains depolarized. However, the Na⁺ channels start closing down spontaneously after a few milliseconds (Fig. 11.1) *even if the membrane remains depolarized*. This process is called **Na⁺ channel inactivation**. They recover from inactivation only after the membrane returns to the normal resting potential. Na⁺ channel inactivation has two important consequences: the **refractory period** and **membrane accommodation**.

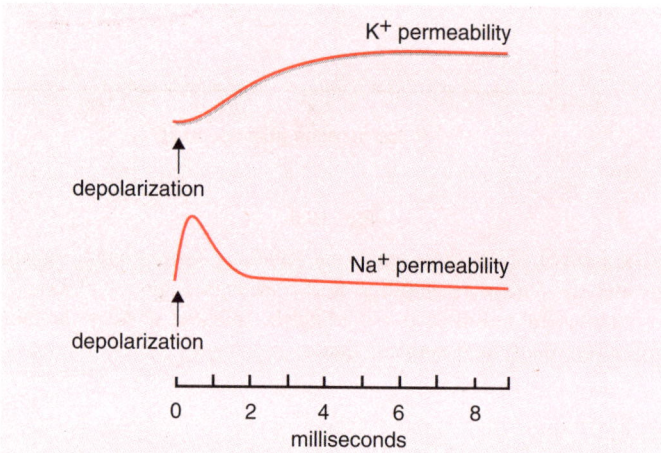

**Fig. 11.1**

## What is the mechanism of Na⁺ channel inactivation?

Na⁺ channels are guarded by two gates: the **activation (m) gate** and the **inactivation (h) gate**. *During depolarization*, the activation gate opens quickly, followed *slowly* by the closure of inactivation gate. This results in a brief interval during which the channel remains open. *During repolarization*, the activation gate closes first followed by the opening of the inactivation gate, so that the channel remains obliterated (Fig. 11.2).

## Why do K⁺ channels have a stabilizing effect on membrane potential?

If the membrane potential depolarizes, K⁺ channels open up in large numbers. The increase in K⁺ permeability hyperpolarizes the membrane. (This can be verified from the Goldman Equation). The membrane potential is thereby restored to its original value. Conversely, if the membrane hyperpolarizes, a large number of K⁺ channels closes down. The fall in K⁺ permeability depolarizes the membrane and restores the membrane potential to its original value. Thus, *whenever there is a change in membrane potential,*

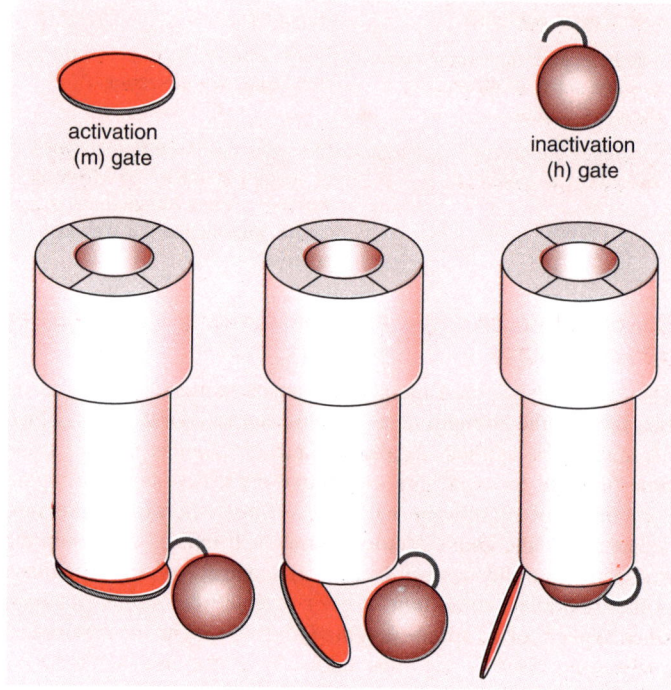

**Fig. 11.2**

*the activated K⁺ channels tend to restore the membrane potential to the original level*. Hence, K⁺ channels are said to have a **stabilizing (negative feedback) effect** on the membrane potential, i.e., they tend to prevent any change in membrane potential (Fig. 11.3).

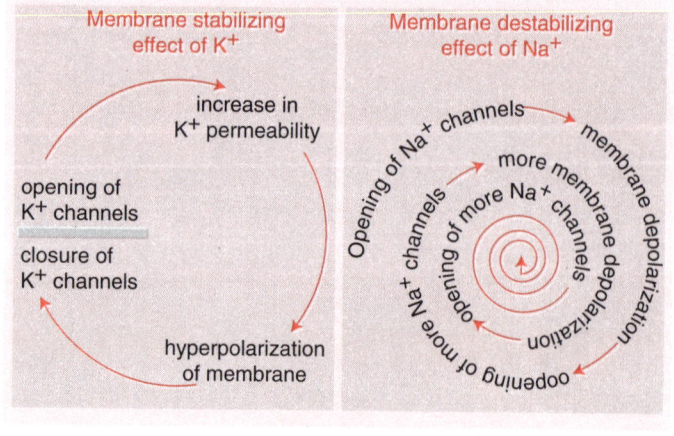

**Fig. 11.3**

## Why do Na+ channels have a destabilizing effect on membrane potential?

When the membrane potential depolarizes, the Na+ channels start opening up. The opening of the Na+ channels depolarizes the membrane further (in accordance with the Goldman equation), leading to the opening of larger number of Na+ channels. Thus, there is a **positive feedback cycle** (the **Hodgkin cycle**) resulting in a very rapid change in membrane potential and opening of nearly all the Na+ channels. Since the opening of even a few Na+ channels can trigger off this vicious cycle resulting in a large change in membrane potential, Na+ channels are said to have a **destabilizing effect** on membrane potential (Fig. 11.3).

## What is the ionic basis of the firing level of a membrane?

Since the resting K+ permeability is much greater than the resting Na+ permeability, the stabilizing effect of K+ is much greater than the destabilizing effect of Na+ channels. Small changes in the membrane potential are therefore promptly restored. However, a large depolarization is associated with a greater increase in Na+ permeability than in K+ permeability. **Firing level** is the potential at which *the destabilizing effect of Na+ ions overrides the stabilizing effect of K+ channels.*

## Name some agents altering channel function.

Two well-known *Na+-channel blockers* are **tetrodotoxin (TTX)** and **saxitoxin (STX)**. These bind to the *outside* of the Na+ channel and prevent the activation of Na+ channels and thereby render the membrane unexcitable. **Pronase** blocks the inactivation of Na+ channel. It does so by binding to intracellular sites on the Na+ channel. A well-known *K+ channel inactivator* is **tetra-ethyl-ammonium (TEA)**. Inactivation of the K+ channel prolongs the action potential. *Local anesthetics* are lipid-soluble substances that bind to intracellular sites on the Na+ channels, e.g. **lidocaine** and **procainamide**.

**Ca2+ ions** act as a *non-specific channel modulator* by altering the charge on the membrane. Normally, cell membranes carry a net negative charge on both the outer and inner surfaces as a result of negatively charged groups in the membrane phospholipids. These positive cations, especially multivalent cations like $Ca^{2+}$, are attracted to these negatively charges on the membrane and repel other cations (Na+ and K+). Lowering concentrations of extracellular calcium ions can cause spontaneous impulse generation, which can be reversed by the addition of calcium ions or other bivalent ions, because of the stabilizing effects of these cations on the channel. Spontaneous impulse generation due to low serum $Ca^{2+}$ levels results in widespread muscle spasms. The condition is called **tetany**, and is commonly seen in hypoparathyroidism. Increasing tissue pH has an effect similar to that of low calcium levels.

# Conduction of Nerve Impulses

## Explain briefly the mechanism of nerve conduction.

When an action potential is produced in a polarized nerve membrane, **local currents** from the action potential spread to the adjacent membrane area and depolarize it to the threshold level, triggering another action potential and the process continues. Thus, there are *two essential components of action potential propagation*: (a) the *flow of local currents*, which depolarizes the adjacent membrane. This **electrotonic conduction** of membrane depolarization, however, tends to fade out very quickly (Fig. 12.1). (b) The *triggering of a fresh action potential* in the adjacent membrane. The new action potential depolarizes the membrane maximally, and thereby restores the depolarization to its original magnitude of ~ 110 mV. Without the first **conductive component**, *an action potential cannot be conducted at all*. Without the second **regenerative component**, *an action potential can be conducted only up to a limited distance* beyond which it will fade out. Before the local currents fade out completely, a fresh action potential must be generated for the action potential to be propagated. The conductive component is very fast and depends on the electrical characteristics of the membrane (called the *cable*

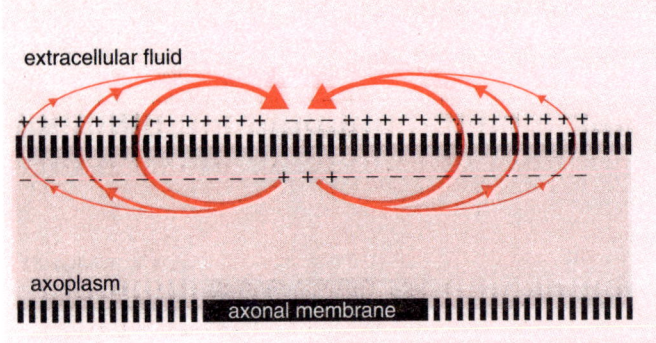

extracellular fluid

axoplasm

axonal membrane

**Fig. 12.1**

*properties* of the membrane). The regenerative component is much slower. *Frequent action potentials along the neuron tend to slow down the conduction velocity.*

## What is saltatory conduction?

In a myelinated neuron, the membrane potential is negligible (-3 mV) in the myelinated segments. The high resting potential of −70mV is present only at the nodes of Ranvier. The action potentials too are produced only at the nodes of Ranvier. When an action potential is produced at a polarized node of Ranvier, the **local currents** from it gets electrotonically conducted to the next node where it triggers another action potential (Fig. 12.2). The action potentials therefore seem to 'jump' from node to node, which is called **saltatory conduction**. Since there are fewer action potentials during saltatory conduction, the conduction velocity is very high. (Frequent action potentials along the neuron tend to slow down the conduction velocity.)

## Enumerate the factors affecting nerve conduction velocity.

The factors affecting nerve conduction velocity are as follows :

(i) *Axon diameter.* An axon with a larger diameter conducts faster. In an unmyelinated fiber, the speed of propagation is directly proportional to the square root of the fiber diameter (D), i.e.,

$$\text{Conduction velocity} \propto \sqrt{D}.$$

(ii) *Myelination and saltatory conduction.* Myelination speeds up conduction. Thus, the action potential travels electrotonically along the long myelinated segments, and fresh action potentials are generated only at the nodes. This is called **saltatory conduction**. In a myelinated neuron, the conduction velocity is directly proportional to the fiber diameter (D).

Conduction velocity $\quad\quad \alpha \quad\quad$ axonal diameter
Conduction velocity (in m/s) $\;=\; 6 \times$ axonal diameter (in μ)

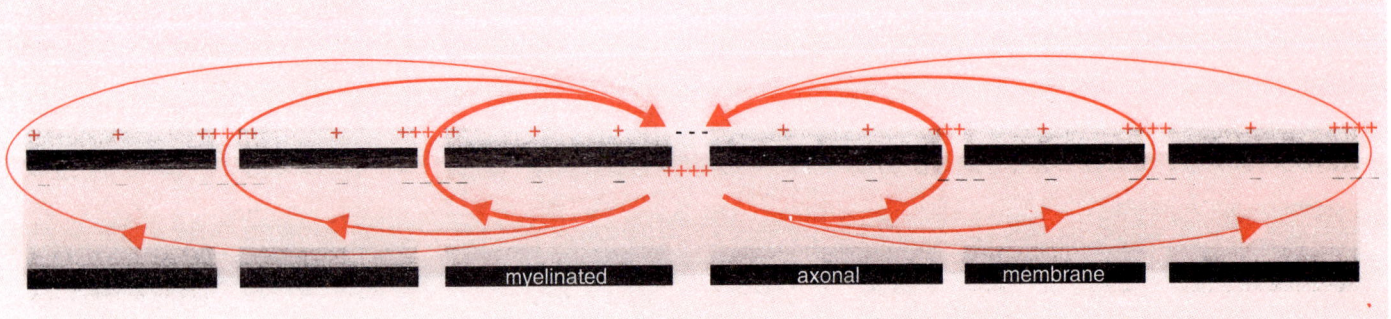

myelinated axonal membrane

**Fig. 12.2**

(iii) *Temperature*. A decrease in temperature slows down conduction velocity. (iv) *Resting membrane potential*. Effect of RMP changes on conduction velocity is quite variable. Usually, any change in the RMP in either direction (hyperpolarization or depolarization) slows down the conduction velocity.

## Enumerate the factors causing conduction failure.

Factors causing conduction failure are: (i) local anesthetics; (ii) pressure; (iii) hypoxia and (iv) demyelination. The susceptibility of the neuron to the first three factors listed above is given below.

| Susceptibility to: | Most susceptible | Intermediate | Least susceptible |
|---|---|---|---|
| Hypoxia | B | A | C |
| Pressure | A | B | C |
| Local anesthetic | C | B | A |

# Neuromuscular Transmission

## Enumerate the steps of neuromuscular transmission.

The steps of neuromuscular transmission (Fig. 13.1) are as follows:
(1) An action potential is conducted down the motor axon to the prejunctional axon terminal. (2) Depolarization of the terminal buttons opens up voltage-gated $Ca^{2+}$ channels in its membranes. $Ca^{2+}$ moves into the terminals along an electrochemical gradient. (3) Elevated $Ca^{2+}$ concentration in the terminal button causes exocytosis of the ACh-containing synaptic vesicles in the terminal button into the myoneural cleft. (4) The acetylcholine released from the axon terminal then diffuses across the myoneural cleft and binds to a specific acetylcholine receptors on the motor end-plate. (5) The binding of ACh with the ACh receptor (ACh-R) increases the conductance of the postjunctional membrane to $Na^+$ and $K^+$, resulting in a transient depolarization of the post-junctional membrane. This depolarization is called the *endplate potential (EPP)*. (6) The EPP is transient because acetylcholine is quickly hydrolyzed by the enzyme *acetylcholinesterase (ACh-E)* into choline and acetate. AChE is present in high concentration in the junctional cleft. (7) The postjunctional membrane cannot generate action potentials. However, the EPP depolarizes the adjacent muscle membrane by electrotonic conduction. When the depolarization exceeds the threshold, an action potential is triggered in the adjacent muscle membrane.

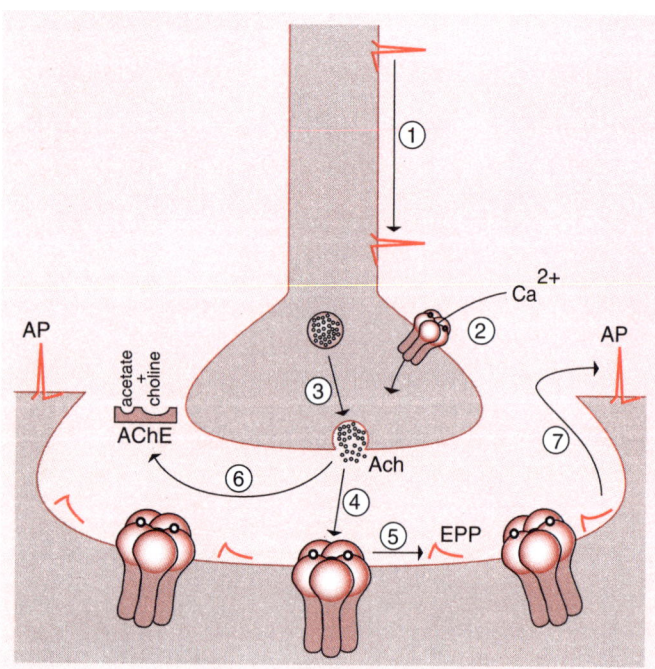

**Fig. 13.1**

## What is MEPP?

Each quantum of ACh released into the synaptic cleft produces a small depolarization called a **miniature endplate potential (MEPP)**, which is ~0.5 mV in amplitude and not enough to trigger an action potential in the adjacent muscle plasma membrane. MEPP's occur spontaneously even if the motor neuron is not stimulated, with an average frequency of about 1 per second.

## What is EPP?

Each action potential reaching the axonal ending results in the release of about *60 quanta* of ACh, with each quantum containing 10,000 ACh molecules. The 600,000 ACh molecules bind to 300,000 ACh-R (2 on each). Opening of ACh-R takes the membrane potential from –90mV to –65mV. This *25mV* change in membrane potential is called the **end plate potential (EPP)** (Fig. 13.2). The EPP gets conducted electrotonically from the end plate to the adjacent muscle fiber membrane which gets depolarized to its firing level and generates an action potential.

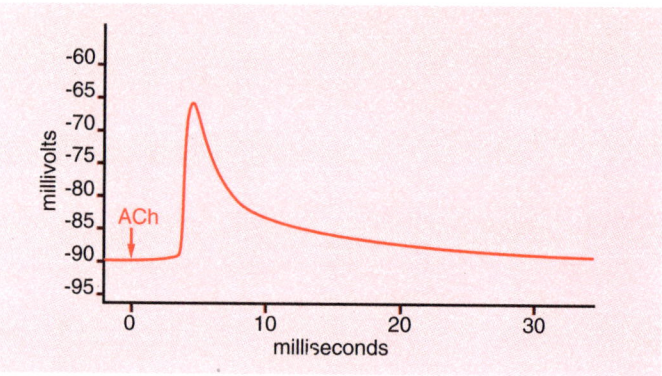

**Fig. 13.2**

## What is the safety factor of neuromuscular transmission?

Only 6 quanta are necessary for the transmission of the action potential across the neuromuscular junction but as many as 60 are released normally. This provides a *10 fold safety factor* of neuromuscular transmission.

## Enumerate the drugs affecting neuromuscular transmission.

*(i) Drugs affecting acetylcholine release* include **botulinus toxin**, which is associated with food-poisoning and interferes with the synthesis or release of ACh. In this way it produces muscular paralysis; **black widow spider toxin**, which stimulates secretion of massive amounts of ACh, leading to its depletion and consequent motor paralysis, and **hemicholiniums**, which block

the choline transport system and inhibit choline uptake (Fig. 13.3). Prolonged treatment with hemicholiniums depletes the store of transmitter and ultimately decreases the ACh content of the quanta.

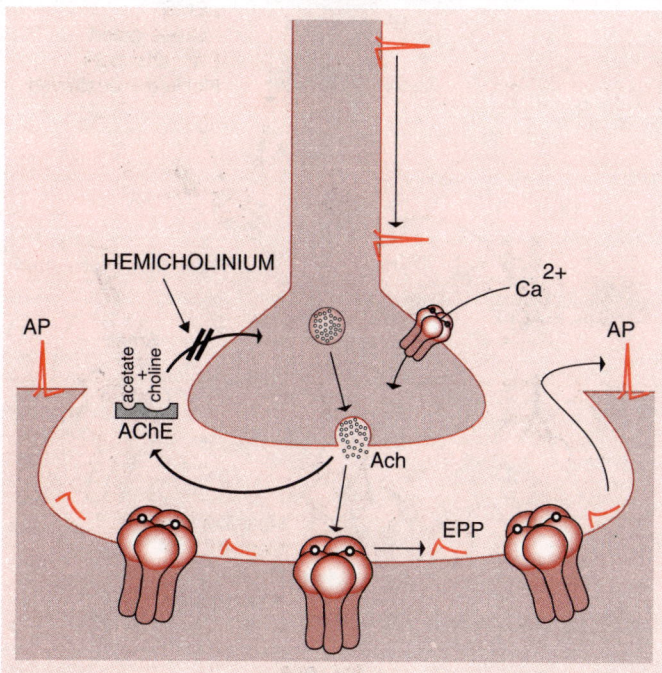

**Fig. 13.3**

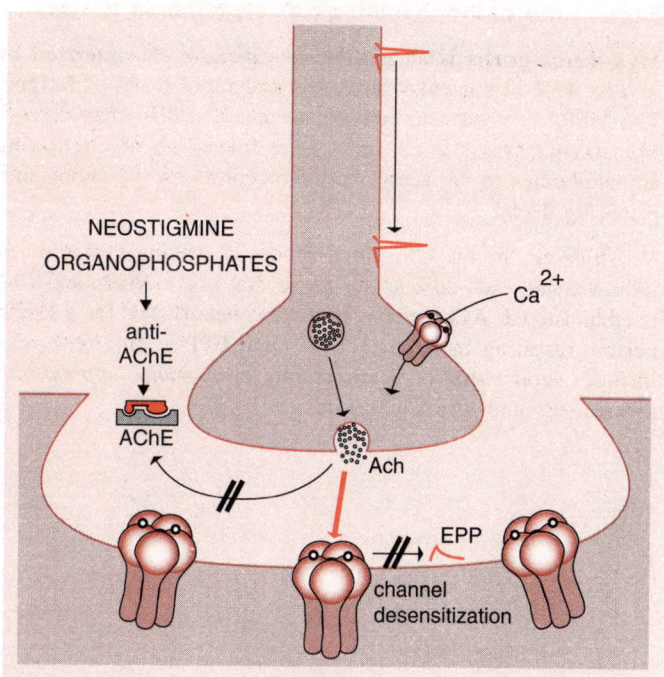

**Fig. 13.4**

(ii) *Drugs inactivating acetylcholinesterase* are called **anticholinesterases (anti-ChE)**. These drugs bind to AChE, thereby preventing ACh from binding to the same sites (Fig. 13.4). The AChE is freed only when the anti-ChE bound to it is hydrolyzed. By inactivating AChE, anti-ChE drugs permit large amounts of ACh to accumulate within the myoneural cleft. In the presence of an anti-ChE, the EPP is larger (more depolarization) and dramatically prolonged. Initially the depolarization results in a persistent muscle contraction (spasm) but after sometime it makes the motor end-plate inexcitable due to *channel desensitization*. Anti-ChE are of two types. Drugs like **neostigmine**, which are hydrolyzed by AChE in a few hours, are called *reversible inhibitors*. Thereafter, the AChE becomes available once again for inactivating ACh. Reversible inhibitors are used in the treatment of myasthenia gravis and in curare poisoning. **Organophosphate** compounds like Malathione and Baygon (insecticides) and diisopropyl phosphofluoridate or DFP (a nerve-gas used in chemical warfare) are poorly hydrolyzed by ACh-E and therefore remain attached to the ACh-E for several weeks. These are called *irreversible inhibitors*. In presence of these irreversible inhibitors, ACh is unable to bind to the inactivated ACh-E. Hence, irreversible AChE inhibitors produces deadly paralysis.

(iii) *Drugs binding to acetylcholine receptors* are of two types. Drugs like **succinylcholine** produce neuromuscular block by depolarizing the end plate (**depolarizing neuromuscular block**). In moderate dosage, these drugs (called **cholinomimetic drugs**) bind to ACh receptors in the motor end-plate and depolarize the end plate resulting in muscle spasm. In high dosage, however, it will induce desensitization of the ACh-gated channels with

consequent paralysis. Succinylcholine, is commonly used during surgery as a muscle relaxant and to reduce movements during electroconvulsion treatment of psychotic patients. Drugs like **d-tubocurarine** bind to the ACh receptors but do not stimulate them, and therefore, do not depolarize the membrane. They therefore block neuromuscular transmission without depolarizing the end-plate (**non-depolarizing neuromuscular block**). They only keep the ACh receptors blocked so that ACh is unable to bind to them (Fig. 13.5). **Bungarotoxin** found in the venom of the krait also produces non-depolarizing block.

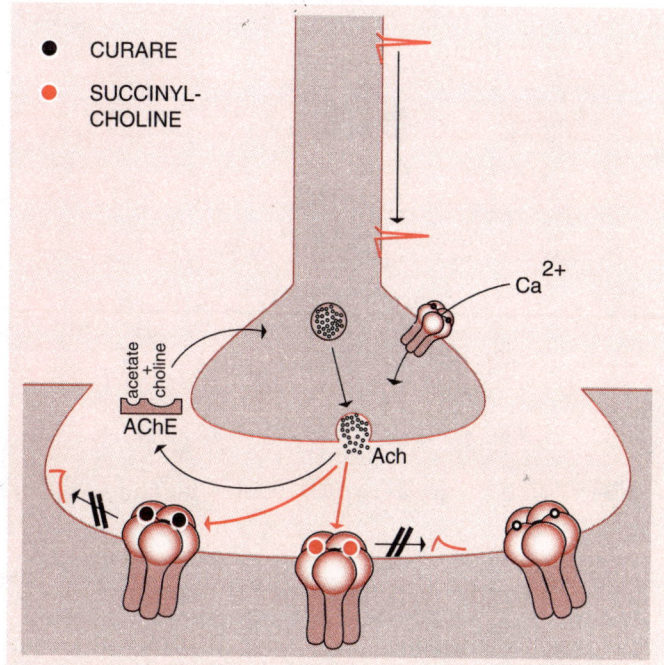

**Fig. 13.5**

### Explain the pathophysiology of myasthenia gravis.

Myasthenia gravis is an *autoimmune disease* characterized by severe skeletal muscular weakness and rapid onset of fatigue. The MEPP in myasthenic muscle are much smaller than normal. Myasthenia gravis is caused by the formation of circulating autoantibodies to the acetylcholine receptors on the motor endplate (Fig. 13.6).

*Neostigmine*, an anti-ChE drug, produces striking symptomatic improvement, each dose acting for several hours. When anti-ChE is administered, ACh persists in the myoneural cleft for a longer period, resulting in larger MEPP's and EPP's. Treatment also includes suppression of autoimmunity by *immuno-suppressants*, *thymectomy* and *plasmapheresis*.

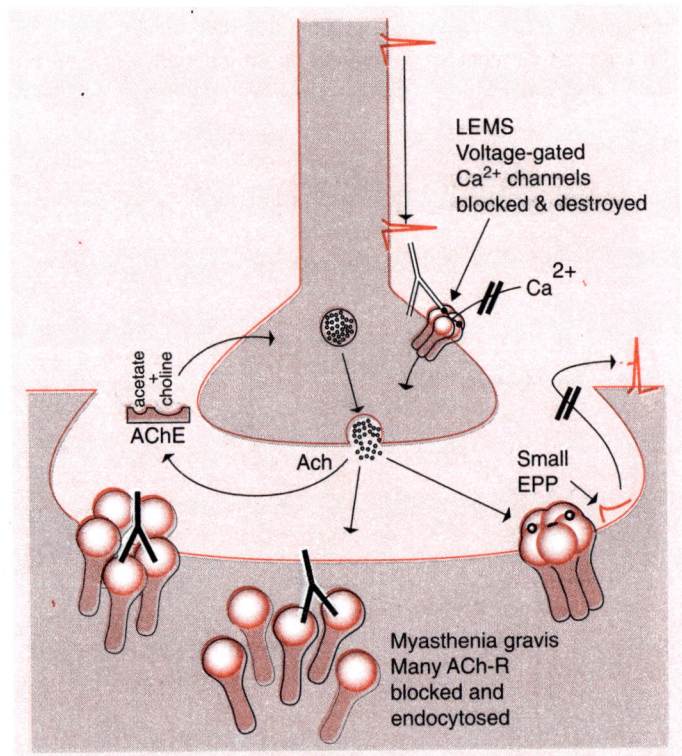

**Fig. 13.6**

# Mechanism & Energetics of Muscle Contraction

### Describe the steps of cross-bridge cycling.

The shortening of a muscle fiber occurs due to the *sliding of actin filaments on myosin filaments*. The repetitive events that bring about this shortening are called the **cross-bridge cycling** (Fig. 14.1). In brief, (i) ATP binds to myosin ATPase present on the myosin head and splits into ADP and $P_i$. The energy released activates the myosin head, which is now ready to bind to actin. (ii) The activated myosin head binds with the active sites of actin filaments forming *actomyosin*. Simultaneously, the myosin head flexes at its hinge (the **power stroke**). As a result, the actin filament slides on myosin filament, bringing the Z-disks closer and shortening the sarcomere. (iii) As the myosin head flexes, the ADP and Pi present on it are cast off, making way for a fresh molecule of ATP. When ATP binds to myosin ATPase, the myosin head detaches from actin, and the cross-bridge cycle is repeated all over again.

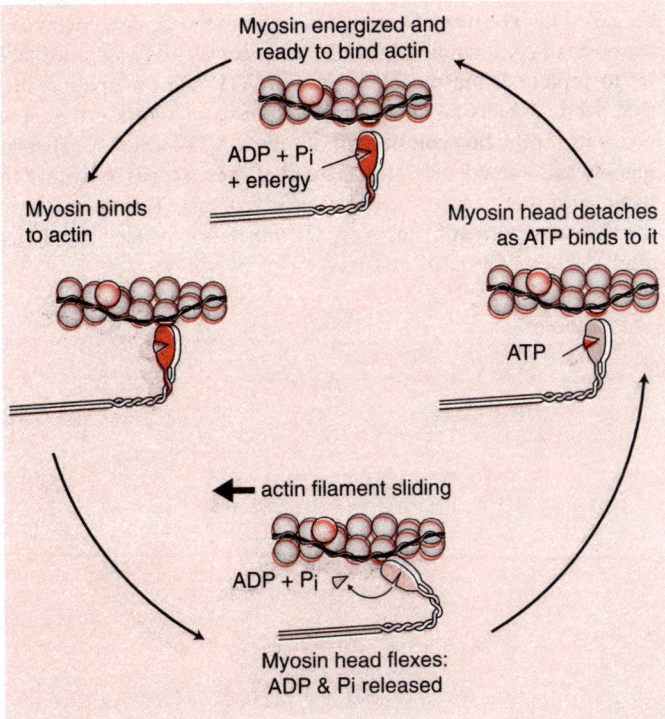

**Fig. 14.1**

### What is the mechanism of excitation-contraction coupling in a skeletal muscle?

The term excitation *contraction coupling* refers to the events between the generation of sarcolemmal action potential and the outpouring of $Ca^{2+}$ from L-tubule cisterns into the sarcoplasm.

Although there is no continuity between the T-tubules and the L-tubules, yet, depolarization of the T-tubules results in an outpouring of $Ca^{2+}$ from the L-tubules. The mechanism involves two membrane receptors: *dihydropyridine receptors (DHP)* and *ryanodine receptor (RYR) channels* (Fig. 14.2), that are mechanically interlocked.

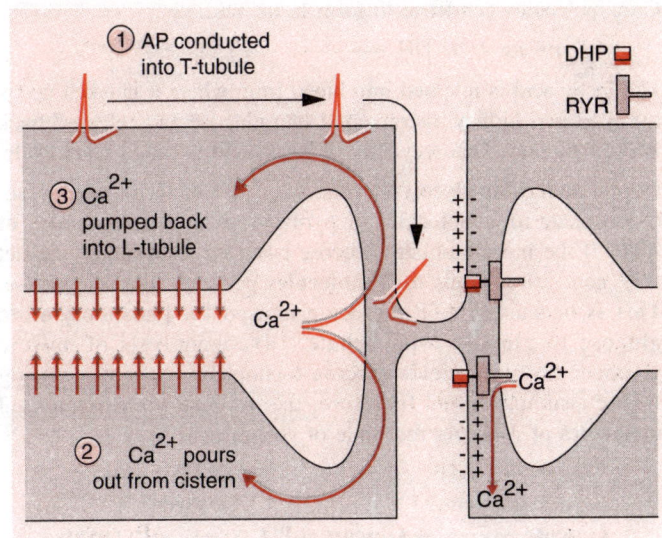

**Fig. 14.2**

### What is the role of ATP in muscle contraction and relaxation?

ATP has three roles in muscle contraction and relaxation: (i) it provides the energy for the power stroke of myosin head; (ii) it brings about a dissociation of myosin head from actin filament; and (iii) it brings about muscle relaxation by pumping out $Ca^{2+}$ from the sarcoplasm into the L-tubules.

### Explain the mechanism of contraction remainder and rigor mortis.

When a muscle gets fatigued, its ATP content decreases. As a result, the *sarcoplasmic $Ca^{2+}$ concentration remains elevated* even when the muscle is not depolarized. In the absence of ATP, therefore, the *active sites of actin remain uncovered* (due to high sarcoplasmic $Ca^{2+}$) and *bound to the myosin heads* (because ATP is also required for the dissociation of myosin heads from actin). The muscle therefore fails to relax completely and remains in a partially contracted state called **contraction remainder** (Fig. 15.5). For identical reasons (i.e. depletion of ATPs), the muscles become contracted and rigid after death, a state known as **rigor mortis**.

## Describe the energy sources for muscle contraction.

ATP is the immediate source of energy for muscle contraction. However, the ATP stores in the muscle can sustain muscle contraction for *up to 3 seconds*. In about 3 sec, all the ATP is depleted from the muscle cell. Thereafter, ATP is regenerated using the energy released by the *dephosphorylation of creatine phosphate* reserves of the muscle fiber.

$$\text{Creatine phosphate + ADP} \longrightarrow \text{creatine + ATP}$$

The creatine phosphate reserves (20 mM/L) of the muscle fiber can sustain contraction for about 5 more seconds, i.e., *up to 8 seconds*. After depletion of creatine phosphate reserves, further supply of energy for regeneration of ATP comes from glycolysis, which can sustain muscle contraction *up to 1 minute*. The end product of glycolysis is pyruvate and ATP molecules. When $O_2$ is available, the acetyl-CoA is metabolized completely through the Kreb's cycle. In absence of oxygen however, the acetyl CoA molecules condense to form lactic acid.

$$\text{Pyruvate + NADH} \longleftrightarrow \text{Lactate + NAD}^+$$

The lactic acid is released into blood from where it is taken up by the liver and kidney, reconverted into glucose and released back into circulation. This recycling of lactic acid is called **Cori cycle**.

During **anaerobic glycolysis**, conversion of 1 molecule of glucose-6-phosphate to 2 molecules of pyruvate releases **3 molecules of ATP**. If the muscle utilizes glucose taken up from blood, the net ATP generation drops to **2 molecules** per molecule of glucose. This is because 1 ATP molecule is used for phosphorylating glucose to glucose-6-phosphate. Glycogenolysis of muscle glycogen however yields glucose-6-phophate without requiring ATP consumption and therefore, the net ATP yield remains **3 molecules of ATP** per molecule of glucose.

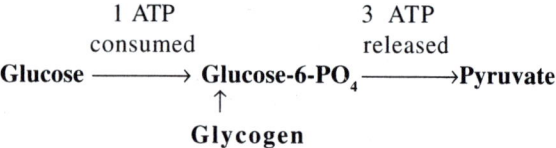

```
          1 ATP              3 ATP
         consumed           released
Glucose ——————→ Glucose-6-PO₄ ——————→Pyruvate
                    ↑
                Glycogen
```

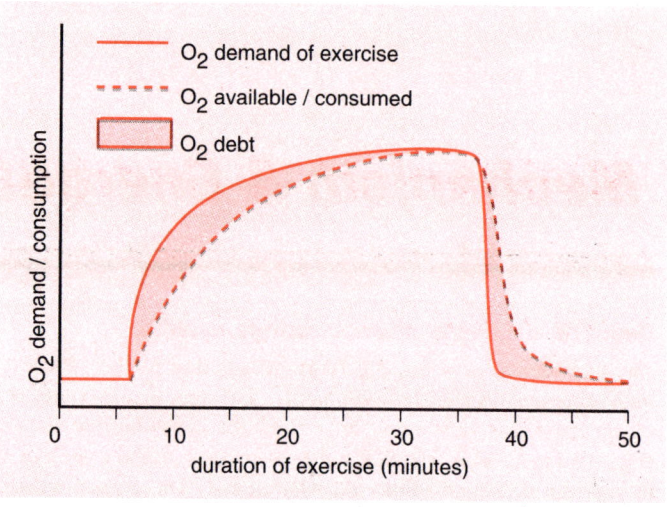

**Fig. 14.3**

Glycolysis alone can sustain contraction for about 1½ minutes only since lactic acid accumulation makes prolonged contraction difficult. In presence of oxygen, the terminal product of glycolysis viz., pyruvate is converted into acetyl CoA and fed into the Kreb's cycle in which 38 molecules of ATP are generated. Kreb's cycle can sustain muscle contraction *for several hours.*

## What is recovery oxygen?

After the muscle stops contracting, it continues to take up extra $O_2$ called the **recovery $O_2$** which is equal to the $O_2$ debt incurred at the onset of contraction (Fig. 14.3). The recovery oxygen is utilized: (i) to replenish the muscle stores of ATP and phosphocreatine that were exhausted in the initial phase of contraction. This accounts for the **fast component** of recovery $O_2$, which is expended quickly and immediately after the end of exercise. (ii) to oxidize the lactic acid that accumulated during glycolysis. This accounts for the **slow component** of recovery $O_2$, which is expended slowly and after the completion of fast oxygen recovery.

# Gross Characteristics of Muscle Contraction

## Explain the difference between isotonic and isometric recording.

In **isotonic** contraction, the *muscle shortens without any change in its tension* (or stiffness). To record isotonic muscle contraction, the *load on the muscle must be zero*. Hence, for isotonic recording, the recording lever should be as light as possible. The muscle tendon is attached to the lever and the muscle is allowed to shorten freely. The shortening is recorded by the lever. On the other hand, for recording **isometric** increase in muscle tension, *the load on the muscle must be immovable*. In practice, however, the muscle is made to produce a very small displacement of a very heavy load. The displacement, which is measured after magnification, gives an indirect measure of the degree of muscle tension. Isometric recording is made using a tension transducer which serves two purposes: (i) it acts like an immovable load, allowing only minimal muscle shortening in response to large contractile forces; (ii) it produces a large, measurable current in response to small muscle shortening. The recorded current serves as an indirect index of isometric contraction (Fig. 15.1).

## Describe the phases of a muscle twitch.

A typical isotonic twitch recorded from a frog's gastrocnemius-sciatic preparation takes about 0.1s and shows 3 phases: (1) The **latent phase** (~0.01s): This is the time taken by (a) the impulse to travel along the nerve to the neuromuscular junction, (b) neuromuscular transmission, (c) excitation-contraction coupling, (d) the initial isometric phase of contraction and (e) the inertia of the recording lever. The latent period is longer when the distance between the point of nerve stimulation and the neuromuscular junction is more, or when a heavier load prolongs the initial isotonic contraction phase. (2) **Isotonic contraction phase** (0.4s) in which the muscle shortens up to 20% of its resting length. *Greater the load, shorter the isotonic contraction phase, and lesser is the shortening.* (3) **Isotonic relaxation phase** (0.5s) in which the muscle is stretched back to its original length by the dead weight suspended from the recording lever.

## What are slow and fast twitch fibers?

Depending on the duration of a single twitch, muscle fibers are categorized into slow twitch and fast twitch muscle fibers. **Slow twitch fibers** rely on oxidative metabolism and are *red* due to their *myoglobin content*. **Fast twitch fibers**, which lack myoglobin, are called *white* fibers. Most muscles contain a varying admixture of both types of fibers and are called **pale muscles** (and *not* white muscle). Examples of pale muscles are the gastrocnemius muscle, extraocular muscles and the dorsal interossei. They help in quick, powerful movements but are easily fatigable. Muscles that contain

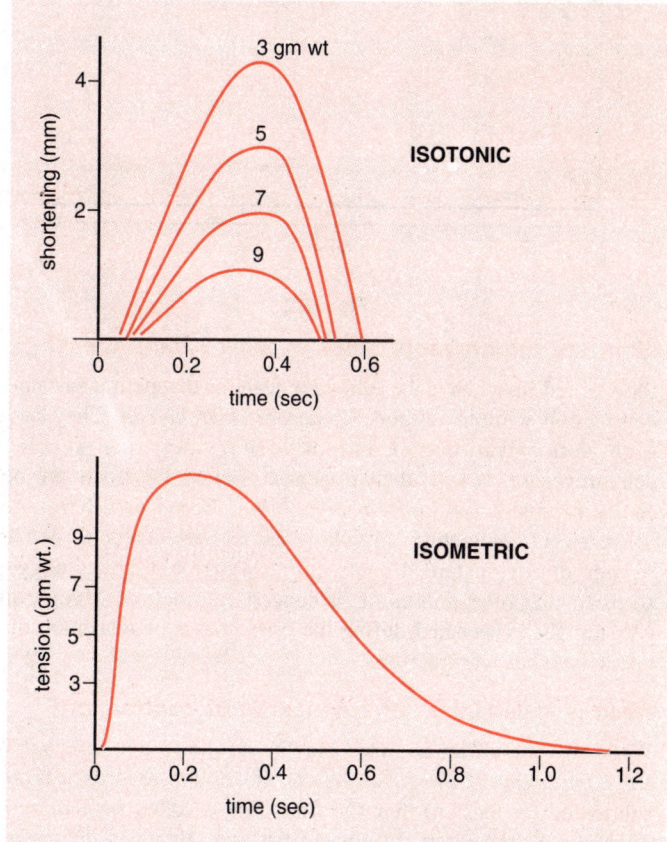

**Fig. 15.1**

only red fibers are called **red muscles**. Examples of red muscles are soleus and the lumbricals. They help in slow, sustained movements and are not easily fatigued (Fig. 15.2).

## What are the characteristics of fast twitch fibers?

Fast or white fibers have the following features which enable quick and powerful contractions but make them easily fatigable: (i) *anaerobic metabolism*; thus, they have a high concentrations of glycolytic enzymes like phosphorylases. (Uptake of oxygen from blood and Kreb's cycle are slow processes). Anaerobic contraction is faster but makes the muscle more prone to fatigue due to lactic acid production. (ii) higher *glycogen* content, providing a ready source of glucose. (Glucose uptake from blood is a slower process.) (iii) *larger* length and diameter, allowing stronger contractions; (iv) more *extensive sarcoplasmic reticulum* with a higher capacity for pumping $Ca^{2+}$, which makes contraction and relaxation quicker. (v) an isoenzyme of myosin ATPase that has faster kinetics. It also has larger amounts of myosin ATPase.

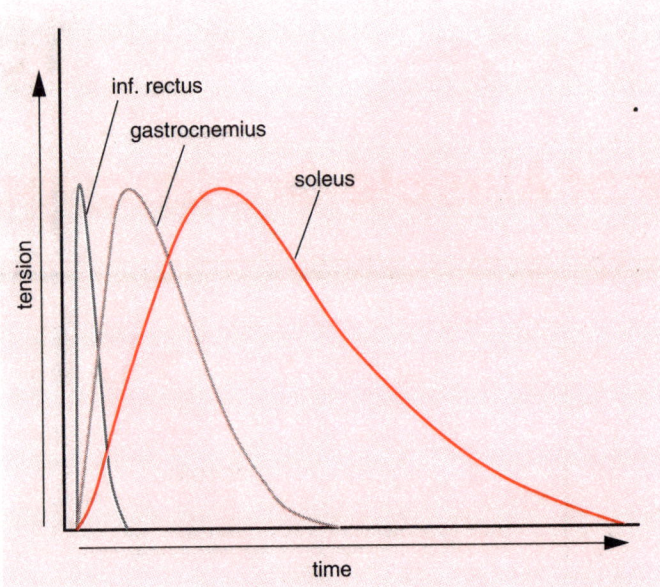

**Fig. 15.2**

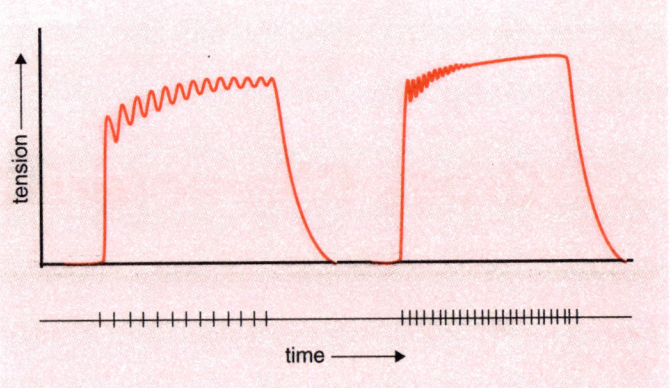

**Fig. 15.3**

## What are the characteristics of slow twitch fibers?

Slow or red fibers have the following features that permit sustained contraction without fatigue. (i) *aerobic metabolism*. They have high concentrations of oxidative enzymes like succinic dehydrogenase, NADH dehydrogenase. Hence, the fibers are not easily fatigued. (ii) *contain myoglobin*. Blood capillaries get squeezed by contracting muscle fibers and are unable to deliver oxygen during sustained contraction. Myoglobin stocks oxygen so as to tide over phases of prolonged contraction. Myoglobin gets rapidly oxygenated during the brief phases of relaxation that occur between contractions.

## What is mechanism of summation of contraction?

When two stimuli are so timed that the second twitch starts *before the completion of the first*, the second twitch records a larger shortening (or tension) than the first. This is called *summation of twitches*. As the interval between the two stimuli is decreased, individual peaks of the two twitches become less discernable till only a single large twitch is observed.

## What is muscle tetanus and what is its mechanism?

When multiple stimuli are delivered in quick succession to produce summation of twitches, the muscle gets tetanized, i.e. it remains contracted and does not relax. If the stimuli are spaced sufficiently close, the individual peaks fuse to produce a *complete tetanus* and the contraction reaches a near-perfect plateau. If the peaks of the individual twitches are discernable, it indicates the presence of brief relaxation in between peaks, and the tetanus is said to be *incomplete tetanus* (Fig. 15.3).

**Tetanic tension** is about 4 times the twitch tension. There are two theories for this higher tension generated during muscle tetanus: (i) One theory assumes that during a single twitch, the amount of $Ca^{2+}$ released into the sarcoplasm is *not enough* to produce tetanic tension. When the muscle is stimulated in rapid succession, $Ca^{2+}$ comes out into the sarcoplasm with each stimulus and there is a progressive accumulation of $Ca^{2+}$ in the sarcoplasm. Tetanic

tension is reached *when sarcoplasmic $Ca^{2+}$ levels reaches its maximum*. Studies with $Ca^{2+}$-sensitive photoprotein aequorin show that sarcoplasmic $Ca^{2+}$ *does* increase on stimulation in rapid succession. (ii) There are experiments to suggest that even during a single twitch, *enough $Ca^{2+}$ is released* into the sarcoplasm to cause complete shortening of its sarcomeres. However, the $Ca^{2+}$ starts moving back into sarcoplasmic reticulum well before the muscle tension is able to rise to tetanic levels. During tetanus, $Ca^{2+}$ is continuously present in the sarcoplasm and the *muscle gets adequate time to reach tetanic tension*. It seems that cumulative rise in sarcoplasmic $Ca^{2+}$ is important only in slow-twitch fibers where the outpouring of $Ca^{2+}$ is slow. In fast-twitch fibers, the time factor may be more important.

## What is beneficial effect?

Summation of twitches is different from the beneficial effect *seen in isotonic recordings*. When a muscle is stimulated twice in quick succession so that a second twitch is produced immediately *after the completion of the first*, the second twitch is greater (more shortening). This is called the **beneficial effect** of the first twitch on the second and occurs due to the *reduction of internal viscoelastic forces* brought about by release of muscle heat.

## What is the effect of temperature on muscle twitch?

The effect of temperature is different in isotonic and isometric contraction. *In isometric contraction, a rise in temperature reduces the twitch-tension of muscles*. A rise in temperature (within physiological limits) promotes the activity of $Ca^{2+}$-ATPase which pumps back $Ca^{2+}$ faster into the sarcoplasmic reticulum and hastens relaxation. Contraction is quicker too, due to faster diffusion of $Ca^{2+}$ from reticulum to sarcoplasm. Since the duration of the $Ca^{2+}$ pulse decreases with rise in temperature, less time is available for the rise of twitch tension. Hence, the strength of an isometric muscle twitch falls at higher temperature. *Isotonic shortening of muscles however tends to increase with rise in temperature*. This is due to the decrease in the internal viscoelastic resistance to shortening which more than compensates for the reduction in muscle tension (Fig. 15.4).

## How does fatigue affect the muscle twitch?

Muscle fatigue is associated with *a fall in muscle tension and an increased time required for relaxation*. The fatigue occurs due to ATP-depletion in the muscle and is most prominently

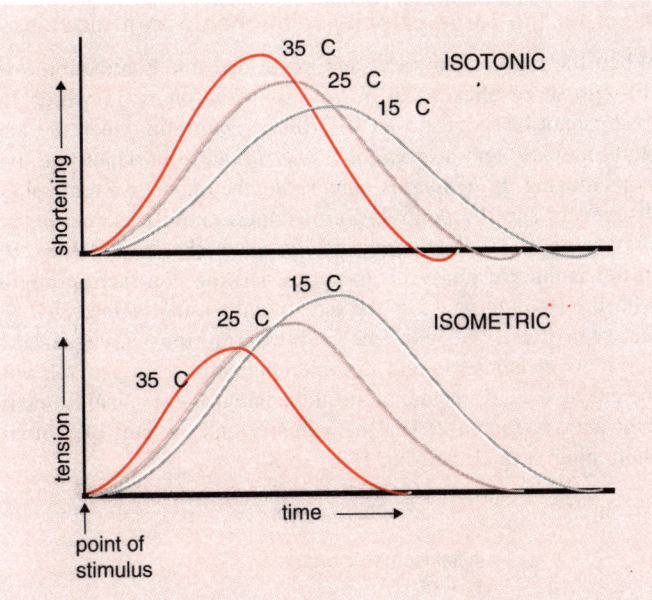

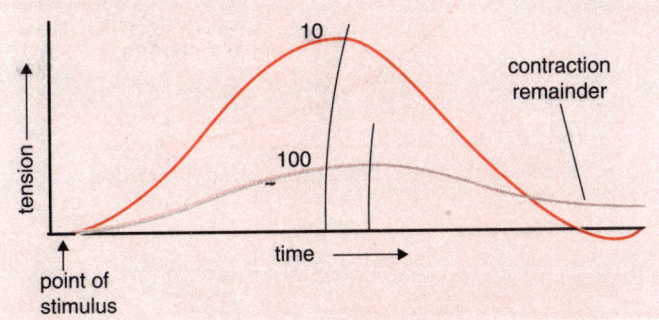

Fig. 15.4

revealed by its **incomplete relaxation** (Fig. 15.5). In a large motor unit, fatigue can also occur at the neuromuscular junction. However, the depletion of acetylcholine occurs only at prolonged, high frequency (>50 Hz) stimulation. Usually, *psychological fatigue* occurs in the central synapses of the brain earlier than in the muscle itself. Such fatigue can be overcome by adequate encouragement and motivation.

Fig. 15.5

### What is the effect of preload and afterload on muscle twitch?

**Preload** is *the load placed on a muscle before the muscle contracts*. It serves to stretch the muscle sarcomeres, thus producing a passive tension across the muscle. This passive tension increases muscle contraction in two ways: (i) It adds an elastic recoil force to the muscle during its contraction. (ii) It stretches the muscle to its resting length, producing the optimum length-tension relationship (Fig. 15.7) for active force generation. In real life situations, it is a common practice to pre-stretch a muscle using antagonist muscles. Through experience, we learn how much force our muscles generate at different lengths and unconsciously, we adjust muscle length before initiating a movement to develop the power we want.

**Afterload** is an opposing force which the muscle encounters immediately after it starts contracting. It is a force that a muscle

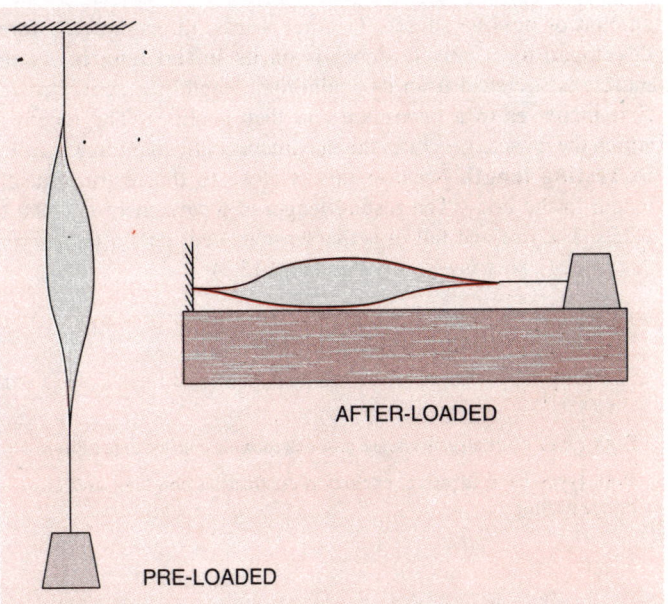

Fig. 15.6

must overcome before an observable shortening of the muscle can occur. The contraction of an after-loaded muscle is comparatively lesser. In real life situations, after-loaded contractions tend to occur in novel situations when the magnitude of the load is not known or during rapid adjustments to unexpected perturbations in load (Fig. 15.6).

### What is the equilibrium length of a muscle?

The length of a muscle when it is detached from its bony attachments is called its *equilibrium length*.

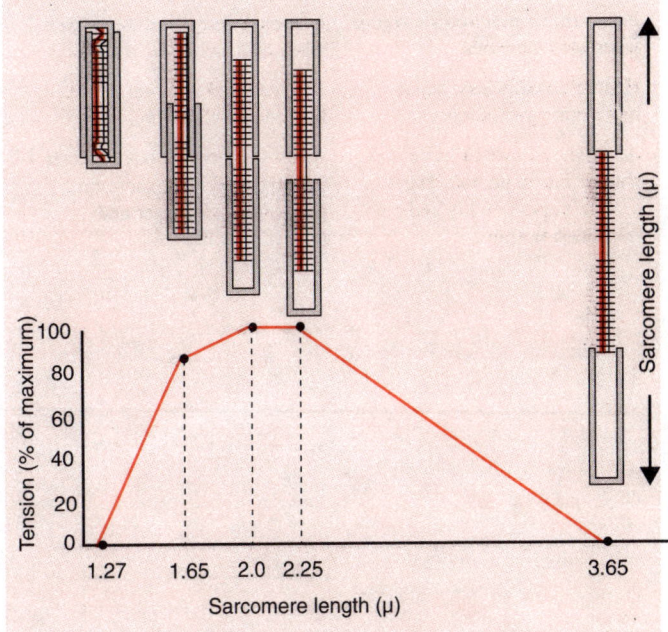

Fig. 15.7

### Describe the length-tension relationship in a muscle.

If the muscle is stimulated after stretching it passively, the contractile force developed by it will vary depending on the amount of passive stretch. In other words, the contractile force developed by a muscle depends on its **initial length**. As the muscle is stretched from its equilibrium length, the active tension first increases to a maximum and then declines. The length at which the muscle generates the maximum contractile force is called its **resting length** because this is close to the resting muscle length in the body. The resting length of a sarcomere is ~2.0 to 2.25μ. The rise and fall of active tension occur due to the *varying degrees of cross-bridge overlap* (Fig. 15.7).

## Enumerate the differences between isotonic and isometric contraction.

**SIMILARITIES**

Both types of contractions are associated with energy expenditure.

Both types have identical excitation-contraction coupling and cross-bridge cycling.

**DIFFERENCES**

| Isometric contraction | Isotonic contraction |
|---|---|
| Occurs when a muscle contracts against an immovable load | Occurs when a muscle contracts against zero load |
| Actin filaments are unable to slide on myosin filaments | Actin filaments easily slide on myosin filaments |
| Tension rises during contraction | Tension remains unchanged during contraction |
| No shortening occurs; hence, no external work is done | Shortening occurs and external work is done |
| Occurs at the beginning and end of all contractions | Occurs in the middle of a contraction |
| Isometric contraction *increases* when load increases | Isotonic contraction *decreases* when load increases |
| Heat released is less; hence, more energy-efficient | Heat released is more; hence, less energy-efficient |
| An isometric twitch has a shorter latent period. The tension peaks quickly and relaxation is slow. | An isotonic twitch has a longer latent period. The shortening peaks somewhat later and relaxation is quicker. |

## Describe the force-velocity relationship in a muscle.

When the muscle contracts against a load, the contraction goes through three phases: an *initial isometric phase* in which the load cannot be moved, a *middle isotonic phase* in which the load starts moving, and a *terminal isometric phase* in which the load stops moving. *If the load is immovable*, the middle iso-tonic phase disappears and the contrac-tion becomes entirely isometric, not shortening at all ($V_0$). Con-versely, *when the load is zero*, the initial isometric phase disap-pears, and the contraction begins with the isotonic phase at the maximum possible velocity ($V_{max}$). Between these two extremes, all contractions have variable durations of isometric and isotonic contractions. In general, with increasing load, (i) the durations of the initial and terminal isometric contractions increase; (ii) the velocity and amount of isotonic shortening keep decreasing (Fig. 15.8).

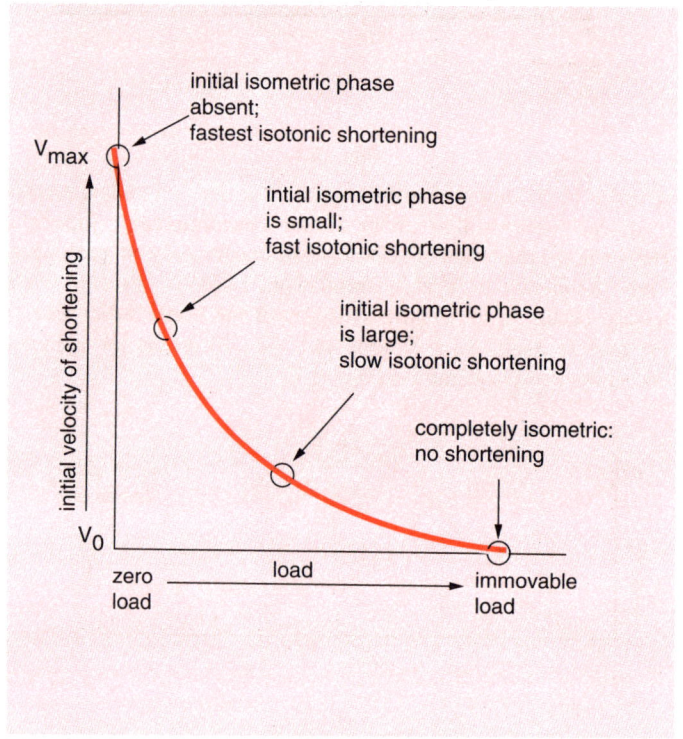

**Fig. 15.8**

# The Motor Unit

## Define a motor unit.

A solitary Aα motor neuron with all its peripheral branches and innervated extrafusal muscle fibers is called a **motor unit**. The term motor unit is sometime extended to multi-unit smooth muscles too.

## What is meant by the innervation ratio of a motor unit?

The number of muscle fibers innervated by a single neuron is called the **innervation ratio** of the motor unit. The ratio is low in muscles concerned with precision movement and high in those not requiring precision. For example, the extraocular muscles have the lowest innervation ratio of less than 6 per axon, while the gastrocnemius muscle has an innervation ratio of up to 2000 per axon.

## Does the motor unit obey the all-or-none law?

Yes, the motor unit as a whole does obey the all-or-none law. When the nerve fiber of the motor unit is stimulated, all the fibers of the motor unit will either contract maximally, or not contract at all, depending upon whether the stimulus is of sub-threshold or threshold intensity.

## What is motor recruitment?

When a muscle begins to contract, only a few units contract first. If the power generated is inadequate, more units are 'recruited'. This process of employing progressively greater number of motor units for muscle contraction is called **motor recruitment**.

## What is the size (Henneman) principle of motor recruitment?

When a muscle begins to contract against a load, the smallest motor units (which have only a few muscle fibers in them) are recruited first. If the force generated is insufficient, then the larger motor units are recruited. This order of recruitment from the smaller to the larger motor units is called the **Henneman principle**. In fact, the largest motor units in a muscle are idle most of the time since such large muscle forces are rarely required.

## What are the differences between Type-I and Type-II motor units?

| Motor unit | Type I | Type IIb |
|---|---|---|
| Names | Slow oxidative Red fibers Tonic fibers S (slow) | Fast oxidative White fibers Phasic fibers F (fast) |
| Metabolism | Aerobic Low glycolytic and high oxidative capacity | Anaerobic High glycolytic and low oxidative capacity. |
| Fatigability | Little or none | Rapid |
| Fiber length | Small | Large |
| Fiber diameter | Small | Large |
| Glycogen content | Low | High |
| Mitochondria | High | Low |
| Sarcoplasmic reticulum (SR) | Normal | Extensive |
| $Ca^{2+}$ pumping into SR | Moderate | High |
| Capillary density | High | Low |
| Blood supply | High | Normal |
| Myoglobin content | High | Low |
| Myosin ATPase activity | Low | High |
| Phosphorylase | Low | High |
| Succinic dehydrogenase | High | Low |
| NADH dehydrogenase | High | Low |
| Number of units in a muscle | Many | Few |
| Number of terminals per axon | Few | Many |
| Axon diameter | Small | Large |
| Conduction speed | Slow | Fast |
| Order of recruitment | Early | Later |
| Twitch duration | Long | Brief |
| Tetanic tension | Small | Large |

# Electromyography & Electroneurography

## Define and describe a motor unit potential.

The motor unit potential (MUP) is a *compound potential* which represents the *sum of the individual action potentials generated in those muscle fibers of the unit* that are within the pick-up range of the recording electrode. Since fibers of several motor units intermingle singly, each EMG electrode records the activity of more than one motor unit. *In the commonly recorded EMG, each vertical line represents a MUP*. When the EMG is recorded at a higher speed, each MUP is usually seen to be biphasic, triphasic or polyphasic.

## What are fasciculation potentials?

**Fasciculation** is an *involuntary contraction of a single motor unit*. It results in jerky, *visible twitching of a group of muscle fibers* that occur in patients with chronic partial denervation, especially when this is due to spinal cord lesions. The motor unit potentials that occur during fasciculation are called **fasciculation potential**.

Fasciculation potentials occur due to the instability of the membrane potential. They originate spontaneously at multiple sites along motor axon or the soma of the diseased motor neuron and in distal immature collaterals sprouts. Potentials originating lower down the neuron spread antidromically by axonal reflex (Fig. 55.1) to the other nerve terminals of the motor units. Fasciculations can occur in normal persons too.

## What are fibrillation potentials?

Fibrillation potentials are action potentials that *arise spontaneously from single denervated muscle fibers*. They occur due to rhythmical oscillations of the resting membrane potential in the denervated skeletal muscle fibers, or due to spontaneous depolarizations originating in the transverse tubular system of the muscle fiber. Fibrillation potentials usually have amplitude between 20 and 300µV (much lesser than a MUP), duration of less than 5 msec, and a firing rate of 2 – 20/s.

## What is a compound action potential?

A peripheral nerve is made of several neurons of different conduction velocities. When a nerve trunk is strongly stimulated, all its neurons get excited. The *record obtained from the nerve surface* some distance away (Fig. 17.1) will show multiple peaks, each peak corresponding to the action potentials of a group of neurons having similar conduction velocities. The record so obtained is called the **compound action potential** (Fig. 17.2).

## Compare and contrast an action potential and a compound action potential.

**SIMILARITIES**

Both are the potentials recorded during depolarization of nerve fibers.

**DIFFERENCES**

| Action potential | Compound action potential |
|---|---|
| Recorded intracellularly | Recorded extracellularly |
| Single peaked | Multipeaked |
| Potentials recorded are higher (in millivolts) | Potentials recorded are lower (in microvolts) |

## Describe the Erlanger & Gasser's classification of nerve fibers.

The Erlanger & Gasser's classification of nerve fibers is given in Table 17.1.

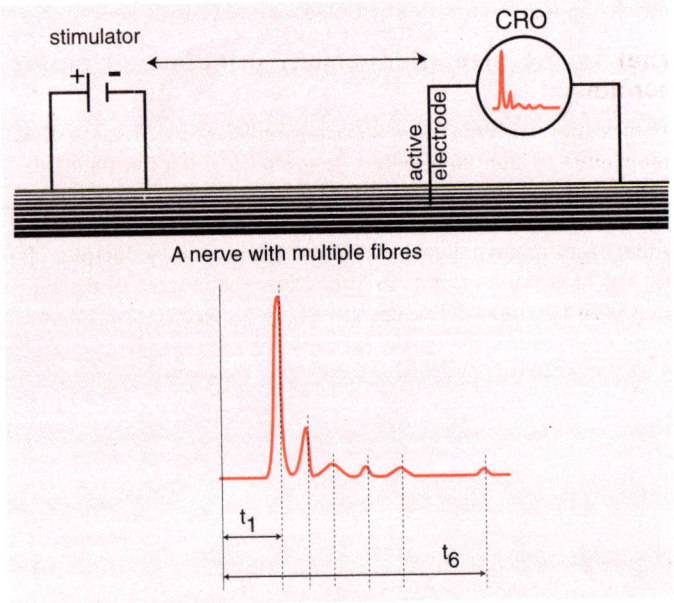

**Fig. 17.1**

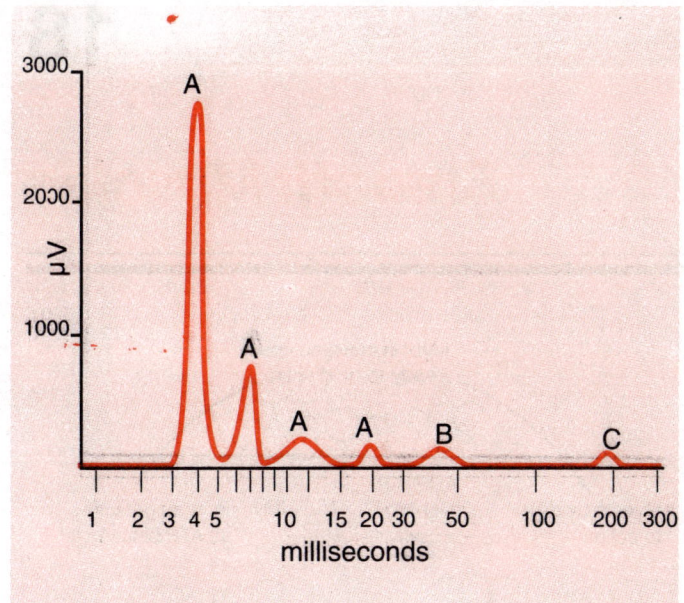

**Fig. 17.2**

| Table 17.1 | | | | |
|---|---|---|---|---|
| | **Function** | **Fiber diameter (μ)** | **Conduction velocity\* (m/sec)** | **Spike duration (millisec)** |
| **Aα** | Somatic motor Proprioception | 12 – 20 | 100 | 0.5 |
| **Aβ** | Touch, pressure | 5 – 12 | 60 | 0.5 |
| **Aγ** | Fusimotor | 3 – 6 | 40 | 0.5 |
| **Aδ** | Pain, temperature Crude touch | 2 – 5 | 20 | 0.5 |
| **B** | Autonomic preganglionic | < 2 | 10 | 1.0 |
| **C** | Sympathetic postganglionic, pain, temperature | < 1 | 2 | 2.0 |
| \* | *range: ± 20%.* | | | |

# Smooth Muscles

## What are the structural differences between skeletal and smooth muscles?

| Skeletal muscle fiber | Smooth muscle fiber |
|---|---|
| Is large, cylindrical and multinucleate | Is small, spindle shaped and uninucleate |
| Has well-developed **T-tubules** | Has **caveoli** which are rudimentary T-tubules |
| Has **Z-disks** | Has **dense bodies** instead of Z-disks |
| Actin and myosin filaments are roughly equal in number | Actin filaments far outnumber the myosin filaments |
| Actin filaments are parallel | Actin filaments radiate from the dense bodies |

## What are the salient features of smooth muscle contraction?

Compared to skeletal muscle, a smooth muscles: (i) has slower onset of contraction and relaxation. The contraction begins about 200 ms after the peak of a spike and ends 500 ms after excitation is over. (ii) has lower energy-requirements for contraction. (iii) can maintain a high tension without actively contracting (**latching**); (iv) has higher percentage of shortening. It contracts up to 30% of its initial length. (v) generates identical shortening (1 nm) and tension ($5 \times 10^{-12}$ Newton) in a single cross-bridge cycle of a single myosin head. (vi) can readjust its resting length, i.e., the length at which it generates maximum active tension (**plasticity**).

## Briefly describe the cross-bridge cycling in smooth muscle.

The cross-bridge cycling in smooth is similar to that in skeletal muscles. However, its regulation is different. *Smooth muscle does not contain tropomyosin or troponin.* One of the light chains of the myosin filament located in the neck region, called the **regulatory chain of myosin**, serves the function of tropomyosin. Similarly a $Ca^{2+}$-binding protein called **calmodulin** serves the role of troponin. When sarcoplasmic $Ca^{2+}$ rises, the $Ca^{2+}$ binds to calmodulin, the $Ca^{2+}$-calmodulin complex activates the enzyme **myosin light chain kinase** (MLCK), which in turn phosphorylates the **myosin regulatory chain**. Phosphorylation of the regulatory chain permits actin-myosin interaction and the cross-bridge cycling starts. The cycling stops when another enzyme - **myosin phosphatase** - dephosphorylates the regulatory chain (Fig. 18.1).

## What are the factors causing excitation and inhibition of smooth muscle?

*Multi-unit* smooth muscles are stimulated *only through nerves*. *Single-unit* smooth muscles are excited by several factors: (i) spontaneous excitation (through pacemaker); (ii) ephaptic

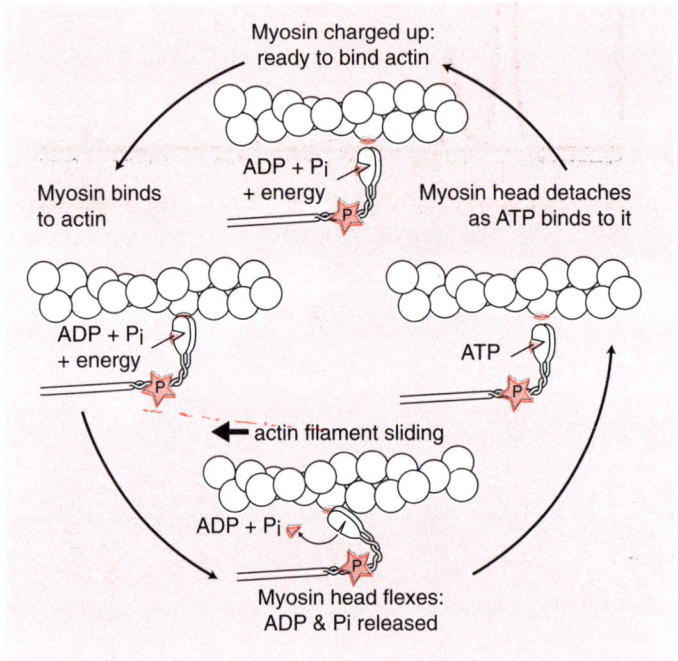

**Fig. 18.1**

excitation (from adjacent cells); (iii) nerves (i.e. by neuro-transmitters); (iv) hormones; (v) stretch; (vi) cold temperature.

## What are tonic and phasic smooth muscles?

Smooth muscles of gastrointestinal and urogenital sphincters remain mostly contracted and relax occasionally in response to inhibitory stimuli. Smooth muscles located in the walls of blood vessels and airways also remain partially contracted. Such muscles are called **tonic smooth muscles**. On the other hand, muscles forming the walls of gastrointestinal and urogenital tracts remain mostly relaxed and contract only in response to excitatory stimuli. These are called **phasic smooth muscles**.

## What are the different mechanisms of excitation-contraction coupling in smooth muscles?

The different mechanisms of excitation contraction coupling in smooth muscle are electro-mechanical coupling, pharmaco-mechanical coupling and mechanomechanical coupling (Fig. 18.2). In **electro-mechanical coupling**, the smooth muscle is excited through sarcolemmal depolarization. When the membrane depolarizes, voltage-gated $Ca^{2+}$ channels present on the sarcolemma open up and $Ca^{2+}$ moves into the sarcoplasm from the extracellular fluid. This $Ca^{2+}$ stimulates the release of more $Ca^{2+}$ from the sarcoplasmic reticulum. This is called *$Ca^{2+}$ induced $Ca^{2+}$*

*release (CICR)*. In **pharmacomechanical coupling**, the muscle is excited by chemical agents in the absence of any membrane depolarization. Neurotransmitters and hormones bind to *ligand-gated $Ca^{2+}$ channels* on the sarcolemma and open them up, letting in $Ca^{2+}$ from the ECF. In **mechanomechanical coupling**, the muscle is excited by stretch, which opens up *stretch-sensitive $Ca^{2+}$ channels* on the sarcolemma, letting in $Ca^{2+}$ from the ECF.

### Why is the RMP of smooth muscles not stable?

Unlike in the skeletal muscle, the RMP of the smooth muscle cell is lesser: approximately –50mV. In single-unit smooth muscles,

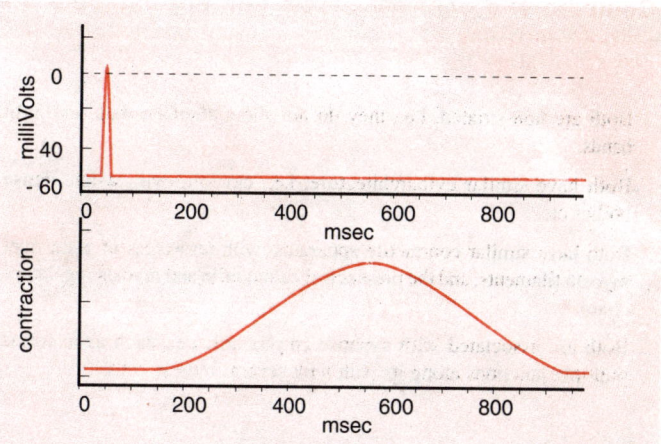

**Fig. 18.3**

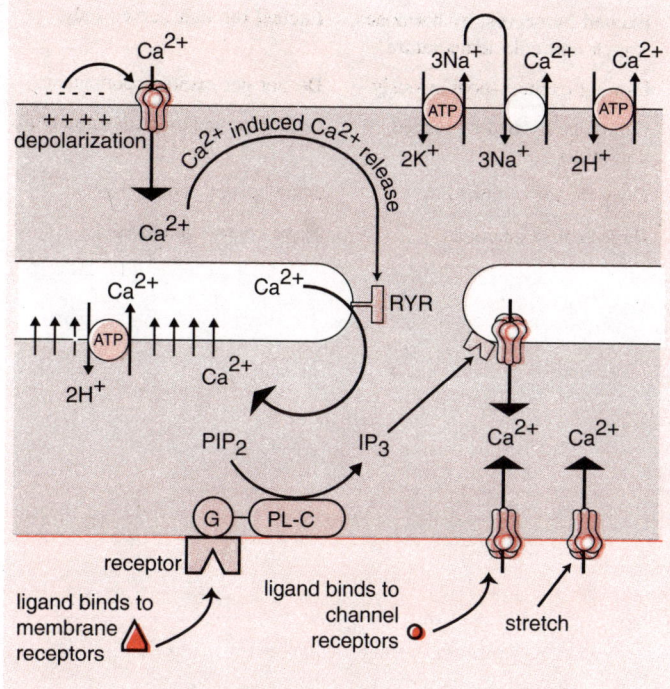

**Fig. 18.2**

the RMP is often unstable, oscillating between –55 mV and –35mV. These oscillations are called **pacemaker potentials**. They occur due to rhythmic changes in either $Ca^{2+}$ channel permeability and / or the activity of $Na^+$-$K^+$ pump.

### What are the different types of action potentials in smooth muscle?

The action potentials in single-unit smooth muscles can be of three types: *spike-potentials* (Fig. 18.3), *spikes superimposed on oscillatory pacemaker potentials* (Fig. 18.4), and *action potential with plateau* (Fig. 18.5).

### Describe the neuromuscular transmission in smooth muscles?

The potentials generated in smooth muscle through neuro-muscular transmission are called **junctional potentials**. They may be *excitatory junctional potential* (EJP) or *inhibitory junctional potential* (IJP) depending on whether the neurotransmitter secreted at the junction depolarizes or hyperpolarizes the smooth muscle membrane. *Acetylcholine* binds to ligand-gated ACh receptors present on smooth muscles and depolarizes the membrane. Acetylcholine receptors present on smooth muscles

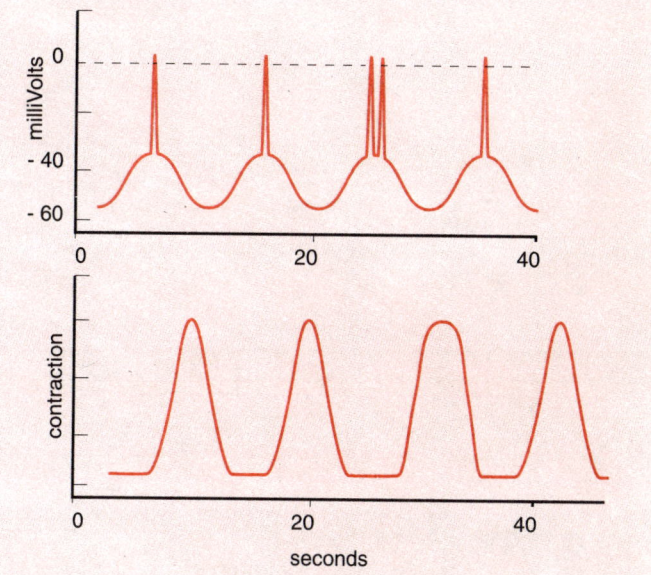

**Fig. 18.4**

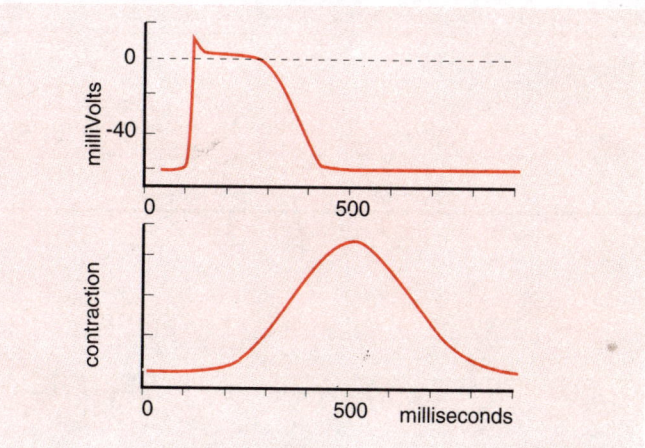

**Fig. 18.5**

are of the *muscarinic* type. The effect of *catecholamines* on smooth muscle depends on the type of receptor stimulated. Adrenergic receptors are of two types: α and β. In general, β adrenoceptors are inhibitory, causing relaxation while α-adrenoceptors may be either excitatory or inhibitory.

# Compare and contrast single unit and multiple unit smooth muscles.

## SIMILARITIES

Both are non-striated, i.e., they do not show alternate dark and light bands.

Both have similar cytoarchitecture, i.e., caveoli, cytoplasmic dense bodies etc.

Both have similar contractile apparatus, with an excess of actin over myosin filaments, and the presence of calmodulin and myosin regulatory chain.

Both are associated with synapse *en passant*, i.e., each axon forms multiple junctions along its path with several muscle cells.

## DIFFERENCES

| Single unit smooth muscle | Multi unit smooth muscle |
|---|---|
| Present in the walls of gastrointestinal tract and genitourinary tract | Present in the intrinsic muscles of the eye, piloerector muscles, vas deferens, and in the walls of large elastic arteries. |
| Can be tonic (remain tonically contracted) or phasic (remain relaxed and contract only when stimulated) | Always phasic. |
| Show ephaptic conduction | Do not show ephaptic conduction |
| Excited by nerves, by hormones, stretch and cold temperature. | Excited through nerves only. |
| Can get excited spontaneously. | Do not get excited spontaneously. |
| Cannot be excited by graded potentials | Can be excited by graded potentials |
| Obey the all-or-none law | Show graded contractions. |
| Have diffuse junctions | Have contact junctions |

# Cardiac Muscle

### Where are automatic and non-automatic cardiac fibers located in the heart ?

Cardiac muscle fibers are broadly of two types: (i) the **non-automatic fibers** are located in the atria and ventricles. They are meant primarily for generating contractile force. (ii) the **automatic fibers** constitute the conducting system of the heart that is spontaneously excitable. They are relatively less contractile as they have fewer myofibrils and mitochondria and have poorly developed sarcoplasmic reticulum.

### What are the major similarities of cardiac muscle with skeletal and smooth muscles ?

Cardiac muscle *resembles skeletal muscle fibers* in that: (i) it contains regular sarcomeres delimited by Z-disks and shows similar length-tension relationship; (ii) its contraction is regulated by troponin-tropomyosin complex. Cardiac muscle *resembles the visceral smooth muscle* in that: (i) it shows automaticity and ephaptic conduction; (ii) its contractility is affected by hormones.

### How is cardiac excitation contraction coupling different from that in skeletal muscles ?

The sarcoplasmic $Ca^{2+}$ pulse is produced predominantly by mobilization of *intracellular* $Ca^{2+}$ when the ryanodine channels on lateral cisterns open up. However, this mobilization is triggered by a smaller amount of extracellular $Ca^{2+}$ that enters through the sarcolemma when the membrane is excited and binds to the ryanodine receptors. This process is called **calcium-induced calcium release (CICR)** (Fig. 18.2). Although cardiac fibers show T-tubules as in skeletal muscle fibers, these T-tubules do little else than to let in extracellular $Ca^{2+}$ like the rest of the sarcolemma.

### Describe the phases of action potential in non-automatic cardiac fibers.

The action potential in a non-automatic cardiac fiber shows a characteristic **plateau**. In all, it has four phases (Fig. 19.1). (i) **Phase 0** is the phase of depolarization that occurs due to the opening of $Na^+$ channels, resulting in a fast inward depolarizing current. (ii) **Phase 1** is the partial repolarization that occurs due to $Na^+$ channel inactivation and a transient increase in $K^+$ permeability (the *transient outward $K^+$ current*). (ii) **Phase 2** is the plateau during which the membrane repolarizes very slowly, or not at all. This prolonged plateau increases the duration of cardiac action potential and also, the duration of its refractory period (Fig. 19.2). Due to its long refractory period, *cardiac muscle cannot be tetanized* like skeletal muscle. (iv) **Phase 3** is the phase of complete repolarization. It occurs due to outward diffusion of $K^+$. (v) **Phase**

**4** is the phase of RMP of ~ –90mV. It is maintained by a resting $K^+$ current, the largest contributor to which is the *inward rectifying $K^+$ current*.

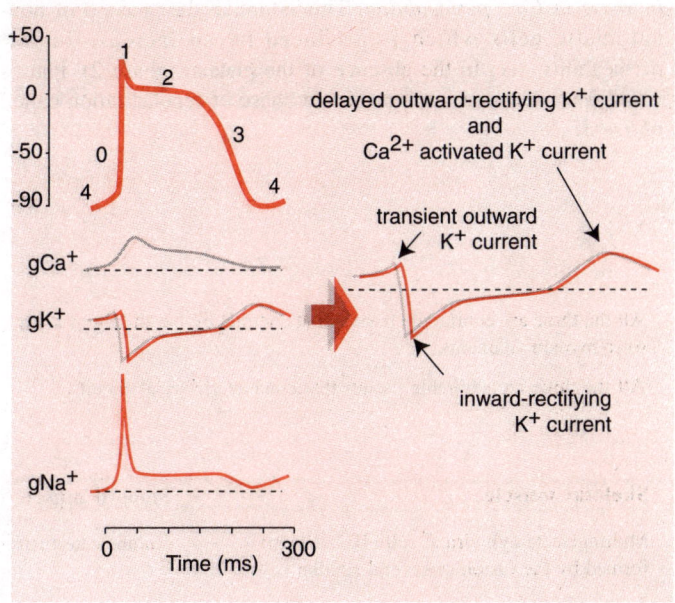

**Fig. 19.1**

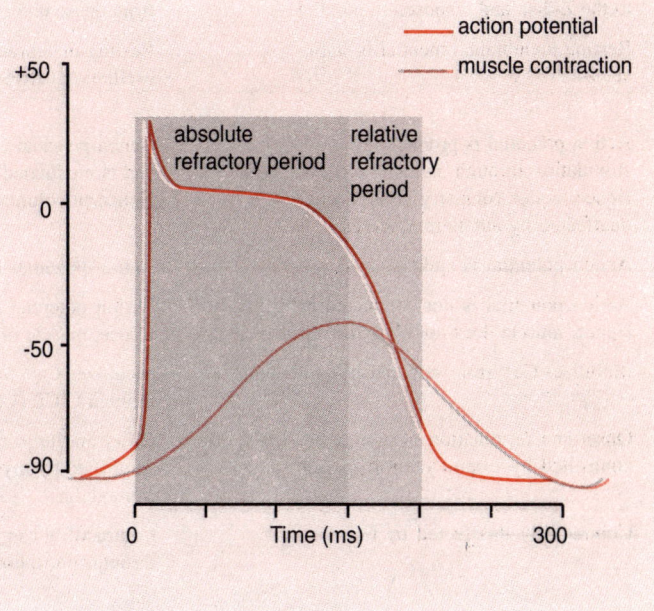

**Fig. 19.2**

## Describe the action potential in automatic cardiac fibers.

Action potentials of automatic cardiac fibers are single spikes on the peaks of an oscillating membrane potential (Fig. 19.3). The action potential of an automatic cardiac fiber shows salient differences from that of a non-automatic fiber: (i) The *RMP* is less negative (–70mV) than in non-automatic cardiac fibers (–90mV). (ii) *Phase 4* of the AP shows a slow drift towards the threshold potential till the phase 0 is triggered. This characteristic phase 4 is also called the *pacemaker potential* or the *diastolic depolarization*. (iii) *Phase 0* is less steep and its peak is less sharp (more rounded) than the phase 0 in non-automatic fibers. This is because the depolarization in phase 0 occurs due to an *increase in Ca²⁺ permeability*. This is unlike the phase 0 of non-automatic cells which is produced by an increase in Na⁺ permeability. (iv) In the absence of the plateau (phase 2), Phases 1 and 3 are blended into one single phase of repolarization called *phase 3*.

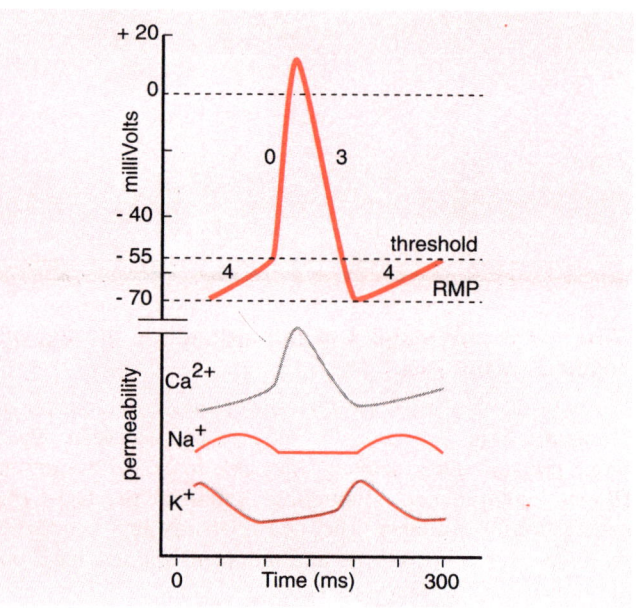

**Fig. 19.3**

## Compare and contrast skeletal, smooth and cardiac muscles.

**SIMILARITIES**

All the three are contractile tissues that contract by the sliding of actin over myosin filaments.

All the three are excitable tissues that conduct electrical signals.

**DIFFERENCES**

| Skeletal muscle | Smooth muscle (single unit) | Cardiac muscle |
|---|---|---|
| Multinucleate cylindrical cell (10 – 30 cm) formed by the fusion of several smaller cells. | Uninucleate fusiform cell (0.02 to 0.5 mm) | Uninucleate, cylindrical cells (0.1mm) that branch and join one another at the intercalated disk. |
| Sarcotubular system well developed. | Sarcotubular system poorly developed. | Sarcotubular system well developed. |
| Fiber is striated. Actin filaments attached to the Z-disk and disposed in parallel. | Fiber is unstriated. Actin filaments radiate from dense bodies. | Fiber is striated. Actin filaments attached to the Z-disk and disposed in parallel. |
| Resting membrane potential is stable at -90mV. | Resting membrane potential unstable, oscillating between –55 and –35mV. | Resting membrane potential is either stable at -90mV (non-automatic) or oscillates between -60 and -55 mV. |
| Action potential is produced by stimulation through somatic nerve. Hence, under voluntary control and unaffected by autonomic nerves. | Action potential is produced spontaneously and is modulated by autonomic nerves. Hence, involuntary. | Action potential is produced spontaneously and is modulated by autonomic nerves. Hence, involuntary. |
| Action potential is spike-shaped. | Action potential is spike-shaped or has a plateau. | Action potential has a plateau. |
| Action potential is not conducted ephaptically. Hence, muscle does not obey the all-or-none law. | Action potential is conducted ephaptically. Hence, muscle obeys the all-or-none law. | Action potential is conducted ephaptically. Hence, muscle obeys the all-or-none law. |
| Mobilizes Ca²⁺ from sarcoplasmic reticulum. | Mobilizes Ca²⁺ from sarcoplasmic reticulum through CICR (Ca²⁺-induced Ca²⁺ release) | Mobilizes Ca²⁺ from sarcoplasmic reticulum through CICR (Ca²⁺-induced Ca²⁺ release) |
| Onset and termination of contraction are controlled by tropomyosin-troponin complex. | Onset and termination of contraction are controlled by myosin regulatory chain and calmodulin. | Onset and termination of contraction are controlled by tropomyosin-troponin complex. |
| Contractility unaffected by hormones. | Contractility can be modulated by hormones through phosphorylation of myosin. | Contractility can be modulated by hormones through phosphorylation of myosin. |

# Blood & Plasma Proteins

## Give the normal counts of the cellular elements of blood.

| Red Blood Cells | Males | 5.5 (±1.0) million/µL | |
|---|---|---|---|
| | Females | 4.8 (±1.0) million/µL | |
| **White Blood Cells** | | | |
| Total Leucocytic Count | | 4000-11,000/µL | |
| Differential Leucocytic Count | Neutrophils | 3000-6000 | (50-70%) |
| | Eosinophils | 150-300 | (1-4%) |
| | Basophils | 0-100 | (0.4%) |
| | Lymphocytes | 1500-4000 | (20-40%) |
| | Monocytes | 300-600 | (2-8%) |
| **Platelets** | | 200,000-500,000/µL | |

## What is the difference between plasma and serum?

The plasma contains innumerable substances, of which proteins (the *plasma proteins*) are the major constituents. The other constituents are electrolytes, proteins, carbohydrates, lipids, minerals, enzymes and metabolites. Plasma contains, among other substances, coagulation proteins. Hence like blood, it too clots on standing. *Plasma without the coagulation proteins* is called **serum**. It is obtained by allowing whole blood to clot. As the clot hardens, it shrinks and extrudes the serum.

Serum has essentially the same composition as plasma except that (i) its fibrinogen and clotting factors II, V, and VIII have been removed, and (ii) it has a higher serotonin content due to the breakdown of platelets during clotting.

## What is the normal plasma protein concentration in the plasma?

| Total proteins | : | 5.5 – 8.0 g% |
|---|---|---|
| Albumin | : | 3.5 – 5.5 g% |
| Globulin | : | 2.0 – 3.5 g% |

Physiological variations are seen in infancy and pregnancy. **Infants** have plasma protein concentrations of 5.0-5.5 g%. In the first 6 months of **pregnancy**, the albumin and globulin levels decrease while the fibrinogen level increases.

## What is the normal specific gravity of blood?

The normal specific gravity of blood is between 1.055 – 1.060. The specific gravity of blood is affected by the hemoglobin concentration as well as the plasma protein concentration.

## What are the properties of plasma proteins?

(1) Plasma proteins are large molecules with molecular weights ranging mostly from 50,000 to 300,000 Daltons. (2) With the notable exception of albumin, *nearly all plasma proteins are glycoproteins*, containing oligosaccharides. The oligosaccharide chains are responsible for certain properties of plasma proteins like solubility, viscosity, charge, denaturation etc. (3) Like most other proteins, their charged residues tend to be located on the surface. (4) Many plasma proteins exhibit *polymorphism*. Polymorphism is a Mendelian trait that exists in the population in at least two phenotypes, neither of which is rare. Plasma proteins showing polymorphism are haptoglobin, transferrin, ceruloplasmin, and immunoglobulins.

Due to the large size of the protein molecules, (5) they can be separated from the plasma by *ultracentrifugation* (unlike electrolytes or other smaller molecules). (6) They are unable to pass across the capillary membrane and consequently exert an *oncotic pressure* of about 25 mm Hg. (7) Owing to their size and particularly their shape, they greatly contribute to *blood viscosity*. The plasma protein fibrinogen is a significant contributor to blood viscosity.

Due to the presence of polar residues on their surfaces, (8) the protein molecules are *soluble* in water. (9) The molecules show *electrophoretic mobility*. (10) The molecules are *amphoteric*. This is because the polar residues comprise both $NH_2$ and COOH groups. (11) They act as efficient *buffers* by virtue of their amphoteric nature. (12) They easily *bind with metallic ions and steroids*. The bonds are formed with the polar residues.

## What are the functions of plasma proteins?

The *general functions* of plasma proteins include (1) holding back the fluid portion of blood inside the blood vessels by virtue of the osmotic pressure it exerts, and (2) buffering the body fluids. They account for 15% of the blood buffering capacity. Besides the general function, different plasma proteins have *specific functions*. Plasma proteins can variously act as nutrients, enzymes, hormones, antibodies, clotting/fibrinolytic factors, and as carrier molecules.

| Function | Plasma protein |
|---|---|
| Nutrients | Lipoproteins |
| Enzymes | Amylase, alkaline phosphatase |
| Hormones | Anterior pituitary hormones, angiotensin |
| Antibodies | Gamma globulin |
| Clotting and fibrinolytic | Fibrinogen, prothrombin, fibrinolysin |
| Carrier | Albumin, ceruloplasmin, transferrin |
| Scavenger | Gel-solin, $G_c$ protein |

### How are plasma proteins classified?

Plasma proteins are classified broadly into albumin and globulin on the basis of their molecular weight. Thus, the different groups of plasma proteins include pre-albumin, albumin, $\alpha 1$ globulin, $\alpha 2$ globulin, $\beta$ globulin and $\gamma$ globulin (Fig. 20.1).

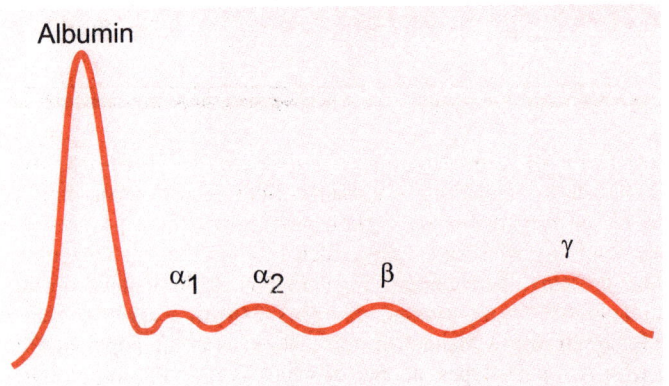

**Fig. 20.1**

### Where are plasma proteins synthesized?

The $\gamma$ globulins or the immunoglobulins are produced by the plasma cells. Most of the other plasma proteins are synthesized in the liver.

### Enumerate the causes of hypoproteinemia?

Hypoproteinemia, i.e., a generalized decrease in plasma proteins occurs in (1) **liver diseases**, because hepatic protein synthesis is depressed; (2) **renal disorders** like the nephrotic syndrome, in which glomerular membrane permeability increases markedly (3) **malnutrition** and starvation; (4) **protein-losing enteropathy**.

### What is A:G ratio and how is it affected in different diseases?

The normal ratio of plasma albumin to plasma globulin (the A:G ratio) is 1.7 : 1. Most cases of hypoproteinemia are due to a reduction in plasma albumin while hyperproteinemia is mostly due to increase in plasma globulin. Hence, in most of these cases, this ratio tends to decrease or even reverse.

### Name some causes of hyperproteinemia.

Increase in plasma proteins are seen in (1) *Acute inflammatory states*. Several plasma proteins increase sharply during any acute inflammation. These are called **acute phase proteins**. They include **C-reactive proteins (CRP)**, so called because it reacts with C-polysaccharide of pneumococci. (2) *Multiple myeloma*. In this condition, the plasma cells secrete large amounts of immunoglobulins resulting in **hypergammaglobinemia**.

### What is ESR and what are the factors affecting it?

When *anticoagulated blood* is allowed to stand in a long vertical tube, its erythrocytes settle down, leaving clear plasma on the top of the tube. The rate at which the erythrocytes settle down in a tube of standard dimensions (2.5 mm inner diameter, 200 mm height) is called the **erythrocytic sedimentation rate (ESR)** and is one of the oldest hematological tests that are still in use.

The most important factor that determines ESR is the extent of **rouleaux formation** by erythrocytes. (1) Rouleaux formation is determined mainly by the nature of plasma. *Increased rouleaux formation occurs when plasma contains increased amounts of fibrinogen (as in pregnancy) and serum globulin (as in inflammatory diseases)*. (2) Red cell characteristics also affect rouleaux formation and therefore the ESR. Hypochromic cells tend to fall more slowly in plasma than normochromic cells. Anisocytosis is usually associated with reduced ESR.

### What are the clinical uses of ESR ?

Two well-known causes of elevated ESR are *tuberculosis* and *rheumatoid arthritis*. However, ESR is elevated in so many diseases that it has little diagnostic utility. It is elevated in almost all *inflammatory disorders* and *collagen diseases*. Its main utility is in *prognosis*, i.e., prediction of the probable course of a disease in an individual and the chances of recovery. Thus, during a 6 to 9 month course of tuberculosis treatment, serial measurements of ESR will indicate if the patient is improving. It has similar use in certain malignancies, esp., Hodgkin's disease.

# Red Blood Cells & Anemia

### What are the advantages of carrying hemoglobin within a cell as against in the free form in plasma?

The advantages of carrying hemoglobin within a cell as against in the free form in plasma are threefold: (1) It prevents the rapid destruction and elimination of the hemoglobin. (2) It prevents a marked increase in the plasma viscosity that would have occurred if hemoglobin existed as a plasma protein. (3) It prevents blood from having a high osmolarity.

### What is the normal life span of an RBC ?

The normal life span of an RBC is about 120 days.

### Describe the normal shape of an RBC.

RBCs are *circular, non-nucleated* cells. It has the shape of a *biconcave* disc with a *large surface-to-volume ratio*, which represents the most efficient shape for rapid gaseous exchange. The red cell is *flexible* and it is readily distorted during its passage in the circulation. Thus as it passes through capillaries, it assumes a *parachute-like configuration* (Fig. 21.1). Excessive variation in the shape of the RBCs is called **poikilocytosis**.

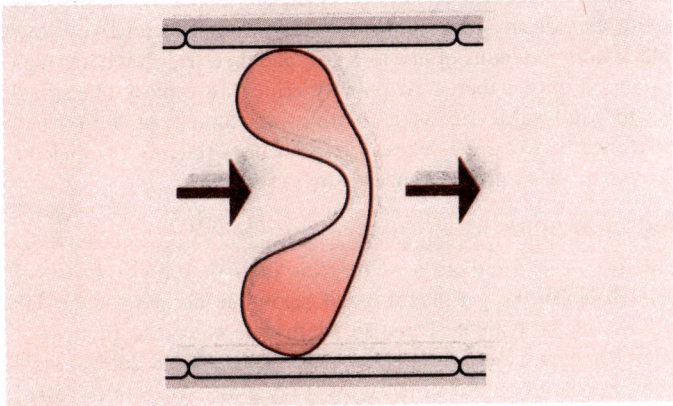

**Fig. 21.1**

### What are the normal variations in size of an RBC?

The mean cell diameter of red cells varies from 6.7 to 7.7 $\mu$m with a mean of 7.2 $\mu$m. The disc thickness is 2$\mu$. Excessive variation in red cell size is called **anisocytosis**.

### How is erythropoiesis regulated?

The production of RBCs is regulated by a hormone called **erythropoietin**. Erythropoietin is a glycoprotein secreted mainly by the kidney (85%) and liver (15%). In the kidney, erythropoietin-secreting cells are found in the interstitium of the inner cortex and outer medulla, lying just outside the tubular basement membrane.

Erythropoietin increases erythropoiesis by acting on the bone marrow as well as the fetal yolk sac, liver and spleen where it promotes (i) *differentiation* of erythropoietic stem cells to proerythroblasts, (ii) *proliferation* of committed stem cells, (iii) hemoglobin *synthesis* by increasing globulin synthesis and potentiating $\delta$-amino levulinic acid synthetase, and (iv) *release* of RBCs from bone marrow.

### What are the factors increasing erythropoietin secretion?

The factors that promote erythropoietin synthesis are (1) *hypoxia*. (2) *alkalosis*. (3) *hormones*: growth hormone, prolactin, thyroid hormones, catecholamines, corticosteroids and androgens. (4) *hemolysates*: (products, mainly nucleotides released following RBC destruction) cAMP, NAD and NADP. The effect of androgens on erythropoietin explains why males have higher RBC count.

Stimulation of erythropoietin by hypoxia is physiological feedback mechanism through which the number of RBCs is increased whenever there is $O_2$ deficiency in the tissues. The increase in RBC count improves tissue oxygenation. The same is true for hemolysates. Whenever there is increased red cell destruction, the hemolysates bring about increased red cell production.

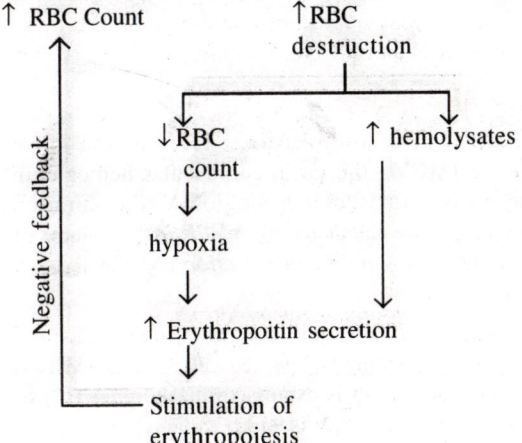

### How is red cell fragility measured? Name the conditions in which it is increased or decreased.

The red cell can become more rigid as a result of pathological changes in the membrane or in the cell contents. In these conditions, the **mechanical fragility** of the cell increases, i.e. they are less able to tolerate deforming stresses, than is the normal healthy red cell. Also, such cells are removed from circulation in larger numbers than normal cells.

A convenient method for testing red cell fragility is to test for **osmotic fragility**. RBCs are suspended in a series of saline solutions with strengths ranging from 0.9% to 0.3%. Red cells with normal osmotic fragility start showing hemolysis (red cell rupture with loss of hemoglobin) in 0.5% saline and are completely hemolyzed in 0.35% saline.

However, a normal or *low osmotic fragility does not rule out the possibility of a high mechanical fragility*. In sickle cell anemia, the RBCs are sickle-shaped and have a high mechanical fragility. However, the osmotic fragility of the sickled cells is normal or even low.

### What is meant by the terms normochromia, hyperchromia and hypochromia?

Red cell staining is deeper at the periphery and fades at the center (the central pallor). *Cells which stain normally* are assumed to have a normal concentration of hemoglobin and are called **normochromic**.

The term **hypochromia** is used to describe a *decrease in the intensity of staining*. Hypochromia is nearly always *associated with a decrease in the MCHC*, i.e. a decrease in the concentration of hemoglobin in the red cells. However, cells that are thinner than normal (as in thalassemia) may appear slightly hypochromic even though the MCHC is normal.

The term **hyperchromia** is used to describe an *increase in the intensity of staining* of the red cell, in which the cell stains more deeply and the central area of pallor is not apparent. Such an appearance is usually *due to an increase in the thickness of the cell*, and not to an increase in MCHC. (1) Spherocytosis have both an increase in red cell thickness as well as an elevated MCHC. They certainly are hyperchromic. (2) In megaloblastic anemia, the red cell diameter is increased but MCHC remains normal. Whether or not the cells should be called hyperchromic depends on what is meant by the term hyperchromia. Considering its ambiguity, *the term hyperchromia is best abandoned* in favor of the more objective terms like MCH and MCHC.

### Name the three RBC indices.

The *red cell indices* or *absolute values* refer to the mean corpuscular volume (MCV), the mean corpuscular hemoglobin (MCH) and the mean corpuscular hemoglobin concentration (MCHC). These indices are calculated from *VPRC* (the volume of packed red cells), the *hemoglobin concentration* and the *red cell count* as follows.

The **mean cell volume (MCV)** is the average volume of the red cells. It is calculated by dividing the packed cell volume (VPRC) by the red cell count. The result is expressed in femtoliter (fL) or cubic micrometer ($\mu^3$). Normal MCV is 90 $\mu^3$ (78-94 $\mu^3$).

$$MCV = \frac{\text{Volume of packed red cells (VPRC)}}{\text{red cell count (in 1L)}}$$

The **mean cell hemoglobin (MCH)** is the average weight of hemoglobin contained in each cell. The MCH is calculated by dividing the amount of hemoglobin in 1 L blood by the number of red cells present in 1 L of blood (the red cell count). The result is expressed in picograms. Normal MCH is 30 pg (28-32 pg).

$$MCH = \frac{\text{Hemoglobin concentration in g / dL}}{\text{red cell count (in 1 L)}} \times 10$$

The **mean cell hemoglobin concentration (MCHC)** is the average concentration of hemoglobin in the red cells. It is calculated by dividing the amount of hemoglobin in 1 L of blood by the volume of packed red cells in 1 L blood. The result is expressed in g/dL. Normal MCHC is 33 g% (32-38 g%).

$$MCHC = \frac{\text{Hemoglobin concentration in g / dL}}{\text{Volume of packed red cells (VPRC) (in 1 dL)}}$$

The three indices are related by the formula :

$$MCHC = \frac{MCH}{MCV}$$

### What is VPRC? Name the clinical significance of VPRC.

VPRC is total volume of packed red cells in 1 dL of blood and is determined by centrifuging blood at 3000 rpm in a graduated centrifuge tube. It was earlier called **packed cell volume (PCV)**. However, since cells other than red cells are not considered, this term has been abandoned. VPRC is also called the **hematocrit**.

The VPRC is a useful clinical test that is used for detecting anemia, polycythemia (increase in the number of red cells), hemodilution or hemoconcentration (i.e., relatively less or more red cells as compared to plasma.). *A normal VPRC does not rule out the possibility of a low red cell count*: it might be a case of hemoconcentration.

### How does RBC count vary with age and sex?

The values of red cell count and VPRC are higher on the first day of life than at any time subsequently. They fall to relatively low values from 3 months of age to 1 year and then rise slowly through childhood until puberty. At puberty there is a rapid and marked rise to adult values in males, with establishment of the normal difference between the sexes. These changes roughly parallel the changes in hemoglobin concentration (Fig. 22.1).

### Define anemia.

Anemia is defined as a *reduction in the concentration of hemoglobin* in the peripheral blood below the normal for the age and sex of the patient. Thus, an adult male is said to be anemic when his hemoglobin falls below 13.0 g/dL, and an adult female when her hemoglobin falls below 11.5 g/dL. Anemia is called *moderate when it falls below 9g/dL* and *severe when it falls below 6g/dL*.

The fall of the hemoglobin below normal values is usually, but not always, accompanied by a fall of the red cell count. Thus occasionally, esp. in the hypochromic microcytic anemia of iron deficiency, the red cell count is normal although the hemoglobin is significantly reduced. This is due to the low hemoglobin content of the individual cells.

### How are anemias classified?

There are two main classifications of anemia: (1) the *etiological classification*, based on the cause of the anemia;

(2) the *laboratory classification*, based on the characteristics of the red cell as determined by blood examination.

The **laboratory (or morphological) classification of anemias** is based on two features, namely, the average cell volume (MCV) and the mean corpuscular hemoglobin concentration (MCHC). The following main types are recognized: (1) **Normocytic anemias**, in which the MCV is within the normal range (76-96 fl). Most normocytic anemias are also normochromic with a normal MCHC (30-35 g/dl), but in some mild hypochromia may occur. (2) **Microcytic anemias**, in which the MCV is reduced (less than 76 fl). Microcytic anemias are mostly hypochromic with the MCHC reduced (less than 30 g/dl). (3) **Macrocytic anemias**, in which the MCV is increased (greater than 96 fl). Most macrocytic anemias are normochromic but in some a mild hypochromia (reduced MCHC) may occur.

The **etiological classification** of anemias is based on the cause, which can be a deficiency of nutrients, increased destruction of erythrocytes or acute/chronic blood loss. Accordingly, anemias may be (1) **Deficiency anemias**, which occur due to impaired red cell formation that can occur when there is deficiency of iron (iron-deficiency anemia) or due to vitamin $B_{12}$ or folate deficiency (megaloblastic anemia). (2) **Hemolytic anemias**, which are due to increased red cell destruction. They are relatively uncommon. Red cells are destroyed in large numbers either due to some defect in the red cell itself (intracorpuscular defect), or due to some defect in its immediate environment (extracorpuscular defect). **Intracorpuscular abnormalities** include (a) *Membrane defects* like hereditary spherocytosis; (b) *Hemoglobin defects* like sickle cell anemias, thalassemias; (c) *Enzyme defects* like glucose-6-phosphatase dehydrogenase (G6PD) deficiency. **Extracorpuscular abnormalities** include (a) *Immunological damage* caused by the presence of antibodies which lyse RBCs e.g., autoimmune hemolytic anemias and hemolytic disease of the newborn; (b) *Mechanical damage*: Microangiopathic hemolytic anemia; (c) *Others*: Hemolytic anemias due to infection, burns, chemicals and drugs.

**Hemorrhagic anemia** occurs due to blood loss, both acute and chronic. It is a common cause of anemia. Anemia following acute blood loss (acute post-hemorrhagic anemia) results in hemodilution. This is because the *plasma is restored much faster than the cellular elements*. The result is a normocytic, normochromic anemia. Anemia due to chronic blood loss (chronic post-hemorrhagic anemia) tends to show features of iron deficiency, i.e., a microcytic, hypochromic anemia.

## What are the general signs and symptoms of anemia?

Anemia results in reduced $O_2$-carrying capacity of blood, resulting in *tissue hypoxia*. The hypoxia causes symptoms like easy fatigability (due to muscle hypoxia) and faintness (due to cerebral hypoxia), especially on exertion.

The hypoxia brings about several compensatory responses. While alleviating tissue hypoxia, some of these responses add to the symptoms like *breathlessness* due to compensatory stimulation of respiratory center and *palpitation* due to compensatory increase in cardiac output. Signs include *cardiac murmurs* due to turbulence of blood while passing through the cardiac valves — another consequence of the raised cardiac output.

# Hemoglobin & its Reactions

## What is the normal hemoglobin concentration in adults? How does it change after birth?

The adult values of hemoglobin are 15.5 ± 2.5g/dL (for men) and 14.0 ± 2.5g/dL (for women). In infants, it is higher. The average hemoglobin concentration of blood from the umbilical cord averages 16.5 g/dl. The **cord blood** is representative of the infant's blood before birth. Shortly after birth the hemoglobin value of normal infants increases rapidly. The hemoglobin on the first day of life is ~18.5 g/dL. This is due to (1) the '**transfusion**' of cells from the placenta to the infant and (2) the **hemoconcentration** caused by rapid reduction of plasma volume. After the 2 days, there is marked fall for 2 weeks, stabilizing by the third month at 12.0 g/dL. It starts rising again at the end of 1 year towards the adult level. An adolescent spurt occurs in boys (Fig. 22.1).

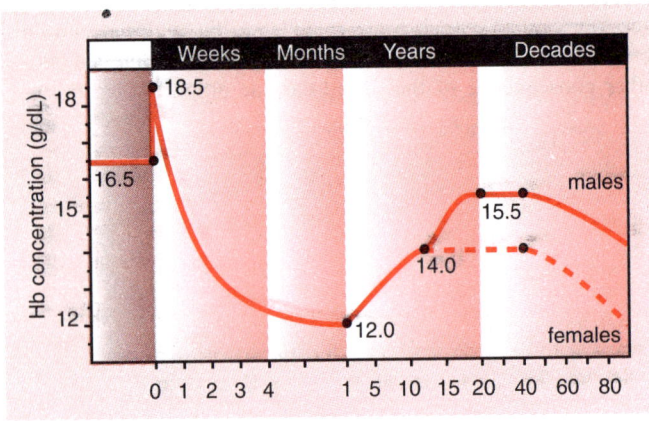

**Fig. 22.1**

## Briefly outline the structure of hemoglobin.

**Hemoglobin**, (molecular weight of 64,450) is a globular molecule made up of 4 subunits. Each subunit is made of a polypeptide chain containing **heme** – an iron-containing porphyrin (Fig. 22.2). The four polypeptide chains present in a hemoglobin molecule are collectively called **globin**. The polypeptide chains may be of different types. However, hemoglobin A, which comprises 97% of the normal hemoglobin, is made of **two ∝ chains**, containing 141 amino acid residues, and **two β chains**, containing 146 amino acid residues. The **iron** atom of heme is attached between the histidine residues. In the deoxygenated state, the iron atom is located between the plane of the ring and a histidine residue.

## Enumerate the important physiological reactions of hemoglobin.

(1) **Oxygenation**. Oxygen binds reversibly with hemoglobin to form oxyhemoglobin. A total of four $O_2$ molecules bind to a molecule

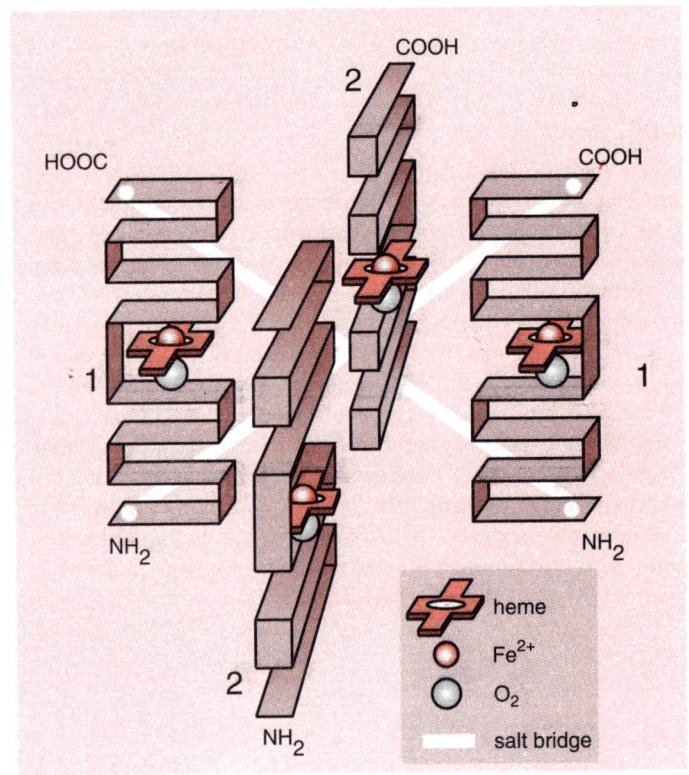

**Fig. 22.2**

of hemoglobin – one each to a heme molecule. 1 g of hemoglobin contains *3.4 mg of iron*, and can carry up to *1.34 ml of oxygen*. Formation of oxyhemoglobin is more difficult in the presence of $CO_2$ (the Bohr effect). (2) **Buffering of $H^+$ ions.** $H^+$ ions are buffered by the $NH_2$ of the intermediate histidine residues to form $NH_3^+$. The buffering of $H^+$ ions is important for transport of $CO_2$ in plasma as bicarbonates. *Oxygenation of hemoglobin reduces the buffering capacity of hemoglobin.* (3) Reaction with $CO_2$ to form **carbaminohemoglobin**. $CO_2$ binds to the terminal $\alpha$-$NH_2$ groups of the $\alpha$ and $\beta$ polypeptide chains to produce carbamino-hemoglobin and releases $H^+$ which are buffered by hemoglobin. (4) **Reaction with 2,3 diphosphoglycerate (DPG)**. DPG binds to $NH_3^+$ groups on the $\beta$ polypeptide chains. Binding of DPG makes it difficult for $O_2$ to bind to hemoglobin (Bohr effect). (5) Reaction with carbon monoxide forming **carboxyhemoglobin**. Carbon monoxide reacts with hemoglobin to form carboxyhemoglobin. The affinity of hemoglobin for CO is 200 times higher than its affinity for $O_2$. It binds exactly where $O_2$ binds to heme. (6) **Oxidation** of heme iron to form **methemoglobin**. The ferrous iron of hemoglobin is susceptible to oxidation to ferric iron by superoxides and other oxidizing agents, forming methemoglobin that cannot carry oxygen. When more than 10% of the normal hemoglobin changes to methemoglobin, it causes a dusky discoloration of the skin resembling cyanosis. (7) **Glycosylation** of hemoglobin. Hemoglobin is nonenzymatically glycosylated by the glucose that enters the erythrocytes.

## What is the clinical importance of glycosylated hemoglobin?

The amount of glycosylated hemoglobin (HbA$_{1C}$), normally about 5%, is proportionate to the blood glucose concentration. The HbA$_{1C}$ level reflects the average blood glucose concentration over the preceding 6 – 8 weeks and serves as *an index of long-term control of diabetes mellitus*. Thus, a patient who is mostly careless about controlling his hyperglycemia and takes an insulin injection only before visiting his doctor would have normal blood glucose but his HbA$_{1C}$ will be elevated.

## Enumerate the different types of normal hemoglobin in the body.

The different types of normal hemoglobin in the body are given below.

| HbA | $\alpha_2\beta_2$ | Comprises about 97% of the hemoglobin of adult red cells. Small amounts of Hb-A are detected in the fetus as early as the eighth week of life. During the first few months of post-natal life, Hb-A almost completely replaces Hb-F. |
|---|---|---|
| HbA$_2$ | $\alpha_2\delta_2$ | Is present in small amounts (about 1.5-3.2 % in normal adults) |
| HbF | $\alpha_2\gamma_2$ | It is the predominant form of hemoglobin in the fetus. It has greater affinity for oxygen. It is more resistant to acid denaturation; hence, it is measured by the alkali denaturation method. |
| Hb-Bart's | $\gamma_4$ | Present in the fetus in small amounts. |
| Hb-Gower 1 | $\zeta_2\varepsilon_2$ | Embryonic forms of hemoglobin. |
| Hb-Gower 2 | $\alpha_2\varepsilon_2$ | |
| Hb-Portland | $\xi_2\varepsilon_2$ | |

Fetal hemoglobin is the main oxygen binding protein in intra-uterine life (after the first 12 weeks). Fetal hemoglobin usually disappears from the red cells of normal infants after the age of 4 to 6 months, although very small amounts (less than 2%) can be detected in the cells of most children and adults.

## Define hemoglobinopathy.

Hemoglobinopathies refer to *abnormalities in the aminoacid sequence of the polypeptide chains of hemoglobin*. Examples are Hb-S, Hb-C, Hb-E and Hb-D Punjab. They occur due to a defect in the gene that directs the synthesis of these polypeptide chains. Several abnormal hemoglobins, however, have no harmful effects.

## What is sickle cell anemia?

In **hemoglobin S**, the $\alpha$ chains are normal but in the $\beta$ chains, the *glutamic acid residue at position 6 is replaced by valine*. This substitution results in the *polymerization of HbS* forming long, fibrous precipitates. *The precipitates distort the erythrocyte, making it sickle shaped*. Sickle cell *anemia results from increased destruction of sickled red cells*.

Sickling occurs *only when the oxygenation of hemoglobin is low*. Sickling is less in cells that have higher HbF. HbF prevents the formation of long polymers of HbS.

## Briefly explain the pathophysiology of sickle-cell anemia.

Sickling of red cells causes two types of problems: (1) sickled cells are hemolyzed in large numbers, resulting in **hemolytic anemia**. The hemolysis is both intravascular and extravascular. *Intravascular hemolysis* occurs due to the fragmentation of the rigid cells due to mechanical stress as it tries to pass through narrow capillaries. *Extravascular hemolysis* occurs due to excessive phagocytosis of the IgG-coated sickle cells by macrophages in splenic sinusoids. (2) Sickled cells *obstruct capillary microcirculation*. The occlusion has two effects: (a) It causes **stagnant hypoxia**. The hypoxia produces sickling of more cells and initiates a vicious cycle. (b) It causes severe **ischemic pain**, causing **vasoocclusive crisis**.

## Define thalassemia. Briefly explain the pathophysiology of thalassemia.

Thalassemias are disorders in which the hemoglobin polypeptide chains are produced in decreased amounts or are absent because of defects in the regulatory portion of the globin genes. *Decreased or absent $\alpha$ and $\beta$ polypeptides* are called $\alpha$ and $\beta$ thalassemia respectively. Decreased polypeptide chain synthesis has two effects: (1) a general reduction in the amount of hemoglobin synthesized and (2) an imbalance between the amounts of different chains. In $\alpha$ **thalassemia** for example, in the absence of $\alpha$ chains, four $\beta$ chains aggregate to form $\beta_4$, called **Hb-H**. These aggregates precipitate in the cytoplasm and cause membrane damage. *Red cells with these aggregates are removed in large numbers by splenic macrophages*, causing **hemolytic anemia**.

# Hemoglobin Degradation & Jaundice

## Explain the terms intravascular in extravascular hemolysis.

Aged RBCs are phagocytosed by macrophages, mostly those lining the hepatic and splenic sinusoids. Hemoglobin is broken down and *bilirubin is formed within the macrophages*. The bilirubin formed inside macrophages is released into blood. *Liver cells take up the bilirubin from circulation and conjugate it with glucuronide*. Iron is released into circulation. *Conjugated bilirubin is excreted into the intestine* through the bile ducts. (1) When there is excessive removal of RBCs by macrophages (**extravascular hemolysis**), the capacity of liver cells to conjugate bilirubin may be exceeded, resulting in **hyperbilirubinemia**. (2) When there is excessive breakdown of RBCs inside the blood vessels (**intravascular hemolysis**), the free hemoglobin enters into circulation (**hemoglobinemia**). It also results in hyperbilirubinemia and may result in **hemoglobinuria**.

## Briefly outline the formation of bilirubin.

Inside the macrophage, the heme molecule is cleaved off globin. Globin is degraded into aminoacids and reused. Next, the iron in the porphyrin is converted into $Fe^{3+}$ form. The ring is broken to release the iron and carbon monoxide, resulting in the formation of **biliverdin**, a green pigment. These reactions are catalyzed by *heme oxygenase*, an enzyme complex present in the microsomes of macrophages. Biliverdin is then converted into **bilirubin**, a yellow pigment, by *bilirubin reductase*.

## Briefly outline the excretion of bilirubin.

Bilirubin is poorly soluble in water and is transported in plasma bound to albumin. In the hepatic sinusoids, bilirubin dissociates from albumin to enter the liver cell through facilitated diffusion. Bilirubin is lipid soluble and would tend to persist inside the cell. The hepatocytes conjugate bilirubin with **uridine diphosphate glucuronic acid**, making it water-soluble so that it can be excreted in bile. The reaction is catalyzed by the enzyme **gluconosyl transferase** present in hepatic microsomes (i.e. the smooth endoplasmic reticulum of the liver cells). The reaction occurs in two stages.

| UDP-glucuronic acid + bilirubin | *UDP-glucuronosyl-transferase* ——————————→ | bilirubin monoglucuronide + UDP |
|---|---|---|
| UDP-glucuronic acid + bilirubin monoglucuronide | *UDP-glucuronosyl-transferase* ——————————→ | bilirubin diglucuronide + UDP |

The conjugated bilirubin is excreted into the hepatic canaliculi through active transport. This active transport is the rate-limiting step in the entire process of bilirubin excretion.

## Briefly outline the formation of and excretion of urobilinogen.

The conjugated bilirubin excreted in bile is acted upon by intestinal bacteria in the terminal ileum and the large intestine. The bacterial enzyme *β-glucuronidase* splits off the glucuronide and converts bilirubin into **urobilinogen**, a colorless compound. The urobilinogen formed is reabsorbed from the intestine and

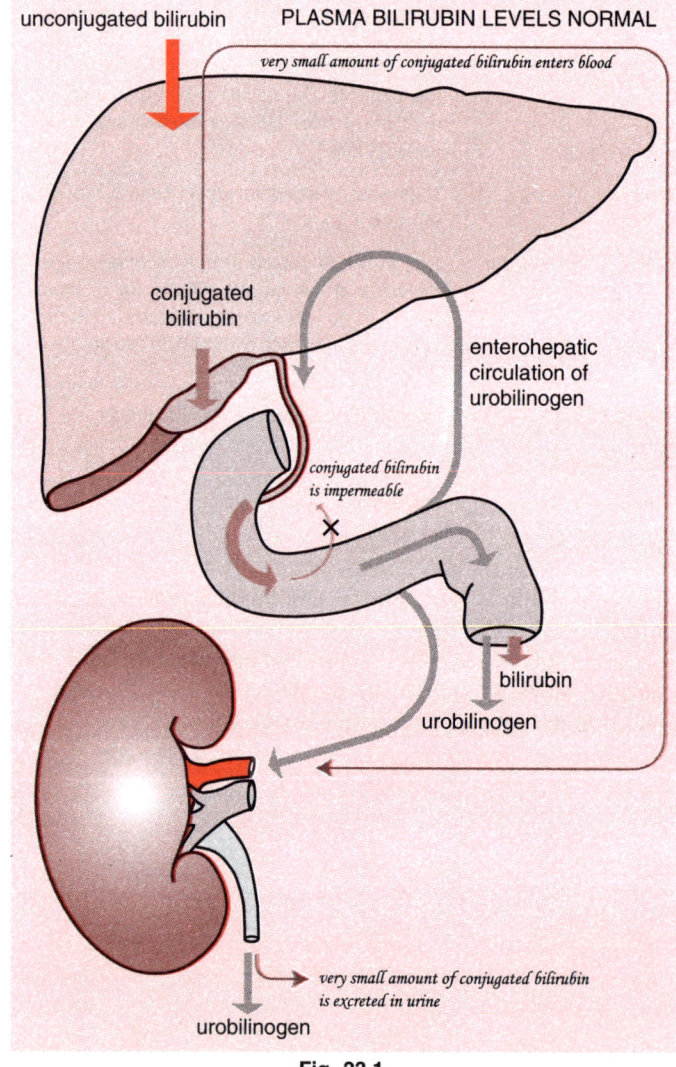

unconjugated bilirubin

PLASMA BILIRUBIN LEVELS NORMAL

*very small amount of conjugated bilirubin enters blood*

conjugated bilirubin

enterohepatic circulation of urobilinogen

*conjugated bilirubin is impermeable*

bilirubin

urobilinogen

*very small amount of conjugated bilirubin is excreted in urine*

urobilinogen

**Fig. 23.1**

reexcreted by the liver into the intestine through bile. This constitutes the **enterohepatic cycle** of urobilinogen. A relatively small amount of urobilinogen that is absorbed from the intestine is excreted in urine (Fig. 23.1).

### Why does stool darken on standing in air?

Most of the urobilinogens (colorless) formed in the intestine are further oxidized to **urobilins** (colored compounds) and excreted in feces. The darkening of feces on standing in air is due to conversion of the residual urobilinogens to urobilins.

### Define hyperbilirubinemia and jaundice.

The normal serum bilirubin level ranges from 0.3 mg – 1.0 mg/ 100ml. Most of this bilirubin is in the unconjugated form. The term **jaundice** or **icterus** refers to the yellowish discoloration of the skin and mucous membranes caused by an excessive accumulation of bilirubin in blood (**hyperbilirubinemia**). Clinical jaundice is apparent *when serum bilirubin exceeds 2 mg/100ml.* In hypothyroid states, the serum carotene is elevated, and the skin becomes yellow. This skin condition differs from that observed in jaundice in that the *sclera of the eye is not yellow.* The excess

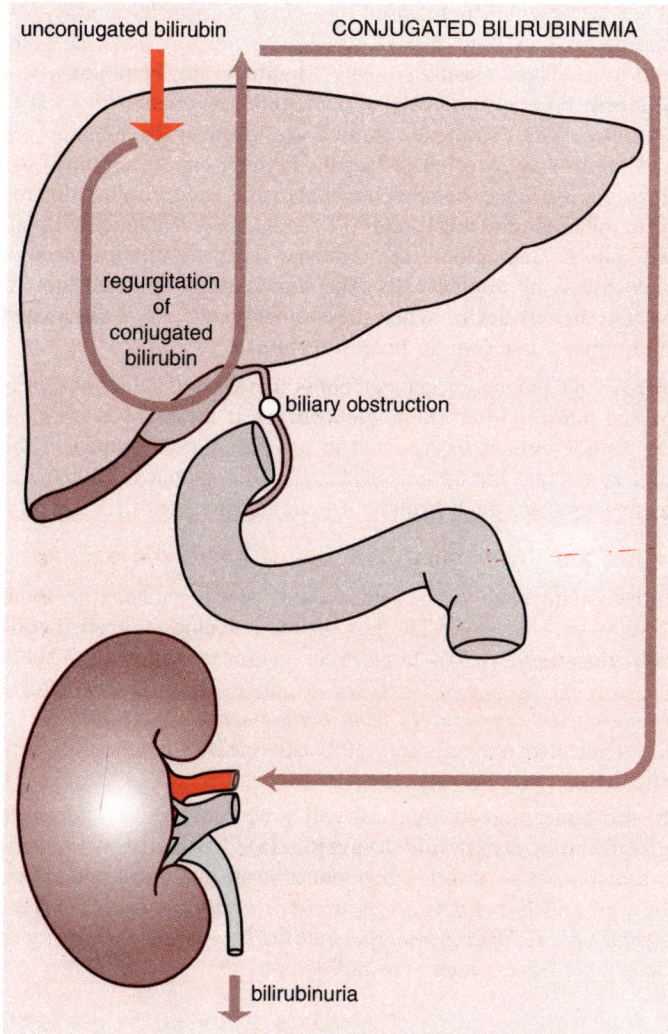

**Fig. 23.2**

bilirubin in blood may be mostly conjugated or mostly unconjugated. Accordingly, it is called *predominantly conjugated* or *predominantly unconjugated hyperbilirubinemia.*

### What is the difference between choluric and acholuric jaundice?

When jaundice is associated with the presence of bile pigments in urine, it is called choluric jaundice. If jaundice is not associated with the presence of bile pigments in urine, it is called acholuric. *Conjugated hyperbilirubinemia* is always **choluric** while *unconjugated hyperbilirubinemia* is always **acholuric**. Unconjugated bilirubin is poorly soluble in water and is transported in plasma bound to albumin. Hence, the bilirubin is not filtered into urine. Conjugated bilirubin is water-soluble and therefore it is transported in plasma in dissolved form. Hence, in conjugated hyperbilirubinemia, the bilirubin appears in urine.

### What is prehepatic jaundice? Why does it result in unconjugated hyperbilirubinemia?

When the jaundice occurs due to increased formation of bilirubin, as in *hemolytic anemias*, it is called prehepatic jaundice. The liver is unable to conjugate the large amounts of bilirubin produced, resulting in unconjugated hyperbilirubinemia.

### What is post hepatic jaundice? Why does it result in conjugated hyperbilirubinemia?

Posthepatic jaundice occurs due to *biliary obstruction.* As a result, the conjugated bilirubin produced in the liver regurgitates back into blood instead of flowing out into the duodenum. This results in conjugated hyperbilirubinemia.

### What is hepatic jaundice? Why does it usually result in conjugated hyperbilirubinemia?

The commonest cause of hepatic jaundice is *infective hepatitis.* In this condition, there is impairment of all the steps, i.e., hepatic uptake of bilirubin from blood, conjugation of bilirubin and finally, the excretion (of bilirubin) into biliary canaliculi. While reduced uptake and conjugation tend to produce unconjugated hyperbilirubinemia, reduced excretion produces conjugated hyperbilirubinemia. Since the *excretion of bilirubin is the worst affected in infective hepatitis*, it results in conjugated hyperbilirubinemia.

### What are the differences between prehepatic, hepatic and posthepatic jaundice?

The differences between these three types of jaundice are largely due to the type of hyperbilirubinemia they produce (conjugated or unconjugated). Prehepatic jaundice results in unconjugated hyperbilirubinemia while posthepatic jaundice is associated with conjugated hyperbilirubinemia. *Hepatic jaundice may be associated with either of the two depending on the cause.* Unconjugated bilirubinemia occurs in **neonatal jaundice** and in genetic defects of UDP glucuronosyl transferase, as in **Gilbert syndrome** (mild form) or **Crigler-Najjar syndrome** (severe form). Conjugated bilirubinemia occurs in more generalized disorder of the liver, e.g., **infective hepatitis**.

The other differences are really the characteristics of the cause of the jaundice and are unrelated to hyperbilirubinemia. These differences help the diagnostician to ascertain the cause of the jaundice but strictly speaking, cannot be considered as differences in the type of jaundice itself. For example, preheptatic jaundice is due to excessive hemolysis and therefore shows all the evidences of **hemolytic anemia**. Similarly, hepatic jaundice may be associated with all the features of impaired hepatic functions. For example, if the hepatic canalicular cells are damaged, there is rise in serum alkaline phosphatase. If the hepatitis is associated with hypergammaglobinemia, addition of thymol barbitone to the serum produces turbidity (**thymol turbidity test**). Finally, posthepatic jaundice occurs due to biliary obstruction and therefore is associated with features of fat indigestion (**steatorrhea**). The biliary obstruction results in damage to biliary canaliculi in the liver with consequent large increase in **serum alkaline phosphatase** level.

### Compare and contrast conjugated and unconjugated hyperbilirubinemia.

**SIMILARITIES**

Both types of hyperbilirubinemia are associated with jaundice, i.e., yellowish discoloration of the skin and mucous membranes.

**DIFFERENCES**

| Conjugated hyperbilirubinemia | Unconjugated hyperbilirubinemia |
|---|---|
| Jaundice is choluric | Jaundice is acholuric |
| Jaundice is mostly due to posthepatic causes. Hepatic causes include infective hepatitis. | Jaundice is mostly due to prehepatic causes. Hepatic causes include neonatal jaundice, Gilbert syndrome and Crigler - Najjar syndrome |
| Kernicterus can never occur | Kernicterus can occur |
| Stool may be clay-colored | Stool is never clay-colored |
| Van den Berg reaction is direct | Van den Berg reaction is indirect |

### What is kernicterus?

Kernicterus is a neurological condition that *occurs in infants with severe unconjugated bilirubinemia*. Since the blood-brain barrier in infants is more permeable than in adults, the free bilirubin is able to cross it and gets deposited in the basal ganglia, resulting in neurological signs and symptoms.

### What is the cause of neonatal jaundice and how is it treated?

In neonatal jaundice (also called **physiologic jaundice of the newborn**), up to 5 mg/dL of hyperbilirubinemia may be seen normally in the newborn. It appears within 2 – 5 days of birth and subsides in 2 weeks. In the fetus, bilirubin is removed from circulation by the placenta. At birth, all of a sudden, the newborn has to excrete its own bilirubin, but its *hepatic conjugation of bilirubin is inadequate due to reduced UDP-glucuronosyl transferase activity*. As a result, hyperbilirubinemia occurs which subsides when the newborn's liver 'matures'.

### How is neonatal jaundice treated and prevented?

The jaundice can be reduced by **phototherapy**. Exposure of the skin to white or blue lights causes photoisomerization of bilirubin to water-soluble **lumirubin**, which is rapidly excreted in bile without requiring any conjugation. The jaundice can be prevented by administration of **phenobarbital** to the pregnant mother or the newborn. Phenobarbital belongs to a group of drugs called **hepatic microsomal enzyme inducers**. Microsomal inducers *increase the activity of glucuronyl transferase*.

### Describe the Van den Berg test.

The Van den Berg test is used for estimating conjugated as well as unconjugated bilirubin levels in plasma. When Ehrlich's diazo reagent is added to conjugated bilirubin, a reddish brown coloration is obtained. It is called the **direct** Van den Berg reaction. Unconjugated bilirubin, which is water-insoluble, has to be dissolved in methanol before adding the reagent. Hence, the reddish violet coloration obtained after adding the reagent is called **indirect** Van den Berg reaction.

### Enumerate the consequences of intravascular hemolysis.

When hemoglobin is released into circulation in large amounts, plasma proteins bind to it so that iron is not lost from the body into urine. Three plasma proteins – **haptoglobin**, **hemopexin** and **albumin** bind successively to hemoglobin or heme, till each is saturated. The complexes formed are taken up by hepatocytes and the iron is recycled. When the binding capacities of all the three are exceeded, hemoglobin starts circulating in blood in free form (**hemoglobinemia**) and is filtered into the renal tubules. Small amounts of hemoglobin are removed from the tubules through endocytosis by tubular cells. The iron is stored in renal tubular cells as **hemosiderin**. When these tubular cells are desquamated into tubules, it results in **hemosiderinuria**.

When large amount of hemoglobin is filtered into the tubules, it is passed into the urine (**hemoglobinuria**). If the urine is alkaline, the hemoglobin is oxygenated to oxyhemoglobin (**pink**) in the urinary tract. If the urine is acidic, the hemoglobin is oxidized to methemoglobin (**dark brown**). The urine color varies accordingly.

### What are the clinical features of hemolytic anemia?

In hemolytic anemias, the reticulocyte count is increased to about 5 –20% or even more. The less mature reticulocytes (called **shift reticulocytes**) are 30% larger than mature reticulocytes. This is because *in response to increased demand, erythropoietin delivers reticulocytes prematurely from bone marrow to circulation*. A few nucleated red cells (erythroblasts released prematurely into circulation) may also be seen.

In the bone marrow, the red cell precursors show excessive proliferation (**erythroid hyperplasia**). Normally, white cell precursors are 3 – 4 times more numerous than red cell precursors. In erythroid hyperplasia, *the myeloid: erythroid ratio becomes roughly 1 : 1*. The *marrow-space in the bone widens*, resulting in detectable bone changes in radiographs.

## What is the role of iron in the body?

The role of iron in the body lies in the synthesis of hemoglobin (cytoplasmic maturation of RBCs), myoglobin and cytochromes (intracellular enzymes).

## What is the dietary form of iron: $Fe^{2+}$ or $Fe^{3+}$?

The dietary form of iron is the ferric ($Fe^{3+}$) form.

## How much is the daily requirement of iron?

The daily requirement of iron is 10 – 20 mg in diet (only 10% of the dietary intake is absorbed).

## What are the dietary sources of iron?

The dietary sources of iron are meat, liver, egg, leafy vegetables, whole wheat and jaggery.

## What is the mechanism of iron absorption?

Dietary iron, which is in the $Fe^{3+}$ state, gets dissolved in gastric hydrochloric acid and form soluble complexes with reducing agents like **ascorbic acid**, which reduces it to $Fe^{2+}$ Reduction to $Fe^{2+}$ also occurs at the brush border of the ileum which have **$Fe^{3+}$ reductase** on it. The $Fe^{2+}$ is transported into the ileal cells by facilitated diffusion. Heme molecule, if present in the diet, also enters the mucosal cell through facilitated diffusion.

Once inside the cell, heme is split by *heme oxidase*, releasing the iron. The iron binds to **mobilferrin** present in the cytoplasm. Mobilferrin transfers the iron molecule to the transferrin receptor present on the basolateral membrane of the mucosal cells. The transferrin receptor transfers the iron to transferrin present in blood (Fig. 24.1).

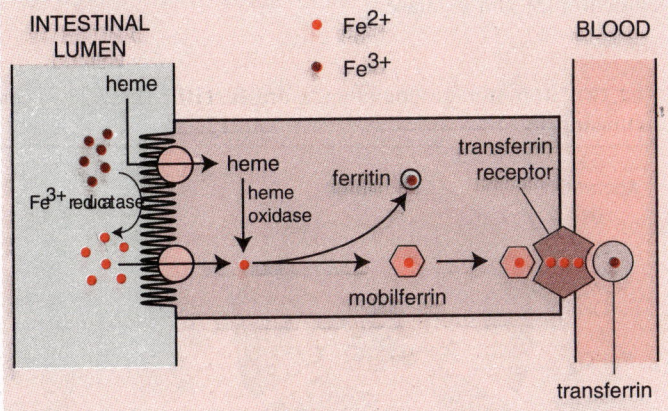

**Fig. 24.1**

## How is iron absorption regulated?

When the intestinal mucosal cell is presented with excess dietary iron, the mobilferrin transport system in the cell gets saturated. The iron absorbed into the cell therefore binds to apoferritin forming ferritin. Ferritin molecules do not release the iron into the blood. Ferritin remains inside the mucosal cell till they are shed into the intestinal lumen (Fig. 24.2). The excess iron that is absorbed into the mucosal cell is thus lost with the shedding of the ferritin-loaded mucosal cell.

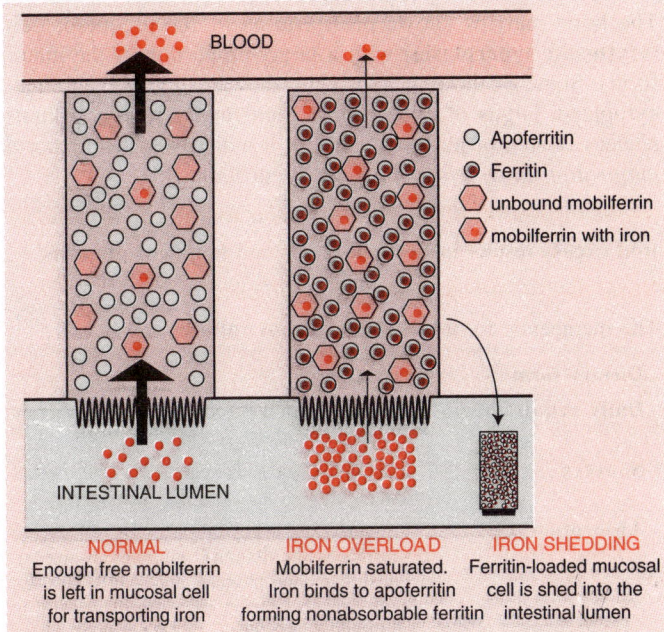

**Fig. 24.2**

## What is the site of iron absorption?

Most of the iron is absorbed in the *duodenum and upper jejunum*. Very little is absorbed in the stomach. Yet, *partial gastrectomy causes marked reduction in iron absorption*, which shows the importance of gastric hydrochloric acid in iron absorption.

## What are the factors increasing iron absorption?

Two major dietary enhancers of nonheme iron absorption are **ascorbate** and **meats**. Ascorbate exerts its effect by reducing ferric iron to the absorbable ferrous form. Other reducing agents, such as cysteine exert similar effects. **Human breast milk** improves iron absorption.

## What are the dietary factors inhibiting iron absorption

**Phytates**, which are natural components of grains and some other vegetable foods, form stable, poorly absorbable complexes with iron. Bran and other fibers inhibit iron absorption mainly because of their phytate content. **Polyphenols** present in legumes, tea, coffee, and wine cause poor absorption of iron. **Phosphates** inhibit absorption of iron from egg yolks. **Calcium** inhibits iron absorption. **Egg white** and bovine **milk proteins** also inhibit iron absorption.

The acid gastric juice favors absorption of nonheme iron by causing its solubilization. Hence, the absorption of ferric iron is impaired in subjects with **gastrectomy** or **achlorhydria**.

### What is the transport form of iron in blood?

Iron is transported as $Fe^{3+}$ bound to **transferrin**, and also as **ferritin** (ferric hydrophosphate) bound to apoferritin.

### What is the blood picture of iron deficiency anemia?

The RBCs are typically **microcytic** and appears **hypochromic** in blood film. Both MCH and MCHC are reduced. The red cell count is also reduced.

### What is the bone marrow picture of iron deficiency anemia?

The bone marrow shows proliferation of the precursor cells (**erythroid hyperplasia**) with a larger proportion of the mature forms. Some of the precursor cells show scanty, polychromatic cytoplasm (signs of cytoplasmic immaturity) with a pyknotic nucleus (a sign of nuclear maturity). It indicates that *cytoplasmic maturation lags behind nuclear maturation*.

### What happens when there is iron excess in the body?

Iron excess results in **hemosiderosis** and **hemochromatosis**.

### What is the therapeutic form of iron?

The therapeutic form of iron is **ferrous sulfate**.

| Dietary form | Ferric ($Fe^{3+}$) |
|---|---|
| **Daily requirements** | 10 – 20 mg in diet (only 10% of the dietary intake is absorbed). |
| **Sources** | Meat, liver, egg, leafy vegetables, whole wheat and jaggery |
| **Absorption** | $Fe^{3+}$ is reduced to $Fe^{2+}$ by gastric HCl. Reducing substances like vitamin C enhances absorption. Phosphates and phytates (present in cereals) decrease absorption by forming insoluble complexes with iron. |
| **Site of absorption** | Duodenum and upper jejunum |
| **Body resources** | 5g (in the liver, spleen, bone marrow, lymph node and the RES cells). |
| **Storage forms** | 2/3 as ferritin and 1/3 as hemosiderin. |
| **Transport forms** | As $Fe^{3+}$ bound to transferrin; as ferritin (ferric hydrophosphate) bound to apoferritin |
| **Role** | Synthesis of Hb (cytoplasmic maturation of RBCs), myoglobin and cytochromes (intracellular enzymes). |
| **Causes of deficiency** | Decrease in dietary intake or absorption; Increased demand (pregnancy) or losses (hemorrhage). |
| **Effects of deficiency** | Iron deficiency anemia |
| **Effects of excess** | Hemosiderosis and hemochromatosis. |
| **Diagnosis of deficiency** | Serum iron level (Normal = 120µg/dl) and Total iron-binding capacity (Normal = 250-450µg/dl). |
| **Therapeutic form** | Ferrous sulfate |

### What is the iron cycle?

The term *iron cycle* refers to the uptake of iron from plasma into RBCs, and its eventual return to the plasma after the death of the RBCs. Each day, about 30 mg of iron goes through this cycle. About 2 mg iron enters the cycle from diet, and the same amount leaves the cycle into the tissues (Fig. 24.3).

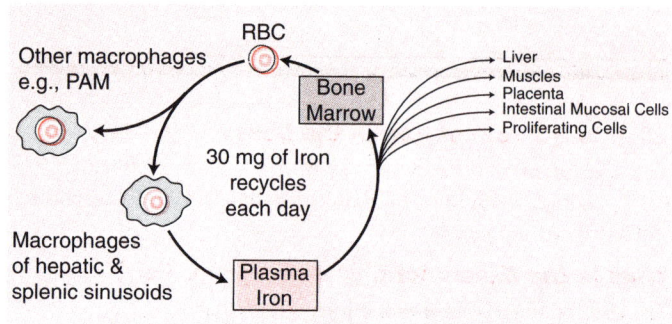

**Fig. 24.3**

Iron travels from plasma to the bone marrow where it is incorporated into hemoglobin. At end of their life span, RBCs are engulfed by macrophages. After phagocytosis, the red cell membrane is lysed, heme is released from hemoglobin and iron liberated by the *heme oxygenase* reaction. *Macrophages lining the sinuses of liver and spleen release the iron into circulation*, where it becomes bound to transferrin, completing the cycle.

Other *macrophages like the pulmonary alveolar macrophages (PAM) lack the ability to return the iron to the circulation*. They store the iron. These iron-loaded macrophages may remain in the tissues, or may enter the circulation to leave the body through the intestine.

Less than 2 mg iron is taken up each day by many tissues for the synthesis of non-hemoglobin, iron-containing enzymes and proteins like *cytochromes*, *catalase*, and *myoglobin*. These tissues include the **liver**, which takes up the largest amount of iron 5% next to RBCs; the **placenta**, which transfers the iron to fetus; the **intestinal mucosal cells**, which store iron as ferritin, thereby regulating iron absorption; the **skeletal muscles**, which produce myoglobin; and the **proliferating cells** that requires excess cytochromes and catalases.

### What are the iron storage proteins?

The two iron storage compounds are **ferritin** (Fig. 24.4) and **hemosiderin**.

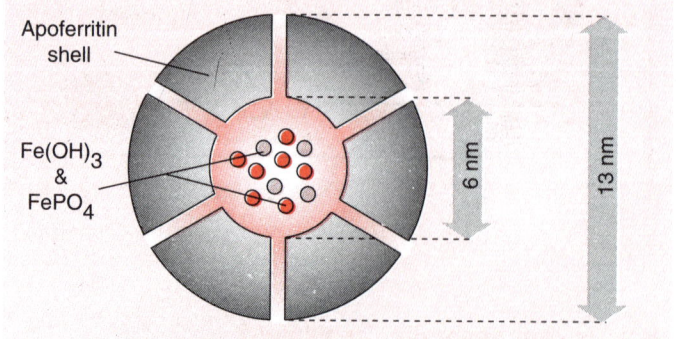

**Fig. 24.4**

# Compare and contrast ferritin and hemosiderin.

## SIMILARITIES

Both are iron storage compounds.

## DIFFERENCES

| Ferritin | Hemosiderin |
|---|---|
| Composition fairly consistent | Composition highly variable |
| Not enclosed by membrane | May be enclosed by membrane |
| Iron content lesser (~20%) | Iron content greater (~30%) |
| Iron in the form of $Fe(OH)_3$ and $FePO_4$ | Iron in the form of $Fe_2O_3$ |
| Water-soluble | Water-insoluble |
| Stains with Prussian Blue | Does not stain with Prussian Blue |

# Folic Acid & Vitamin B$_{12}$

### What is the dietary form and active form of folic acid?

Dietary folic acid is present in the form of **polyglutamates**. The active form is **tetrahydrofolate (THF)**.

### What are the dietary sources of folic acid?

The dietary sources of folic acid are leafy vegetables, yeast, pulses and liver.

### What is the mechanism of absorption of folic acid?

Polyglutamates are first reduced to monoglutamates by the carboxypeptidases present in the pancreatic juice. Monoglutamates are further converted into absorbable methytetrahydrofolates.

### How are folic acid and vitamin B$_{12}$ stored in the body?

About 500 mg of folic acid remains stored in liver, RBCs and WBCs. About 5 mg of vitamin B$_{12}$ is stored in the liver.

### What is the therapeutic form of folic acid?

The therapeutic form of folic acid is **pteroylglutamic acid**.

### What are the causes of folate deficiency?

The common causes of folate deficiency are (1) *Inadequate intake:* unbalanced diet (common in alcoholics, teenagers, some infants); (2) *Increased requirements:* as in pregnancy, infancy, malignancy, increased hematopoiesis (chronic hemolytic anemias); (3) *Malabsorption:* due to sprue; (4) *Folate inhibitors:* methotrexate.

### What is the laboratory test for diagnosis of folate deficiency?

Folate deficiency is detected by the **FIGLU test**. In folate deficiency, there is a marked rise in the urinary excretion of FIGLU (**formiminoglutamate**) after oral administration of histidine. The test is however not specific for folates: it is positive in vitamin B$_{12}$ deficiency too.

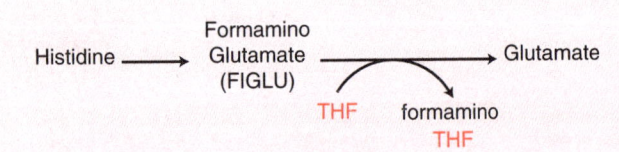

**Fig. 25.1**

### What are the effects of folate deficiency?

Because folic acid is important for DNA synthesis and cell division, specially affected are those cells that multiply rapidly, like the hemopoietic cells. Erythropoiesis, leucopoiesis and thrombopoiesis – all are affected. In general, *the nuclear maturation in the cell lags behind the cytoplasmic maturation.* Defective erythropoiesis results in **megaloblastic anemia**.

| | Cobalamin | Folic acid |
|---|---|---|
| **Dietary form** | Deoxyadenosyl-cobalamin | Polyglutamates. |
| **Daily requirements** | 2µg | 200µg. |
| **Sources** | Animal products (meat, liver, fish, meat, egg) | Leafy vegetables, yeast, pulses and liver |
| **Absorption** | Intrinsic factor secreted by the parietal cells binds to B$_{12}$ as well as to the ileal receptors thereby facilitating diffusion. | Carboxypeptidases reduce poly- to mono-glutamates. Jejunal mucosal cells convert monoglutamates to absorbable methyl-THF. |
| **Site of absorption** | Ileum | Ileum |
| **Body resources** | 5mg (in liver). | 500 mg (in liver, RBCs & WBCs). |
| **Storage forms** | Deoxyadenosylco-balamin | 5-methyl THF |
| **Transport form** | As methylcobalamin bound to transco-balamin | 5-methyl THF |
| **Role** | DNA synthesis in blood cells. | DNA synthesis in blood cells. |
| **Causes of deficiency** | Low intake/absorption; High demand (pregnancy) or losses (fish tapeworm infestation). | Decreased dietary intake or absorption; increased demand (pregnancy) |
| **Effects of deficiency** | Megaloblastic anemia | Megaloblastic anemia |
| **Effects of excess** | Water-soluble. Excess is excreted. | Water-soluble. Excess is excreted. |
| **Diagnosis of deficiency** | Serum B$_{12}$ level (Normal= 50µg/dl); Methylmalonic acid test (increased urinary excretion) | Serum folic acid level (normal = 200ng/dl); FIGLU Test (increased urinary excretion of formaminoglutamic acid). |
| **Therapeutic form** | Hydroxycobalamin | Pteroylglutamic acid |

### What is the active form of vitamin B$_{12}$?

The active forms of cobalamin are **methylcobalamin** and **deoxyadenosylcobalamin**. These active forms are formed inside the cells from cobalamin.

### What is the daily requirement of folic acid and vitamin B₁₂?

The daily requirement of folic acid is 200μg while that of vitamin B$_{12}$ is 2μg.

### What are the dietary sources of folic acid and vitamin B₁₂?

The dietary sources of vitamin B$_{12}$ are animal products (meat, liver, fish and egg). Dietary sources of folic acid are leafy vegetables, yeast, pulses and liver.

### What is the site of absorption of folic acid and vitamin B₁₂?

Both are absorbed from the ileum.

### What is the mechanism of absorption of vitamin B₁₂?

The **intrinsic factor** secreted by the parietal cells of gastric glands binds to B$_{12}$. In the ileum, intrinsic factor binds to receptors on ileal mucosal cells, thereby anchoring vitamin B$_{12}$ to the mucosal cell and resulting in its absorption through *facilitated diffusion* (Fig. 25.2).

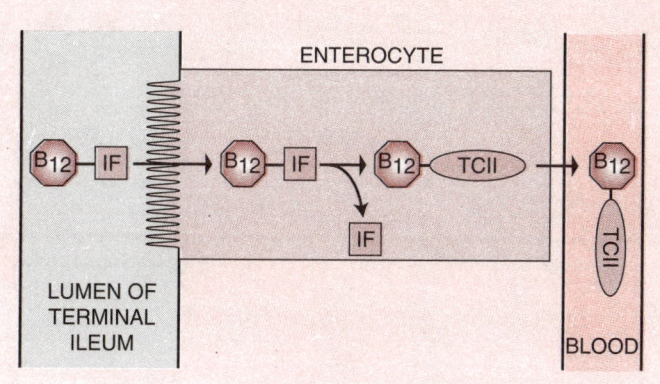

**Fig. 25.2**

### What is the therapeutic form of vitamin B₁₂?

The therapeutic form of vitamin B$_{12}$ is **hydroxycobalamin**.

### How is vitamin B₁₂ absorbed and stored?

Cobalamin is stored in liver, bound to **transcobalamin-I**. Vitamin B$_{12}$ is the only water-soluble vitamin to be stored in the liver.

### What are the actions of vitamin B₁₂?

Vitamin B$_{12}$ serves as a co-factor to folic acid in *DNA synthesis*. It also helps in the *maintenance of myelin sheath* in the neuron.

### What are the causes of vitamin B₁₂ deficiency?

Although it is reasonable to expect that vegetarians would be prone to vitamin B$_{12}$ deficiency, it is rare, possibly because *milk* provides adequate amounts of vitamin B$_{12}$ to vegetarians. Most cases of vitamin B$_{12}$ deficiency are because of a *reduction in intestinal absorption* of vitamin B$_{12}$, the causes of which could be (1) *inadequate production of intrinsic factor (IF)*, as in **pernicious anemia**, **gastrectomy** and congenital deficiency of IF (rare). (2) *Disorders (sprue, enteritis) or resection of terminal ileum;* (3) *Competition for cobalamin* with **fish tapeworm** and

with bacteria in the **blind loop syndrome**. Fish tapeworm and bacteria consume most of the cobalamin in the intestine, leaving behind little for absorption.

### What is the laboratory test for diagnosis of vitamin B₁₂ deficiency?

The laboratory test is the **methylmalonic acid test**. Increased amounts of this acid are excreted in urine in vitamin B$_{12}$ deficiency because vitamin B$_{12}$ is required for the conversion of methylmalonyl CoA to succinyl CoA.

### What is megaloblastic anemia?

It is a deficiency anemia due to inadequate intake of folic acid and/or vitamin B$_{12}$. It owes its name to the presence of abnormal normoblasts called **megaloblasts** in the bone marrow.

### What is the blood picture in megaloblastic anemia?

In megaloblastic anemia, there is marked *macrocytosis, anisocytosis* and *poikilocytosis*. There is also *neutropenia* with hypersegmented (aged) neutrophils and *thrombocytopenia*. This is because the production of other blood cells is also affected due to impaired DNA synthesis.

### What is the bone marrow picture in megaloblastic anemia?

In megaloblastic anemia, all the red cell precursors (proerythroblasts and erythroblasts) show megaloblastic changes and are respectively called **promegaloblasts** and **megaloblasts**. Compared to their erythroblastic counterparts, megaloblasts have the following features: (1) The cell is larger with a larger nucleus and more cytoplasm. (2) The chromatin is more reticular than the corresponding erythroblast, which has a more clumped chromatin. Clumping of chromatin occurs as the cell matures. (3) Hemoglobinization of cytoplasm proceeds normally. Thus, nuclear maturation (indicated by the state of chromatin) can be said to be lagging behind cytoplasmic maturation (indicated by hemoglobinization). (4) There is a greater proportion of the more primitive precursor cells (like promegaloblast) than there is in normal erythropoiesis. This occurs due to *maturation arrest*.

### What is pernicious anemia and what are its clinical features?

It is an *autoimmune disease* that destroys most of the gastric mucosa, abolishing almost completely the secretion of not only IF but also gastric HCl (**achlorhydria**) and pepsin. Abolition of IF secretion causes vitamin B$_{12}$ deficiency by impairing its absorption. There are three main effects of the deficiency vitamin B$_{12}$. These are (1) **megaloblastic anemia**, (2) **glossitis** (sore tongue) and (3) neurological manifestations: there is **demyelination** and axonal degeneration of peripheral nerves and posterolateral columns of the spinal cord.

### Compare and contrast folic acid, vitamin B₁₂ and iron deficiency anemias.

**SIMILARITIES**

All the three anemias are associated with low hemoglobin concentration, resulting in hypoxic symptoms in severe cases.

**DIFFERENCES**

| Iron deficiency anemia | Folic acid deficiency anemia | Vitamin $B_{12}$ deficiency anemia |
| --- | --- | --- |
| Inadequate intake is a common cause | Inadequate intake is a common cause | Inadequate intake is rarely the cause. |
| Erythrocytes are microcytic and hypochromic. | Erythrocytes are macrocytic | Erythrocytes are macrocytic. |
| Nuclear maturation in erythrocytes is normal. | Nuclear maturation is impaired. | Nuclear maturation is impaired. |
| Bone marrow shows hyperplasia of red cell precursors (erythroid hyperplasia) | Bone marrow shows megaloblastic changes and presence of erythroblasts. | Bone marrow shows megaloblastic changes and presence of erythroblasts. |
| White cells are unaffected. | Associated with neutropenia and thrombocytopenia. | Associated with neutropenia and thrombocytopenia. |
| No associated neurological problems. | No associated neurological problems. | Associated with neurological signs. |

# 26

# *Blood Grouping & Transfusion*

### Define Landsteiner's law.

Landsteiner's law states that (a) when a blood contains a particular agglutinogen, its corresponding agglutinin is always absent in that blood, and (b) when a particular agglutinogen is absent in the blood, its corresponding agglutinin is always present in the blood. The first clause of the law is always true but the second clause is valid only for the ABO blood groups.

### Enumerate some of the major, minor and familial blood groups.

The major blood groups are ABO and the Rhesus groups. Minor blood groups are MN and P groups. Examples of familial blood groups are the Kell, Duffy, Deigo, Lewis, Lutheran, Kidd etc.

### What is the population distribution of blood groups on India?

In India, 40% belong to O group, 33% to B, 22% to A and the rest 5% to AB. As for the distribution of Rhesus Groups, over 99% of Asians are positive.

### How are blood groups inherited?

The ABO phenotypes are controlled by a pair of 3 alternative alleles: A, B and O. For example, A blood group has A and O alleles while B group has B and O alleles. Group AB has A and B alleles while group O has two O alleles. Inheritance follows the classical Mendelian pattern. The A and B antigens are inherited as **Mendelian codominants** (Fig. 26.1). For example, an individual who has inherited an A-antigen from one parent and a B-antigen from the other parent will have AB blood group. Thus, an individual whose *phenotypic* blood group is B may have either the *genotype BB (homozygous)* or *BO (heterozygous)*.

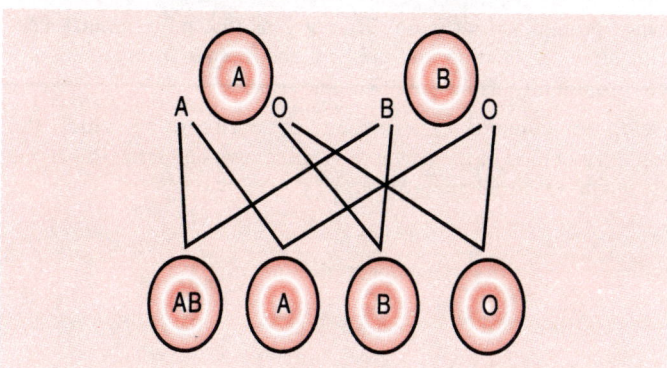

**Fig. 26.1**

### Enumerate the clinical importance of blood groups.

Blood groups are important in **transfusion medicine** (for avoiding mismatched transfusion), in medicolegal cases of **disputed paternity**, and occasionally, in predicting the propensity for some diseases.

### Explain the terms universal donors and recipients

In emergency situations, there may be no time for finding out the blood group of the patient, and even when known, the blood of the same group may not be available. In such situations, blood group O may be transfused indiscriminately to all patients in dire need of transfusion. This is because *O group blood has no agglutinogens* and the chances of fatal reactions occurring following a mismatched transfusion (O group blood donated to persons with A, B or AB blood groups) are the lowest with it. Persons with O blood group are therefore called **universal donors**. In the same way, a person with AB blood group is a **universal recipient**. In emergency situations, he or she can be transfused with any of the ABO blood groups. This is because AB group blood has neither α nor β agglutinins.

### Describe the laboratory determination of blood groups.

For ABO blood grouping, the test sample of blood or RBC suspension is reacted with sera containing α and β (called *antisera-A* and *antisera-B*). The sample is grouped according to the sera that agglutinates it.

Unlike in the ABO system, addition of anti-D serum to D+ (Rhesus+) RBC suspension does not immediately produce agglutination of RBCs. Visible agglutination will be produced by the subsequent addition of either albumin or Coomb's serum (anti-IgG) to the RBC-sera mixture (Fig. 26.2).

### What is cross matching and what is its importance?

Transfusion of blood of the same group *does not guarantee* a reaction-free transfusion, and the blood of donor and recipient must always be directly tested against each other (*cross-matching*) to see if they are compatible.

For example, if O group blood is transfused to a recipient with A, B or AB blood group, the transfusion is considered safe. However, the O group donor may have very high titers of α and β agglutinins, and these may cause hemolysis of the recipient's RBCs. Such O group donors are called *dangerous universal donors*.

Moreover, there are an endless number of minor and familial blood groups and it is not practically feasible to find out whether or not a blood sample belongs to any of those groups, or contains any agglutinins reacting with them. The donor's and recipient's blood may be ABO and Rhesus compatible, but it may so turn out that the donor has P agglutinogens and the recipient has anti-P agglutinins. Hence, *blood grouping alone is never adequate*.

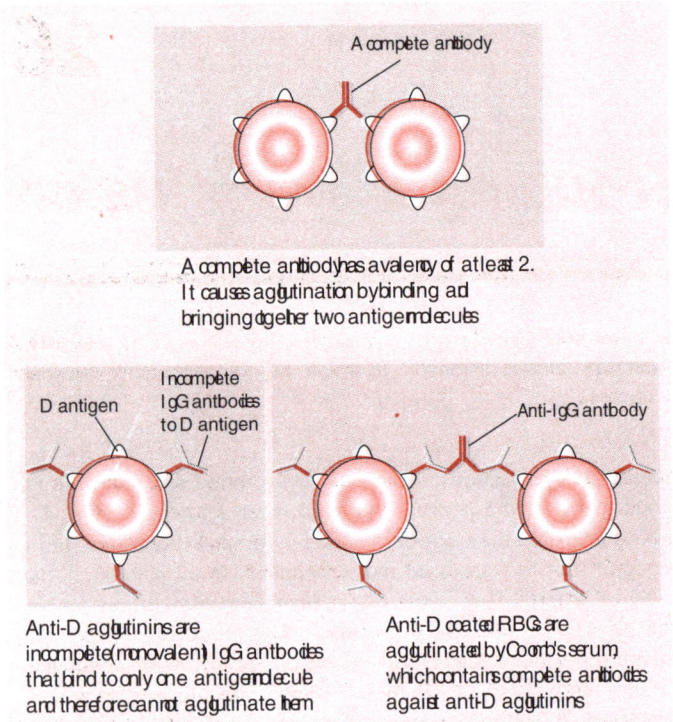

A complete antibody

A complete antibody has a valency of at least 2. It causes agglutination by binding and bringing together two antigen molecules

D antigen

Incomplete IgG antibodies to D antigen

Anti-IgG antibody

Anti-D agglutinins are incomplete (monovalent) IgG antibodies that bind to only one antigen molecule and therefore cannot agglutinate them

Anti-D coated RBCs are agglutinated by Coomb's serum, which contains complete antibodies against anti-D agglutinins

**Fig. 26.2**

Cross matching may be major or minor. **Major cross matching** involves testing the donor's RBCs against recipient's serum. **Minor cross matching** involves testing the recipient's RBCs against donor's serum.

### What are the complications of blood transfusion?

The most feared complication of transfusion is (1) **hemolytic reactions** due to mismatched transfusion. Other complications include: (2) **Febrile reactions** due to destruction of leukocytes and platelet by antibodies against them. (3) **Circulatory overload** can develop if transfusion is too rapid. (4) **Hemosiderosis** is caused by repeated blood transfusions, as in thalassemic patients. (5) **Hyperkalemia** occurs because in stored blood, the RBCs leak out intracellular $K^+$ into the plasma and therefore the plasma $K^+$ concentration in stored blood is high. (6) **Hypocalcemia** occurs because stored blood contains citrates as anticoagulant. When transfused into recipient, the citrates get metabolized. However, if the rate of transfusion exceeds the rate of citrate metabolism, the citrates chelate $Ca^{2+}$ in recipient's blood and cause hypocalcemia. (7) **Reduced tissue oxygenation**. Red cells in stored blood have very low amounts of DPG in them. Hence, stored blood has high affinity for $O_2$ and consequently, tends to give off less $O_2$ to the tissues. In patients receiving large amounts of transfusion, this reduced release of $O_2$ to tissues can cause serious problems,

(8) **Transmission of diseases** like hepatitis B and AIDS constitute a serious risk.

### What is the management of hemolytic transfusion reactions?

When reactions occur, transfusion must be stopped immediately and the patient is intravenously injected with rapid-acting corticosteroids.

### Describe the pathogenesis of erythroblastosis fetalis.

If two consecutive Rh+ babies are born to an Rh- mother, the second baby is liable to develop neonatal jaundice. This happens because during the first pregnancy, the mother is sensitized to Rh agglutinogens of the fetus due to leakage of fetal RBCs into the maternal circulation. *The leak occurs late in the third trimester or during parturition* when the maternal and fetal bloods come in contact for the first time. However, *agglutinins are not formed quickly* or in significant titers on first exposure and the first Rh+ fetus usually escapes unharmed. A second Rh+ fetus however evokes rapid formation of anti-Rh agglutinins in the third trimester, which cross over to fetal circulation, hemolyzing the fetal RBCs. The hemolytic disease can also occur if the Rh- mother is sensitized to Rhesus antigens by a prior Rh+ blood transfusion.

As a result of the hemolysis of fetal RBCs, there is appearance of immature erythroblasts in the fetal circulation (**erythroblastosis fetalis**) due to compensatory hyperactivity of the fetal erythropoietic organs. Depending on its severity, erythroblastosis fetalis takes one of the following forms. In severe cases, the fetus looks like a bag of water due to edema and often dies *in utero* (**hydrops fetalis**). Less severe cases result in jaundice of the newborn (**icterus neonatorum gravis**). The jaundice is much lesser till birth when the mother conjugates and excretes most of the fetal bilirubin load but exacerbates immediately after birth. The mildest cases result only in anemia of the newborn (**congenital anemia of the newborn**).

### Outline the prevention and treatment of fetal rhesus hemolytic disease.

Prevention of the condition is possible by preventing the mother from getting sensitized to Rh antigens during the first pregnancy. This is done by administering a single dose of **anti-Rh antibodies** *during the post-partum period in the first 72 hours*. The antibodies promptly destroy any Rh antigens that might gain access to maternal circulation and prevents the mother from developing active immunity against the Rh antigen.

Treatment consists of **exchange transfusion** in which the hemolyzed blood of the newborn is withdrawn and fresh Rh- blood is transfused simultaneously.

# 27

# Blood Platelets

## What are the major steps of hemostasis?

The term **hemostasis** means the stoppage of bleeding. It occurs in three major steps. (1) **Constriction of the damaged vessel**, slowing down the bleeding. Unless the blood flow is slowed down, any clot formed will be washed away. The immediate constriction occurs mainly due to the direct *response of vascular smooth muscle* to injury. A little later, further constriction is induced by the *serotonin released from platelets* that adhere to the site of injury. (2) **Formation of a temporary hemostatic plug**, arresting the bleeding. Formation of the plug begins when platelets come in contact with the subendothelial tissues of blood vessels that get exposed as a result of injury. It occurs in three steps (Fig. 27.1): (a) *Platelet adhesion*, in which integrins present on platelets anchor them to the collagen of the subendothelial tissues. (b) *Platelet activation*, in which platelet metabolic activity is stimulated by the contact of platelets with collagen. Activated platelets develop pseudopodia, discharge their granules, and stick to other platelets. (c) *Platelet aggregation*, in which more and more activated platelets accumulate at the site of injury by sticking to each other. It results in the formation of the *temporary hemostatic (platelet) plug*. (3) **Consolidation of the temporary plug** by formation of fibrin threads. This involves the enzymatic conversion of the plasma protein *fibrinogen* into *fibrin* through an elaborate process called *coagulation* or *clotting*. The fibrin threads bind to platelets through *integrin* (glycoproteins), anchoring the platelets tightly together. (4) The clot formed ultimately undergoes retraction and dissolution. **Clot retraction** occurs due to the contraction of platelets. It pulls the edges of the wound together, making wound healing easier. **Fibrinolysis** or dissolution of the clot is necessary for the restoration of normal blood flow to the healed tissue. Fibrinolysis is produced by a substance called *plasmin*, which splits fibrin enzymatically.

## Describe the structure of platelets.

The platelets or **thromboplastids** (Fig. 27.2) are anucleate thin biconvex discs, which are round or ovoid granulated bodies 2 – 4 μm in diameter. Platelets are produced in the bone marrow by fragmentation of very large nucleated cells called **megakaryocytes**. Platelets are released into the blood where they have a life span of ~10 days. Platelets have 1 – 2 mitochondria and consume oxygen. However, they lack a nucleus and therefore unable to synthesize proteins. Platelets exhibit two concentric zones. The **hyalomere** is a thin pale-blue peripheral zone of the platelet. It contains no organelles but has a great concentration of actin and myosin proteins. The **granulomere** is the thicker central region of the platelet, and contains a canalicular system, secretory granules and scattered particles of glycogen.

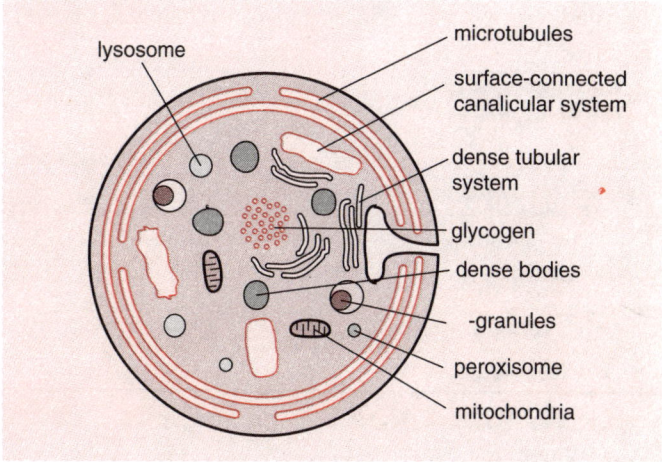

**Fig. 27.2**

The **platelet granules** are of three types: **lysosomal granules**, dense granules and α granules. **Dense granules** secrete ADP, which amplifies platelet activation. The **α-granules** secrete: (i) *Platelet factor 4*, which neutralizes the anticoagulant activity of heparin. (ii) *Thrombospondin*, which brings about platelet aggregation. (iii) *Platelet-derived growth factor* (*PDGF*) and *Transforming growth factor-β* (*TGF-β*) which are chemoattractants for white blood cells, smooth muscle cells, and fibroblasts. They also stimulate mitosis of these cells and thus contribute to the

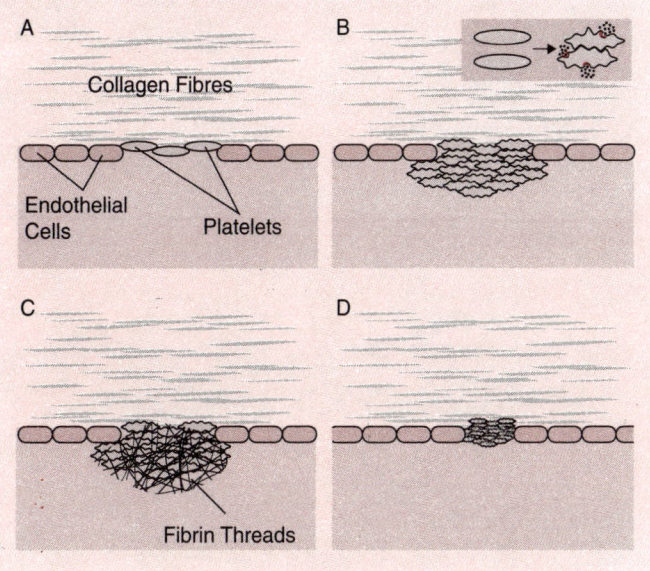

**Fig. 27.1**

processes of inflammation and wound healing. (iv) *Fibronectin*, which helps in platelet adhesion to the site of injury.

### What are the functions of platelets?

Blood platelets have the following functions. (1) When the endothelium is disrupted, the breach is closed by a mass of platelets called the platelet thrombus or the **platelet plug**. (2) Phospholipids present on the surface of platelets are essential for some of the key reactions of **blood coagulation** that take place only on the surface of platelets. (3) Platelets secrete certain **growth factors** (*Platelet-derived growth factor* or *PGDF* or *Transforming growth factor-β* (*TGF-β*) that are useful in the process of tissue healing. (4) It releases granules that are **chemotactic** for neutrophils. (5) Platelets have a weak **phagocytic** activity.

### What is the normal platelet count?

The normal count: 150,000 – 400,000 / mm³ of blood.

### What is thrombocytopenia and what are its causes?

When the platelet count falls below 150,000 / mm³, it is called **thrombocytopenia**. Thrombocytopenia can occur without any obvious cause in which case it is called **primary thrombocytopenia**. Where the cause is identifiable, it is called **secondary**

**thrombocytopenia** and occurs (1) following *drug* administration (e.g., aspirin), (2) in malignancies e.g., *leukemias*, aplastic anemia and bone marrow infiltration, and (3) *hypersplenism* in which an abnormally hyperactive spleen destroys platelets (as also other blood cells) in larger than usual numbers.

When the platelet count is low, clot retraction is deficient and there is poor constriction of ruptured vessels. The resulting clinical syndrome is called (**thrombocytopenic purpura**) and is characterized by easy bruisability and multiple subcutaneous hemorrhages. Purpura may also occur when the platelet count is normal, but the platelets are abnormal. Such purpura is called **thrombasthenic purpura**.

### What is thrombocytosis and what are its causes?

Thrombocytosis is a rise of platelet count above 400,000 /mm³. Individuals with thrombocytosis are predisposed to thrombotic events. Common causes of thrombocytosis include (1) *hemorrhage*. A moderate increase in the platelet count may follow acute hemorrhage; (2) *surgery* and *trauma*, particularly bone fractures may cause a moderate rise in platelet count and (3) *splenectomy* causes thrombocytosis by reducing the number of platelets that are removed from circulation.

# Blood Coagulation

## Name the various coagulation factors. Which of these belong to the extrinsic, intrinsic and the common pathway?

| COAGULATION FACTORS | | |
|---|---|---|
| **FactorSymbol** | **FactorName** | **Pathway** |
| I | Fibrinogen | Common |
| II | Prothrombin | Common |
| III | Thromboplastin | Common |
| IV | Calcium ions | All |
| V | Labile Factor | Common |
| VI | Dropped. Earlier called Accelerin | |
| VII | Stable Factor | Extrinsic |
| VIII | Antihemophilic Globulin | Intrinsic |
| IX | Christmas Factor | Common |
| X | Stuart-Prower Factor | Common |
| XI | Plasma Thromboplastin Antecedent (PTA) | Intrinsic |
| XII | Hagerman Factor | Intrinsic |
| XIII | Fibrin Stabilizing Factor or Laki-Lorand Factor | Common |
| HMWK | High molecular Weight Protein | Intrinsic |
| Pre-K | Prekallekrein | Intrinsic |
| Ka | Kallekrein | Intrinsic |
| PPL | Platelet Phospholipids | Common |

The activated form of a factor is denoted by the suffix 'a'. E.g., Va is activated Factor V.

## Briefly describe the coagulation cascade.

The coagulation cascade is shown in Fig. 28.1.

## How is the intrinsic pathway initiated?

The intrinsic pathway begins with the activation of factor XII to XIIa. This activation occurs when factor XII comes in contact with negatively charged surface. The formation of factor XIIa is greatly enhanced through feedback activation by prekallekrein (Fig. 28.2). Factor XIIa activates prekallekrein to kallekrein, which in turn activates factor XII to XIIa (Fig. 28.2).

## How is the extrinsic pathway initiated?

The extrinsic pathway is initiated by the release of **tissue factor (TF)**, which is a glycoprotein released by fibroblasts and smooth muscle cells of the vessel wall. In the presence of $Ca^{2+}$ and

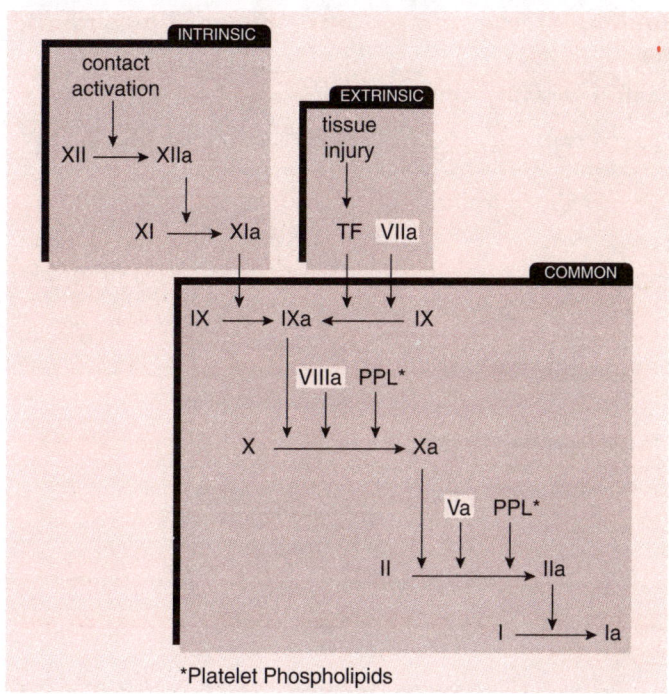

*Platelet Phospholipids

**Fig. 28.1**

membrane phospholipids, TF binds to factor VII and activates it to factor VIIa.

## What is the role of factor XIII in coagulation?

The action of thrombin on fibrinogen results in the formation of **fibrin monomers**. These monomers polymerize spontaneously through *weak non-covalent bonds* to form long **fibrin threads**. However, these threads are weak. They are *made stronger and more resistant* to fibrinolysis by factor XIIIa. In the presence of $Ca^{2+}$, factor XIIIa polymerizes the fibrin monomers through *strong covalent bonds*.

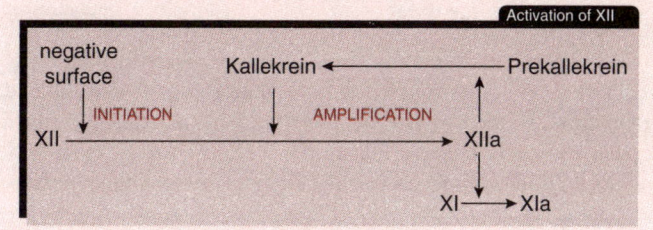

**Fig. 28.2**

# Pro- & Anti-Hemostatic Mechanisms

## Enumerate the various anti- and pro-hemostatic mechanisms.

| Anti-Hemostatic Mechanisms | |
|---|---|
| *Factors preventing platelet aggregation:* | Prostacyclin (PGI$_2$) (endogenous), Aspirin (exogenous) |
| *Factors preventing coagulation:* | Protein C pathway (protein C, thrombomodulin, and protein S), heparin – antithrombin-III system (endogenous); calcium chelators, coumarin derivatives, heparin (exogenous). |
| *Factors causing fibrinolysis:* | Plasmin (endogenous), Streptokinase and staphylokinase (exogenous) |
| **Pro-Hemostatic Mechanisms** | |
| *Fibrinolysis inhibitors* | Plasminogen Activator Inhibitor (PAI), Anti-plasmin (endogenous); ε-aminocaproic acid (exogenous) |

## Explain why aspirin minimizes platelet activation and aggregation.

Aspirin irreversibly (for the remaining life of the platelet) *inhibits the cyclooxygenase pathway of arachidonic acid oxidation* and thereby minimizes platelet activation and aggregation. This makes aspirin it a valuable drug for the prevention of thrombosis.

## What is the mechanism of action of heparin?

Heparin sulfate is an anticoagulant present on the luminal surface of vascular endothelium. (1) It prevents the activation of prothrombin to thrombin. (2) It inhibits the action of thrombin on fibrinogen. (3) It potentiates the action of antithrombin III. Antithrombin III is present in plasma as well as in vascular endothelium. It inactivates a number of coagulation factors including thrombin.

## What is plasmin? What is its significance?

**Plasmin** (fibrinolysin) is the principal fibrinolytic factor in blood. While clotting of blood is important for arresting bleeding, fibrinolysis is important for wound healing and restoration of blood flow. In the absence of plasmin, there is extensive fibrin deposition in the tissues. Plasmin is also important for growth and fertility, since it plays a role in cell movement and in ovulation.

## How is plasmin activated?

Plasmin is formed from its inactive precursor **plasminogen**. The activators may be intrinsic, extrinsic or exogenous. *Intrinsic activators* are Factor XIIa, kallekrein and thrombin. *Extrinsic activators* are called **plasminogen activators** and are found in endothelial cells, renal cells and even tumor cells. Several bacterial proteins are *exogenous activators* of plasmin. These include the bacterial enzymes **streptokinase** and **staphylokinase**. These are used in the treatment of early myocardial infarction.

Plasmin lyses both fibrin and fibrinogen. The products of fibrinogen breakdown (called **fibrinogen degradation products** or **FDP**) inhibit the activity of thrombin. Thus, there is a negative feedback which controls plasmin generation. Interestingly, the same thrombin that is involved in the final steps of coagulation also initiates the pathway for fibrinolysis (Fig. 29.1).

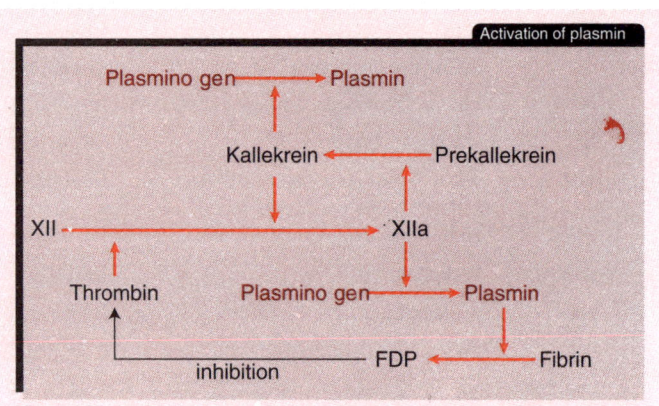

**Fig. 29.1**

## Why does blood become incoagulable following violent death?

In violent deaths, the blood is fluid and incoagulable due to fibrinolysis. This is due to the large amounts of adrenaline released into blood before death. The adrenaline causes rapid release of plasminogen activators from endothelial cells causing massive fibrinolysis.

# Hemorrhagic & Thrombotic Disorders

### Enumerate the difference between coagulation disorders and platelet/vascular disorders.

The characteristics of bleeding due to vascular and platelet disorders are similar. They tend to cause spontaneous bleeding, resulting in purplish patches on the skin or mucous membranes. The condition is called **purpura**. *The term purpura comes from the word purple*, which denotes the color of the bleeding patches. Coagulation disorders do not cause purpura. Spontaneous bleeding, when it does occur in severe coagulation disorders, occurs in joints and muscle.

| Vascular / platelet disorders | Coagulation disorders |
| --- | --- |
| Bleeding usually confined to the skin | Bleeding usually in deeper tissues |
| Bleeding usually takes the form of confluent petichae and small echymosis | Bleeding usually takes the form of large ecchymoses |
| Spontaneous bleeding is common | Spontaneous bleeding is uncommon |
| Wound bleeding: | Wound bleeding: |
| is excessive | is less profuse |
| is immediate | is delayed for several hours |
| stops quickly on application of local pressure | does not stop quickly on application of local pressure |
| lasts < 48 hours | continues > 48 hours |
| rarely recurs | tends to recur |

### Enumerate the confirmatory tests for vascular / platelet disorder

(1) **Tourniquet test** is positive in most cases of thrombocytopenia. It is performed by placing the sphygmomanometer cuff around the upper arm and raising the pressure to halfway between the systolic and diastolic pressures. The idea is to permit arterial flow but occlude the venous return so as to severely increase the capillary hydrostatic pressure. The pressure is kept elevated for 5 minutes. After the cuff is deflated and the congestion disappears, the number of petichiae in the cubital fossa is counted. If *more than 20 petichiae are present in an area of 3 cm diameter*, the test is positive and suggests thrombocytopenia. (2) **Bleeding time** is estimated by pricking the finger or the earlobe to a measured depth and mopping the blood that flows out once every 15 seconds. The *normal bleeding time is 2 – 6 minutes*. (3) **Clot retraction time.** Fresh blood is taken in a test tube and incubated in a water bath at 37°C. Clot retraction is indicated by the pulling

away of the clot from the sides of the tube. Normally, clot retraction should begin in 1 hour and be complete in 24 hours. Also, the volume of serum left behind after complete clot retraction is normally 45 – 65% of the volume of blood.

### Enumerate the confirmatory tests for coagulation disorders.

(1) **Clotting time** tests the factors of the *intrinsic* and *common* pathways. It is the time taken for blood to clot spontaneously in a glass tube. *Normal clotting time is 5 to 11 minutes*. The test is not sensitive: *clotting time is prolonged only in severe coagulation disorders*. However, it remains a useful and simple test for controlling the dose of heparin during anticoagulant therapy. (2) **Partial thromboplastin time (PTT)** assesses the *intrinsic* and *common* pathways of coagulation. It is the time taken by plasma, previously incubated with kaolin or other contact factors, to clot in the presence of $Ca^{2+}$ and platelet lipid substitute. Normally, the *plasma clots in 35 to 45 seconds*. If the clotting time is prolonged by more than 10 minutes, the result is considered abnormal. (3) **Prothrombin time (PT)** assesses the *extrinsic* and *common* pathways of coagulation. It is the time taken by plasma to clot after tissue factor (usually an extract of brain tissue) and $Ca^{2+}$ are added. Since the time taken varies with the type of tissue factor used, the test is always performed simultaneously on patient's plasma and normal plasma. If the time taken for the patient's plasma to clot is 40% less or 20% more than that of a normal subject, it is considered abnormal. (4) **Thrombin time** estimates the *fibrinogen concentration* in plasma. It is the time taken by plasma to clot after addition of thrombin to it. With a standardized thrombin solution, *plasma clots in 15 seconds*. Prolongation to 18 seconds or more is regarded as abnormal.

### What is the difference between thrombocytopenia and thrombasthenia?

**Thrombocytopenia** is a reduction in the platelet count below 150,000/mm$^3$. **Thrombasthenia** is an impairment in the platelet functions.

### Name two well known vascular causes of bleeding due to vascular cause.

Two well known vascular causes of bleeding are **scurvy** and **Cushing's syndrome**.

### Classify coagulation disorders giving examples.

Coagulation disorders can be classified as : (1) **deficiency of coagulation factors** due to (a) defective synthesis, e.g., in hemophilia, vitamin K deficiency and severe liver disease, or due to (b) excessive utilization, as in defibrination syndrome.

(2) inhibition of coagulation due to appearance of **abnormal inhibitors**. (3) **increased fibrinolysis**. (4) **platelet disorder**.

### What are hemophilia A and hemophilia B?

Hemophilia occurs due to a genetic deficiency of Factor VIII (**hemophilia A** or **classical hemophilia**) or of Factor IX (**hemophilia B** or **christmas disease**).

### How is hemophilia inherited?

Hemophilia is inherited as a sex-linked (on X chromosome) disorder mostly transmitted by females who themselves have no symptoms (Fig. 30.1). To have frank hemophilia, a female has to be homozygous for the hemophilic gene. Female carriers of hemophilia, who are heterozygotes, usually produce sufficient factor VIII for normal hemostasis.

### What are the sources of Vitamin K?

Vitamin K is obtained in part from food, especially green leafy vegetables (as **vitamin $K_1$** or **phylloquinone**), and partly from the bacterial flora in the intestine that synthesize the vitamin (as **menaquinone**). When one source is deficient, the other compensates. **Dietary vitamin $K_1$** is fat-soluble vitamin and requires bile salts for its absorption. **Bacterial vitamin menaquinone** is water-soluble and is absorbed even in the absence of bile.

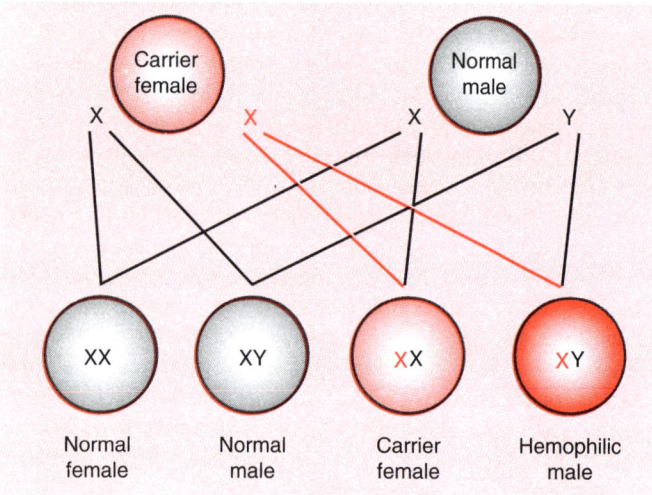

**Fig. 30.1**

### What is the active form of vitamin K?

The physiologically active form of vitamin K is **vitamin $KH_2$** (**reduced hydroquinone**) (Fig. 30.2). In the liver, vitamin K is converted to this active form in the endoplasmic reticulum (microsomes) of liver cells. Liver cells also store vitamin K – enough for about a month.

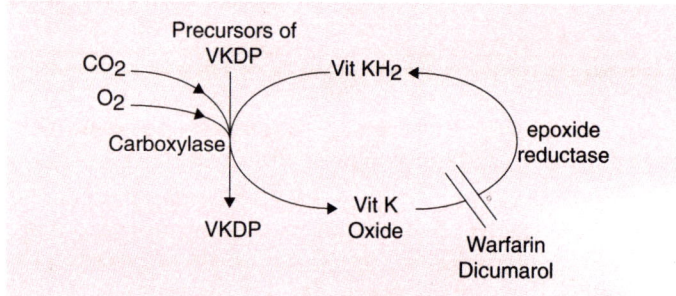

**Fig. 30.2**

### What are the causes of vitamin K deficiency?

There are three major causes of vitamin K deficiency: (1) *inadequate dietary intake* (2) *intestinal malabsorption* e.g., in obstructive jaundice. Due to absence of bile, absorption of fats and fat-soluble vitamins are impaired. (3) *hepatocellular disease*.

### Why does Vitamin K deficiency cause bleeding tendency?

Vitamin K deficiency results in low plasma levels of both procoagulants as well as some anticoagulants. These proteins are called **vitamin K dependent proteins (VKDP)** The procoagulants are factors 2, 7, 9 and 10. The anticoagulants are **protein C** and **protein S**.

# 31

# Neutrophils, Eosinophils & Basophils

## Name the different granulocytes and briefly describe their morphology.

The granulocytes are neutrophils, eosinophils and basophils (Fig. 31.1). All granulocytes contain secretory granules that readily take up Romanowsky-type stains. Hence, they are called granulocytes. The **neutrophil** is 10 – 14 μ in diameter. Its nucleus is multilobed and hence is also called **polymorphonuclear leukocyte**. The number of lobes is related to the age of the neutrophils, with the younger ones having a single-lobed horseshoe shaped nucleus and the older ones having a multilobed nucleus. The **eosinophil** contains a bilobed nucleus and distinctive large granules that stain orange-red using Wright's stain. The granules pack the cytoplasm densely. The **basophil** has a lighter staining nucleus than the neutrophil, and seldom contains more than two lobes. The cytoplasm is pink and contains a varying number (usually not very numerous) of large, deeply staining *basophilic granules*. The granules do not pack the cytoplasm but overlie the nucleus and obscures its detail.

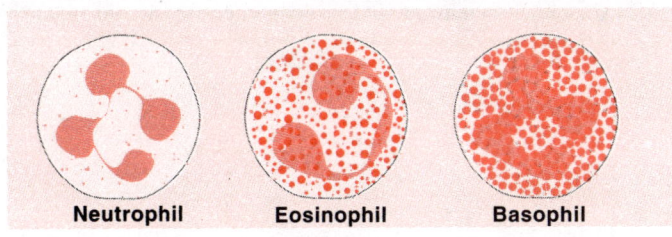

| Neutrophil | Eosinophil | Basophil |

**Fig. 31.1**

## What is Arneth count?

The frequency distribution of neutrophils with different number of lobes is called the **Arneth count** and was done to assess the average age of neutrophils in circulation. Nearly 45% of the neutrophils are trilobed and in the right stage of maturity for optimum functioning. 20% are over-aged with 4 or 5 lobes and 35% are under-aged with less than 3 lobes. A preponderance of immature cells is called a *shift to the left*, while a preponderance of the older cells is called a *shift to the right*.

## What are the different types of neutrophilic granules?

As in all granulocytes, neutrophils have two types of granules: the primary or **azurophilic granules** that are also present in other granulocytes, and the secondary or **specific granules** which are peculiar to neutrophils alone.

The *azurophilic granules* include are **myeloperoxidase** (which imparts a greenish color to the pus, and **defensins**, a group of cationic proteins that kills a variety of bacteria, fungi and viruses. The *specific (secondary) granules* include **apolactoferrin** (an iron-binding protein) and **collagenase**.

## What is the normal neutrophilic count and what are its physiological variations?

The normal leucocytic count is $2.0 - 7.5 \times 10^9/L$, which accounts for 40 – 75 % of the total leucocytic count. An increase is called **neutrophilia** and a decrease is called **neutropenia**. *At birth*, there is leukocytosis (25,000/mm³) that is mainly neutrophilic. It returns to normal after 1 week. The neutrophilic count also show a transient increase due to mobilization of neutrophils from the marginal pool. The phenomenon is called the **shift-leukocytosis**. Most cases of shift-leukocytosis are due to the *stimulation of corticosteroids* from the adrenal cortex, and are seen (1) *after physical exercise*. Marked neutrophilia and leukocytosis occur after strenuous exercise. (2) *during pregnancy*. The leukocytosis increases till term and peaks at parturition. (3) *in anxiety* or stress of any kind. (4) *diurnal*. It increases slightly in the afternoon (the **afternoon-tide**).

## What are the causes of neutrophilia and neutropenia?

**Neutrophilia** is seen in (1) *infections and septicemia* esp. with pyogenic cocci (like *Staphylococci*) and bacilli (like *Escherichia coli*) but also with non-pyogenic organisms (like diphtheria and cholera). (2) *hemorrhage and trauma*, as in surgery, fractures, crush injuries, and burns (3) *malignancies* like myeloid leukemia (4) *cardiac disorders* like myocardial infarction, paroxysmal tachycardia (5) *metabolic disturbances* like renal failure and diabetic coma (6) *drugs* like adrenaline. **Neutropenia** is seen in (1) *viral infections* like influenza, measles, infective hepatitis, (2) *bacterial infection*, like typhoid fever, (3) *aplastic anemia and (4) hypersplenism*.

## What is margination?

When a neutrophil flowing inside a capillary approaches an area of inflammation, it gets marginated, i.e., it gets attracted to the capillary endothelium and starts rolling along its surface. Margination usually occurs in the **postcapillary venule**. Nearly half the circulating neutrophils normally remain marginated.

## What is diapedesis?

Neutrophils can insinuate themselves through the walls of the capillaries between endothelial cells by a process called **diapedesis**. Thereby, the neutrophils migrate to the tissues.

## What is respiratory burst?

Within seconds of stimulation, neutrophils sharply increase their oxygen uptake, a phenomenon known as the **respiratory burst**.

## What are the contents of the eosinophilic granules?

A material called **major basic protein** (MBP) makes up about 50% of the mass of the large granules. MBP is thought to play a key role in the eosinophil's ability to damage the larva-tissue stage of helminthic parasites and is an extremely potent tissue toxin. A potent bactericidal and tissue toxin called **eosinophilic cationic protein** (ECP), a **neurotoxic protein**, and an **eosinophil peroxidase** are also present in the large granules.

### What is the normal eosinophilic count are what are the physiological variations in it?

The normal eosinophilic count is 150-300 /mm$^3$ (1-4 % of TLC). It shows diurnal fluctuations. Being lowest at 10 am, and highest at midnight. *The count at 8:00 am represents basal level.* Emotional stress decreases the count. The count also decreases progressively during the intermenstrual period.

### What are the causes of eosinopenia and eosinophilia?

**Eosinophilia** occurs in (1) *allergic disorders*, which are the commonest cause of eosinophilia. Allergic causes include asthma, drug allergy and food sensitivity. (2) *parasitic infestations*, like hookworm, tapeworm, hydatid and filaria. In general, eosinophilia is more with parasites causing tissue infection than with those causing intestinal infections. (3) *skin diseases*, like eczema, dermatitis and scabies. **Eosinopenia** occurs in (1) *endocrine disorders* like Cushing's disease and in (2) *stress*, as in acute infection, traumatic shock, surgical operation, severe exercise, burns, acute emotional stress or exposure to cold.

### What are the contents of basophil granules?

Basophils granule contents include the allergic mediator, **histamine**. Basophils also contain the proteoglycan **chondroitin sulfate**.

### Compare and contrast mast cells and basophils.

| SIMILARITIES |
| --- |

- Both are derived from a marrow stem cell
- Both can be stimulated to grow by IL-3
- Both are heavily granulated, with the granules containing histamine;
- Both have surface membrane receptors for IgE and degranulate when an antigen interlinks the IgE on its surface.

| DIFFERENCES | |
| --- | --- |
| **Basophil** | **Mast cell** |
| Present in blood stream | Present in tissues |
| Has a multilobed nucleus | Has a round nucleus |
| Its granule contains the proteoglycan chondroitin sulfate. | Its granules contain the proteoglycan heparin |

### What are the functions of the mast cells/basophils?

Mast cells are responsible for triggering **immediate hypersensitivity reactions**. They also participate in inflammatory responses and tissue repair.

### What are the causes of basophilia and basopenia?

**Basophilia** occurs in (1) chronic myeloid leukemia and (2) hypersensitivity states. **Basopenia** commonly occurs (1) when there is neutrophilic leukocytosis, as in infections, and (2) in Cushing's syndrome and prolonged corticosteroid therapy.

# 32

# Monocyte, Lymphocyte & Lymphoid Organs

## Describe the morphology of a monocyte.

Monocytes (Fig. 32.1) are spherical cells that measure 14 – 18µ in diameter in dried blood smears. It has a relatively abundant dull gray-blue cytoplasm, which may have a ground-glass appearance. The cytoplasm contains a few azurophilic granules. The nucleus is eccentric and kidney-shaped. Its chromatin stains less intensely than that of lymphocytes, and there are one or two nucleoli.

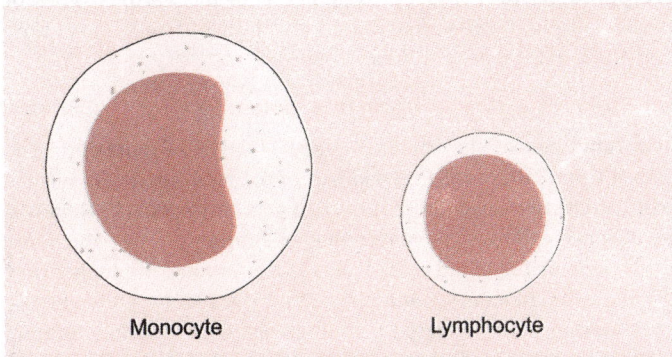

Monocyte  Lymphocyte

**Fig. 32.1**

## What are the functions of a monocyte?

Monocytes originate in the bone marrow and circulate in the blood for about 3 days and then migrate *through the walls of post-capillary venules* into the connective tissue of organs throughout the body. There, they differentiate into **tissue macrophages**. Tissue macrophages do not reenter the circulation. Circulating monocytes *perform no essential function* and are simply a mobile reserve of cells capable of migrating into tissues and developing into macrophages.

## What are the causes of monocytosis?

Monocytes are normally 3-8% of the circulating leukocytes. Some of the causes of monocytosis are: (1) *bacterial infections like* tuberculosis and typhoid, (2) *Protozoal infections like* malaria and kala azar, (3) *rickettsial infections* e.g., oriental sore, (4) *neoplastic diseases like* infectious mononucleosis, Hodgkin's disease and monocytic leukemia, (5) *rheumatoid arthritis and collagen diseases and (6) ulcerative colitis* and *regional enteritis*

## Define the mononuclear phagocytic system (MPS) and enumerate the cells constituting it.

Monocytes enter the blood from the bone marrow and circulate for about 3 days. They then enter the tissues and become **tissue macrophages** and survive for another 3 months. Tissue macrophages settle at several strategic locations in the body and constitute the **tissue-macrophage system**. Monocytes and macrophages together constitute the **mononuclear phagocytic system**. The MPS includes (1) precursor cells from the bone marrow (2) promonocytes from the bone marrow (3) monocytes from the bone marrow and blood (4) macrophages in liver (**Kuppfer cells**), spleen, lymph node, bone marrow, lung (**pulmonary alveolar macrophages** or PAM also called **dust cells**), connective tissue (**histiocytes**), pleura and peritoneum, bones (**osteoclasts**) and central nervous system (**microglial cells**).

The criteria for identifying the cells of MPS are (1) vigorous phagocytosis and pinocytosis and (2) ability to attach firmly to a glass surface. According to these criteria, reticulum cells of the spleen and lymph nodes, endothelial cell and fibroblasts do not belong to MPS although they did so originally when they were called the reticulo-endothelial system (RES).

## What are the functions of MPS ?

The functions of MPS include (1) **Inflammation and healing**. MPS cells ingest cell debris, broken down RBCs, fibrin and bacteria. (2) **Defense against bacteria**. Bacteria entering through blood or lymph are sequestered and destroyed by the RE organs. (3) **Immune response**. (a) *Processing of antigen* by macrophages is essential before an antigen can evoke cell-mediated immunity. (b) Monocytes and macrophages are very efficient in phagocytosing antigen-antibody-complement complexes. This is because MPS cells have receptors for immunoglobulins and complements. (4) **Removal of weak RBC's**. The MPS cells, especially those in the spleen, remove effete (weak) RBCs. The heme moiety is *divested* of its iron, which is stored in the MPS cells where it combines with apoferritin to form *ferritin*. In case of massive *breakdown of RBC's,* e.g. following a local extravasation, the iron binding protein is supersaturated with ferric iron and forms *hemosiderin*. (5) **Storage**. MPS cells store excess lipids and mucoprotein and becomes swollen.

## Describe the morphology of a lymphocyte.

Lymphocytes (Fig. 32.1) are small round cells 7-12µ in diameter, with a deeply staining, slightly indented nucleus and a thin rim of clear blue cytoplasm. They contain no specific granules but may have a few small azurophilic granules. On the basis of their diameter and relative amount of cytoplasm, lymphocytes are described as **large** (11 – 15µ), **medium** (7 - 11µ) and **small** (4 – 7µ).

## What is the functional difference between small and large lymphocytes?

Large and small were earlier believed to be the successive stages of development from the lymphoblast, which is larger than the lymphocyte. However, it is now known that the large lymphocytes are actually the **natural killer (NK) cells**, which constitute about 10 – 20% of the lymphocytes in peripheral blood.

## What is the normal lymphocytic count?

Lymphocytes are the second most numerous leukocytes, accounting for 20-35% of the circulating white blood cells (1500-4000/mm³). Children have higher counts.

## Enumerate the causes of lymphocytosis and lymphopenia.

**Lymphocytosis** occurs in (1) *viral infections* e.g., mumps, measles, chicken pox, influenza, viral hepatitis, (2) *bacterial infections* e.g., typhoid, tuberculosis, whooping cough, (3) *parasitic infections* e.g., toxoplasmosis, (4) *malignancies* e.g., lymphocytic leukemia, lymphocytic lymphoma and (4) *autoimmune diseases* e.g., myasthenia gravis, thyrotoxicosis. **Lymphopenia** occurs in (1) *acquired immunodeficiency syndrome* (AIDS) (2) *pancytopenia* from any cause (e.g., aplastic anemia, bone marrow infiltration, hypersplenism) and (3) *corticosteroid* administration

## What are the functional subtypes of lymphocytes?

Small lymphocytes can be broadly classified into 3 subtypes: B-cells, T-cells and killer cells based on their developmental background, life span, and functions. **B cells** mediates humoral immunity. **T cells** mediates cell mediated immunity (CMI). **Natural killer(NK) cells** are highly cytotoxic for tumor cells. Their action is non-specific and facilitated by *antibody dependent cell-mediated cytotoxicity (ADCC)*.

These subtypes are not morphologically distinguishable, but they have distinctive surface molecules that are *identifiable by immunocytochemical methods*. NK cells lack identifying surface markers.

## How are B and T lymphocytes distributed in the body?

B lymphocytic stem cells are *processed* (rendered mature and immunocompetent) in the bone marrow (B for **bursa of fabricus**, the site of B cell processing in birds). Committed T lymphocytic stem cells are processed in the **thymus**. Following processing, the mature T and B cells enter the circulation where they are present in an approximately 70:30 ratio. Most of them leak out through the venules to settle in the **peripheral lymphoid tissues** (lymph nodes, spleen, and lymphoid tissues associated with the alimentary, respiratory and urinary tracts). Some of the lymphocytes return again to the circulation through the lymphatics draining these peripheral lymphoid tissues.

## What are the functions of lymphocytes?

Lymphocytes are the principal cells responsible for the immune response. When exposed to suitable antigen, lymphocytes become larger, and come to resemble a lymphoblast. This process is called **blast transformation**. Some of the lymphocytes however proliferate without blast transformation to form **memory cells** that respond vigorously to subsequent challenge by the same antigen. After blast transformation, B-lymphocytes transform into **plasma cells** and produce antibodies while T-lymphocytes transform into 2 different types of cells, **cytotoxic T cells** and **helper T cells** ($T_C$ and $T_H$) that are responsible for **cell-mediated immunity**, i.e., combating the antigen without antibody formation.

## What is a lymphoid organ?

Lymphoid organs are tissues that are concerned with the growth, development and deployment of lymphocytes. They include **bone marrow, thymus, lymph nodes, spleen,** and **mucosa-associated lymphoid tissue (MALT)**. Together with the various types of immunological cells distributed through out the body, they *constitute the immune system.*

## What are the functions of the spleen?

The functions of the spleen include (1) **RBC formation**: The spleen form RBCs in the second half of the fetal life. It can resume RBC production in adult life if the BM gets destroyed. (2) **Removal of defective RBCs** by macrophages lining splenic sinusoids. (3) **Reservoir for blood cells**: It acts as a reservoir for lymphocytes, plasma cells, monocytes and platelets. It does so by preferentially sequestering newly released cells from the bone marrow, forming a reservoir inside it. In lower animals (but not in man), it acts as a reservoir for whole blood also. (4) **Antibody production**: Without the spleen, the antibodies are formed late and in lower titers. (5) **Defense against blood borne infections**: Splenectomy renders the body vulnerable to fatal septicemia. (6) **Storage**: The macrophage cells in spleen perform the usual storage functions. The conditions in which RBCs are removed in excessive numbers, splenectomy is helpful in elevating the RBC count. These conditions include *spherocytosis* and *autoimmune hemolytic anemias.*

# 33

# Immune Response, Tolerance & Hypersensitivity

### Define immunity.

It is a highly specific defense mechanism of the body that is targeted *specifically* at any foreign material (called **antigen**) introduced into the body. The defense mechanism includes production of substances called **antibodies** that react specifically with the antigen.

### What is natural immunity?

It includes the *non-specific defense mechanisms* of the body like (1) **phagocytosis** by leukocytes and the monocyte-macrophage system cells; (2) destruction of ingested microbes by **gastric acid**; (3) **resistance of the skin** to microbial infection; (4) **plasma enzymes** like (a) lysozymes which lyses bacteria, (b) basic polypeptides which inactivates certain gram positive bacteria and (c) complements which have lytic and several other effects on foreign substances. (5) **Natural killer (NK) cells** which are the *large lymphocytes that non-specifically destroy foreign cells, tumor cells and infected cells.*

### What is the difference between active immunity and passive immunity?

Both are forms of acquired immunity. **Active immunity** is mostly acquired actively, which involves a direct encounter with the antigen. An essential aspect of active acquired immune response is the development of **immunological memory** of the antigen so that on subsequent encounters, the response to the same antigen is more vigorous (**secondary response**).

**Passive immunity** is acquired passively, as when the mother passes its antibodies to the fetus through the placenta or colostrum, or when antibodies are injected for therapeutic purposes. Passively acquired immunity *does not confer immunological memory.*

### What is the difference between an antigen and a hapten?

An **antigen** is usually a high molecular weight protein. But it may also be low molecular weight protein (e.g. insulin) or a high molecular weight polysaccharide (e.g. dextran). Immunogenic molecules require some degree of chemical complexity. Large substances lacking chemical complexity, such as nylon, polyacrylamide and teflon, are not immunogens. The specificity of an antigen is due to specific areas of its molecule called **determinant sites** or **epitopes**. One protein can have several epitopes and these may differ from each other not only in their specificity but also in their antigenic potency.

A **hapten** is usually a *non protein substance* which has little or no antigenic property by itself but *which combines with a protein to form a new antigen* which is capable of stimulating production of specific immunoglobulins. The specificity of the immunoglobulin produced depends upon the hapten fraction rather than the carrier protein. A secondary response can be obtained by subsequent challenge by the same carrier hapten complex but not by the hapten combined with a different carrier. The hapten however does not require the protein carrier to react with the antibody produced. Lipids and simple carbohydrates that are not antigenic and the more complex polysaccharides that are poorly antigenic produce powerful antigens when they are combined with protein.

### What are the differences between primary and secondary immune responses?

When an antigen is introduced into an animal for the first time, there is an interval varying from 4 days to 4 weeks before any immunoglobulin can be detected in the serum. Then follows a rise in the antibody titer which reaches maximum at a time which may vary from 6 days to 3 months. The titer of antibody is also low. This is called the **primary response**.

When the same antigen is injected into the body on a second occasion, there is an immediate drop in the circulating antibody titer due to its neutralization by the injected antigen. However, after 2 – 3 days, a rapid exponential rise in titer is noted which reaches a peak after 7 – 14 days and again falls off rapidly at first and later more slowly. The final level of the antibody is usually above the previous one. This is the **secondary response**, the salient features of which are: (i) a smaller dose of antigen is required to produce it; (ii) the lag is shorter; (iii) there is a greater antibody production (Fig. 33.1).

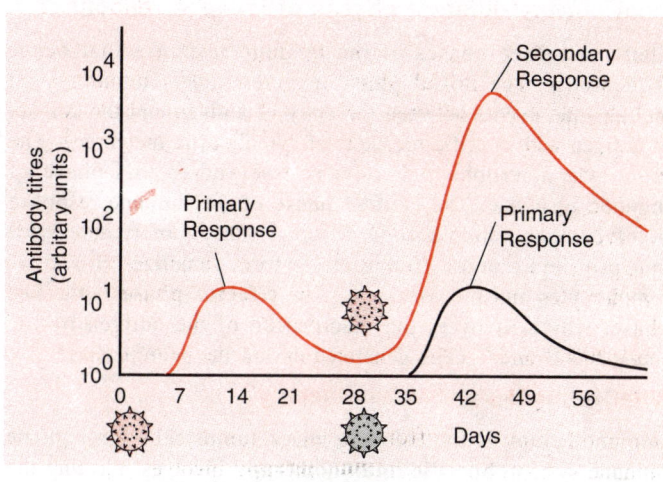

**Fig. 33.1**

| | Primary response | Secondary response |
|---|---|---|
| Responding B cells | Unsensitized B cells | Memory B cells |
| Latent period | 5 – 10 days | 1 – 3 days |
| Peak antibody titer | Smaller | Larger |
| Persistence of antibody titer | Short | Long |
| Predominating antibody class | IgM is more than IgG | IgG |
| Induced by | All immunogens including T-cell independent antigens | Only T-cell dependent protein antigens. |
| Dose of antigen required | High | Low |

## What is the difference between active and passive immunization?

**Active immunization** against a microbe can be achieved by injecting its antigens into the body. When the microbe invades the body, a secondary response is elicited by its antigens and it is quickly destroyed before it can multiply and infect the body. Subsequent attacks by the same microbe only helps in boosting the secondary response and prolonging the immunity.

**Passive immunization** is conferred by injecting preformed antibodies (produced in animals or in another person) against specific microbial antigens. When the microbe subsequently invades the body, it is quickly eliminated by the injected antibodies. Such summary disposal of the microbes however preempts the development of active immunity.

## What is the difference between humoral and cell-mediated immunity?

Humoral and cell-mediated immunity are two components of active immunity. **Humoral immunity** is a *major defense against bacterial infections*. It is mediated by γ-globulin plasma proteins (**immunoglobulins**) that are produced by B-lymphocytes. There are five types of immunoglobulins (Ig): IgM, IgG, IgA, IgE and IgD.

**Cell-mediated immunity** is mainly responsible for *defense against tumor and transplant cells and infections due to viruses, fungi,* and certain *bacteria like Mycobacterium tuberculosis*. It is mediated by **T lymphocytes**. There are two types of T lymphocytes: cytotoxic T cells ($T_C$), and helper T cells ($T_H$).

## What are the different phases of immune response?

There are three phases of the immune response that occur sequentially. The **initial phase** involves innate immunity and includes the events between the entry of antigen and the contact of antigen with specific receptors on lymphocytic membrane. The monocyte-macrophage system is essential to this phase of immune response. The **central phase** of the immune response involves cooperation among different subsets of lymphocytes that proliferate and differentiate to form sensitized T and B-lymphocytes and memory cells. The **effector phase** is the last phase, which involves the inactivation of the antigen by the sensitized B and T cells generated during the central phase.

## What is meant by immunotherapy?

Immunotherapy is the effort to attack tumor cells through the immune system. **Specific immunotherapy** involves injecting the patient with tumor cells in order to induce immunity against tumor antigens. It is often supplemented by injection of cytokines so as to stimulate the differentiation of helper T cells, which are usually not formed in large numbers in antitumor immune responses. Monoclonal antibodies directed against tumor antigens have been used in immunotherapy to treat cancer. However, *most cancer cells undergo antigenic modulation*, rendering the antibodies ineffective. Efforts are therefore on to combine the selectivity of monoclonal antibodies with the killing power of cancer drugs. The technical name for the agents that combine these two activities is **immunotoxins** – which has been called the *magic bullet*. Antitumor toxins are linked to monoclonal antibodies that destroy targeted tumor cells but leave normal cells unharmed. When the antibody binds to the tumor cell, the cell internalizes the antibody along with the toxin. **Nonspecific immunotherapy** relies on the activation of immune responses that are not tumor-specific but inhibit tumor growth. This is done by injecting cytokines like tumor necrosis factor (TNF).

## What is immune tolerance and when is it seen?

It is defined as the *acquired inability* of a host to express specific humoral or cell-mediated immunity to an antigen to which it should normally respond. Tolerance is the opposite of secondary immune response.

## What is hypersensitivity? Give examples.

When an immune reaction results in considerable damage to the body it is called **hypersensitivity**. There are four types of hypersensitivity reactions: **Type-I (anaphylaxis)** occurs due to *mast cell degranulation* and is caused by antigens that evoke a strong IgE response. Examples are allergic rhinitis (hay fever), atopic dermatitis (eczema) and acute urticaria (hives). It occurs within minutes after a second exposure to the offending *allergen* (antigen). Mast cell degranulation occurs when the antigen interlinks the IgE molecules present on the basophils and mast cells (Fig. 33.2). The mediators include *histamine and slow-reacting substance of anaphylaxis* (SRS-A) and cause dilatation and leakage, sensory nerve stimulation (itching, sneezing and coughing).

**Type II (antibody mediated cytotoxicity)** is also an immediate reaction that damages the antigen-bearing blood cells like RBCs, WBCs and platelets. Example of this is seen in *incompatible blood transfusion* and *hemolytic disease of the newborn*. When antibodies react with the antigens, they *also damage the cells (RBC, WBC or platelets) on which the antigens are located*. **Type III (immune complex disorders)** is characterized by the deposition of the *antigen-antibody complex in various normal*

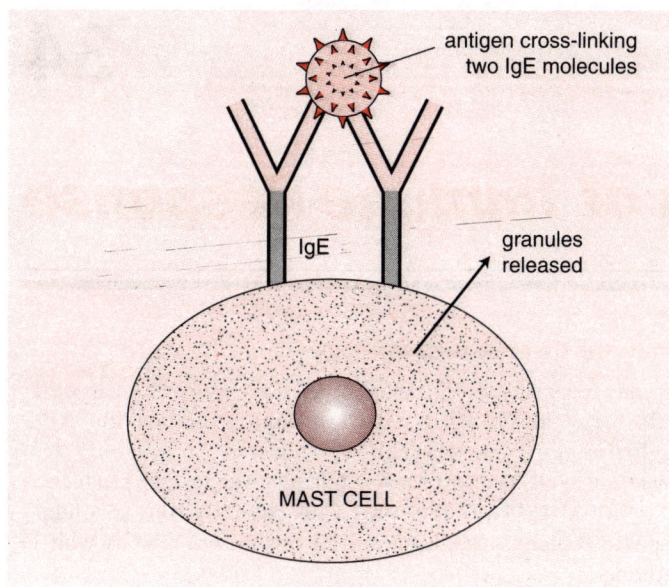

antigen cross-linking two IgE molecules

IgE

granules released

MAST CELL

**Fig. 33.2**

*tissues* of the body where it *fixes complement*. Complement activation *damages the tissue cells in the vicinity* (damage of *innocent bystanders*). A form of *glomerulonephritis* (damage to the glomeruli of the kidney) is an example of this form. **Type-IV (delayed-type hypersensitivity or DTH)** differs from the preceding types in two ways: (a) It is not mediated by antibodies; rather, they are mediated by macrophages that have been activated by T-cells. The cytokines secreted do most of the damage. (b) The hypersensitivity starts after several hours and peaks at 48 to 72 hours. DTH is characteristically associated with **granuloma formation**. *A granuloma is a collection of lymphocytes and macrophages.* The typical example of DTH is typically seen in **Koch phenomenon** – the hypersensitivity to **tuberculin**, which is the antigen present in *Mycobacterium tuberculosis*.

## What is autoimmunity and why does it occur?

**Autoimmunity** occurs when the body's immune response gets directed against its own tissues, which are normally exempted as 'self'. The possible mechanisms of autoimmunity are as follows. (1) A 'self antigen which did not come in contact with the body's immune system during fetal life elicits an immune response in the adult if it comes in contact with immunocompetent cells. This appears to the mechanism of cataract following lens injury. Lens proteins are enclosed in a capsule and do not come in contact with the immune system unless they leak out following injury or surgery. (2) An antibody formed in response to some foreign antigen cross reacts with some tissue of the body itself. This occurs in rheumatic heart disease where the heart is damaged by antibodies formed against streptococcal infections. (3) With age, some tissues of the body undergo an antigenic change that is not recognized as self. (4) The $T_s$ cells (**suppressor cells**, a subpopulation of T-cells) fail to check the immune process adequately.

Examples of autoimmune diseases include *Hashimoto's disease* and *Grave's disease* (autoantibodies against the thyroid), *insulin-dependent diabetes mellitus* (autoantibodies against the B-cells of the pancreas), *myasthenia gravis* (autoantibodies against the acetylcholine receptors on the motor end-plate), *rheumatoid arthritis* (autoantibodies against the joints) *pernicious anemia* (autoantibodies against the gastric mucosa), *autoimmune hemolytic anemia* (autoantibodies against the erythrocytic membrane), *thrombocytopenic purpura* (autoantibodies against the platelets) and *rheumatic fever* (autoantibodies against the endocardium).

# Mechanism of Immune Response

## What is meant by the term blast transformation?

Normally, a lymphocyte develops from a lymphoblast, which is larger in size. However, when stimulated by a suitable antigen, the *lymphocyte becomes larger and looks once again like a lymphoblast*. This is known as **blast transformation**. The B-lymphoblast further differentiates into a **plasma cell**, which produces immunoglobulins. The T-lymphocytes further differentiates into 2 different effector T cells: $T_H$ (*H* for **helper**) cells, and $T_C$ (*C* for **cell mediated cytotoxicity**).

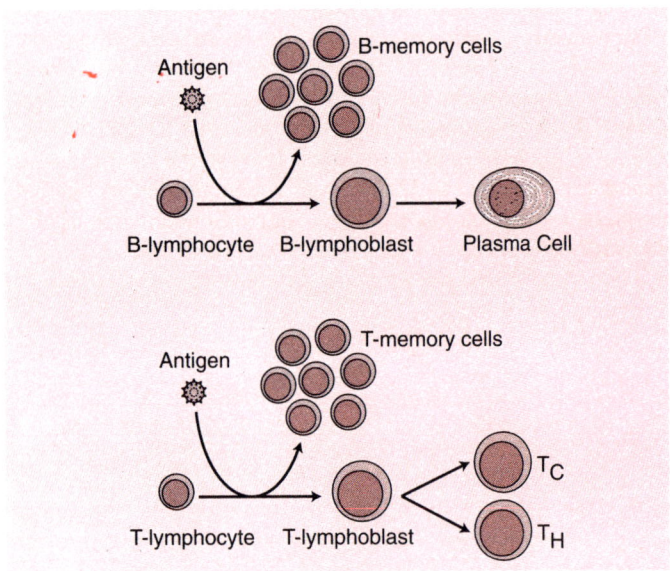

**Fig. 34.1**

## What are memory cells?

Some of the B-lymphocytes and T-lymphocytes do not enlarge or undergo blast transformation when exposed to antigen. Instead, they only proliferate forming a large number of small-sized **memory cells** (Fig. 34.1). It is these memory cells that are responsible for the secondary response.

## What are T-B cooperation and T-T cooperation?

Helper T cells are of two types - $T_H1$ and $T_H2$. The $T_H1$ **cells** are called **inflammatory cells**. They secrete cytokines which (a) stimulate macrophages and produce DTH and (b) helps in the differentiation of cytotoxic T cells (**T-T cooperation**). $T_H2$ **cells** are primary concerned with enabling B-cells to produce antibodies (**T-B cooperation**). They secrete several interleukins.

## What are thymus independent (TI) antigens?

Thymus independent (TI) antigens do not require the help of $T_H$ cells for stimulating B cells. Examples include the **ABO agglutinogens** and **dextran**. *TI antigens induce only IgM formation* with *no class switch* (changeover to IgG production after initial IgM production). Consequently, the secondary response (which is dependent on IgG production) is weak with TI antigens.

## What are the theories of immune specificity?

The antibody produced in response to an antigen is highly specific, i.e. it reacts with only the antigen that has evoked its production and not with any other antigen. Such specificity also implies that since there are innumerable antigens to which the body can be possibly exposed, there must be an equal number of antibodies in the body to match them. However the ultimate origin of all these antibodies is a solitary hemopoietic stem cell and somewhere down the line of differentiation, the cells or the antibodies acquire a bewildering range of specificity. The crucial question is that *at what stage of differentiation does the specificity develop*. The possibilities are: (1) The **template (instructive) theory of Pauling**. It suggests that antibody specificity does not develop during the course of differentiation but develops only following antigenic stimulation. The antigen acts as a template and the antibody moulds itself to fit with it. Thus, it suggests that the antigen "instructs" the production of its antibody and that *immunoglobulins present in the body are non-specific prior to antigenic exposure*. (2) The **germline theory (selective) of Ehrlich**. It suggests that a complete range of antibodies exists in the body and *the antigen has only to select and stimulate the production of one of the antibodies*. It further suggests that each B cell produces the complete set of antibodies, which are present on its surface. In other words, the *B cell itself is non-specific but produces specific antibodies*. It however seems unlikely that so many genes are devoted only to antibody production. (3) The **somatic mutation (selective) theory of Burnet, Jerne and Talmadge** differs from Ehrlich's theory in suggesting that the complete set of antibodies is produced, not by just one non-specific B cell but by a complete set of *specific B cells*. It explains that during the processing of lymphocytes in the central lymphoid tissues, the cells mutate frequently during proliferation giving rise to many genetically diverse B cells, each capable of producing a different antibody. Each specific B cell multiply and establish a population of genetically and immunologically identical B cells called a **clone**. An *antigen has only to select and stimulate its specific clone* (hence the name **clonal selection theory**).

# Immune Effectors

## What are the various immune effector mechanisms?

The final inactivation of the antigen occurs through several mechanisms, all of which are ultimately dependent on the activation of B and T lymphocytes. These mechanisms are (1) **phagocytosis** of the cell on which it is present, (2) **cytolysis** of the cell on which it is present. (3) **bacteriostasis**, in case of bacterial antigens, and (4) **neutralization**, in case of toxic antigens.

Processes that make antigens and antigen-bearing cells susceptible to the above fate are as follows. (5) **Agglutination** causes clumping of antigens, rendering them increasingly susceptible to phagocytosis. (6) **Opsonization** is the coating of antigens with antibody and complements. It helps phagocytes to bind and phagocytose the antigen. This is because phagocytes have receptors for the Fc of IgM, IgG, IgA and complements. (7) **Antibody-dependent cell-mediated cytotoxicity (ADCC)** is a form of cytotoxicity in which NK cells recognize and kill antibody coated target cells, which are identified by the stem (Fc portion) of the antibody molecules coating the target cells. Opsonization is to phagocytosis as what ADCC is to cytolysis.

The above events require that immune cells are able to reach the site where antigens are located. That is made possible through (8) **vasodilatation**, which causes increased movement of phagocytic cells and immunoreactive proteins from the blood vessels into the extravascular spaces, and (9) **chemotactic factors**, which attract the cells to the site of the antigen. Many if not all the factors producing vasodilatation and chemotaxis are released by mast cells. (10) **Mast-cell degranulation** occurs when the antigen interlinks the IgE molecules present on the basophils and mast cells. The mediators include **histamine** and **slow-reacting substance of anaphylaxis (SRS A)**.

## Briefly describe the structure of an immunoglobulin molecule.

An immunoglobulin molecule is made of two heavy and two light chains. Disulphide bonds anchor the light chain to the heavy chain and also holds the two heavy chains together. The heavy chains are of five subtypes: $\mu$, $\gamma$, $\alpha$, $\varepsilon$ and $\delta$ (constituting respectively IgM, IgG, IgA, IgE and IgD). The light chains are only of two types: **kappa** and **lambda**. The $NH_2$ terminal half of each chain (designated as $V_L$ in the light chain and $V_H$ in the heavy chain), has a variable sequence of aminoacids and is therefore called the **variable region**. The COOH terminal half has a relatively constant sequence and is called the **constant region**. The variable regions bind to the antigen.

Disulphide bonds fold each chain into incomplete loops (Fig. 35.1). There are four loops in the heavy chain of which only one (designated as VH) lies in the variable region and the three others (designated as $CH_1$, $CH_2$ and $CH_3$) lie in the constant region. Each light chain however has only two loops, one in the variable region (designated as VL) and one in the constant region (designated as CL). The $CH_2$ in IgG binds to complement C1q. The $CH_3$ attaches to macrophages. In IgM, it also binds to complement.

The immunoglobulin molecule can also be split enzymatically by papain or pepsin. Papain yields **Fab (antigen binding fraction)**, which bears all the variable regions, and **Fc (crystallisable fraction)**. Fc determines such properties of the immunoglobulin as diffusibility, placental transfer, complement fixation, opsonization etc.

## Name the different types of immunoglobulins and enumerate their salient characteristics.

**Immunoglobulin-M** (IgM). (1) It comprises about 10% of the total plasma immunoglobulins. (2) It is *the predominant immunoglobulin produced in the primary response*. It appears early in the secondary response but its level does not rise significantly thereafter. (3) Because of its large size, it is

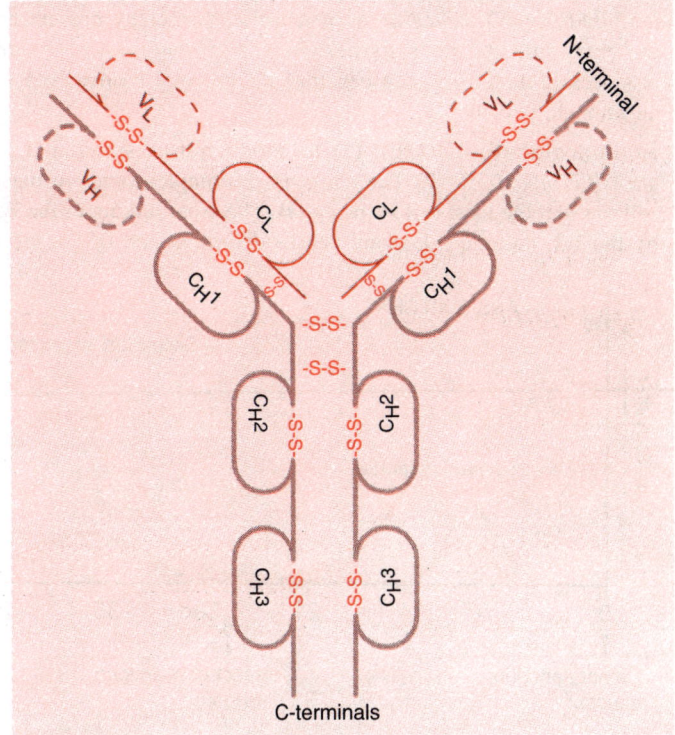

**Fig. 35.1**

*predominantly intravascular*. This, coupled with its early production makes it *important in bacteremias*. (4) IgM is the only immunoglobulin that is *produced before birth*. Natural antibodies like anti-A and anti-B agglutinogens are therefore of the IgM type. (5) It has a theoretical valence of 10. (6) It has much more affinity and avidity of binding for large antigens with multiple epitopes than for small haptens. (7) IgM causes *very effective agglutination*. It produces *complement fixation* by the classical pathway and the *lysis* it causes thereby is very effective. Its opsonizing power is however rather weak.

**Immunoglobulin-G** (IgG). (1) It is the *most abundant immuno-globulin*, comprising about 70% of the total immunoglobulins. (2) It is the major immunoglobulin to be synthesized during the *secondary response* in which the initial IgM production gives way to IgG production (**class switch**) (Fig. 35.2). (3) Unlike IgM, it is *able to cross the placenta*. Thus it is able to provide passive immunity to the neonate in its first few weeks. The protection is further reinforced by the *transfer of colostral IgG across the gut mucosa* of the neonates. (4) IgG readily *diffuses out into the extravascular spaces* where its concentration is same as that in the plasma. It is also *found in milk, saliva, nasal and bronchial secretions*. (5) IgG causes *opsonization, ADCC* and *neutralization of toxins*. Although it fixes complements by the classical pathway, the lysis it produces through complement fixation is weak. The IgG antigen complex binds to platelet through Fc receptors causing *platelet aggregation*.

**Immunoglobulin-A** (IgA). (1) It is secreted in *colostrum, saliva, nasal* and *lung secretions, tears, genitourinary* and *gastrointestinal fluids*. (2) IgA causes *opsonization* and *neutralization*. It also *fixes complement by the alternate pathway*. (3) The *intestinal mucosa secretes IgA* bound to a secretory protein that stabilizes it against proteolysis. (4) It *coats the microbes and inhibits their adherence to the mucosal cells* thereby preventing the entry into the body tissues. *Neisseria gonorrhoea*, which produces IgA protease, can penetrate the mucosal barrier even in an immune person.

**Immunoglobulin-E** (IgE). (1) Its production is stimulated in *parasitic infections*. (2) The antigen IgE complex binds to mast cell through the mast cell Fc receptors. The cross linking of the Fc by the IgE antigen IgE chain causes *degranulation of the mast*

cells with the *release of anaphylotoxins* like histamine, slow reacting substance of anaphylaxis (SRS-A), mast cell chemotactic factor, eosinophil chemotactic factor etc.

**Immunoglobulin-D** (Ig D) is present on the surface of B cells and is known to act as the antigen receptors for the B cells.

## What are cytokines?

Cytokines are small proteins that usually act in an autocrine (on the cell that produced them) or paracrine (on cells close by) manner. Some cytokines have systemic effects like fever. Cytokines are secreted not only by lymphocytes and macrophages but also by endothelial cells, neurons glial cells, and other types of cells. Most of the cytokines are initially named for their actions e.g., the B-cell-differentiating factor. However, once the amino acid sequence of a factor is known, its name is changed to **interleukin.** Thus, for example, the name of B cell-differentiating factor was changed to interleukin-4. Some common cytokines are interleukins (IL), interferons (IFN), tumor necrosis factor TNFα, TNFβ, growth factors, colony-stimulating factors, migration inhibition factor, macrophage chemotactic factor, etc.

## What are complements?

The complement system is a system of nine **enzymatic proteins** designated C1 to C9 present in the blood as plasma proteins. Normally in the inactive state, their activity is triggered *when C1 binds to the antigen-antibody complex*. The activated C1 in turn activates the other complements in cascade reactions. While the *final product* of complement activation (**C5b-C6-C7-C8-C9**) *is cytolytic*, many of the byproducts causes *vasodilatation, chemotaxis, opsonization, immune adherence* and *mast cell degranulation*. The antibodies that can 'fix' (activate) complements are IgM and IgG. IgA also fixes complement but does so by the *alternate pathway* and not by the *classical pathway* as in the case of IgM.

The *activation of C3* to C3a and C3b occupies a central position in complement activation, just as activation of factor IX occupies a central position in the coagulation pathway. The important products of complement activation are given below.

| C2b | A patent vasodilator |
|-----|----------------------|
| C3a | An opsonin |
| C3b | Causes mast cell degranulation |
| C5b | Causes chemotaxis and mast cell degeneration |
| C5b-C6-C7 | Chemotaxis |
| C5b-C6-C7-C8-C9 | Membrane-attack complex. |

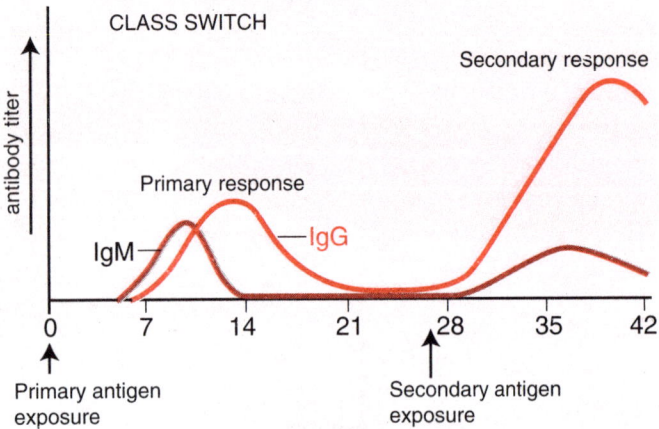

**Fig. 35.2**

# *Immunomodulation*

### What is an adjuvant? Give examples.

**Adjuvants** (L. *adjuvere,* to help) are substances that are mixed with an antigen before injection for nonspecifically enhancing the antibody or cell-mediated immune response. The first adjuvant to be discovered was the **Freund's adjuvant**. It contains heat-killed *Mycobacterium tuberculosis,* mineral oil and lanolin (a detergent for emulsifying the oil). Another adjuvant that is in wide use is the **Bacillus Calmette-Guerin (BCG)**.

### Enumerate the different methods of immunosupression.

Immunosupression disarms the immune system. Its main applications are in (1) reducing inflammation, (2) organ transplantation prolongation, (3) reduction of autoimmune disorders, (4) reduction of Rh blood antigen sensitization, and (5) cancers of the hemopoietic system. Immune suppression may be specific or nonspecific. **Specific immunosuppression** is a form of immunologic tolerance. **Nonspecific immunosuppression** again is of two types: *artificially induced* immunosuppression is produced by the destruction of lymphocytes by physical means such as irradiation or inoculation of chemical or biologic agents. *Naturally induced* immunosuppression is a biologic form of suppression and is primarily exemplified by immunodeficiency diseases.

*Physical methods* of immunosuppression include thoracic duct drainage, thymectomy, splenectomy and irradiation. *Chemical immunosuppessants* are generally antiproliferative agents like corticosteroids, antimetabolites, and antibiotics. *Biologic methods of immunosuppression* include antigen-induced suppression (which is used for **allergen desensitization**), antibody-induced suppression (e.g., prevention of Rh blood antigen sensitization in susceptible pregnant women by administration of anti-D serum), and administration of antilymphocyte serum reacts (using antilymphocyte serum concomitantly with donor cells facilitates induction of tolerance to skin allografts).

### Outline the pathophysiology of AIDS.

Acquired immunodeficiency syndrome (AIDS) was first identified in 1981. It is characterized by dramatic weight loss, night sweats, swollen lymph nodes, and high susceptibility to opportunistic infections. It is also associated with neuropsychiatric abnormalities. Death is inevitable, sooner or later. **Acquired immunodeficiency syndrome (AIDS)** is (1) *acquired* because victims do not inherit the disease; (2) is an *immunodeficiency* because there is a breakdown of their immune system, and (3) is a *syndrome* because of its association with several diseases that take advantage of the body's collapsed defenses.

AIDS is a contagious disease which spreads by intimate homosexual or heterosexual contact, by exposure to infected blood or blood products, or from mother to child during pregnancy. It is caused by an RNA retrovirus called the **human immunodeficiency virus type 1 (HIV-1)**. *AIDS patients have lymphopenia – primarily the CD4$^+$ cells* which are the precursors of T$_H$1 cells. This is because CD4$^+$ molecule acts as a specific receptor that binds with high affinity to the HIV's envelope glycoprotein called **gpl20**. The number of circulating NK cells in AIDS patients is not significantly reduced, but their *cytotoxic ability is diminished*. The humoral dysfunction associated with AIDS is an *inability to produce an adequate IgM response*.

HIV virus does not kill the infected CD4$^+$ cells. Instead, they activate them to T$_H$1 cells. This leads to a widespread activation of the immune system, which causes immunological destruction and eventually gets exhausted itself. Monocytes also express CD4$^+$ molecules and therefore get infected with HIV virus. Monocytes are more refractory to the cytopathic effects of the virus – the virus can survive in these cells and thus be transported to different parts of the body, such as the brain and lung. Thus, monocytes serve as a major reservoir for HIV in the body. HIV-1 also invades brain cells, causing dementia in over half the patients. This may be due to factors released from infected microglia.

# Hemopoiesis & Bone Marrow

## What are the various sites of hemopoiesis?

In *the fetus* all blood cells originate in the mesenchyme. During the first 2 months of fetal life blood formation takes place in the yolk sac. Thereafter, the liver becomes the main site of hemopoiesis until about the 7th month, and the spleen makes a small contribution (Fig. 37.1).

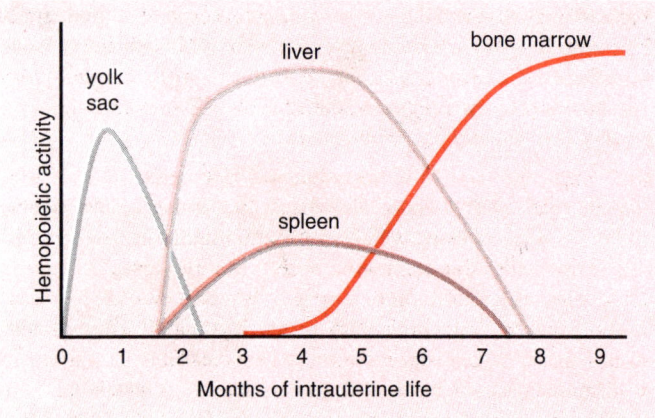

**Fig. 37.1**

**Intramedullary hemopoiesis** (hemopoiesis in the bone marrow) commences in the 3rd month, and by the 7th month it is the major site of hemopoiesis. Shortly after birth, it is the only site of formation of red cells, granulocytes and platelets. Although some lymphocytes and monocytes are formed in the liver and bone marrow, the main sites for their production are the spleen, lymph nodes and other lymphoid tissues. *After birth, (1)* red cells, granulocytes and platelets are formed only in the bone marrow. (2) Lymphocytes are formed mainly in the lymph nodes and other collections of lymphoid tissues in the spleen, gastrointestinal tract, tonsils and other sites. The marrow makes only a small contribution to lymphocyte production. (3) Monocytes are formed partly in the spleen and lymphoid tissue, but the bone marrow makes the major contribution.

**Extramedullary hemopoiesis** is the term applied to blood formation in organs other than the marrow. After birth the spleen, liver and lymph nodes normally play no part in the formation of blood cells. However, when there is an increased demand for blood cells that cannot be met by the hyperactivity of the bone marrow alone, these organs revert to their fetal role of hemopoiesis, as the stem cell retains its potential hemopoietic activity. It occurs most commonly in infants and young children in whom the whole of their marrow cavity is occupied by red (hemopoietic) marrow and there is little space for expansion of the marrow cavity.

## What are the precursor cells of the mature RBC and what are the changes associated with erythropoiesis?

All blood cells, *including lymphocytes*, originate from the **pluripotent stem cell**. Lymphocytes mature and proliferate outside the marrow, in the thymus and peripheral lymphoid tissues. All other blood cells are collectively called **myeloid cells**. Hemopoietic stem cells comprise only 0.01% of the total marrow population. A small numbers also circulate in the blood. Stem cells possess two fundamental properties: **self-renewal**, i.e., the ability by cell division to give rise to more stem cells, and **differentiation and commitment**, i.e. the ability to differentiate into mature specialized blood cells. There are three functionally different stem cells: (1) the **pluripotent stem cell**, which can give rise to any blood cell, (2) the **myeloid stem cell** giving rise to erythrocytes, granulocytes of all types, monocytes, and platelets; and (3) the **lymphocyte stem cell** which gives rise only to lymphocytes.

## What are progenitor cells and how are they different from stem cells?

With time, the capability of a stem cell for self-renewal diminishes and its commitment to a particular line of differentiation increases. When the self-renewal capability is lost, the cell is no longer called a stem cell but is termed a **progenitor cell**. Progenitor cells are *committed to one or at the most two lines of development.*

Progenitor cells are more numerous than stem cells and like stem cells, are present in both the bone marrow and the circulating blood. *Stem cells and progenitor cells cannot be differentiated morphologically.* They both look like a large lymphocyte. However, they can be separated by immunological techniques, taking advantage of the different types of molecules present on their cell membrane. Progenitor cells are recognized by their ability to give rise to **clones** (colonies, or a group of cells) of differentiated cells in the presence of growth factors. Hence, progenitor cells are also called **colony-forming cells** (**CFC**) or **colony-forming units** (**CFU**). Progenitor cells may be multipotent or unipotent. An example of **multipotent progenitor cells** is the **CFU-GEMM** (colony-forming unit: granulocyte, erythroid, megakaryocyte, macrophage). Examples of unipotent progenitor cells are **CFU-E** (erythroid) and **Meg-CFU** (megakaryocytes). The erythroid series has two types of erythroid progenitor cells, burst forming units-erythrocyte (**BFU-E**) and colony forming units-erythrocyte (**CFU-E**). BFU-E forms large colonies whereas CFU-E forms much smaller colonies (Fig. 37.2).

## Describe a reticulocyte. What is the normal reticulocyte count and what is its significance?

The reticulocyte is a flat, disc-shaped, non-nucleated cell, of

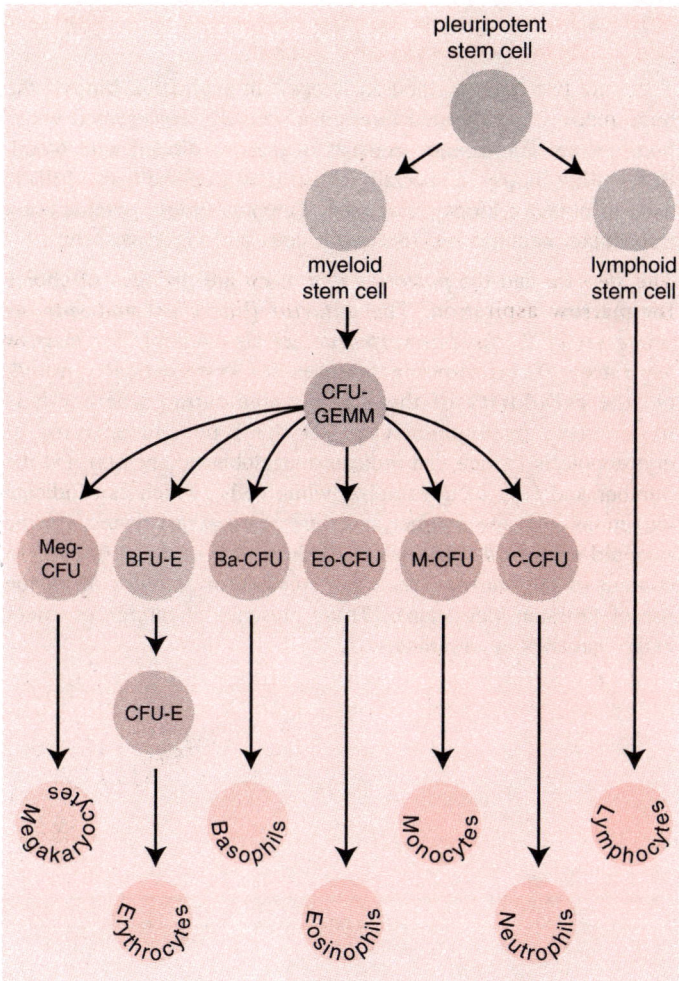

**Fig. 37.2**

slightly larger volume and diameter than the mature erythrocyte. The hemoglobin content is about the same as that of the mature cell. The cytoplasm still contains small amounts of RNA. With Romanowsky stains, it shows a faint *polychromatic tint*. With supravital stain such as brilliant cresyl blue, the RNA appears in the form of a **fine reticulum**. As the reticulocyte matures, the RNA is catabolized and ribosomes disintegrate. The reticulocyte takes about 1 to 2 days to mature to an erythrocyte. Reticulocytes are present in circulation too where they *comprise 0.2 – 2.0% of the RBC count*. Their number *increases in hemolytic anemia and following treatment of deficiency anemias*.

### Name the precursor cells in granulopoiesis.

The first recognizable cell of the granulocytic series is the **myeloblast**, from which the mature granulocytes develop through a series of cells, namely the **promyelocyte**, **myelocyte**, **metamyelocyte** and **stab form**.

It is at the *myelocyte stage* that the cell develops the **specific granules** that determine the nature of the mature cell, i.e., whether it is a neutrophil, eosinophil, or basophil. Apart from the difference in granules, the myelocyte, metamyelocyte and band form have the same structural characteristics for all the granulocytes. The maturation of the granulocytes is characterized by (1) the

development of specific granules in the cytoplasm; (2) loss of basophilia of the cytoplasm; (3) progressive ripening of the nucleus, which ultimately becomes segmented, and (4) the development of motility and ability to act as a phagocyte. (5) Mitotic division occurs up to the stage of the myelocyte, in which it is most active. The metamyelocyte is not capable of mitotic division.

### Name the precursor cells in the course of lymphopoiesis and monopoiesis.

The **lymphoblast** resembles the myeloblast morphologically. Lymphoblasts give rise to the **large lymphocytes** and **small lymphocytes**, both of which are found in circulation. Monopoiesis begins with the **monoblast**, from which develops the **promonocyte** and the mature **monocyte**.

### Name the precursor cells in the course of thrombocytopoiesis.

Thrombopoiesis begins with the **megakaryoblast**, which matures successively into the **promegakaryocyte** and the **megakaryocyte**. The megakaryocyte is a large cell from 30 to 90 μm in diameter. It has large amounts of light-blue cytoplasm containing fine azurophilic granules. It has a single multilobed nucleus with coarse chromatin. The cell margin shows pseudopodia. **Platelets** are formed by the breaking off of small fragments of the cytoplasm of these megakaryocytes.

### What is the difference between red marrow and white marrow?

The bone marrow is liquid in consistency. It appears either *red or yellow*. An adult has about 3 – 4 liters of bone marrow. Hemopoiesis occurs in the **red marrow**, which owes its color to the hemoglobin in the red cells precursors and to the blood in the blood vessels. The **yellow marrow** is composed principally of fat with a small number of capillaries and reticulum cells interspersed. The *reticulum cells are potentially hemopoietic* and form *part of the marrow reserve*, which can be called on when there is an increased demand for blood formation.

### What are the changes in bone marrow with age?

At birth, the marrow in all the bones of the body appears red and contains no fat. At the age of about 4 to 5 years, fat cells begin to appear in the red marrow, which begins to recede from the long bones and is replaced by yellow fatty marrow. By the age of 20 years, only the upper parts of the femur and humerus contain red marrow. Thus, in adult life red marrow is found only in the bones of (1) the thorax (ribs, clavicles, scapula and sternum), (2) vertebra (3) skull (4) pelvis and (5) upper parts of the femur and humerus, occupying up to one-third of the shafts (Fig. 37.3).

### What is meant by the bone marrow reserve?

The bone marrow has a large reserve hemopoietic capacity, which enables it to significantly increase output in response to increased demands. The reserve capacity of the marrow is made up of two elements: (1) the **functional reserve** of the hemopoietic cells which can start proliferating and differentiating on receiving appropriate stimulus. (2) the **anatomical reserve**, in the form of the fat cells, which can be readily replaced by active hemopoietic cells. The

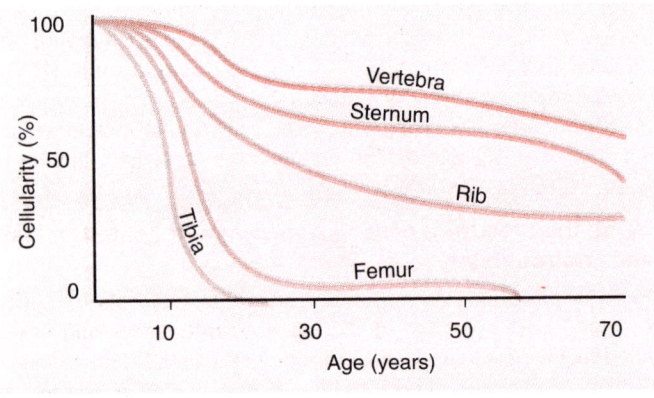

**Fig. 37.3**

replacement of fat cells occurs initially in the red marrow itself, which become *redder* in color. Later, yellow marrow is transformed into red marrow, either by activation of the dormant stem cells in the yellow marrow, or by migration of stem cells from red cells. Still later, the bone may be eroded by the expanding marrow cavity.

### How is bone marrow biopsy performed and what are the important observations made?

There are two main methods of biopsy. In **aspiration biopsy**, the bone marrow is aspirated through a specially constructed wide-bore needle. The aspirate consists of marrow diluted with blood. In **trephine biopsy**, a specially constructed trephine (saw, drill) is used to obtain a biopsy specimen. Trephine biopsy obtains bony trabeculae, hemopoietic tissue, fat cells and blood vessels.

The *sternum* and the *posterior iliac crest* are the sites of choice for marrow aspiration. The *anterior iliac crest* and *spinous processes of the lumbar vertebrae* are also suitable for marrow aspiration. The following features are systematically noted: (1) the **cellularity** of the marrow (indicating whether it is hyperactive or hypoactive); (2) the type and activity of erythropoiesis (which can indicate megaloblastic anemia); (3) the number and type of developing white cells (which can indicate leukemias); (4) the number and type of megakaryocytes; (5) the **myeloid-erythroid ratio** (normally about 3:4 or 4:1); (6) the iron content of the marrow (seen as hemosiderin granules or by the use of Prussian blue stain); (7) the presence of foreign or tumor cells, parasites or organisms.

# 38

# Principles of Electrocardiography

### What is measured in an ECG: current or potential?

ECG records potential. The potentials recorded are indicative of the magnitude and direction of body currents set up by the activity of heart.

### Explain the terms unipolar and bipolar leads.

A **bipolar limb lead** has two electrodes that measure the potential difference between any two limbs. The **unipolar limb lead** is similar except that *one of the electrodes is kept at zero potential* while the other is placed either on a limb or on the chest.

### Define the terms Einthoven's triangle, Einthoven's law and indifferent electrode.

**Einthoven's triangle** (Fig. 38.1) is the imaginary triangle formed around the heart by the proximal ends of the two arms and the left leg. **Indifferent electrode** is the name given to the junction formed by connecting leads from the three limbs: the two arms and the left leg. The **Einthoven's law** states that the indifferent electrode formed by connecting the three ends of the Einthoven's triangle is always at zero potential.

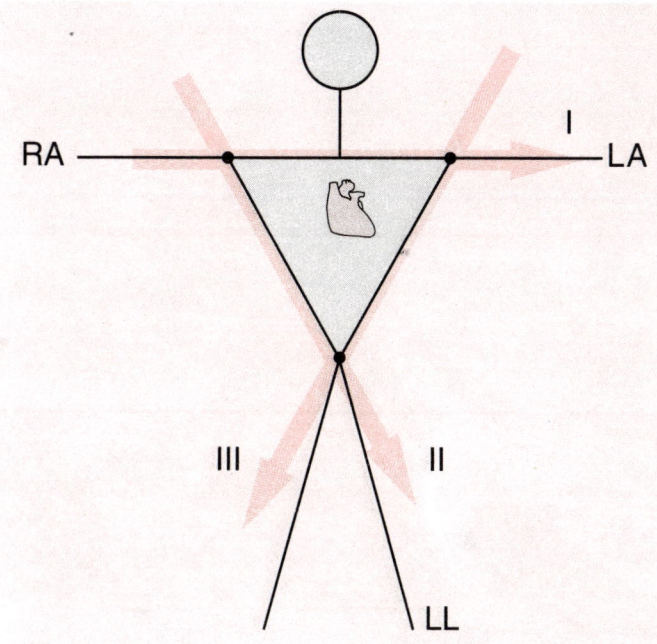

**Fig. 38.1**

### Enumerate the standard limb leads and mention their axes.

**Standard limb** leads are bipolar leads that record the potential difference between any two corners of the Einthoven's triangle.

**Lead I** records the potential difference between left arm (active electrode) and right arm (reference electrode). Its axis is 0°. **Lead II** records the potential difference between left leg (active electrode) and right arm (reference electrode). Its axis is 60°. **Lead III** records the potential difference between left leg (active electrode) and left arm (reference electrode). Its axis is 120° (Fig. 38.2).

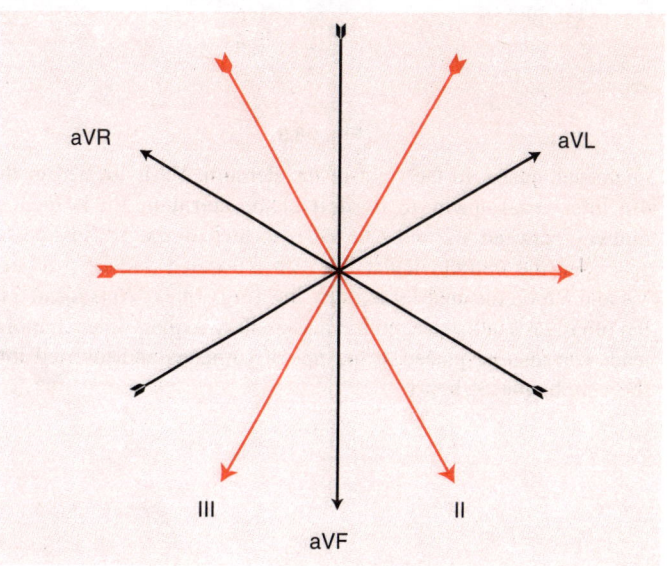

**Fig. 38.2**

### Enumerate the augmented limb leads and mention their axes.

**Augmented limb leads** are unipolar leads that record the potential difference between one corner of the Einthoven's triangle and the average potential of the other two corners. **Lead aVF** records the potential difference between the left leg (active electrode) with respect to the average of right arm and left arm (reference electrode). Its axis is 90°. **Lead aVL** records the potential difference between the left arm (active electrode) with respect to the average of right arm and left leg (reference electrode). Its axis is –30°. **Lead aVR** records the potential difference between the right arm (active electrode) with respect to the average of left arm and left leg (reference electrode). Its axis is 210°. *In augmented limb leads, the potential recorded gets 50% amplified, and hence the name 'augmented'.*

### Enumerate the chest leads and mention their sites.

These are leads that are placed on the chest *in a transverse plane at the level of the heart.* They are disposed at regular angular intervals – with at least one in every 30°. V1 is located in the 4th

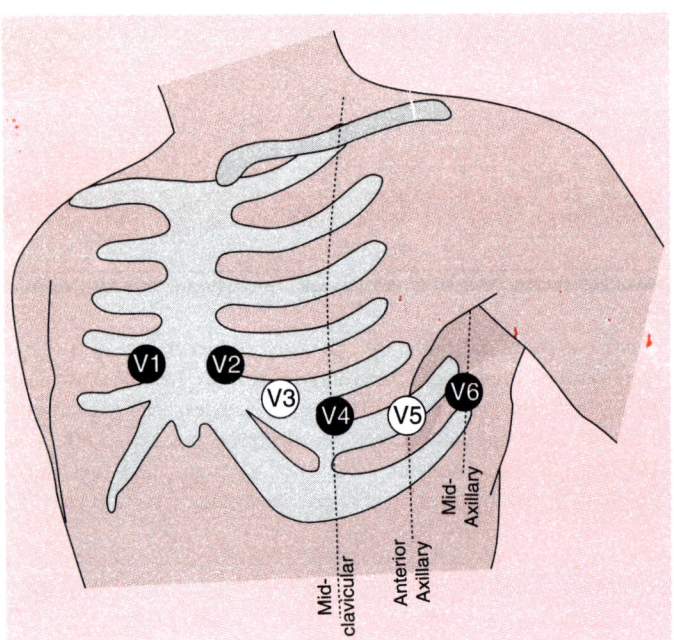

**Fig. 38.3**

intercostal space, to the right of the sternum. V2 is located in the 4th intercostal space, to the left of the sternum. V3 is located midway between V2 and V4. V4 is located in the 5th intercostal space, on the mid-clavicular line. V5 is located midway between V4 and V6 on the anterior axillary line (Fig. 38.3). V6 is located in the 6th intercostal space, on the mid-axillary axillary line. Unipolar leads can also be placed at the tips of catheters and inserted into the esophagus or heart.

# 39

# Electrocardiogram

## Briefly describe the spread of excitation in the heart.

**Atrial depolarization** is complete in about 0.1 s. The excitation spreads through the atria to reach the atrio-ventricular node in two different ways: by a radial spread of excitation from the sinoatrial (SA) node, and by spread of excitation from the interatrial pathways. **Ventricular depolarization** is completed in 0.08 – 0.1s. It *begins at the upper part of the interventricular septum* and spreads in the following sequence: (i) along the left surface of the interventricular septum; (ii) across the thickness of the septum from its left to right surface; (iii) down the septum towards the apex; (iv) along the endocardial surface, back towards the base of the heart; (v) radially outward, from the endocardial towards the epicardial surface; (vi) The left ventricle, which has a larger muscle mass than the right ventricle, is slightly slower to depolarize. *The base of the left ventricle and the pulmonary conus are the last portions to depolarize.*

## How does the direction of the instantaneous electrical axis of the heart change through the cardiac cycle?

During the initial part of systole, the electrical axis is directed downwards and to the right. This is responsible for the Q-wave.

Thereafter, through most part of the systole, the axis is directed downwards and to the left, which results in the R-wave. Towards the end of the systole, the axis swings upwards and to the left, resulting in the S-wave (Fig. 39.1).

## What is the law of the heart?

The SA node has the highest discharge rate (72/min). All other parts of the conductive system have lower rates of discharge, e.g., atrioventricular (AV) node discharges at 40/s. Hence, discharges from the SA node spreads to all parts of the heart and determines the overall heart rate. It is only when the SA node ceases to discharge that pacemakers like the AV node with lower frequency take over. This is known as the **law of the heart**.

## Describe the normal ECG waves and mention the state of the myocardium.

The **P wave** is produced by atrial depolarization. The **QRS complex** is produced by ventricular depolarization. The **T wave** by ventricular repolarization. The **U wave** is only occasionally recorded, and is due to the repolarization of the papillary muscles. *There is no ECG wave corresponding to atrial repolarization* because the same is obscured by the large QRS complex.

## Draw a labelled diagram of the electrocardiogram.

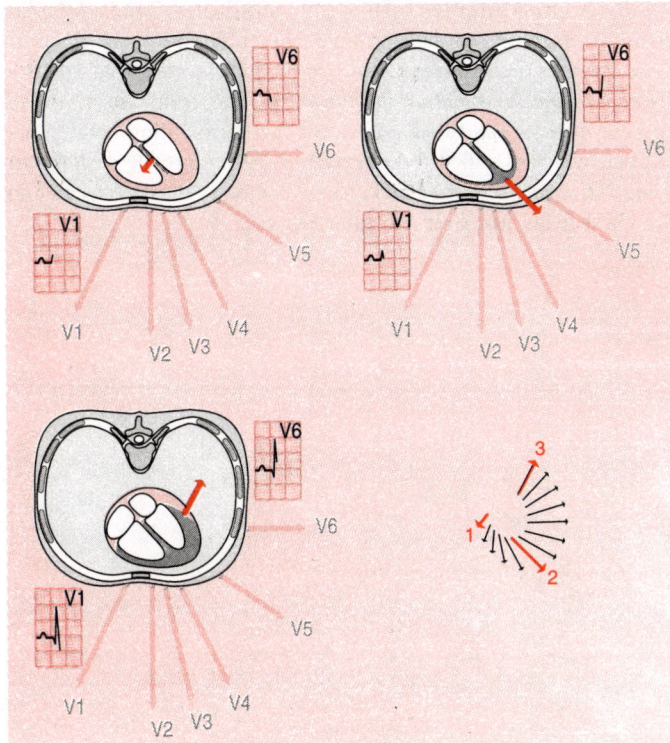

**Fig. 39.1**

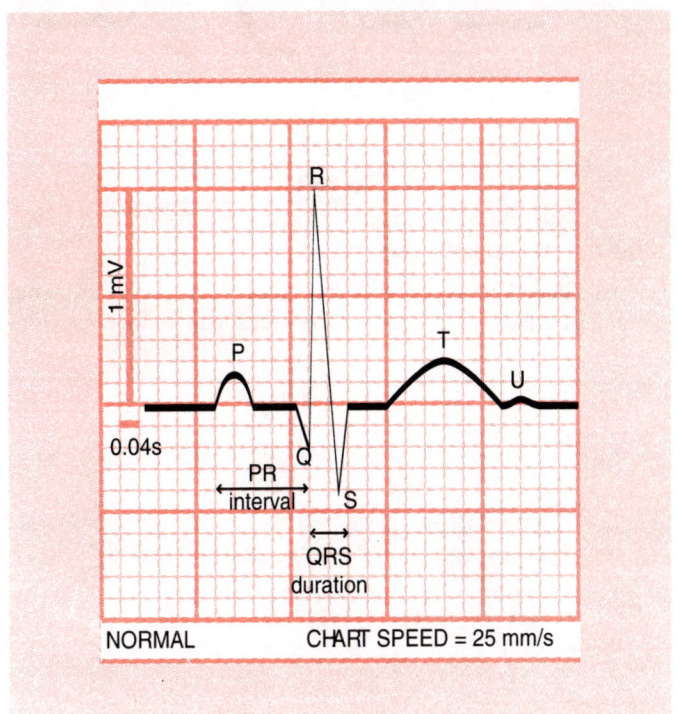

**Fig. 39.2**

## What are the normal duration and amplitudes of the ECG waves and intervals?

| | Duration (mm)* | Range of Duration (mm)* | Amplitude (mm)# | Amplitude Range (mm)# |
|---|---|---|---|---|
| P wave | 2.5 | 1 – 3 | 2.5 | |
| P-R interval | 5 | 3 – 5 | | |
| QRS complex | 2.5 | 2 – 2.5 | | |
|   Q-wave | | | 1 | 0 – 4 |
|   R-wave | | | 7 | 2 – 17 |
|   S-wave | | | 1 | 0 – 5 |
| ST interval | 8 | | | |
| T wave | 5 | | 4 | 1 – 6 |
| QT interval | 10 | 10 – 11 | | |

\* To obtain duration in milliseconds, multiply by 0.04.
\# To obtain amplitude in millivolts, multiply by 0.1.

## What is the J-point and what is its significance?

**J-point** is the point where the S-wave ends. It is one point on the ECG that is always at zero potential (Fig. 39.3).

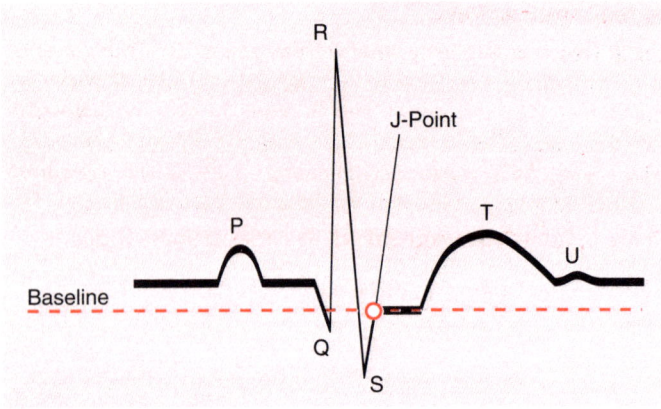

**Fig. 39.3**

## What is the mean electrical axis of the heart and what is its normal range?

The magnitude and direction of the cardiac vector keeps changing continuously through out the cardiac cycle. The average direction

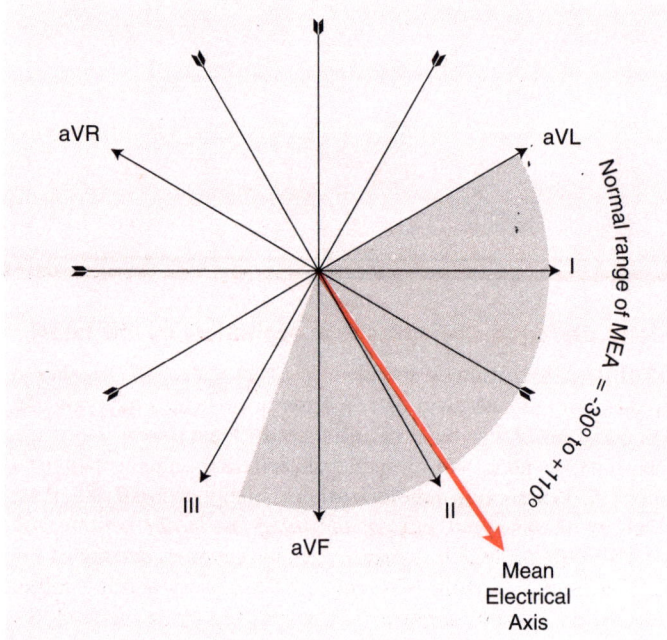

**Fig. 39.4**

and amplitude of this swinging instantaneous cardiac vector is called the **mean electrical axis**. The normal direction of the mean QRS vector is generally said to be -30 to +110 degrees (Fig. 39.4).

## What are the ECG changes associated with myocardial infarction?

The ECG changes of myocardial infarction results primarily from three basic abnormalities of the cardiac muscle: *rapid repolarization* (occurs seconds after the infarction), *decrease in RMP* (occurs minutes after the infarction) and *delayed depolarization* (occurs half an hour after infarction). All three of these changes *make the external surface of infarcted area positive relative to the surrounding normal area*. This results in a *flow of current into the infarcted area* from the surrounding areas. This current, which is called the **current of injury** produces *elevation of the ST segment* in the ECG. The elevation is most noticeable in the chest leads just over the infarcted area.

# 40

# Abnormalities of Cardiac Excitation

## What is sick sinus syndrome?

When a dysfunction of the sinus node results in marked bradycardia with symptoms like dizziness and repeated episodes of syncope, it is called sick sinus syndrome. It can occur due to (i) a reduction of SA node discharge frequency to 60/min or lesser (sinus bradycardia) that does not improve with sympathetic stimulation or vagal inhibition; (ii) due to blockade of impulse conduction from the SA node to the atria (**sinoatrial block**); or (iii) due to the complete stoppage of sinus discharge (**sinus arrest**).

## What is heart block? What is meant by first, second and third degree atrioventricular block?

Any block or slowing down of the conduction of cardiac impulses along the cardiac conductive pathway is called **heart block**. In **1st degree** atrioventricular block (Fig. 40.1), there is a slowing of impulse conduction from the atria to the ventricle across the AV node. Hence the ECG shows a *prolongation of the PR interval*. In **2nd degree** atrioventricular block (Fig. 40.2), in addition to the slowing of conduction, there is atrioventricular conduction failure at regular intervals, i.e., *some of the impulses fail to reach the ventricle*. In **3rd degree** atrioventricular block (Fig. 40.3), the atrioventricular conduction failure is complete, i.e., *none of the impulses that originate in the SA node reach the ventricle*.

## What is Wenckeback phenomenon?

It is a variant of the 2nd degree atrioventricular block in which the *PR interval increases progressively till a ventricular beat is dropped* (Fig. 40.4).

## What is idioventricular rhythm?

In 3rd degree heart block, ventricular depolarization is initiated by the AV node and the ventricles beat at a rate determined by the AV node frequency of ~ 40/s. This is called the **ideoventricular rhythm**. The atria however continue to beat at the normal sinus rhythm of 72/min. Thus, the atrial and ventricular rhythms become entirely independent, each contracting at its own rate. This is called **atrioventricular dissociation**.

## What are the ECG changes associated with bundle branch block?

Conduction blockade of any of the branches of the conductive system of the heart results in slower depolarization of the part of the ventricle that is supplied by the branch. As a result, the total *QRS duration gets prolonged* and *becomes multipeaked*. Also, the mean electrical *axis deviates to the side of the block*. Thus, left bundle branch block is associated with left-axis deviation while right bundle block is associated with right-axis deviation.

## What is an extrasystole?

If the SA node or AV node fails to excite the heart, **latent pacemakers** lower down in the conduction system take over. In diseased states, even atrial and ventricular muscle fibers can discharge spontaneously although normally, they do not show any prepotential. Any site in the heart other than the SA node or AV node that shows spontaneous discharge is called an **ectopic focus**, and the contraction resulting from its discharge is called an **extrasystole**.

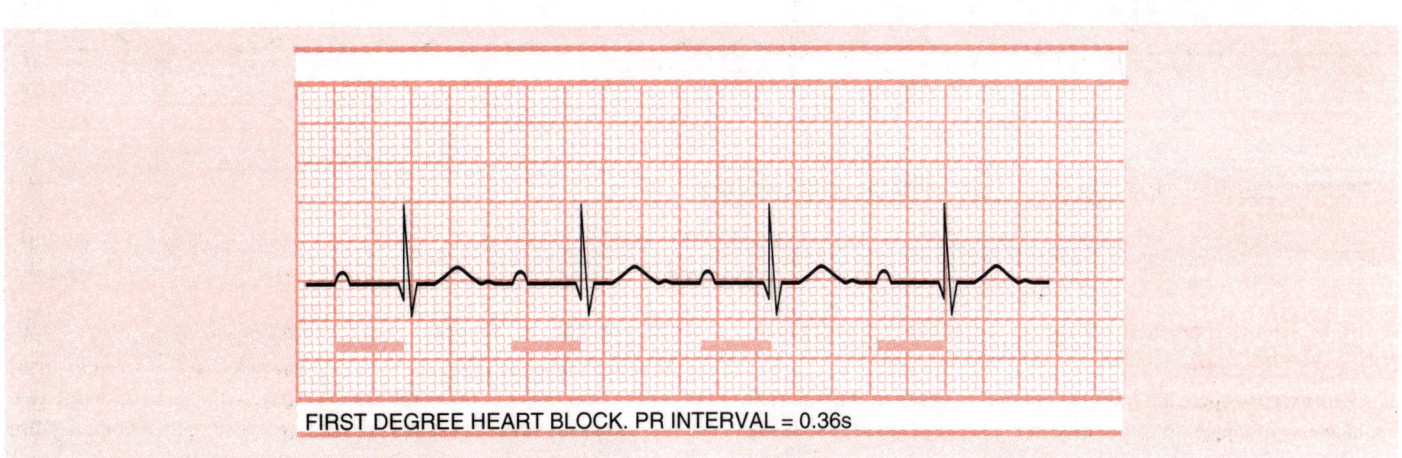

FIRST DEGREE HEART BLOCK. PR INTERVAL = 0.36s

**Fig. 40.1**

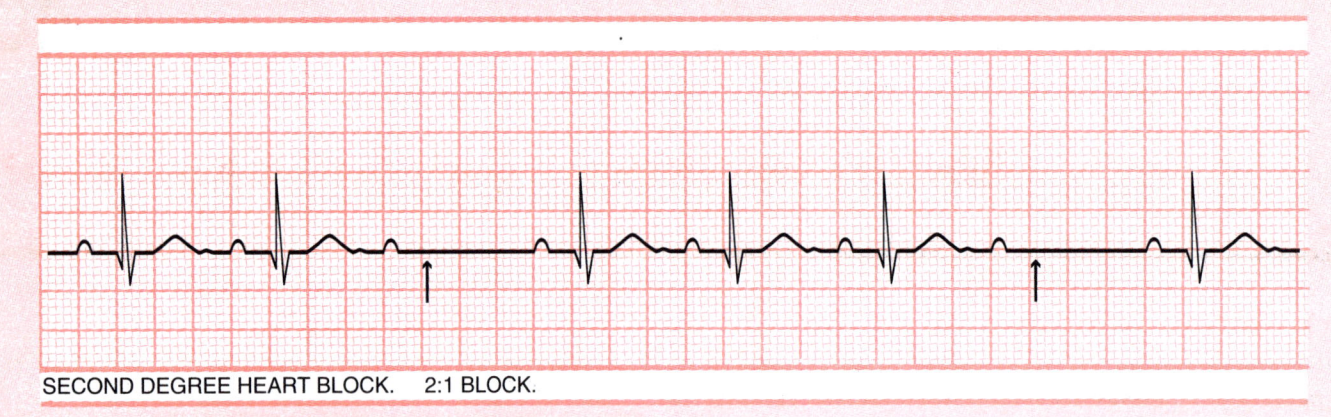

SECOND DEGREE HEART BLOCK.    2:1 BLOCK.

**Fig. 40.2**

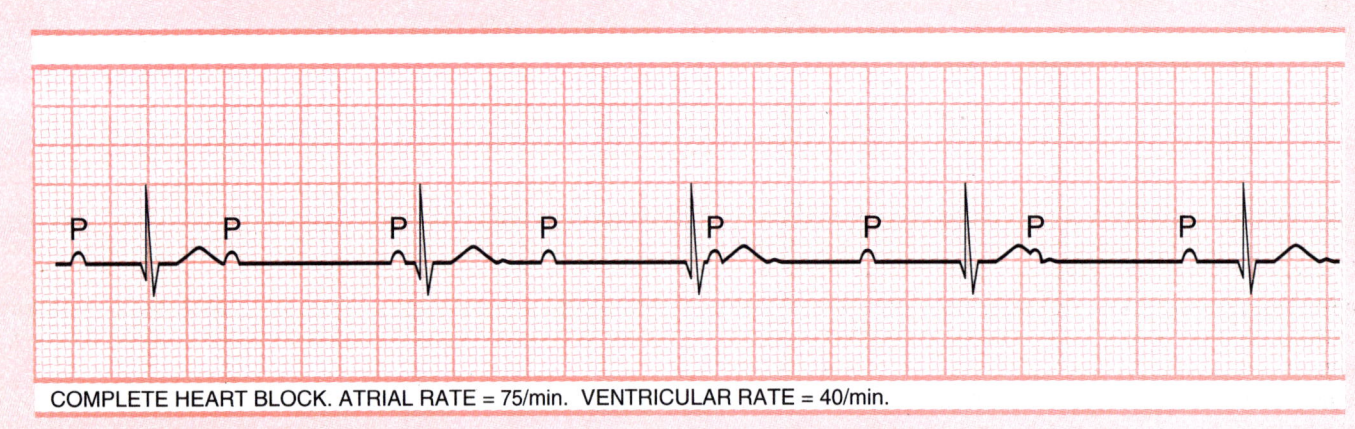

COMPLETE HEART BLOCK. ATRIAL RATE = 75/min.  VENTRICULAR RATE = 40/min.

**Fig. 40.3**

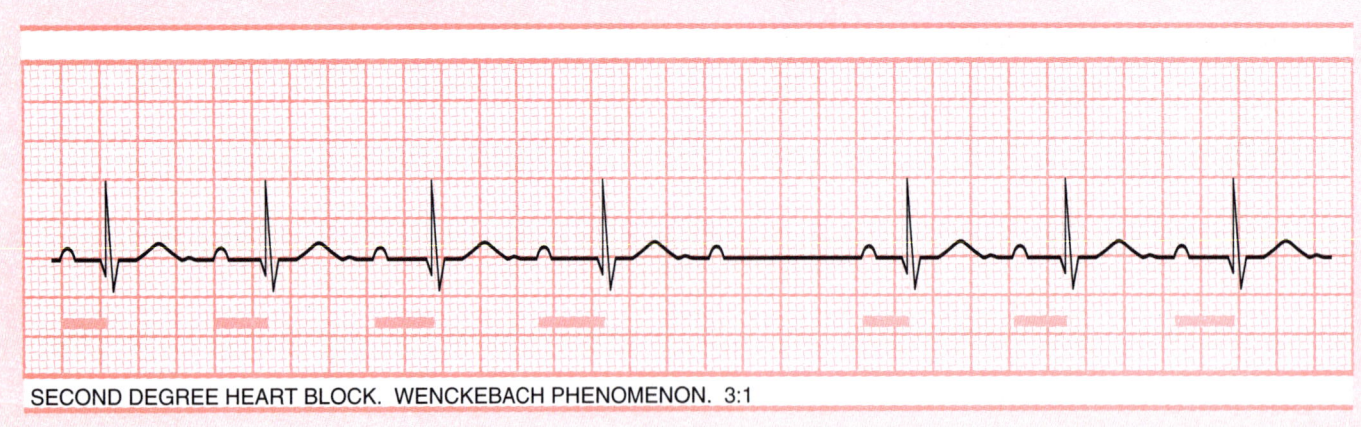

SECOND DEGREE HEART BLOCK.  WENCKEBACH PHENOMENON. 3:1

**Fig. 40.4**

## What is the difference between an atrial extrasystole and a ventricular extrasystole?

In **atrial extrasystole**, the impulse not only spreads to the ventricle but also travels back to depolarize the sinoatrial node and in the process, resets the sinoatrial node. After the extrasystole, the sinoatrial node discharges again only after the normal R-R interval has elapsed.  Hence, there is *no compensatory pause* (Fig. 40.5).

A **ventricular extrasystole** is not preceded by a regular atrial contraction. Also, it does not usually activate the atria or depolarize the sinoatrial node and therefore the regular sinoatrial node rhythm is not disturbed. However, the regular sinus impulse which follows the extrasystole fails to activate the ventricle, which is still

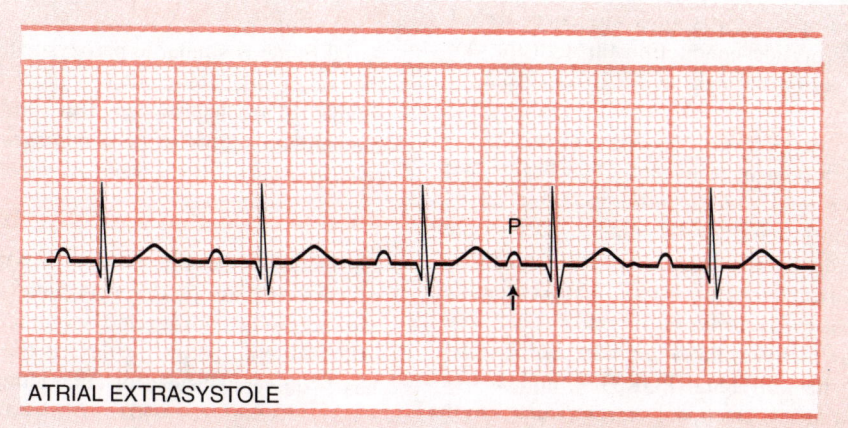

ATRIAL EXTRASYSTOLE

**Fig. 40.5**

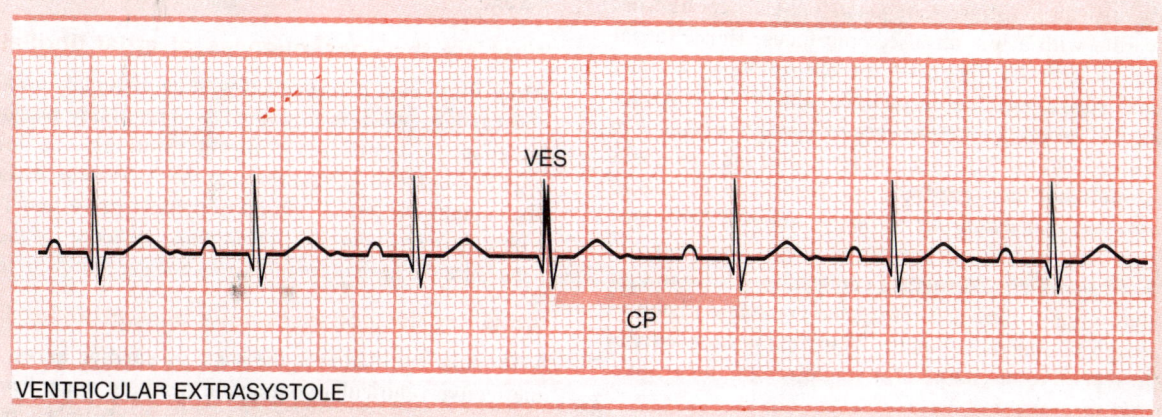

VENTRICULAR EXTRASYSTOLE

**Fig. 40.6**

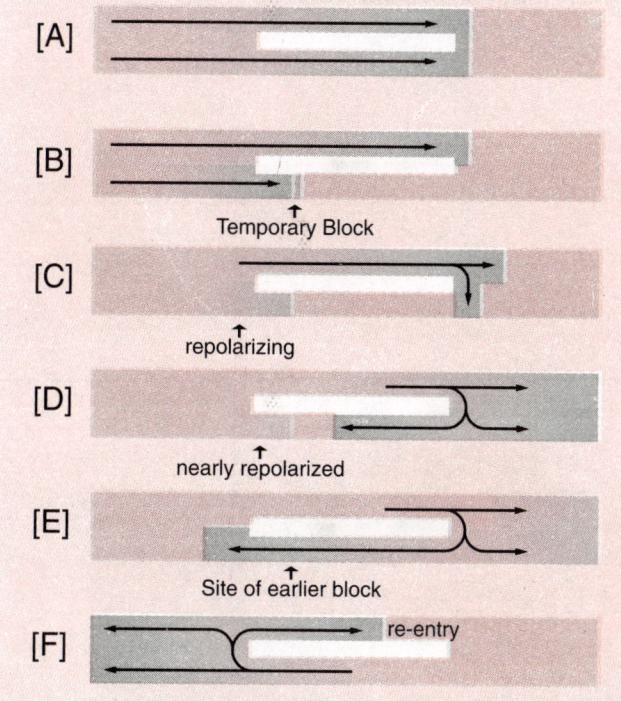

**Fig. 40.7**

refractory from the premature contraction. Instead, the ventricle responds to the next normal sinus impulse. Hence, there is a slight pause – the **compensatory pause** – following the ventricular extrasystole, and *the interval between the two sinus beats preceding and following the extrasystole is exactly twice the normal R-R interval* (Fig. 40.6).

## What are the pathophysiological mechanisms of tachyarrhythmias?

One cause of tachyarrhythmias is the *occurrence of repeated extrasystoles*. Another cause of tachyarrhythmias is the **reentrant circuit** that is a closed-circuit pathway in the heart along which impulses are repeatedly conducted without cessation. In a normal heart, impulses flow in more or less parallel pathways. However, any inhomogeneity in conduction velocity or excitability of any part of the myocardium can result in the formation of reentrant circuits. This is explained diagrammatically below (Fig. 40.7). The temporary block referred to in the diagram could be an ectopic focus that is still refractory after having discharged once. Alternatively, it could be a site that permits only unidirectional conduction so that the forward conduction is blocked but the retrograde conduction is permitted. The reentrant pathways may be of two types: a **microreentrant circuit** that is localized to a very small area in the sinus node, atrium or the AV node. Microreentrant circuits are made possible by local inhomogeneity in cardiac excitability and conductivity or a **macroreentrant circuit** that involves anterograde conduction through the AV node and retrograde conduction through an AV bypass tract.

## What is paroxysmal tachycardia?

Paroxysmal tachycardia is a bout of tachycardia that begins and ends suddenly (*paroxysm = a sudden outburst*). A bout of paroxysmal tachycardia can last for several minutes. Depending on the site of the ectopic focus, the tachycardia may be: **paroxysmal atrial tachycardia** (atrial rate = 160 – 220 per minute), **atrioventricular junctional tachycardia** (atrial rate = 120 – 200 per minute), or **ventricular tachycardia** (ventricular rate = 140 – 220 beats per minute). The individual PQRST complexes in paroxysmal tachycardia of atrial, junctional or ventricular origin are similar to those in atrial, junctional and ventricular extrasystoles respectively.

It is clinically difficult to differentiate *junctional* tachycardia from *atrial* tachycardia with a low atrial ectopic focus. Hence, atrial and junctional tachycardia together are often cautiously termed as **paroxysmal supraventricular tachycardia** (PSVT). **Atrial tachycardia** could be due to the presence of *multiple ectopic foci* or a *microreentrant circuit*. Microreentry seem to be the commoner mechanism. **Junctional tachycardia** is mostly (70% cases) due to a *macroreentrant circuit within the AV node*. Another 20% cases occur due to a *macroreentrant circuit involving the aberrant* **Bundle of Kent** in which anterograde conduction into ventricles occurs through the AV node and retrograde conduction back to the atria, through the aberrant bundle. **Ventricular tachycardia** occurs due to repetitive discharge of a single *ectopic focus*, or a *microreentrant circuit*.

## What is atrial flutter?

Atrial flutter is similar to paroxysmal atrial tachycardia except that the rate of atrial contractions is much higher at 220 – 350 beats per minute. Its mechanisms are also similar. However, the commonest mechanism seems to be a *macroreentrant circuit around the tricuspid valve or the vena caval opening*.

## What is fibrillation and why does it occur?

Fibrillation of the atria and ventricles results from random excitation of various parts of the atria and ventricle respectively. In the absence of a coordinated sequence of excitation, there is no effective contraction of any of the cardiac chambers, and the heart 'quivers' instead of contracting. Fibrillation occurs due to *numerous microreentrant circuits*. There are numerous depolarized patches all over the heart, and the impulse just wanders along the repolarized areas in between the depolarized patches.

## What are the consequences of atrial fibrillation?

Atrial fibrillation is associated with an extremely erratic pulse rate and rhythm, which is described as **irregularly irregular**. This is because the ventricles contract randomly, as and when the impulses in the atria pass through the A-V node. Atrial fibrillation also makes the atrial contraction ineffective and is associated with a *loss of about 30% of the pump function of the heart*. This is because the atria normally act as booster pumps to the ventricles.

## What are the consequences of ventricular fibrillation?

Ventricular fibrillation is the same as **cardiac arrest**. It results in ineffective ventricular contraction resulting in cardiac failure. It is a medical emergency and results in death unless treated within minutes. Its management involves **DC cardioversion** followed by appropriate **antiarrhythmic drugs**.

# 41

# Cardiac Cycle

### What are the different phases of the cardiac cycle and what are their duration?

| Diastole 0.5 sec | | |
|---|---|---|
| | Isovolumetric relaxation | 0.05s |
| | Rapid filling | 0.05s |
| | Diastasis | 0.30s |
| | Atrial systole | 0.10s |
| Systole 0.3 sec | | |
| | Isovolumetric contraction | 0.05s |
| | Rapid ejection | 0.20s |
| | Protodiastole | 0.05s |

### Why is the mid-phase of diastole called diastasis?

During diastasis, blood flows slowly and smoothly from the pulmonary veins, through the left atrium, into the ventricle. There is no turbulence anywhere along the path.

### Why are the initial parts of systole and diastole isovolumetric?

As the ventricle starts contracting, the intraventricular pressure rises. The rising pressure shuts close the mitral valve but the pressure is not enough to push open the semilunar valves. With both the outlets (mitral and aortic valves) momentarily closed, the pressure inside the ventricle rises steeply as the ventricle contracts.

### What is the dicrotic notch and what is its cause?

During isovolumetric relaxation, there is a sharp drop in ventricular pressure. Hence, blood in the aorta tries to rush back into the ventricle, only to collide against the closed aortic valve. The collision causes a small but sharp rise in aortic pressure. This sharp pressure rise is recordable even from peripheral arteries and is called the **dicrotic notch**.

### What are the timings of the first and second heart sounds in the cardiac cycle?

The **first heart sound (S1)** is a low, slightly prolonged 'lub' sound, caused by vibrations set up by the sudden *closure of the A-V valves* (mitral and tricuspid) at the onset of ventricular systole. It has a duration of about 0.15 s and a frequency of 25–45 Hz. It is soft when the heart rate is low, and loud when the heart rate is high.

The **second heart sound (S2)** is a shorter, louder high-pitched 'dup' sound, caused by vibrations associated with *closure of the semilunar valves* just at the onset of ventricular diastole. The second sound lasts about 0.12 s, with a frequency of 50 Hz. Like the S1, it is louder when the heart rate is high.

### Draw a labelled diagram to show the different phases of the cardiac cycle.

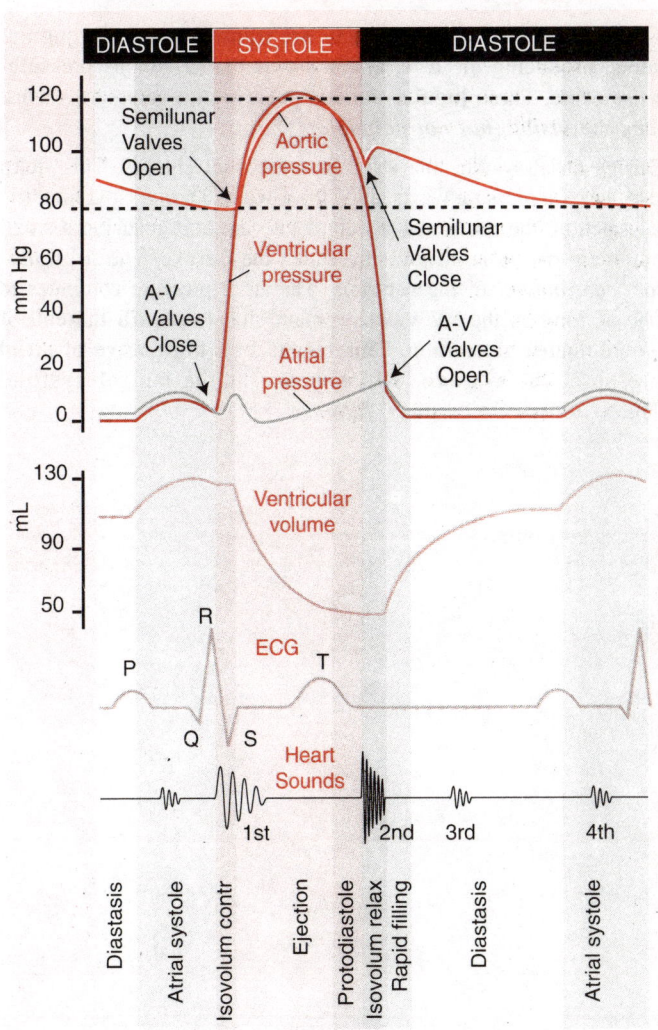

Fig. 41.1

### What is the timing of the third and fourth heart sounds in the cardiac cycle?

The third **heart sound (S3)** is a soft, low-pitched sound heard during the first-third of the diastole in many normal young individuals. It coincides with the period of *rapid ventricular filling* and is probably due to vibrations set up by the inrush of blood. It has a duration of 0.1 s.

The fourth **heart sound (S4)** can sometimes be heard immediately before the first sound when atrial pressure is high or the ventricle is stiff in conditions such as ventricular hypertrophy. It is *due to ventricular filling against resistance* and is rarely heard in normal adults.

### What is the timing of the ECG waves in relation to the cardiac cycle?

Atrial systole starts after the P wave of the ECG. Ventricular systole starts at the peak of the R wave and ends just after the T wave. The end of the T-wave coincides with the end of systole.

### What are the three jugular venous waves and when do they occur in the cardiac cycle?

The variations in atrial pressure are transmitted to the jugular veins, producing the **a**, **c**, and **v** waves of the venous pressure-pulse curve. These **jugular venous pulse** are low-pressure waves: they are *visible but not palpable*.

During atrial systole, the atrial pressure rises sharply. This sharp rise causes a pressure wave called the **a-wave**. During isovolumetric contraction, the mitral valve bulges into the atria, causing a small but sharp rise in atrial pressure called the **c-wave**. The *'c' stands for 'contraction'* of the ventricle. The atrial pressure continues to rise as long as the AV valves remain closed i.e., till the end of isovolumetric relaxation. This results in a third wave of atrial pressure, the **v-wave**, which peaks at the end of systole. The *'v' stands for 'venous' filling.*

### What happens to the duration of systole and diastole when the heart rate increases?

When the heart rate increases, the duration of all the phases decrease. However, the *duration of diastole decreases much more than the duration of the systole*. The decrease in diastole occurs due to greater automaticity of the sinus node. The decrease in systole is associated with a decrease in the duration of cardiac action potential caused by quicker repolarization.

The marked reduction in diastolic time with increase in heart rate has important clinical implications. It is during diastole that most of the ventricular filling occurs. Also, it is during diastole that most of the cardiac muscle, especially the subendocardial portions of the left ventricle gets adequately perfused by the coronary blood flow. Hence at heart rates greater than 150/min., there is a *reduction of both ventricular filling* (which tends to cause cardiac failure) *and cardiac perfusion* (which tends to cause myocardial ischemia and infarction).

| Duration | HR 75/min | HR 200/min |
| --- | --- | --- |
| Cardiac cycle | 0.8s | 0.30s |
| Systole | 0.3s | 0.15s |
| Diastole | 0.5s | 0.15s |

# 42

# Cardiac Output and its Regulation

## Enumerate the indices of cardiac pump function.

**End-diastolic volume**. It is the volume of the ventricle at the beginning of contraction. It is ~130 ml.

**End-systolic volume**. It is the volume to which the ventricle contracts by end of systole. It is about 50 ml.

**Stroke volume**. It is the amount of blood pumped out by each ventricle per stroke. It is about 80ml.

**Ejection fraction**. It is the percent of the end-diastolic ventricular volume that is ejected with each stroke. It is about 65%. The ejection fraction is a valuable index of ventricular function.

$$\text{Ejection fraction} = \frac{\text{Stroke volume}}{\text{End-diastolic ventricular volume}} \times 100$$

**Cardiac output**. It is the amount of blood pumped by the left ventricle per minute. The normal cardiac output is ~ 5 - 6 L / min. In health, the right and left ventricular outputs are nearly equal. Cardiac output is the product of stroke volume and heart rate.

$$\text{Cardiac output} = \text{Stroke volume} \times \text{Heart rate}$$

**Cardiac index**. It is the cardiac output expressed in relation to the body surface area. The normal cardiac index is about 3.2 L / min./m².

**Venous return**. It is the amount of blood entering the right atrium per minute. In health, cardiac performance is enhanced whenever venous return increases so that *cardiac output equals venous return*.

## What is Fick principle? Describe the method of cardiac output estimation using the Fick principle.

Fick principle states that the blood flow through an organ (F) can be obtained by dividing the amount of substance (Q) that is added or removed from the blood by the arteriovenous concentration difference ($C_A - C_V$) it produces (Fig. 42.1). This principle cannot be applied if the organ takes up the substance from sources other than the arterial blood.

$$F = \frac{Q}{(C_A - C_V)}$$

**Q** is the amount of $O_2$ diffusing from blood into the tissues per minute. It is equal to the amount of oxygen that diffuses into blood from the lungs every minute. This can be estimated from the volume difference of the inspired air and the expired air that is passed through soda lime to remove $CO_2$. $C_A$ ($O_2$ concentration in pulmonary arterial blood) can be estimated in an *arterial blood sample withdrawn from any convenient artery*. All arteries have roughly the same $pO_2$ as in pulmonary venous blood. $C_V$ (the $O_2$ concentration in mixed venous blood) is estimated in *venous*

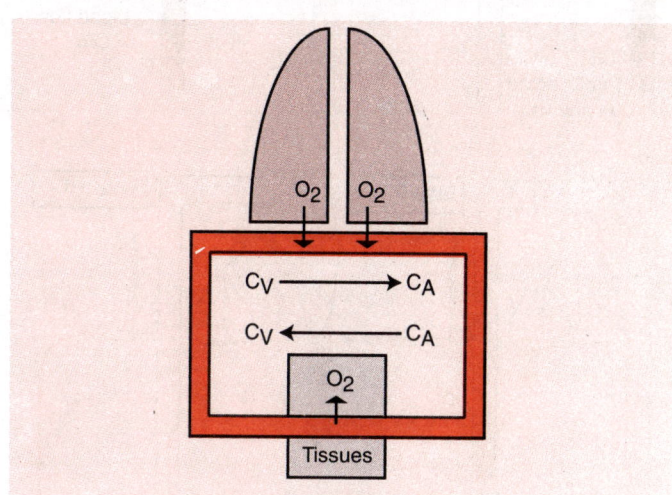

**Fig. 42.1**

*blood sample obtained directly from the pulmonary artery through catheterization.* This is necessary because almost every vein flowing towards the heart brings in blood with different levels of $O_2$ desaturation.

| Example | | |
|---|---|---|
| **Q** | = | 250 mL/min. |
| **$C_A$** | = | 195 mL/L. |
| **$C_V$** | = | 145 mL/L. |
| **CO** | = | 5 L/min. |

## Describe the method of cardiac output estimation using the dye-dilution technique.

A measured amount (A) of indicator dye is injected in any superficial vein in a bolus dose, and blood samples are withdrawn from an artery at regular intervals of a few seconds (Fig. 42.2). The indicator must be a substance that stays in the bloodstream during the test and has no harmful or hemodynamic effects. If the average concentration of the dye in blood is C, and the time taken by the column of dyed blood to flow across the sampling point is T, then

$$\text{Cardiac Output} = \frac{A}{C} \times \frac{60}{T}$$

A graph is plotted between the dye concentration on the Y-axis (in log scale) and time on the X-axis (in linear scale), i.e., on a semi-log paper. The dye-concentration curve is extrapolated to the X-axis. The area under the curve gives the value of C × T (Fig. 42.3).

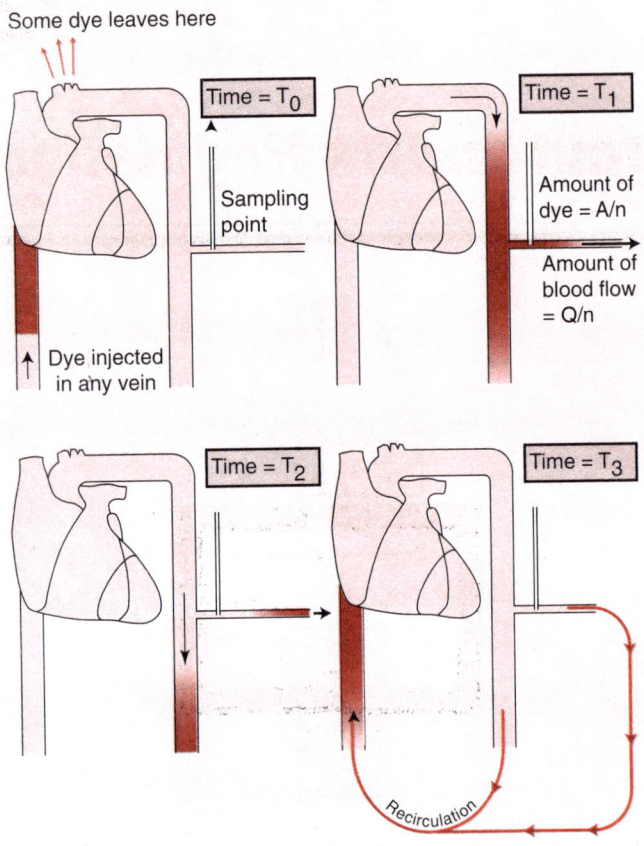

Some dye leaves here

Time = $T_0$

Sampling point

Time = $T_1$

Amount of dye = A/n

Amount of blood flow = Q/n

↑ Dye injected in any vein

Time = $T_2$

Time = $T_3$

Recirculation

**Fig. 42.2**

### Enumerate the various other methods of cardiac output estimation.

**Thermodilution technique.** In this, cold saline is used as an indicator and the temperature of blood is measured instead of the dye concentration. This technique has two important advantages: the saline is completely harmless, and the cold is dissipated in the tissues so that recirculation is not a problem.

**Doppler technique.** In experimental animals, cardiac output can

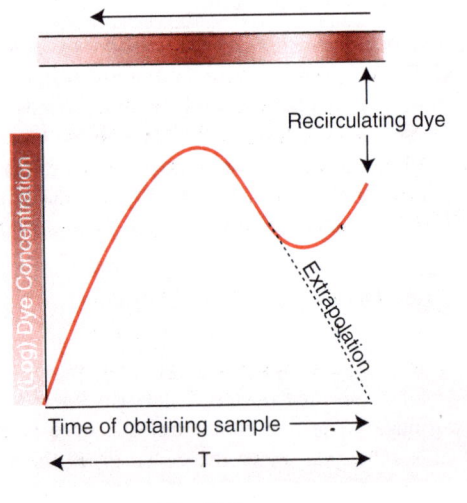

Recirculating dye

(Log) Dye Concentration

Extrapolation

Time of obtaining sample ⟶

⟵ T ⟶

**Fig. 42.3**

be measured with an electromagnetic flow meter placed on the ascending aorta.

**Cineradiographic technique.** It can be measured by injecting radiolabeled red blood cells, imaging the cardiac blood pool at the end of diastole and the end of systole (equilibrium radionucleotide angiocardiography), and then calculating the ejection fraction.

**Ballistocardiography.** The rapid ejection of a large amount of blood through the aorta is associated with a Newtonian reaction in the opposite direction. The reaction is equal in magnitude to the thrust with which blood is pumped through the aorta. This principle is employed to calculate the stroke volume.

### What is Starling's law of the heart?

Starling's law of the heart states that the force of cardiac contraction is proportional to its end diastolic volume (EDV). The law results from this length-tension relationship of striated muscles.

### Briefly describe how cardiac output is regulated to meet the requirements of the body.

Whenever the tissue $O_2$ demand increases, the cardiac output increases to meet the demand. The increase in cardiac output occurs through the following steps:

Increase tissue $O_2$ demand
↓
Tissue hypoxia
↓
Vasodilatation
↓
Increased venous return
↓
Increased diastolic filling
↓ *Starling law*
Increased cardiac output

### Explain why anemia is associated with increased cardiac output.

Anemia is associated with tissue hypoxia, leading to the sequence of events outlined above and culminating in increased cardiac output.

### What is the difference between homometric and heterometric regulation?

When the venous return to the heart increases, the heart can cope with it in two different ways. One is the **heterometric mechanism**, in which the cardiac muscle fibers are stretched to increase their initial length. *Increase in the initial length* increases the force of muscle contraction. This rule is true for all striped muscles: skeletal or cardiac. In the heart, this rule is manifested as the **Starling's law of the heart**. The other is the **homometric mechanism** in which the active tension in cardiac muscle fibers is increased without increasing the initial fiber length. This is possible, for example, by *sympathetic stimulation* of the heart.

### What is the role of sympathetic system in cardiac output regulation?

The role of sympathetic system is to ensure that the heart does not employ heterometric regulation, which in the long run is harmful to the heart. Specifically, sympathetic discharge causes an *increase in the stroke volume*, and even more striking *increase in the ejection fraction*. Sympathetic stimulation also causes an *increase in the heart rate*. Together with an *increased stroke volume*, it has the capability to *increase cardiac output* massively.

## What are the physiological factors controlling venous return?

The venous return to the heart can be considered in two phases: flow of blood from the arterial side to the venous side of circulation, and flow of blood from the veins to the heart. The *first phase* is primarily determined by the degree of vasodilatation in the tissues, which allow arterial blood to flow through to the veins. The *second phase* is determined by the following four factors:

**Muscle pump.** Exercising muscles squeeze the veins, squirting the blood inside in both directions. Since veins have valves, the blood is propelled only forwards. Even if the valves are incompetent, blood is propelled forwards because the larger veins near the heart offer less resistance to the blood flow than the smaller veins of the periphery.

**Respiratory pump.** Respiratory movements of the diaphragm decrease the intrathoracic pressure and increase the intra-abdominal pressure rhythmically. These pressures propel the blood in the intra-abdominal veins upwards into the thorax.

**Sympathetic venoconstriction.** Sympathetic discharge constricts the large veins, reducing their capacitance. As a result, blood tends to squirt towards the great veins.

*Vis-a-fronte.* The vigorously relaxing heart exerts a suction force or 'a pull from the front' *(vis-a-fronte)* on the blood in the great veins. The muscle and respiratory pumps and sympathetic venoconstriction constitute the *vis-a-tergo* or the 'push from behind'.

## What are the other factors affecting venous return?

The flow of blood from the arterial to venous side increases abnormally if there are **arteriovenous shunts** – i.e., channels that allow blood to flow from arteries to veins bypassing the capillaries. Such channels are seen in *Paget's disease* and in *beriberi*. The flow of blood from veins to the heart slows down in case of varicose veins.

## How is central venous pressure assessed?

Central venous pressure (CVP) can be measured directly by inserting a catheter into the thoracic great veins. A peripheral vein that is at the level of the right atrium also gives a fair indication of the CVP. The peripheral venous pressure in the antecubital vein is ~ 7 mm Hg, which is about 4 mm Hg greater than the normal CVP.

Clinicians assess the CVP by examining the **jugular venous pulse**. All veins above the level of the heart are in a collapsed state since the blood pressure inside them is less than zero (i.e., the atmospheric pressure). The jugular vein rises straight up from the right atrium and acts as a manometer for the CVP. When the CVP is more than zero, blood is pushed up some distance into the collapsed jugular vein, which then gets distended. A prominent pulse (the jugular venous pulse) is visible at the upper limit of the blood column in the jugular vein. The vertical height of the distended segment of the jugular vein gives the **jugular venous pressure** (JVP). *CVP, and therefore JVP is elevated in cardiac failure.*

# 43

# Factors affecting Cardiac Output

### Enumerate the factors resulting in a hypereffective heart

Factors resulting in a **hypereffective heart** are *sympathetic stimulation* of the heart, and *inotropic drugs, i.e.,* drugs that increases cardiac contractility, e.g., digitalis.

### Enumerate the factors resulting in a hypoeffective heart.

Factors resulting in a **hypoeffective heart** are: (i) Decrease in pump power, as occurs in *reduced sympathetic discharge,* or *myocardial damage* from any cause – ischemia or inflammation. (ii) Inefficient pumping, as in *valvular or septal defects* of the heart. (iii) Reduced pump filling, as in *pericardial effusion* or *cardiac tamponade* (filling of the pericardial space with blood). Both these conditions restricts diastolic enlargement of the heart. (iv) Increased load on the pump, as in *hypertension.*

### What are the factors affecting peripheral resistance?

Peripheral resistance is mainly controlled by the *sympathetic tone* of blood vessels. Additionally, peripheral resistance decreases in *arteriovenous (A-V) shunts* and *fistulae; thyrotoxicosis,* due to the increased $O_2$ demands of the tissues; and in *wet beriberi,* due to reduced tissue utilization of nutrients which results in compensatory vasodilatation.

### What is meant by the mean circulatory filling pressure? How much is it?

Mean circulatory pressure is the *mean pressure in the vascular system after the circulation is stopped completely.* It is the pressure at which blood is filled into blood vessels and is the same in all parts of the vascular system: arteries, veins, and capillaries. *Normally, it is 11 mm Hg.*

### How does sympathetic discharge affect cardiac output?

Sympathetic discharge increases the cardiac output by making the heart hypereffective. It also increases the mean systemic filling pressure. This too increases the cardiac output. However, it causes vasoconstriction, increasing the peripheral resistance. This tends to decrease the cardiac output.

### What are the factors causing cardiac failure?

Cardiac failure occurs *when cardiac performance falls too low* to cope with the normal venous return (*see* factors causing a hypoeffective heart). It also occurs *when venous return increases beyond the limits of cardiac performance.* The rise in venous return can occur due to increase in filling pressure or a decrease in peripheral resistance.

### What are the salient clinical features of cardiac failure?

The clinical features of cardiac failure are as follows : (i) **Cardiomegaly**, i.e. cardiac enlargement. It occurs as the heart resorts to heterometric mechanism (increased diastolic filling) for maintaining the cardiac output. (ii) **Prolonged circulation time** due to ineffective cardiac pumping. (iii) **Raised** jugular venous pressure due to accumulation of blood behind a hypoeffective heart. (iv) **Pulmonary congestion**. It occurs due to a rise in pulmonary capillary venous pressure, which may result in transudation of fluids in the alveoli causing pulmonary edema. (v) **Hepatomegaly**. Hepatic enlargement occurs as the increased central venous pressure is transmitted backwards into the hepatic portal vein. (vi) **Edema**. It occurs as the raised central venous pressure is transmitted all the way backwards to the systemic capillaries. It is prominent in the dependent portions of the body where the capillary pressures are normally much higher due to hydrostatic effect. (vii) **Dyspnea on exertion** is a prominent symptom. It occurs because during exertion, the left ventricular output fails to rise adequately, leading to an increase in pulmonary venous pressure.

### What is high output cardiac failure?

Cardiac failure can occur if the cardiac output is high but inadequate for providing adequate tissue perfusion (**high-output cardiac failure**). It is seen in *thyrotoxicosis, large A-V fistulae* and *wet beriberi.*

### What is the difference between compensated and decompensated cardiac failure?

**Compensated cardiac failure**, A reduction of cardiac output decreases the blood pressure and the venous return, inhibiting the baroreceptors and volume receptors respectively. These bring about reflex sympathetic discharge, restoring the cardiac output. The result is a **compensated cardiac failure**, which occurs only at a higher central venous pressure. The higher central venous pressure represents an accumulation of blood behind the pumping heart (**backward failure**). However, because of the compensation, the forward failure subsides.

A major contributor to the pathogenesis of cardiac failure is the retention of salt and water in the body by the kidneys with consequent increase in blood volume. The kidneys retain fluid and $Na^+$ ions when the *renal blood flow (RBF) decreases* and/or when there is *increased discharge of renal sympathetic nerves.* The mechanism of renal fluid and water retention involves renin, angiotensin and aldosterone.

If the cardiac function is severely impaired, sympathetic discharge fails to restore cardiac output. This starts off a vicious cycle in which the sympathetic discharge keeps increasing in an effort to restore cardiac output but fails. Rather, *the sympathetic discharge leads to an increase in blood volume through renal mechanisms, which imposes a greater load on the heart.* The retention of large amounts of fluid and electrolytes causes edema of the myocardium, further impairing myocardial function. This is known as **decompensated cardiac failure**.

### What is the difference between forward and backward cardiac failure?

Cardiac failure begins with a reduction in the cardiac output. This is called **forward failure**. Compensation, when it occurs, is possible only at a higher central venous pressure, which also reduces the venous return and results in systemic or pulmonary edema. This is known as **backward failure**.

### What is the difference between cardiogenic shock and forward cardiac failure?

A forward cardiac failure is associated with a reduction in cardiac output that may or may not be severe enough to precipitate a cardiogenic shock.

### What is the treatment of cardiac failure?

The aim of treatment is two-fold: improving cardiac contractility by giving **digitalis**, and reducing the load on the heart. By giving **diuretics** and **ACE inhibitors** (inhibitors of angiotensinogen converting enzyme). Both reduce the blood volume. ACE inhibitors additionally reduce the peripheral resistance, reducing the load on the heart further.

### How is cardiac output graphically analyzed?

The graphic analysis of cardiac output was developed by Arthur Guyton. It consists of two curves: the cardiac function curve and the venous return curve, both drawn as a function of the right atrial pressure (Fig. 43.1). The intersection of the two curves gives the cardiac output (on the y-axis) and the right atrial pressure (on the x-axis). The cardiac function curve is different for a hypoeffective heart and a hypereffective heart. Similarly, venous

return decreases when the mean systemic filling pressure is low and increases when the mean systemic filling pressure is high. Venous return increases when the peripheral resistance is low and decreases when peripheral resistance is high. The effect of these factors on cardiac output and right atrial pressure can be readout easily from the graph.

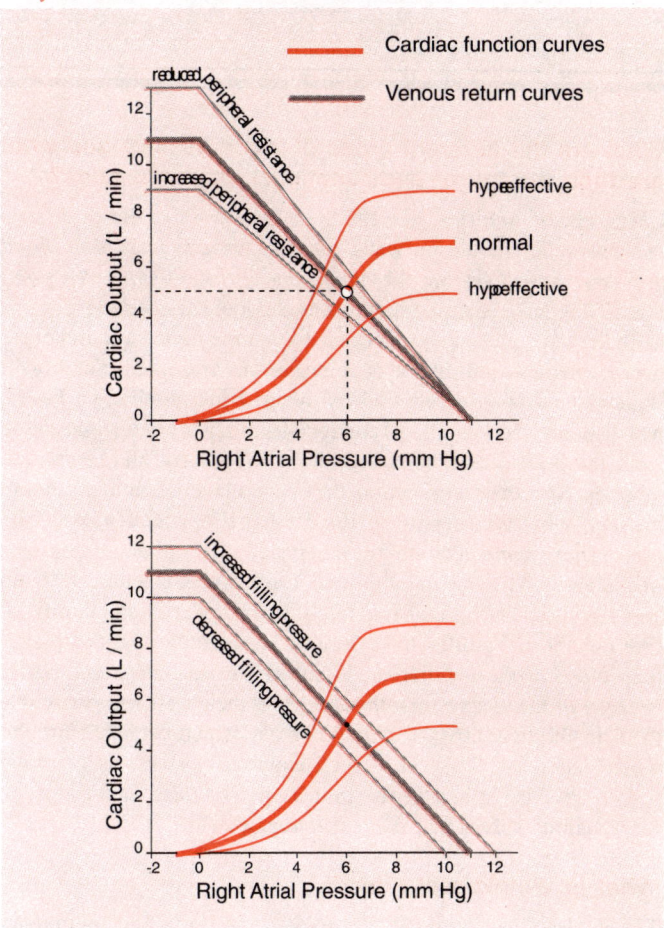

**Fig. 43.1**

# 44

# Circulatory System. Structure Function & Hemodynamics

## What are the different types of blood vessels and what are their structural and functional characteristics?

**Large elastic arteries**, like the aorta have a lot of elastic tissues in their wall. The elastic walls *prevent abrupt changes in blood pressure*. **Arterioles** are the *major site of the resistance to blood flow*. They have mainly smooth muscles (and less elastic tissues) in their wall, and are innervated by sympathetic noradrenergic nerve fibers which constrict them. Some arterioles, notably in skeletal muscles are supplied by sympathetic cholinergic fibers, which dilate the vessels. **Metarterioles** branch off at right angle from the arterioles. Their walls have irregularly placed smooth muscles. Near their termination, they have a layer of circular smooth muscle which constitutes the precapillary sphincter. The *precapillary sphincters* are not innervated. They dilate or constrict in response to local metabolites. **Capillaries** branch off from metarterioles. They are of two types: true capillaries and thorough-fare channels. **Venules** have walls that are only slightly thicker than those of the capillaries. **Veins** are *easily distensible*, partly because of the sparse smooth muscles in their wall and partly due to their elliptical cross-sectional contour which becomes circular when distended. They are called **capacitance vessels** or blood reservoirs. The intima of the limb veins is folded at intervals to form **venous valves** that prevent retrograde flow.

## What is Windkessel effect?

The walls of large elastic ateries like the aorta and pulmonary trunk are stretched during systole, preventing sudden rise in blood pressure. During diastole, they recoil back, preventing sudden drop in blood pressure. This is known as the Windkessel effect.

## What is the difference between true capillaries and capillary thoroughfare channels?

The **true capillaries** form an anastomotic network before reuniting and draining into a venule. Their origin is guarded by the precapillary sphincter. The **capillary thoroughfare vessels** are present in vascular beds of skeletal muscles. They directly *connect the metarteriole with the venule, bypassing the precapillary sphincter.*

## What are arteriovenous shunts and where are they found?

**Arteriovenous shunts** are short channels that *connect arterioles to venules, bypassing the capillaries*. They are present in the *fingers, palms, and ear lobes*. The arteriovenous (A-V) shunts have thick, muscular walls and are abundantly innervated by vasoconstrictor nerve fibers.

## Which vessel has the largest total cross-sectional area?

Capillaries have the highest total cross-sectional area of ~ $4500cm^2$ followed by veins with an area of ~$4000cm^2$.

## Which vessel offers the maximum resistance?

Arteries (total cross-sectional area ~ $20cm^2$) offer the maximum resistance. However, in the presence of sympathetic discharge, **arterioles** (which normally have a total cross-sectional area of ~$400cm^2$) constrict and offer the maximum resistance. Although the aorta has the least cross-sectional area ($4cm^2$), it offers less resistance than the arteries because of its elasticity and its short length.

## Which type of vessel has the largest capacitance?

Veins have the largest capacitance.

## Describe a simple way of estimating the circulation time.

Clinically, the velocity of the circulation can be measured by *injecting a bile salt preparation into an arm vein* and timing the first *appearance of the bitter taste* it produces. The average normal arm-to-tongue **circulation time** is 15 seconds.

## What is the normal central venous pressure?

In the right atrium, the pressure (**central venous pressure**) is ~ 4 mm Hg. The pressure in the venules is ~15 mm Hg. This produces a pressure gradient of 11mm Hg which propels the venous blood towards the heart (the **venous return**).

## What is venous pooling?

Peripheral venous pressure, like arterial pressure, is affected by gravity. It increases by 0.77 mm Hg for each cm below the right atrium and decreases by the same amount for each cm above the right atrium the pressure. Thus, *during standing, venous pressure at the ankle is ~90 mm Hg*. If the venous valves are incompetent, as in varicose veins, it results in **venous pooling**, i.e., accumulation of blood in the lower parts of the body.

## Why are dural sinuses prone to air-embolism?

Venous pressure about 5 mm above the heart is zero. Hence, veins in the head and neck are in a collapsed state. The pressure is less than zero i.e. subatmospheric (about -10 mm Hg) in the dural sinuses which *have rigid walls* and therefore cannot collapse. If a dural sinus is opened during a neurosurgical procedure with the patient seated, air is sucked into the sinus, resulting in **air embolism.**

## What are the consequences of air embolism and why?

The efficient circulation of fluid is possible because fluid is incompressible. Had it been compressible, the cardiac pumping would have caused the blood to get reduced in volume instead of flowing. Gases, however, are highly compressible. When air gains access into circulation (air embolism), it has serious consequences. Large amounts of air fill the heart and effectively stop the circulation, causing sudden death. Small amounts of air flow as bubbles inside blood. In the heart and large vessels, they do not cause any problems, but the bubbles lodge in the small blood vessels, where they stop the flow, causing ischemia.

### How is the Ohm's law relevant to hemodynamics?

The relationship between the mean flow of blood, its mean pressure, and the resistance offered by blood vessels is similar to the relationship between the current, electromotive force, and resistance in an electrical circuit expressed in Ohm's law:

Voltage = Current × Resistance
Pressure = Flow Rate × Resistance

$$\text{Flow in a vascular bed} = \frac{\text{Effective perfusion pressure}}{\text{Resistance of the vascular bed}}$$

The unit of fluid resistance is dyne-s/cm⁵. A simpler alternative is to express fluid resistance in **R unit.** 1 R unit is the resistance which will cause a flow of 1 mL/s when the pressure is 1 mm Hg. Thus, if the mean blood pressure is 100 mm Hg and the cardiac output is 6 L/min (100 mL/s) the total peripheral resistance is

$$\frac{100 \text{ mm Hg}}{100 \text{ ml/s}} = 1 \text{ R unit}$$

### How is the Bernoulli's principle relevant to hemodynamics?

When a constant amount (Q) of fluid flows through a tube, the total fluid energy, i.e., – the sum of its kinetic energy, pressure energy, and potential energy – is constant. This is known as **Bernoulli's principle.** The Bernoulli's principle *explains why arteriolar vasoconstriction causes a rise in arterial blood pressure.* The vasoconstriction reduces the velocity of blood flow, and therefore, there is a rise in blood pressure. Bernoulli's consideration is an important consideration during direct blood pressure measurement. It *explains why end pressure is greater than lateral pressure.*

Bernoulli's principle also has a relevance in pathophysiology. When a vessel is narrowed, the velocity of flow in the narrowed portion increases and the distending pressure decreases. Therefore, when a vessel is narrowed by a pathologic process such as an arteriosclerotic plaque, the *lateral pressure at the constriction is decreased and the narrowing tends to maintain itself.*

### What is the Poiseuille-Hagen formula? How is it relevant to hemodynamics?

The relation between the flow in a long narrow tube, the viscosity of the fluid, and the radius of the tube is given by the **Poiseuille-Hagen formula:**

$$F = (P_A - P_B) \times \frac{\pi}{8} \times \frac{1}{\eta} \times \frac{R^4}{L}$$

Since resistance inversely with the fourth power of the radius,

small changes in arteriolar diameter causes large variations in blood flow through them, enabling effective regulation of blood flow through vascular beds.

The role of viscosity and length is best brought out by the differences in the blood flow in the renal cortex and the renal medulla which are supplied by vasa recta: 90% of the renal blood flow goes to the renal cortex, 9% goes to the outer medulla and 1 % goes to the inner medulla. The factors responsible for the low inner medullary blood flow are: (a) The long length of the vasa recta (vascular resistance is proportional to the length of the vessel). (b) The high viscosity of blood in the inner medulla (due to the loss of large amounts of water into the hyperosmolar interstitium). (c) The low capillary hydrostatic pressure in the vasa recta (because the efferent arterioles of the juxtamedullary nephrons have smaller diameter).

### What is the critical closing pressure?

In blood vessels, a minimum pressure is required to keep the blood flowing. If the pressure falls below this **critical closing pressure**, the vessel collapses, its lumen closes and the flow stops. This minimum pressure is required to force the slightly oversized red cells through the capillaries and also to overcome the pressure of the adjacent tissues that compress upon the blood vessels.

### Why is the viscosity of blood said to be anomalous?

A **Newtonian fluid** is one in which the viscosity is independent of the shear rate. The *viscosity of blood decreases with an increase of shear rate.* This is specially marked at low shear rates. This anomalous viscosity of blood is attributable to axial streaming of blood cells at high shear rates. **Axial streaming** means that the cells occupy the central axis of the tube through which blood is flowing. This *leaves a 5mm wide cell-free zone immediately adjacent to the vessel wall.* This cell free zone produces lesser friction with the vessel wall and therefore, the viscosity is lower.

### What is the Fåhreus-Lindqvist effect and what is its relevance to hemodynamics?

Fåhreus-Lindqvist effect refers to the *fall in blood viscosity with a decrease in tube diameter.* This also is attributable to axial streaming of cells. Since the cell-free zone has a constant width of about 5mm, expressed as a percentage of the tube diameter, is much greater for smaller tubes. This results in a lower viscosity. The effect explains why blood viscosity is lower in capillaries.

### What is plasma skimming?

Because of the cell-free zone in the periphery of flowing blood, a vessel that branches off from the main blood vessel at a large angle carries way more plasma than cells. This phenomenon is called **plasma skimming**. It explains why the *hematocrit of capillary blood is about 25% lower than the whole-body hematocrit.*

### What is the effect of hematocrit on blood viscosity?

In large vessels, increases in hematocrit cause appreciable increases in viscosity. However, in vessels smaller than 100mm in diameter, i.e., in arterioles, capillaries, and venules, the viscosity is much less affected by hematocrit. This is why hematocrit changes have relatively little effect on the peripheral resistance except when the changes are large. The reason is related to the Fåhreus-Lindqvist effect.

### What is the significance of the Reynolds Number? How do you calculate it?

The probability of turbulence is also related to the diameter of the vessel and the viscosity of the blood. This probability can be expressed as:

$$Re = \frac{\rho DV}{\eta}$$

where Re is the **Reynolds number**, $\rho$ is the density of the fluid; D is the diameter of the tube (in cm); V is the velocity of the flow (in cm/s) and $\eta$ is the viscosity of the fluid (in poise). The higher the value of Re, the greater the probability of turbulence.

When Re < 2000, flow is usually not turbulent whereas if Re > 3000, turbulence is almost always present. Constriction of an artery increases the velocity of blood flow through the constriction, producing turbulence, and consequently sound, beyond the constriction. Examples are **bruits** heard over arteries constricted by atherosclerotic plaques and the **Korotkoff sounds** heard when measuring blood pressure.

In humans, the critical velocity is usually exceeded only when an artery is constricted. Turbulence occurs more frequently in anemia because the viscosity of the blood is lower. This is why **systolic murmurs** that are common in anemia.

### What is the law of Laplace and what is its relevance in Physiology?

The **law of Laplace** states that tension in the wall of a cylinder (T) is equal to the product of the transmural pressure (P) and the radius (R).

$$P = \frac{2T}{R}$$

(1) The Laplace law helps explain how the *thin-walled capillaries are able to withstand a pressure as high as 25 mm Hg* (which is the normal capillary hydrostatic pressure). This is possible because capillaries have a very small radius (R). Even though the wall tension is low, the small value of (R) in the denominator makes a very high (P) possible. (2) The law of Laplace *puts the dilated hearts at a disadvantage*. When the radius (R) increases, the wall tension (T) must go up proportionately if the pressure (P) is to be maintained. (3) In accordance with Laplace law, *lower the functional residual capacity of the lungs, the more difficult it is to inflate it*. (4) Because of Laplace law, *greater the gastric filling, slower is the pressure that causes gastric emptying*. This is obviously beneficial to the process of digestion. (5) Laplace law explains why *reduction in detrusor muscle tension prevents rise of intravesicular pressure* even as the baldder fills up to greater volume.

### Compare and contrast windkessel vessels and resistance vessels.

**SIMILARITIES**

Both belong to the arterial system

**DIFFERENCES**

| Windkessel vessels | Resistance vessels |
|---|---|
| These have lot of elastic tissues in their wall. | These have mainly smooth muscles and less elastic tissues in their wall. |
| Prevent abrupt changes in blood pressure. | These are the major sites of resistance to blood flow, and are the main contributors to blood pressure |
| Examples are large arteries like the aorta. | Examples are the arterioles. |

# 45

# Measurement of Blood Flow & Pressure

## What are the different methods of blood flow measurement?

**Electromagnetic flow meters**. These depend on the principle that a voltage is generated in a conductor moving through a magnetic field and that the magnitude of the voltage is proportionate to the speed of movement. Since blood is a conductor, a magnet is placed around the vessel, and the voltage, which is proportionate to the volume flow, is measured with an appropriately placed electrode on the surface of the vessel. **Doppler flow meters**. Ultrasonic waves are sent into a vessel diagonally from one crystal, and the waves reflected from the red and white blood cells are picked up by a second, downstream crystal. The frequency of the reflected waves is higher by an amount that is proportionate to the rate of flow toward the second crystal because of the Doppler effect. **Plethysmography**. The forearm is sealed in a watertight chamber (plethysmograph). The changes in the volume of the forearm reflect the changes in the amount of blood and interstitial fluid in the forearm. When the venous drainage of the forearm is occluded, the rate of increase in the volume of the forearm is a function of the arterial blood flow (venous occlusion plethysmography). **Fick principle** and **indicator dilution**. Indirect methods like the Fick and indicator dilution techniques can be used for regional blood flow measurements. The Kety N$_2$O method for measuring cerebral blood flow and the estimation of renal blood flow by measuring the clearance of paraaminohippuric acid are based on the Fick principle.

## Give examples of direct manometry in clinical practice.

Direct blood pressure measurement is performed clinically for **central venous pressure monitoring** during circulatory shock, and for **pulmonary wedge pressure measurement** in pulmonary hypertension.

## What is the difference between lateral pressure and end pressure?

When an artery is tied off beyond the point at which the cannula is inserted, the pressure recorded is called the **end pressure**. Flow in the artery is interrupted, and all the kinetic energy of flow is converted into pressure energy. If alternatively, a T tube is inserted into a vessel and the pressure is measured in the side arm of the tube, the pressure recorded is called the **lateral pressure**. The *lateral pressure is lower than the end pressure* in accordance with *Bernoulli's principle*.

## What are Traube-Hering waves?

**Traube-Hering waves** are oscillations in blood pressure recordable in anesthetized cats and dogs rendered apneic by paralyzing the respiratory muscles. The *oscillations are synchronous with the respiratory waves*.

## What are Mayer waves?

Mayer waves are slow regular oscillations in arterial pressure that occur at the rate of about one per 20-40 seconds *during hypotension*. These occurs due to oscillations in the feedback correction of blood pressure through chemoreceptor reflex.

## Briefly describe the different methods of indirect manometry.

There are three methods of performing indirect measurement of **sphygmomanometry**: palpatory, auscultatory and the oscillometric methods.

**Palpatory method**. An inflatable cuff attached to a mercury manometer (**sphygmomanometer**) is wrapped around the arm. The lower border of the cuff should be at least 2.5 cm above the cubital fossa. The radial pulse is palpated and the cuff (**Riva-Rocci cuff**) is rapidly inflated until the radial pulse disappears. The cuff pressure is then slowly lowered till the radial pulse reappears. The cuff pressure at which the pulse reappears is taken to be the systolic blood pressure. The measurement obtained is 2-4 mm lower than that measured by the auscultatory method, which is considered to be more accurate. *The diastolic pressure cannot be measured by this method.*

**Auscultatory method**. In this method, the cuff pressure is raised higher than the systolic pressure (as estimated by the palpatory method). The pressure in the cuff is then lowered slowly. At the point at which systolic pressure in the brachial artery just exceeds the cuff pressure, blood spurts through with each heartbeat and produces the characteristic **Korotkov sounds**. This is the point of **systolic blood pressure**. As the cuff pressure is lowered further, the quality of the Korotkov sounds change. Based on the quality of sounds, *four phases of Korotkov sounds* have been described. Finally, when the cuff pressure falls to the level of diastolic pressure, the blood flow in the brachial artery becomes entirely free from turbulence and the Korotkov sounds disappear. This marks the **diastolic blood pressure**. The disappearance of the Korotkov sounds is called the *fifth phase*.

In the **oscillometric method**, the mercury column is observed. As the mercury column falls to touch the systolic pressure, it starts showing small oscillations. The oscillations become largest at the mean blood pressure and abruptly disappear at the diastolic pressure. Visual oscillometric method is rarely used. However, it is commonly employed in electronic devices and gives quite accurate results.

### What should be the level of the manometer during sphygmo-manometry?

The sphygmomanometer should be placed at the *level of the eye* to avoid parallax error while reading out the mercury level. *There is no need to place the manometer at the heart level.*

### In the auscultatory method, which point should be taken as the diastolic pressure?

The beginning of phase-4 is 7-10 mm Hg above the diastolic pressure recorded directly by an intra-arterial needle, whereas the *fifth phase corresponds more accurately to true diastolic pressure.* In individual patients, however, the fourth phase may be detected with greater precision than the fifth phase. Moreover, if however the sounds remain audible till the pressure is lowered to zero (as in aortic regurgitation), the muffling has to be taken as the diastolic pressure. When recording the diastolic pressure, both phases should be noted and recorded (e.g., 120/82/74) if they have been clearly heard. When one of them is not clearly discernable, to avoid confusion, the blood pressure should be recorded as 120/82/__ or 120/__/74.

### What is the auscultatory gap?

During sphygmomanometry, as the cuff pressure is lowered after raising it above the systolic pressure, the Phase-1 Korotkov sounds sometimes disappear briefly and reappear at a lower level. This is called the **auscultatory gap**. This gap is *a potential source of error* in sphygmomanometry. If the cuff pressure is raised to a pressure within the auscultatory gap and then lowered for measuring the blood pressure, a false-low systolic pressure would be recorded. This is prevented by palpating the radial pulse while inflating the blood pressure cuff. The cuff pressure must be raised till the pulse disappears.

### What are the sources of errors in sphygmomanometry?

(1) The manometer should be placed *vertically and at the level of the eye*. If the manometer is not vertical, the result recorded is false high. If it is placed below the eye level, the result read out is false high due to parallax error. (2) The *cuff should be at the level of the heart*. If the arm is raised above the level of the heart, the result recorded will be false low. (3) Cuff-width should be correct. The *standard cuff width for adults is 12.5 cm*. If narrower cuff width is used, the results recorded are false high. In obese patients, wider cuffs should be used. Standard cuffs would give false high reading in obese patients. (4) The *cuff pressure should be raised above the systolic*. Hence, the blood pressure should always be first measured by the palpatory method followed by the auscultatory method. This prevents the errors associated with the auscultatory gap. (5) The *blood pressure should be recorded quickly* since the procedure itself tends to raise the blood pressure due to occlusion of the brachial artery. For the same reason, the *cuff pressure should be lowered to zero between successive readings*. (6) In nervous patients, the first reading may be high due to the rise in blood pressure associated with nervousness. In such patients, *the second reading is lower and should be considered correct.*

# 46

# Capillary Exchange Lymphatic Circulation & Edema

## What are the three types of capillaries?

Capillaries are of three types: continuous, fenestrated and discontinuous. In **continuous capillaries**, the endothelial cells are continuous except at the intercellular junctions where they leave a gap of about 10nm. These intercellular spaces are traversed by channels that are about 4 nm wide. **Fenestrated capillaries** are found *in renal glomeruli* and *vasa recta, in glands* – both exocrine and endocrine, in *choroid plexuses* and in *intestinal villi*. The fenestrations serve as large openings (60 – 70 nm) that permit massive filtration of fluids and the passage of large molecules. **Discontinuous capillaries** are present in *sinusoids* of the bone marrow, liver, and spleen. In these, there are large gaps between individual cells that permit not only the passage of macromolecules but also of erythrocytes.

## What is meant by active and inactive capillaries?

In resting tissues, most of the capillaries are collapsed (**inactive capillaries**) and blood bypasses them to flow through the thoroughfare vessels connecting the metarterioles to the venules. In active tissues, the precapillary sphincters dilate and blood starts flowing through the capillaries (**active capillaries**). The opening and closing of the **precapillary sphincters** is controlled by *local metabolic vasodilators*.

## What are the three different ways in which capillary transport occurs?

The three different ways of capillary transport are filtration of fluids with **bulk flow** of solutes, **diffusion** of solutes, and **pinocytosis**.

## What are Starling forces? What are the different Starling forces that affect capillary exchange?

Filtration and reabsorption of fluid across the capillary membrane is determined by the balance of the following pressures which are called the **Starling forces**.

| | | | |
|---|---|---|---|
| Capillary hydrostatic pressure at arteriolar end | $P_a$ | = 40 mm Hg | pushes fluid out |
| Capillary hydrostatic pressure at venous end | $P_v$ | = 10 mm Hg | pushes fluid out |
| Interstitial hydrostatic pressure | $P_i$ | = 2 mm Hg | pushes fluid in |
| Plasma oncotic pressure at arteriolar end | $\pi_a$ | = 25 mm Hg | pulls fluid in |
| Plasma oncotic pressure at venous end | $\pi_v$ | = 25 mm Hg | pulls fluid in |
| Interstitial oncotic pressure | $\pi_i$ | = 3 mm Hg | pulls fluid out |

The terms 'in' and 'out' are in reference to the capillary lumen. Thus, interstitial hydrostatic pressure pushes fluid into the capillaries while interstitial oncotic pressure pulls out water from the capillaries. From the above figures, the net forces acting on the fluid at the arteriolar and venous end can be calculated separately as follows:

| Arteriolar end | | | Venous end | |
|---|---|---|---|---|
| $P_a$=40 | $p_a$=25 | plasma | $P_v$=10 | $p_v$=25 |
| $P_i$=2 | $p_i$=3 | interstitial fluid | $P_v$=2 | $p_i$=3 |

| arteriolar end | | venous end | |
|---|---|---|---|
| outward forces: | 43 mm Hg | outward forces: | 13 mm Hg |
| inward forces: | 27 mm Hg | inward forces: | 27 mm Hg |
| *net outward forces: 16 mm Hg* | | *net inward forces: 14 mm Hg* | |

It is seen that fluid is filtered out of the capillaries under a filtration pressure of 16 mm Hg while at the venous end, fluid is reabsorbed under a reabsorptive pressure of 14 mm Hg. Thus, there is a *net filtration pressure of 2 mm Hg.*

If the average capillary hydrostatic pressure is taken as $P_C$ and the average plasma osmotic pressure is represented by $\pi_C$, the equation for the net filtration force can then be written as:

$$F = (P_{Cap} + \pi_I) - (P_I + \pi_{Cap})$$

## How does sympathetic discharge affect capillary exchange?

Sympathetic discharge constricts the precapillary sphincter and thereby *favors movement of fluid from the interstitium into the capillary*.

## How do local vasodilators affect capillary exchange?

Local vasodilators dilate the precapillary sphincters and thereby increases the *filtration of fluids from the capillary into the interstitium*.

## What is the difference between paracellular and transcellular transport?

In **paracellular transport**, solutes pass through the junctions between endothelial cells and through fenestrations, when they are present. In **transcellular transport**, solutes pass through the cells by vesicular transport or, in the case of lipid-soluble substances, through the cytoplasm.

## What is the difference between exudate and transudate?

The fluid which enters the interstitial fluid from the capillaries of most organs does not have appreciable amounts of proteins in them. This fluid is called a **transudate**. However, if the permeability of the capillaries increases markedly, as happens during inflammation from any cause, large amounts of proteins diffuse out from the capillaries. This protein rich fluid that comes out of the capillary under conditions of inflammation is called **exudate**.

### How does lymph circulate? How much is the normal lymph flow in 24 hours?

The extra fluid filtered from the capillaries enters the lymphatics as **lymph**. The lymph flows through a system of lymphatic vessels and finally drains into the **thoracic duct** which opens into the junction of the left subclavian and internal jugular veins. Thus *all the lymph is eventually returned to blood*. The normal 24 hour lymph flow is 2-4 L.

### What is the composition of lymph?

The composition of lymph is *similar to plasma* except that its *protein content is usually lower than that of plasma*. The reason is the low permeability of the capillary walls to proteins.

The composition of lymph varies with the region it drains. The *lymph from liver has the highest protein content* (about 6.0g / 100mL) and lymph from the intestine has about 2.0g/100mL of proteins. In the intestine, fats are absorbed into the lymphatics, and the *lymph in the thoracic duct after a meal is milky* because of its high fat content.

### What are agents that increase lymph flow called?

Agents that increase lymph flow are called **lymphagogues.** They include a variety of agents that increase capillary permeability. Agents that cause contraction of smooth muscle also increase lymph flow from the intestines.

### Define edema. How is it different from ascites?

The term **edema** refers to a large increase in **interstitial fluid volume**. **Ascites** is a large increase in the amount of **peritoneal fluid**, which is transcellular and not interstitial fluid.

### Enumerate the factors causing edema.

The causes of edema are as follows: (i) **Increased venous pressure.** An increase in venous pressure is transmitted back to the capillaries, resulting in elevated capillary hydrostatic pressure. Conditions in which venous pressure is elevated include: (a) the *standing posture*, especially for long hours causes ankle edema; (b) *cardiac failure* is also associated with ankle edema; (c) *incompetent venous valves* predisposes to edema in dependent parts on standing; (d) *venous obstruction;* (e) *increased blood volume*. (2) **Decreased plasma protein concentration.** It is one of the common causes of edema. It is seen in: (a) *liver diseases*, because hepatic protein synthesis is depressed; (b) *renal disorders* like the nephrotic syndrome, in which glomerular membrane permeability increases markedly; (c) *malnutrition* and *starvation*; (d) *protein-losing enteropathy*, in which proteins are lost into the intestines. (3) **Anaphylaxis.** In anaphylaxis, there is release of substance P, histamine, kinins, etc. that cause large increase in capillary permeability, leading to *exudation* of large amount of plasma and causing edema. (4) **Inadequate lymph flow.** Edema caused by lymphatic obstruction is called *lymphedema* and is characterized by a high protein content of the edema fluid. Common causes of lymphedema are: (a) *Radical mastectomy*, an operation for cancer of the breast in which removal of the axillary lymph nodes on one side reduces lymph drainage and results in edema of the ipsilateral arm; (b) *Filariasis*, in which filaria migrate into the lymphatics and obstruct them. Over a period of time, massive edema results, usually of the legs or scrotum (elephantiasis).

# 47

# Chemical Control of Cardiovascular System

## How is nitric oxide produced?

Nitric oxide (NO) is produced in endothelial cells by endothelial from L-arginine, which is actively taken up from plasma by facilitated diffusion. The enzyme converting L-arginine to NO is **nitric oxide synthetase** (NOS). NOS is present in three isoforms in three types of tissues: **NOS I** in *nervous tissues*, **NOS II** in *macrophages* and **NOS III** in *endothelium*.

## What is its mechanism of action?

NO activates the guanylate cyclase in vascular smooth muscle and thereby *increases the cGMP concentration*. cGMP acts as a second messenger and *decreases intracellular $Ca^{2+}$ concentrations*, thereby relaxing smooth muscle and inhibiting platelet aggregation.

## How is NO inactivated?

NO has a very short half-life (3-5s). It is inactivated into nitrite ($NO_2^-$) and nitrate ($NO_3^-$) that are excreted in urine. The *plasma and urine concentrations of $NO_3^-$ and cGMP are useful indicators for NO production rates.*

## What are the functions of NO in the body?

(1) NO relaxes vascular smooth muscle cells. NO is released from the endothelium in response to *pulsatile stretch* and *flow-induced shear stress*. When flow to a tissue is suddenly increased by arteriolar dilation, the *large arteries* to the tissue also dilate. This **flow-induced dilation** is due to local release of NO (Fig. 47.1).

Moreover, any luminal narrowing of arterial vessels increases the local blood flow velocity, which stimulates NO release and results in **post-stenotic vasodilatation** (Fig. 47.2). Flow-induced vasodilatation also occurs during physical exercise. Exercise-induced NO formation may explain the *beneficial effects of endurance training on the cardiovascular system.*

(2) NO release is brought about by both vasoconstrictor and vasodilator substances. The vasoconstrictors that act directly on vascular smooth muscle would produce much greater constriction if they did not simultaneously cause the release of NO. Conversely, the vasodilators that have direct actions on vascular smooth muscle produce greater vasodilatation by triggering the simultaneous release of NO. Many of these substances are released during platelet aggregation and blood coagulation. Hence, *aggregating platelets cause vasodilatation if the endothelium is healthy and vasoconstriction if the arteries are atherosclerotic.*

(3) There is a balance in blood between endothelium-derived vasoconstrictors like endothelins and vasodilators like NO. Hence,

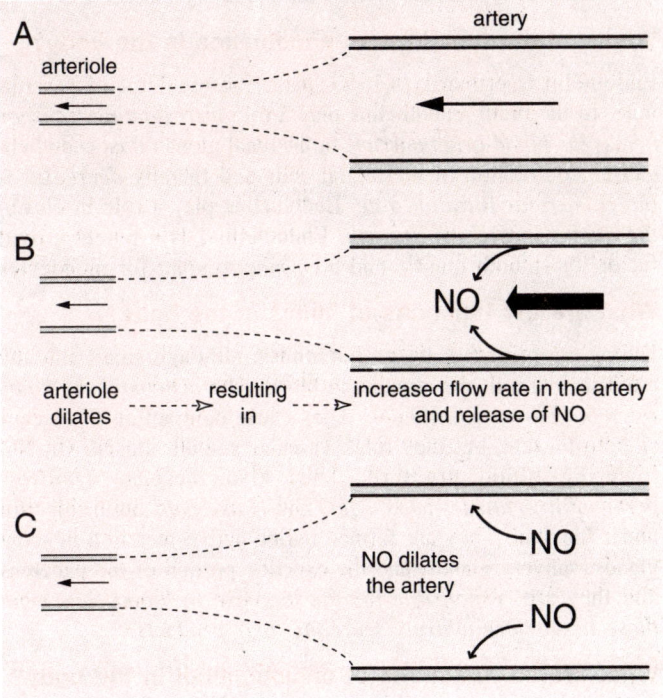

**Fig. 47.1**

a constant release of NO is necessary to *maintain normal blood pressure* and *NO deficiency can cause clinical hypertension.* The drug **nitroglycerin**, which is of great value in the treatment of angina exerts its vasodilator effects by being converted to NO. (4) Penile erection is produced by release of NO, with consequent vasodilatation and engorgement of the corpora cavernosa. The

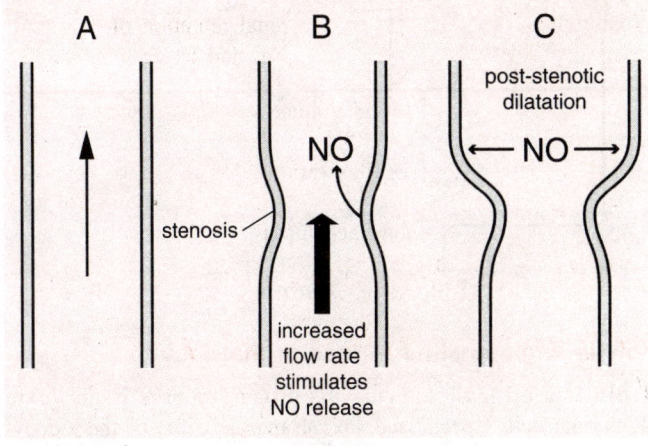

**Fig. 47.2**

drug **Viagra**® (Sildenafil), a selective inhibitor of cGMP-specific phosphodiesterase, acts by *inhibiting the inactivation of* NO. (5) NO *inhibits platelet adhesion and aggregation*. This effect, together with its vasodilator effect, is extremely important for the maintenance of the normal flow of blood. (6) NO decreases LDL oxidation and inhibits superoxide anion production by inhibiting NADPH reductase activity. These actions are related to the strong **anti-atherosclerotic effect** exerted by NO. (7) NO is a mediator of the **inflammatory response**. It is necessary for the cytotoxic activity of macrophages, including their ability to kill cancer cells. Production of NO is elevated in inflammatory diseases.

### What are the functions of endothelins in the body?

Endothelin is primarily a local, paracrine regulator of vascular tone. In the brain, endothelins play a role in *regulating transport across the blood-brain barrier*. In the renal glomerulus, endothelin causes contraction of mesangial cells and thereby *decreases in the glomerular filtration rate*. Endothelins play a role in *closing the ductus arteriosus at birth*. Endothelin-1 is a potent growth factor for smooth muscle and a *chemoattractant* for monocytes.

### What are the functions of kinins in the body?

Kinins are primarily **tissue hormones**, although small amounts are also found in the circulating blood. The *actions of the kinins resemble those of histamine*. They cause contraction of visceral smooth muscle, but they relax vascular smooth muscle via NO, lowering blood pressure. They also *increase capillary permeability, attract leukocytes,* and *cause pain* upon injection under the skin. They are formed during active secretion in sweat glands, salivary glands, and the exocrine portion of the pancreas, and they are *responsible for the increase in blood flow when these tissues are actively secreting their products*.

### What are the functions of angiotensin-II in the body?

Angiotensin II is an extremely potent **vasoconstrictor**. Angiotensin II also *increases water intake* and *stimulates aldosterone secretion*.

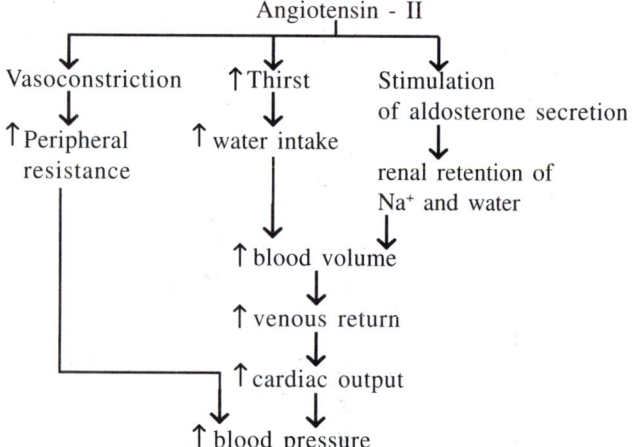

### How is angiotensin-II formed in the body?

**Renin** is a protease enzyme. Its primary source is the juxta-glomerular cells (specialized smooth muscle cells) of the kidneys. It is released in response to *sympathetic discharge to the kidneys*

or in response to circulating catecholamines. It catalyzes the formation of **angiotensin-I**, which is further converted to **angiotensin-II** by **angiotensin converting enzyme** (ACE) found on the surface of *capillary endothelium in the lungs and kidneys*.

$$\text{Angiotensinogen} \xrightarrow{\text{\textit{Renin}}} \text{Angiotensin-I}$$

$$\text{Angiotensin-I} \xrightarrow{\text{\textit{ACE}}} \text{Angiotensin-II}$$

### Compare and contrast the cardiovascular effects of epinephrine and norepinephrine.

**Epinephrine** stimulates both α and β receptors. The α-induced vasoconstriction is more than nullified by the β-induced vasodilatation. Hence, the peripheral resistance and diastolic BP remain unchanged or fall slightly. The β-induced increase in stroke volume and heart rate results in higher cardiac output, a rise in systolic blood pressure and a widening of pulse pressure.

**Norepinephrine** has much greater effect on α than on β receptors. Hence, it produces vasoconstriction with a rise in peripheral resistance and diastolic blood pressure. Due to weak β-activation, direct cardiac stimulation are insignificant. Rather, there is reflex cardio-inhibition due to the rise in diastolic blood pressure.

### Why do the effects of sympathetic discharge on CVS differ from those of catecholamines?

Sympathetic discharge results in the release of norepinephrine from the nerve endings. The norepinephrine released acts only on those structures that are innervated by sympathetic fibers. On the other hand, catecholamines released from the adrenal glands is mostly adrenaline, which acts on all vital tissues.

### What are the effects of acetylcholine on the cardio-vascular system?

Acetylcholine has *negative inotropic, chronotropic, bathmotropic* and *dromotropic* effects on the heart. It also *relaxes vascular smooth muscles*.

### Why do the effects of vagal discharge on CVS differ from those of acetylcholine?

The vagus *does not innervate the blood vessels* and its *innervation of the ventricular myocardium is sparse*. Hence, the cardiovascular effects of the vagus is restricted almost entirely to the atrial muscles, S-A node and A-V node.

### What effect does dopamine have on the cardiovascular system?

The physiologic function of the dopamine in the circulation is unknown. However, its pharmacological effects make it an important drug in the treatment of circulatory shock because (a) it produces *renal vasodilatation* (preventing renal shutdown), acting through dopaminergic receptors, (b) it produces *vasoconstriction elsewhere* (preventing hypotension), probably by stimulating the release of norepinephrine, and (c) it has a positively inotropic effect on the heart by an action on $\beta_1$-adrenergic receptors.

# 48

# Neural Control of Cardiovascular System

### Describe the cardiovascular sympathetic innervation and its functions.

The *sympathetic nerve cells supplying the heart* are located in the intermediolateral horn of T1 – T5 spinal segments. All parts of the heart (SA node, atria, AV node and ventricles) receive sympathetic innervation. The sympathetic innervation on the right side is distributed primarily to the SA node. The sympathetic innervation on the left side primarily to the AV node.

Sympathetic discharge has five effects on the heart: **positive inotropic**: increase in the force of cardiac contraction, **positive chronotropic**: increase the cardiac rate, **positive bathmotropic**: increase in automaticity, **positive dromotropic**: increase in conduction velocity, and **inhibition of parasympathetic effect**, mediated by neuropeptide-Y.

*Sympathetic fibers innervating blood vessels* originate from the intermediolateral horns in T1 – L2 spinal segments. They innervate blood vessels of all calibre except the capillaries and venules which do not have smooth muscles in their wall. Arterioles and resistance vessels are most densely innervated. Most sympathetic fibres produce vasoconstriction and have norepinephrine and sometimes neuropeptide Y as their neurotransmitter. Sympathetic vasoconstrictor fibres show tonic (i.e. continuous) discharge. Hence, sympathectomy produces widespread vasodilatation.

Some sympathetic fibres produce vasodilatation when activated and constitute what is called the **sympathetic vasodilator system**. They supply the resistance vessels of the skeletal muscles and have acetylcholine and VIP as their neurotransmitters.

### Describe the parasympathetic innervation of the cardiovascular system and its functions.

*Parasympathetic fibres to the heart* originate from **nucleus ambiguous**. They reach the heart through the **vagus nerve** and relay in ganglia located within the cardiac muscle. The right vagus is distributed mainly to the SA node; the left vagus mainly to the AV node. *Blood vessels do not have any parasympathetic innervation.*

Parasympathetic discharge to the heart has a **negative chronotropic effect**. It does not have negative inotropic effect, because it does not innervate the contracting myocardial cells in sufficient numbers. When both noradrenergic and cholinergic systems are blocked, the heart rate is approximately 100/min. Since the resting heart rate is ~72/min., it indicates that at rest, the *vagal tone is greater than the sympathetic tone*.

### Describe the receptors and afferents involved in cardiovascular regulation.

The receptors involved in cardiovascular regulation are the mecha-noreceptors and the chemoreceptors. The mechanoreceptors may be baroreceptors or volume receptors.

**Baroreceptors** are the extensively branched and coiled ends of myelinated nerve fibers. They are located in the adventitia of certain arteries at specialized locations like the carotid sinus (**carotid baroreceptors**) and aortic arch (**aortic baroreceptors**). The **carotid sinus** is a small dilation of the internal carotid artery located just above its origin. It is supplied by the **sinus nerve** which is a branch of the **glossopharyngeal nerve**. They terminate in the **nucleus of tractus solitarius (NTS)** in the medulla where they release *glutamate* as the neurotransmitter. The **aortic sinus** is located at the transverse part of arch, adjacent to the root of left subclavian artery. It is supplied by the left aortic (mainly) and right aortic nerves which join the superior laryngeal branch of the vagus. *The sinus nerves (from the carotid sinus) and vagal fibers (from the aortic arch) are together commonly called the* **buffer nerves**.

**Volume receptors** are stretch receptors located in *low-pressure areas of circulation*, e.g., in the walls of the right and left atria (at the entrance of the superior and inferior venae cavae and the pulmonary veins), as well as in the pulmonary circulation. Collectively, they are called **cardiopulmonary receptors**. Structurally, they are identical to baroreceptors: it is their location in low-pressure areas that make them detect blood volume rather than blood pressure.

**Chemoreceptors** are located in the carotid and aortic bodies. They detect the $P_{O_2}$, $P_{CO_2}$ and pH of blood. Their location may be **central** (within the central nervous system) or **peripheral** (attached to the peripheral nervous system). They bring about reflex changes in the rate and depth of breathing. The carotid bodies are located near the carotid bifurcation on each side. The aortic bodies, two or more in number, are located near the arch of the aorta (Fig. 65.2). Afferents neurons innervating the carotid bodies are thinly myelinated Aδ fibers. They ascend to the medulla via the carotid sinus and glossopharyngeal nerves, and fibers from the aortic bodies ascend in the vagi.

### Describe the brainstem centers involved in cardio-vascular regulation.

The brain centers involved in cardiovascular regulation are the medullary sympathetic center (**vasomotor center**), the medullary parasympathetic center (**cardioinhibitory center**) and the medullary relay station for cardiorespiratory afferents.

The **spinal sympathetic center** is located in the **intermediolateral horn** of the spinal cord (T1 – L2). It has two parts: the **pressor area**, containing the intermediolateral (**IML**) cells from which the sympathetic fibers actually originate, and the **depressor area** located a little medially containing the intermediomedial (**IMM**) cells that inhibit the pressor area.

The **medullary sympathetic center** is better known as the **vasomotor center**. It controls the output of the spinal sympathetic center. It has two parts: the **pressor area** located in the rostral ventrolateral medulla (RVLM) which increases the spinal sympathetic output, and the **depressor area**, located in the caudal ventrolateral medulla (CVLM) which reduces the spinal sympathetic output. The **medullary parasympathetic center** gives rise to the vagal parasympathetic fibers to the heart. It was earlier called the **cardioinhibitory center**, and now called by its specific name **nucleus ambiguus**.

The **medullary relay station** for all cardiorespiratory afferents is the **nucleus of tractus solitarius (NTS)**. All peripheral afferents – baroreceptors and chemoreceptors – end here. The afferents release the excitatory neurotransmitter glutamate. Cells of the NTS in turn relays the information to other centers that control parasympathetic and sympathetic output.

### Describe the higher centers for cardiovascular control.

The **hypothalamic autonomic center** controls the lower sympathetic and parasympathetic centers. It has two parts: the **pressor area**, also called the **defense area** which increases the sympathetic output and reduce the parasympathetic output, and the **depressor area** which decreases the sympathetic output and increases the parasympathetic output.

The **subthalamic movement centre** initiates sympathetic discharge simultaneously with the onset of motor activities. It is probably important for the augmented sympathetic discharge that occurs during exercise.

### Describe the baroreceptor reflex arc.

At normal blood pressure levels, the fibers of the buffer nerves (afferents from carotid and aortic sinuses) discharge at a low rate. When the pressure inside the sinus or aortic arch rises, the discharge rate increases. The discharge rate reaches a plateau at 150 mm Hg. When the pressure falls, the rate declines and becomes zero when the blood pressure decreases to 30 mm Hg. The carotid receptors respond both to the mean pressure and the pulse pressure.

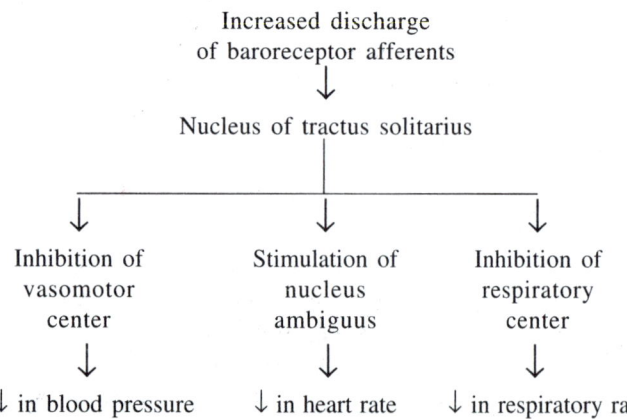

The impulses reach the NTS from where they bring about an inhibition of the vasomotor center and stimulation of the nucleus ambiguus. Hence, *when there is increases in baroreceptor afferent discharge, there is sympathetic stimulation with parasympathetic inhibition,* resulting in decrease in blood pressure and heart rate. There is also a weak inhibition of respiration. The effects on blood pressure are exaggerated by vagotomy which abolishes similar 'buffering effects' of the aortic and cardiopulmonary mechanoreceptors.

### Describe the chemoreceptor reflex arc.

Stimulation of the chemoreceptors afferents results in the activation of the vasomotor center pressor area and inhibition the nucleus ambiguus. Thus, chemoreceptor stimulation causes a rise in blood pressure and heart rate. Chemoreceptor afferents also stimulate the medullary respiratory neurons. The stimulated respiratory neurons inhibit (i.e., gate) the nucleus ambiguus, contributing thereby to the rise in heart rate.

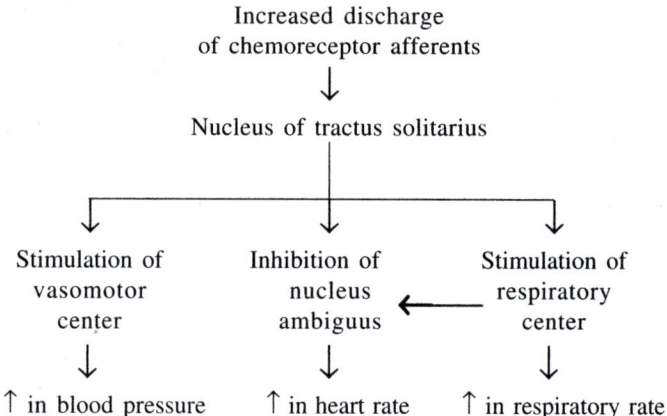

### What are the experimental ways in which the baroreceptor and chemoreceptor reflexes are studied?

The baroreceptor reflex can be stimulated by *clamping of the carotid arteries distal to the carotid sinus.* The chemoreceptor reflex can be stimulated by *perfusing the carotid with perfusate containing 5% oxygen.* Clamping the carotid sinus proximal to the carotid sinus stimulates the carotid chemoreceptors and inhibits the carotid baroreceptors.

### What is Bainbridge reflex?

Bainbridge reflex refers to the tachycardia brought about by the distension of the right atrium. The reflex serves to prevent accumulation of blood in the right atrium when the venous return increases. The Bainbridge reflex however may not be a true reflex. The tachycardia could be due to the direct effect of stretching of the sinoatrial node.

# 49

# Blood Pressure Regulation & Hypertension

## What is the normal blood pressure?

The blood pressure in the brachial artery in young adults in the sitting or lying position at rest is approximately 120/80 mm Hg. It is appreciably lower at night and is lower in women than in men. When the systolic pressure is lower than 130 mm Hg and a diastolic pressure lower than 85 mm Hg, the blood pressure is considered normal. In healthy humans, both the systolic and the diastolic pressures rise with age. A convenient empirical formula as to what should be considered as normal blood pressure at various age is given below.

Systolic blood pressure $= 110 + 3/5$ Age

Diastolic blood pressure $= 70 + 2/5$ Age

## What are the two main determinants of arterial blood pressure?

Arterial blood pressure is the product of the cardiac output and the peripheral resistance.

Arterial BP = Cardiac output × Peripheral resistance

Blood pressure is therefore affected by conditions that affect either or both of these factors. A rise in stroke volume increases the systolic pressure more than the diastolic pressure. A rise in peripheral resistance increases the diastolic pressure more than the systolic pressure. Systolic pressure rise is also related to the distensibility of the arteries. For the same cardiac output, systolic blood pressure is higher if the arterial distensibility is low, as in aged people with atherosclerosed arteries.

## Define pulse pressure and mean blood pressure.

**Pulse pressure** is the difference between the systolic and diastolic pressures. It is normally about 40 mm Hg.

The **mean pressure** is the average pressure throughout the cardiac cycle. Because systole is shorter than diastole, the mean pressure is slightly less than the simple average of the systolic and diastolic pressures.

Mean blood pressure = Diastolic blood pressure × 1/3 Pulse Pressure

For example, if the systolic blood pressure is 120 mm Hg and diastolic blood pressure is 90 mm Hg, the mean blood pressure is 100 mm Hg (and not 105 mm Hg).

## What determines tissue perfusion: systolic, diastolic, pulse or mean blood pressure?

It is the mean blood pressure that determines tissue perfusion.

## Describe briefly the short, intermediate and long-term mechanisms of blood pressure regulation.

The various mechanisms that maintain a near-constant blood pressure in the body can be categorized into **short-term** mechanisms (baroreceptor reflexes), **intermediate-term** mechanisms (stress-relaxation and capillary fluid shift mechanism) and **long-term** mechanisms (pressure diuresis/natriuresis and renin-angiotensin mechanism).

**Baroreceptor reflex** prevents *erratic fluctuations in blood pressures*. Whenever the blood pressure changes rapidly, the baroreceptor reflex quickly brings about a negative feedback, correcting the initial change in blood pressure. In the absence of the reflex, the blood pressure would fluctuate wildly during postural changes, emotional changes or the Valsalva maneuver associated with defecation and coughing.

The *baroreceptor reflex however fails if the change in pressure is slow and sustained*. This is because of **baroreceptor resetting**, wherein the baroreceptor adjusts itself to a different 'resting' blood pressure. The reset baroreceptor reflex then tries to maintain blood pressure at the new resting blood pressure. Because of baroreceptor resetting, this reflex is *useless for the long-term regulation* of blood pressure.

The **capillary fluid shift mechanism** regulates blood pressure by *filtering out more fluid into the interstitial spaces* when the blood pressure rises. Conversely, when the blood pressure falls, interstitial fluid moves into the capillaries and opposes the fall in blood pressure.

The **stress-relaxation mechanism** is based on the *plasticity of vascular smooth muscles*. When there is a sustained increase in arterial blood pressure, the *arterial and arteriolar smooth muscles*

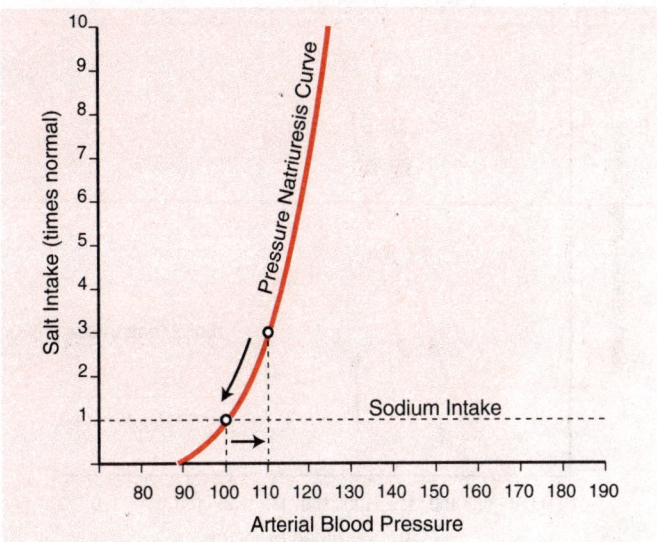

**Fig. 49.1**

*yield to the sustained distending pressure*, leading to a dilatation of these vessels. This leads to an increase in the capacity of the arterial system with a concomitant fall in blood pressure.

**Pressure diuresis and natriuresis** together constitute the most effective mechanism of long term regulation of blood pressure. *Whenever blood pressure increases, there is increased output of salt and water in urine.* The consequent reduction in body fluid and electrolytes restores the blood pressure to normal.

The **renin-angiotensin** mechanism is activated by sympathetic discharge. When blood pressure falls, it results in reflex increase in sympathetic discharge. The sympathetic discharge to the kidneys causes renin-degranulation. Renin catalyzes the formation of angiotensin I which is further converted into angiotensin II by angiotensin-converting enzyme (ACE). Angiotensin II is a powerful vasoconstrictor and therefore helps to restore blood pressure by *increasing the peripheral resistance*. Angiotensin II also brings about an *increase in blood volume*. It thus increases the cardiac output which helps in restoring the blood pressure. The increase in blood volume is brought about in two ways. Angiotensin is a *powerful stimulator of thirst*. It leads to consumption of large volumes of water, leading to a rise in blood volume. Angiotensin also *stimulates the secretion of aldosterone* from the renal medulla. Aldosterone leads to fluid and water retention through renal mechanisms.

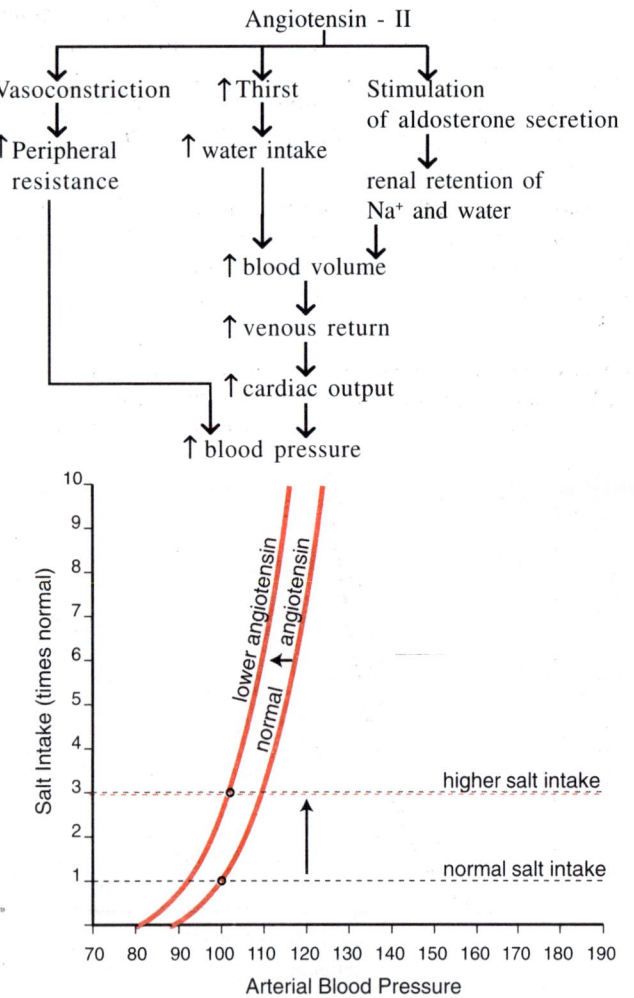

Fig. 49.2

### What is Goldblatt hypertension?

Goldblatt hypertension is a form of experimental hypertension. In this, sustained hypertension is achieved by ablating one kidney and clamping the artery of the other kidney. Hypertension is produced due to impairment of pressure diuresis and natriuresis and is called **one-clip one-kidney Goldblatt hypertension**. A variation of this experiment is in which the renal artery of one kidney is clamped while sparing the second kidney is spared. This is the **one-clip two-kidney Goldblatt hypertension** in which, in addition to the impairment of pressure diuresis and natriuresis, high levels of angiotensin-II contributes to the cause of hypertension.

### How is hypertension graded?

| Classification of Blood Pressure* | | |
|---|---|---|
| **Category** | **Systolic (mm Hg)** | **Diastolic (mm Hg)** |
| Normal | < 130 | < 85 |
| High Normal | 130 – 139 | 85 – 95 |
| Mild Hypertension | 140 – 159 | 90 – 99 |
| Moderate Hypertension | 160 – 179 | 100 – 109 |
| Severe Hypertension | 180 – 209 | 110 – 119 |
| Very Severe Hypertension | ≥ 210 | ≥ 120 |

\* *When systolic diastolic BP are in different categories, the higher category is selected.*

### What are the common causes of hypertension ?

The various causes of hypertension include: (1) **Preeclampsia** and **eclampsia**. The hypertension may be caused by a pressor polypeptide secreted by the placenta. (2) **Hyperaldosteronism** and **Cushing's Syndrome** produces hypertension due to salt and water retention. (3) **Pheochromocytomas**. These are catecholamine-secreting tumors of adrenal medulla. (4) **Renal hypertension** is due to narrowing of the renal arteries. (5) **Coarctation of the aorta**, a congenital narrowing of a segment of the thoracic aorta, increases the resistance to flow, producing severe hypertension in the upper part of the body. The blood pressure in the lower part of the body is usually normal but may be elevated due to increased renin secretion. (6) **Pill hypertension**. Oral contraceptives containing estrogens produces significant hypertension when consumed over prolonged periods. The hypertension is due to an increase in circulating levels of angiotensinogen, the production of which is stimulated by estrogens. (7) **Essential hypertension**. This constitutes the largest group (90%) in which the cause is unknown. It is probably due to **autonomic hyperreactivity** so that there are exaggerated hypertensive responses to stimuli such as cold and excitement. The frequent spasms of the arterioles lead to hypertrophy of their musculature so that at later stages, the hypertension becomes sustained.

### Enumerate the detrimental effects of hypertension.

Hypertension has harmful effects on the heart, nervous system and the kidney. *Cardiac effects.* Hypertension imposes a sustained high afterload on the left ventricle, leading to **left ventricular hypertrophy**. Ultimately, left ventricular function deteriorates, leading to left ventricular failure. There is also **myocardial ischemia** due to increased myocardial $O_2$ demand without a commensurate increase in coronary blood flow. Myocardial $O_2$ demand rises as the high afterload requires development of greater intraventricular pressure and myocardial tension. Most deaths of hypertension are due to myocardial infarction or cardiac failure. *Neurologic effects.* Hypertension is commonly associated with occipital headache, particularly in the morning. Hypertension is associated with characteristic **retinal changes** – narrowing of arterioles, retinal hemorrhages, exudates and papilledema. The high blood pressure also tends to cause **cerebral hemorrhage**. There may be **cerebral infarction** due to the increased incidence of atherosclerosis that is seen in hypertensive patients. *Renal effects.* About 10% of deaths in hypertension occur from **renal failure**. The atherosclerosis associated with hypertension affects the afferent and efferent renal arterioles and thereby decreases glomerular filtration and impairs tubular functions.

### Briefly outline the treatment of hypertension.

Antihypertensive drugs include:(1) **α-adrenergic receptor blocking drugs** that act either in the periphery or in the central nervous system; (2) **β-adrenergic receptor blockers**; (3) **ACE inhibitors** (drugs that inhibit the activity of angiotensin-converting enzyme); and; (4) **calcium channel blockers** that relax vascular smooth muscle; (5) Some patients show marked increase in blood pressure when fed a high-sodium diet, whereas do not. Since there is no easy test to distinguish salt-responsive from salt-resistant humans, **salt-restriction** is advised to all patients of hypertension.

# 50

# Circulatory Shock

### Define circulatory shock.

Shock is a state in which there is widespread, **serious reduction of tissue perfusion**, which if prolonged, leads to general impairment of cellular function. *Shock is triggered by hypotension.* However, hypotension does not always result in shock. Conversely, *shock can get triggered in the absence of hypotension.* This can happen in a hypertensive patient whose blood pressure suddenly drops to normal.

### What is non-progressive (compensated) shock?

Also called the **compensated stage**, the blood pressure in this stage is essentially normal. The cardiac output too is normal or is slightly reduced. The blood pressure is maintained at a normal level by a high rate of **sympathetic discharge**. The *high pulse rate reflects the augmented sympathetic discharge.*

### What are the compensatory reflexes activated in non-progressive shock ?

The compensatory increase in sympathetic discharge is brought about by three reflexes: (1) **Baroreceptor reflex**. Even a slight lowering of the mean blood pressure inhibits the afferent baroreceptor discharge. This in turn disinhibits the vasomotor center. *The utility of the baroreflex ends when the baroreceptors get completely inhibited*, and therefore no further disinhibition of the vasomotor center is possible. This occurs *at ~ 70 mm Hg* of blood pressure. **Chemoreceptor reflex**. This reflex is *activated when the mean blood pressure drops below 70mm Hg.* Stimulation of chemoreceptors occur due to severe stagnant hypoxia and anemic hypoxia (in hemorrhagic shock). **CNS ischemic response**. This reflex is *activated when the mean blood pressure drops to below 55 mm Hg.* It is stimulated by ischemia of CNS tissue and brings about a last bout of the most intense sympathetic discharge.

Sympathetic discharge increases cardiac contractility and peripheral resistance. Also, it increases the blood volume by numerous mechanisms including fluid shift into capillaries, renal conservation of water and increased thirst (see flow chart).

### How much hemorrhage can the body withstand before going into progressive shock?

Approximately *10% of the total blood volume can be removed with no significant effect* on either arterial pressure or cardiac output. Greater blood loss usually diminishes the cardiac output first and later the pressure, both of these falling to zero when about 35 to 45% of the total blood volume has been removed.

### Which is better compensated in shock and why: the blood pressure or the cardiac output?

As shock progresses, the *cardiac output deteriorates more than the blood pressure*. The reason why the blood pressure is better maintained than the cardiac output is that sympathetic discharge, which is the main compensatory mechanism, increases both cardiac output and peripheral resistance. Since blood pressure is the product of both, it increases markedly. On the other hand, the increase in cardiac output is partly thwarted by the increase in peripheral resistance.

### How does shock affect coronary and cerebral blood flow?

Sympathetic stimulation does not cause significant constriction of either the cerebral or the cardiac vessels. In addition, both these vascular beds have excellent local autoregulation which prevents any moderate fall in arterial pressure from significantly affecting their blood flows. Therefore, *blood flow through the heart and brain is maintained essentially at normal levels as long as the arterial pressure does not fall below about 70 mm Hg*, despite the fact that blood flow in many other areas of the body might be decreased to as little as one-quarter normal by this time due to vasoconstriction.

### What are the factors that make shock progressive?

In the progressive stage, there is **hypotension** indicating that *even the maximum compensatory responses are inadequate.* Moreover, the blood pressure falls continuously, which indicates that a **vicious cycle** has started. Somewhere along this vicious cycle is a **point of no return**. Therapeutic interventions before this point can restore normalcy. However, beyond this point, all interventions are ineffective and the shock is called **irreversible**. The vicious cycle occurs due to the following reasons.

**Cardiac Depression.** When the arterial pressure falls low enough, *coronary blood flow decreases below that required for adequate nutrition of the myocardium* itself. This weakens the heart and thereby decreases the cardiac output still more. Thus, a positive feedback cycle develops whereby the shock becomes more and more severe.

**Vasomotor Failure.** In the late stages, the diminished blood flow to the vasomotor center depresses the center itself so that it becomes progressively less active and sympathetic discharge decreases.

**Thrombosis and sludging.** The sluggish blood flow during shock leads to **thrombosis** in the microvessels. The cells stick to each other makes it more difficult for blood to flow through the microvasculature (**sludging of blood**).

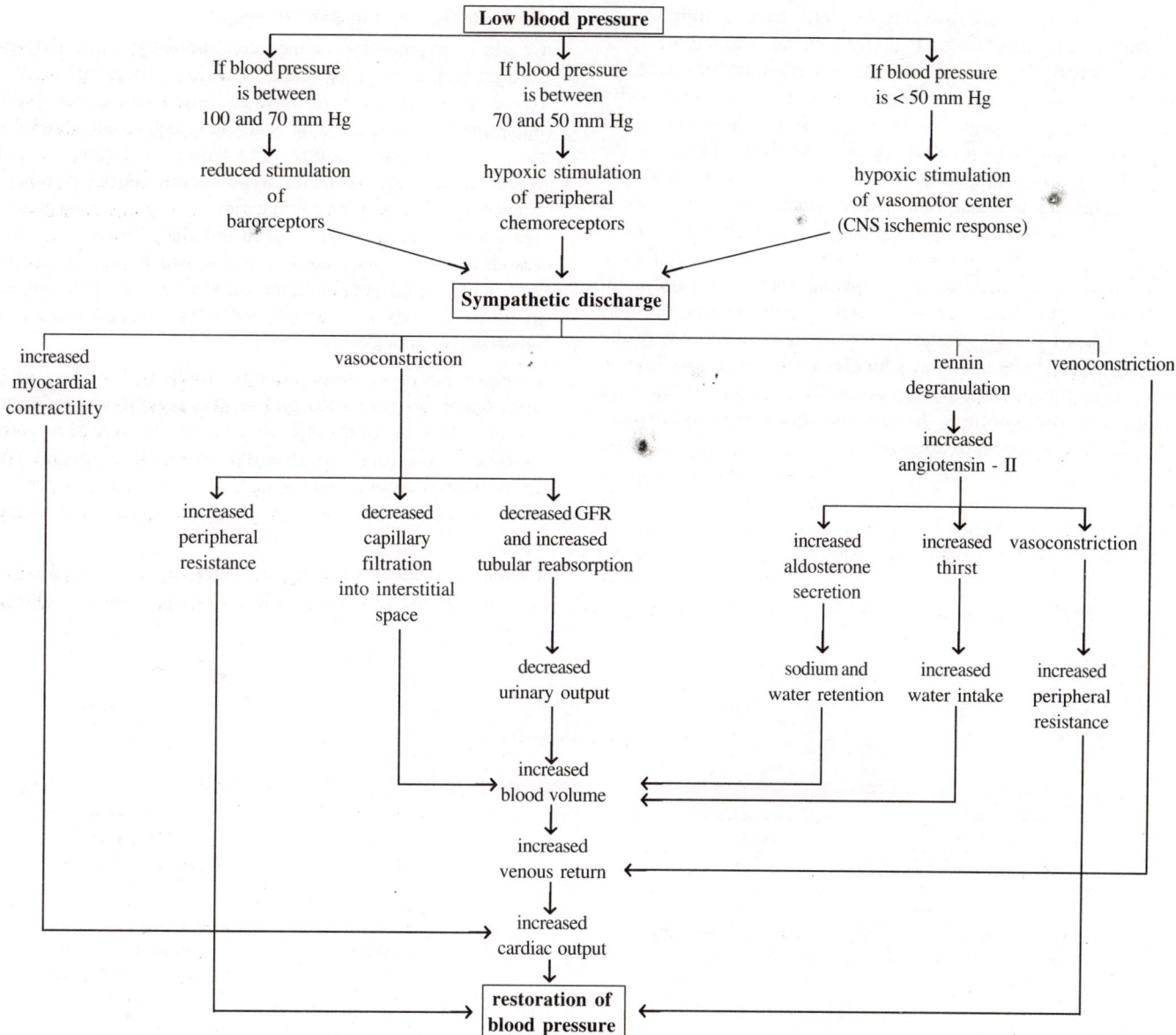

**Increased capillary permeability.** Prolonged capillary hypoxia results in increase in capillary permeability, and large quantities of fluid begin to transude into the tissues. This further decreases the blood volume, aggravating the shock.

**Release of toxins by ischemic tissues.** Endotoxin is a toxin released from dead gram-negative bacteria in the intestines. Diminished blood flow to the intestines causes enhanced formation and absorption of this toxic substance. Endotoxin causes extensive vascular dilatation, increased cellular metabolism despite the inadequate nutrition of the cells, and cardiac depression. It plays a major role in septic shock.

**Acidosis in shock.** The poor delivery of oxygen to the tissues greatly diminishes oxidative metabolism and the cells switch to anaerobic glycolysis. This leads to accumulation of **lactic acid** in the blood. Moreover, the sluggish blood flow through tissues also result in accumulation of $CO_2$ in tissues. The $CO_2$ dissolves in water to produce $H^+$ ions and causing acidosis. Acidosis causes

vasodilatation which aggravates the shock, which in turn causes more acidosis. Thus, another vicious cycle is initiated.

### What are the factors that make shock irreversible?

Shock is made irreversible by generalized cellular deterioration, tissue necrosis and depletion of cellular adenosine. (1) **Generalized cellular deterioration.** In severe shock, there is generalized cellular deterioration throughout the body. Active transport through the cell membrane is greatly diminished. As a result, *sodium and chloride accumulate in the cells and potassium is lost from the cells.* In addition, the cells begin to swell. Mitochondrial activity in the liver cells as well as in many other tissues of the body becomes severely depressed. Lysosomes begin to split in widespread tissue areas, with *intracellular release of hydrolases* that cause further intracellular deterioration. Cellular metabolism of nutrients, such as glucose are depressed. The activities of some hormones are depressed as well, including a marked suppression of insulin action. These changes are specially severe in the **liver** because hepatic cells have a high rate of metabolism and therefore particularly vulnerable to any decrease in blood supply. The liver is also the first organ to be exposed to toxins from the intestine through the portal vein. Also badly affected are the **lungs** (pulmonary edema) and the **heart** (myocardial ischemia). (2) **Tissue necrosis.** Not all cells of the body are equally damaged by shock because some tissues have better blood supplies than others. For instance, the hepatic cells adjacent to the arterial ends of capillaries receive better nutrition than the cells adjacent to the venous ends of the same capillaries. Thus, there is necrosis in the peripheral zone of hepatic acini while the central zone is less affected. Similar punctate lesions occur in heart muscle. Deteriorative lesions also occur in the kidneys, especially in the tubules (**acute tubular necrosis**), leading to acute renal failure and uremic death. Deterioration of the lungs often leads to respiratory distress the **shock lung syndrome**. (3) **Depletion of cellular adenosine.** The single-most important event that marks the point of irreversibility is the *depletion of cellular adenosine*. ATP is degraded to ADP, AMP and eventually to adenosine. The adenosine diffuses out of the cells into the circulating blood and is converted into uric acid. New adenosine is synthesized rather slowly so that, once depleted, the high-energy phosphate stores of the cells are difficult to replenish.

## Enumerate the causes of shock.

Causes of hypotension include conditions causing a reduction in cardiac output and conditions in which peripheral resistance is reduced. A reduction in cardiac output can occur due to an impairment of cardiac pump function (**cardiogenic shock**) or due to a reduced venous return. The commonest cause of reduced venous return is hypovolemia (**hypovolemic shock**). Another cause is excessive peripheral vasodilatation. It is called **vasogenic, low-resistance shock**. It is also called **distributive** shock since vasodilatation is associated with a redistribution of blood flow, with more blood accumulating on the venous side. Obstruction to blood flow is also associated with reduced venous return (**obstructive shock**).

Common causes of **hypovolemic shock** include **loss of blood** (external or internal bleeding), **loss of plasma** (burns and exudative lesions), **loss of fluids** (dehydration due to excessive vomiting, diarrhea, sweating). **Traumatic shock** is a special type of **hypovolemic shock** in which there is associated neurogenic shock too, caused by the severe pain which inhibits the vasomotor center.

Common causes of **cardiogenic shock** are myocardial infarction, arrhythmias and valvular disorders. Common causes of **obstructive**

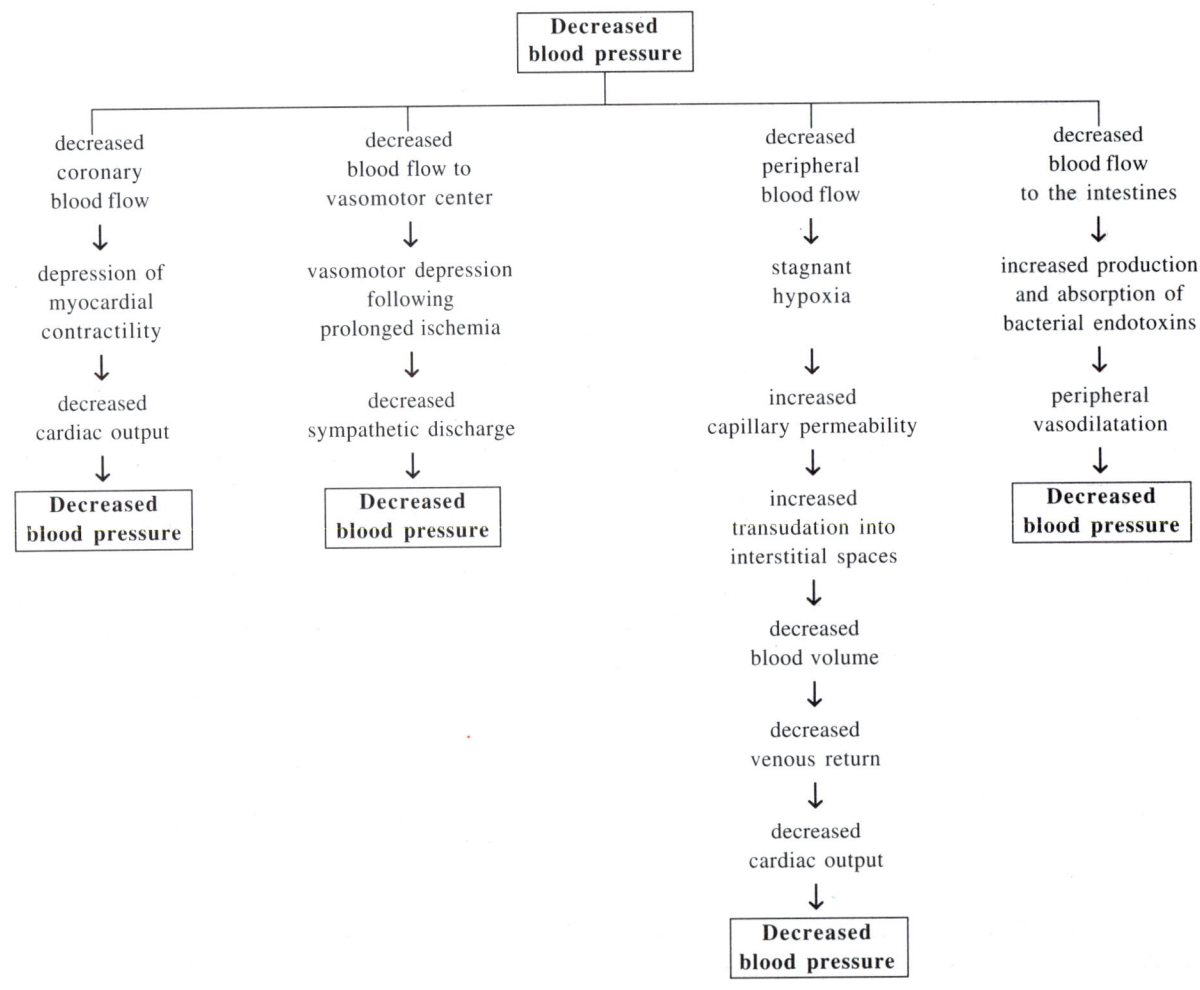

**shock** are pulmonary embolism, cardiac tamponade and tension pneumothorax. **Distributive shock** are of four types: neurogenic, anaphylactic, septicemic and endotoxic. In **neurogenic shock**, there is a marked reduction in sympathetic vasomotor tone. Its causes include deep general anesthesia and spinal anesthesia which affects the thoracolumbar sympathetic outflow, spinal injury, brain concussion or contusion of the basal regions of the brain. In **anaphylactic shock**, there is reduced peripheral resistance due to the release of histamine which causes vasodilatation. Moreover, there is also **hypovolemia** due to increased capillary permeability resulting in excessive exudation. In **septicemic shock**, there is vasodilatation in the infected tissues. The shock occurring in gram-negative septicemia is also known as **endotoxin shock**. The gram-negative bacteria release a toxin called **endotoxin**. Endotoxin shock is similar in mechanism to anaphylactic shock. Additionally, endotoxin depresses myocardial contractility.

### What are the clinical effects of shock?

Shock is characterized by hypotension and tachycardia with a *weak, thready pulse*. It is associated with signs of dehydration like *loss of skin turgor*, *dry tongue* and *sunken eyeball*. The skin *is cold and clammy*, partly due to increased sweating and party due to depression of metabolism. The hypothermia is however absent in septic shock in which the infection may cause fever. There is severe *muscle weakness*. There is *drowsiness* which progresses to stupor and coma. The GFR decreases in the early stages of shock which helps in restoration of blood volume. In the late stages of shock, the renal tubular epithelial cells are damaged. Certain parts of the tubule are particularly vulnerable as they have a very high metabolism but receive only a moderate blood supply. The result is **acute tubular necrosis** with tubular cell death and sloughing and blockage of the tubules. The damage often subsequently causes renal shutdown, with death occurring a week or so later because of **uremia**.

### Shock causes hypothermia but the patients are kept in cold room. Explain why ?

Patients of shock is kept in a cold room so that there is no further hypovolemia from sweating. Temperature regulation is a pre-potent reflex. If exposed to warmth, there would be sweating even at the risk of aggravating shock further. Shock patients are usually hypothermic and therefore naïve attendants might be inclined to cover them with blankets. This should never be done.

### Briefly outline the treatment of shock.

Depending on the cause of hypovolemia (loss of blood, plasma or fluids), the patient is transfused respectively with blood, plasma (or plasma expanders like dextran solution) or isotonic saline solutions (**replacement therapy**). Dextran molecules do not pass through the capillary pores. It therefore promotes osmosis of water from the interstitial to the intravascular spaces, thereby increasing the plasma volume.

*In neurogenic shock*, **sympathomimetic drugs** fulfill the physiological role of the sympathetic nervous system which is severely depressed. In anaphylactic shock, sympathomimetic drugs act as **physiological antagonists** to histamine which is largely responsible in the pathogenesis of the shock. *In hemorrhagic shock*, the sympathetic system is already maximally active, and therefore, *sympathomimetic drugs have limited value*. The sympathomimetic drug of choice is **dopamine** because it *produces renal vasodilatation* and at the same time, produces *vasoconstriction elsewhere in the body*. It also has a positive inotropic effect on the heart.

When the pressure falls too low especially hemorrhagic and neurogenic shock, placing the patient with the head 30 cm lower than the feet (the **Trendelenberg position**) helps in promoting venous return and thereby increasing cardiac output.

**Oxygen therapy** may be beneficial in some instances. However, the response is not marked because the hypoxia of shock is of the anemic and/or stagnant type. *Oxygen is beneficial mostly in hypoxic hypoxia*.

**Glucocorticoids** are frequently given to patients in severe shock for several reasons. They *increase the strength of the heart* in the late stages of shock. They *stabilize the lysosomal membranes* and prevent release of lysosomal enzymes into the cytoplasm of the cells, thus preventing deterioration from this source. They also aid in the *metabolism of glucose* by the severely damaged cells.

# 51

# Coronary Circulation

### How is coronary blood flow measured?

Kety method is used for estimating coronary blood flow. It is based on Fick principle. In this method subject breathes air containing 15% $N_2O$ for 10 minutes, which is sufficient time (T) for equilibration of $N_2O$ between myocardial tissues and blood leaving the heart. Simultaneous samples of arterial blood (from any artery) and coronary venous blood (collected by inserting a catheter into the **coronary sinus**) are taken at the beginning and every 1-minute interval, till 10 minutes. From these data, coronary blood flow can be calculated by Fick equation.

$$CBF = \frac{\text{Amount of } N_2O \text{ taken up by the heart in T minutes}}{\text{AV difference of } N_2O \text{ across heart in T minutes}}$$

Regional distribution of coronary blood flow can be assessed by **radionucleotide scanning**. Radionucleotides like thallium 201 is taken up by the myocardium in direct proportion to their activity. Conversely, technetium 99 is selectively taken up infarcted myocardium and stand out as *hot spots* in a scan.

### Enumerate the determinants of myocardial oxygen demand.

The resting heart has an $O_2$ consumption of 8 ml/min/100g, which is the highest of all organs. The most important determinant of myocardial oxygen demand is the mechanical work performed by the myocardium. *Heart rate, myocardial wall tension,* and *myocardial inotropic state* are the major determinants of the work done and therefore of myocardial oxygen demand.

### How does coronary blood flow vary with the cardiac cycle?

The coronary blood flow in the different phases of cardiac cycle depends on the **pressure gradient** between the **aortic pressure**, which tends to perfuse the coronary capillaries, and the **ventricular pressure**, which tends to prevent perfusion by compressing the coronary capillaries. *In diastole, the intraventricular pressure is zero in both the ventricles* and hence the coronary perfusion pressure is approximately equal to the aortic pressure. The intraventricular pressure however rises high during systole, compressing the coronary vessels. The *compression is most intense in the subendocardial layers of the left ventricle* because the left ventricular pressure (121mmHg) slightly exceeds the aortic pressure (120mm Hg) during systole. Hence, the *subendocardial portion of the left ventricle is not perfused at all during systole.* The *compressive effect of the left ventricular pressure decreases towards the subepicardial layers,* permitting some amount of blood flow does during systole.

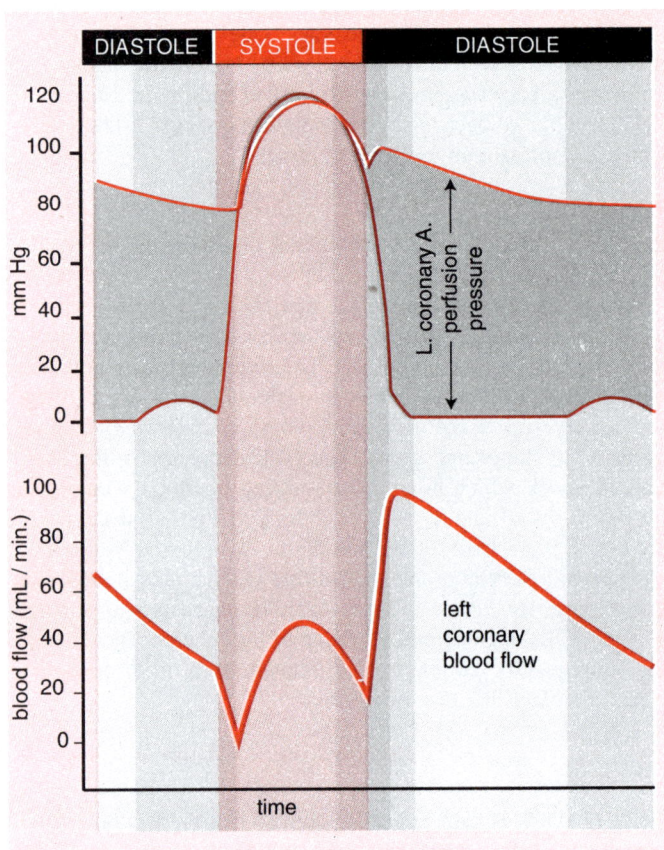

**Fig. 51.1**

However, in the right ventricle, the perfusion pressure remains adequate throughout systole because the right ventricular pressure rises to a maximum of 25 mm Hg, which is 95 mm Hg lower than the peak aortic pressure.

### How is coronary blood flow autoregulated?

As in most other tissues, the autoregulation is largely of **myogenic** origin. The myogenic tone of the vessel wall increases when pressure increases and decreases when pressure decreases, thereby keeping the coronary blood flow nearly constant over a range of perfusion pressure from 60 to 120 mmHg. **Metabolic** regulation also contributes. Whenever there is an increase in blood flow, the vasodilatory metabolites are washed away, producing vasoconstriction. *Adenosine* is a major component of myocardial metabolic regulation of flow. $P_{O_2}$, pH, and $K^+$ also contribute to metabolic regulation of flow.

### How do autonomic nerves affect coronary blood flow?

**Sympathetic stimulation** through $\alpha$-receptor causes coronary vasoconstriction, whereas stimulation of β receptors causes coronary vasodilatation. Since the norepinephrine released from sympathetic fibers acts predominantly on α receptors, sympathetic stimulation causes coronary vasoconstriction. However, sympathetic stimulation of the heart increases its oxygen demand and the metabolites produced causes coronary vasodilatation. This *indirect (metabolic) vasodilatory effect overrides the direct vasoconstrictive effect (through adrenergic receptors)* so that the net effect *in vivo* is *vasodilatation*.

**Parasympathetic stimulation** has *variable effects* due to its multiple modes of action. It *tends to cause vasoconstriction* because (i) it slows down the heart and reduces its oxygen demand; (ii) the acetylcholine released from parasympathetic fibers acts directly on muscarinic receptors on vascular smooth muscles to produce vasoconstriction. On the other hand, parasympathetic

stimulation *tends to cause vasodilatation* because (i) the acetylcholine released acts on sympathetic nerve varicosities to *inhibit norepinephrine release*; (ii) acetylcholine acts on the endothelium, inducing **nitric oxide (NO)** release and (iv) the **vasoactive intestinal polypeptide (VIP)** co-released with acetylcholine exerts a significant vasodilator effect.

## What are the consequences of myocardial ischemia?

Myocardial ischemia is associated with *pain, metabolic changes* in the myocardium, and *modification of cell gene expression*. The pain of myocardial ischemia is usually substernal, radiating to the left shoulder and is therefore called **angina pectoris**. The pain occurs due to accumulation of metabolites, especially the **P-factor**, which is now believed to be $K^+$.

# Cerebral Circulation

## What are the methods of estimation of cerebral blood flow?

**Kety Method** is used for estimating total cerebral blood flow. It is based on Fick's Principle. In this method, the subject breathes air containing 15% $N_2O$ for 10 minutes, which is sufficient time (T) for equilibration of $N_2O$ between brain tissues and blood leaving the brain. Simultaneous samples of arterial blood (from any artery) and mixed venous blood (from internal jugular vein) are taken at 1 minute intervals. From these data cerebral blood flow can be calculated by Fick's equation

$$CBF = \frac{\text{Amount of } N_2O \text{ taken up by} \times \text{brain in T minutes}}{\text{A-V difference of } N_2O \text{ across brain in T minutes}}$$

Regional cerebral blood flow can be estimated by **SPECT** (Single photon emission computed tomography), **PET** (Positron emission tomography), and **MRI** (Magnetic resonance Imaging).

## What are the factors regulating cerebral blood flow?

**Extracranial factors** regulating cerebral blood flow are (i) arterial perfusion pressure, (ii) blood viscosity and (iii) sympathetic discharge. **Intracranial factors** regulating cerebral blood flow include (i) metabolites like $H^+$, $CO_2$, $K^+$ and adenosine, and (ii) the intracranial pressure.

## What is the Monro Kallie doctrine?

It states that there are three elements i.e. **brain**, **CSF** and **blood**, enclosed in rigid cranial cavity. *If any one of them increases, it is at expense of the other two.* For example, if the CSF pressure is increased, either the brain or the blood vessels are compressed. Similarly, if the venous pressure increases, it decreases the cerebral blood flow by decreasing the effective perfusion pressure and by compressing cerebral vessels.

This relationship helps to *maintain constancy of cerebral blood flow*. If the body accelerates upwards (positive 'g' ), the blood moves towards feet and the arterial pressure at level of head decreases. Consequently, the venous pressure and intracranial pressure also fall, and the pressure on intracranial vessels decreases. Thus, the blood flow is less severely compromised. The reverse happens with negative 'g'. With downward acceleration (-ve 'g'), the arterial pressure increases at head level. The intracranial pressure also rises. Hence, the pressure differential across the intracranial vessel walls is not increased and the vessels do not rupture.

The same mechanism helps in circulatory adjustments to posture. When a person stands up from lying down position, there is sudden venous pooling and the arterial pressure at the head level decreases. But at the same time, the intracranial pressure also decreases, which reduces the compression of the intracranial blood vessels. Thus, the cerebral blood flow remains more or less unchanged.

## What is the Cushing's reflex?

When the intracranial pressure is elevated over a short period, the cerebral blood flow is reduced, leading to ischemia. This causes *stimulation of the vasomotor area leading to a rise in the blood pressure*. The reflex helps to maintain cerebral blood flow. The rise in blood pressure causes reflex bradycardia and slowing of breathing.

## What is the mechanism of autoregulation of cerebral blood flow?

Autoregulation operates in the pressure range of 60 – 140 mm Hg. Pressure below 60 mm Hg causes reduced cerebral blood flow and syncope, while above 140 mm Hg causes disruption of blood brain barrier and cerebral edema.

As elsewhere in the body, autoregulation of cerebral blood flow is either metabolic or myogenic in origin. When blood flow decreases, metabolites, mainly $CO_2$, accumulate and the tissue pH falls. The fall in pH produces vasodilatation and restores the cerebral blood flow (**metabolic autoregulation**). An increase in blood flow stretches the vascular smooth muscles. The stretch stimulates the vascular smooth muscles to contract, thereby causing vasoconstriction and restoring the blood flow (**myogenic autoregulation**).

## What is syncope? What are its causes?

Cardiac syncope can occur due to: (i) **obstruction to cardiac output**, e.g., aortic stenosis. It is precipitated by exertion and therefore called **effort syncope**. (ii) **arrhythmias** like sinus arrest, heart block, and Stokes-Adam syndrome. These occur more suddenly are not related to exertion. (iii) **myocardial infarction** in which fainting is the presenting symptom in about 7% of the patients.

**Noncardiac syncope** can be due to (i) **Vasovagal syncope**. It is also called neurocardiogenic syncope – or the common faint. (ii) **Postural syncope**. It is the fainting associated with the assumption of the upright posture. It occurs due to inadequate vasomotor response to the change in posture. (iii) **Carotid sinus syncope**. It occurs due to excessive sensitivity of the carotid sinus to compression, as by a tight collar. They are common in elderly patients. (iv) **Situational syncopes** occur in association with cough (**tussive syncope**), micturition (**micturition syncope**) or defecation (**defecation syncope**). All these activities are associated with the Valsalva maneuver which increases intrathoracic pressure. (v) **Metabolic syncope**. Syncope may be associated with hypoglycemia or hyperventilation. These cause syncope directly, without causing hypotension. *Hypoglycemia* impair the activity of the vasomotor center while hypocapnia associated with *hyperventilation* causes cerebral vasoconstriction, reducing blood supply to the brain.

# Cerebrospinal Fluid

## Where and how is CSF produced?

About 500 ml of CSF is formed per day (0.2 mL/min.). The CSF is *actively secreted by the choroid plexus*. $Na^+$ is secreted into the CSF with the help of $Na^+$-$K^+$ ATPase. $HCO_3^-$ is secreted into the CSF with the help of carbonic anhydrase. Water moves in by osmosis.

## Describe the circulation and absorption of CSF.

From the lateral ventricles CSF flows through the interventricular foramina (of Monro) into the 3rd ventricle. It then flows through the aqueduct of the midbrain (of Sylvius) into the 4th ventricle, from where it flows out through the median (Magendie) and two lateral (Luschka) foramina to circulate in the subarachnoid space around the brain and spinal cord. The CSF returns to the venous system mostly through small membranous villi, the **arachnoid granulations**, located in the dural sinuses. About 20% of the CSF are absorbed into the veins through *spinal arachnoid granulations* while 80% is through the *cerebral arachnoid granulations*.

## Describe the physical characteristics of CSF.

| Amount | 125 – 150 mL |
|---|---|
| Specific Gravity | 1.007 (close to that of brain tissue) |
| pH | 7.33 |
| Pressure | 150 mm Hg |
| Potential | +5 mV (CSF Positive) |
| Cells | < 5 cells / mm3 (mostly lymphocytes) |

## How much is the protein and glucose content of CSF?

CSF contains about 20 mEq/Kg of proteins that are mostly **albumin**. The **glucose** concentration in CSF is 64mEq/Kg.

## Enumerate the functions of the CSF.

The functions of the CSF include (i) providing **buoyancy** to the brain. The brain weighed in air is about 1500 gm, but it weighs just 50 gm in CSF. This reduction in weight is due to buoyancy which gives a cushioning effect to brain, preventing it from injury. (ii) **protecting** the brain by providing a cushion around the brain and protects it from injury. (iii) maintaining the **milieu intérieur**. The CSF provides an optimum environment to neurons, which are highly sensitive to changes in their external environment. (iv) **Removing proteins** that leak out of capillaries into interstitial fluid is drained by CSF and returned to blood stream.

## Explain the term coup and contracoup injuries.

Despite the cushioning effect of the CSF, the brain does sometimes gets injured. For example, if there is a severe blow on skull, it moves. The brain however lags behind due to inertia. This results in the **coup injury**. After some time when the movement of skull stops, the brain continues moving due to inertia. The brain hits the skull on the opposite side of blow. This is known as **contracoup injury** (Fig. 53.1).

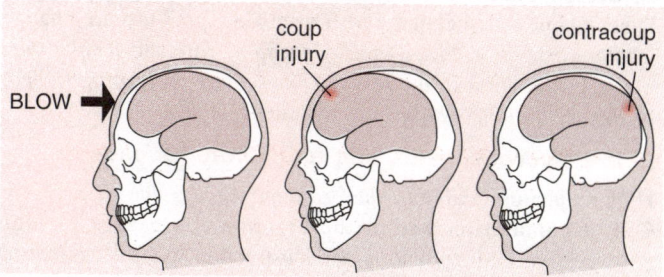

**Fig. 53.1**

## Describe the procedure of lumbar puncture.

Samples of CSF can be drawn by *lumbar, cisternal or verntricular puncture*. The most convenient and commonly used way is by lumbar puncture. It can be done safely between L3 and L4 or L4 and L5 vertebrae, because the spinal cord ends at L1 while the dura and arachnoid continues till S2 vertebrae.

## How much is the normal CSF pressure? How can it be measured?

The CSF pressure can be measured during lumbar puncture by connecting the needle with a manometer. The CSF pressure, as measured through a lumbar puncture is 65 – 200 mm of CSF. It is less in the lying position (5-15 mmHg) and more in the sitting position (265 - 400 mm Hg).

## Enumerate some of the possible abnormalities in the CSF.

Some of the possible abnormalities in the CSF are as follows. (i) **Turbidity** indicates increased protein and cells – indicative of inflammation of meninges. (ii) **Decreased glucose** is seen in meningitis due to utilization of glucose by microbes. (iii) **Neutrophils** in large numbers indicate bacterial meningitis or brain abcess (may reach up to 1000 to 10,000 cells/ml). (iv) **Lymphocytes** in large numbers indicate meningeal syphilis (200-300 cells/ml) (v) **Erythrocytes** in large numbers indicate subarachnoid haemorrhage.

## What is traction headache?

Traction headache occasionally occurs following the withdrawal of CSF by lumbar puncture. This occurs because the brain, due of its reduced buoyancy, *pulls down on the pain-sensitive dura* from which it is suspended by the cerebral veins draining into the dural sinuses. Also, the base of the brain presses upon the interior of the cranium with greater pressure producing pain due to *pressure on the crainal nerves at the base of the brain.*

### Enumerate the features associated with raised intracranial pressure.

Raised intracranial pressure causes neuronal damage in different ways. Some neurons are *damaged directly by the high CSF pressure.* Other neurons are *damaged due to ischemia* resulting from compression of blood vessels. Further damage occurs if there is **herniation** of a part of the brain through openings in the cranial bones or tentorium.

A characteristic sign occurs when the raised intracranial pressure causes *compression of the ophthalmic veins.* Blood can still flow along the arteries and reach the optic disc, but its return is impeded. As a result, there is *swelling of optic disc* known as **papilloedema**. Other features associated with raised CSF pressure are changes in *blood pressure, heart rate, respiratory rate* and *temperature.* There is alteration in the level of consciousness leading to signs of *disorientation, stupor* and eventually *coma.*

### Define hydrocephalus and enumerate its causes.

Hydrocephalus (*water in the cranium*) occurs due to excessive CSF accumulation within the cranium. Its causes include: (i) excessive CSF formation, (ii) obstruction to CSF circulation, and (iii) impaired absorption of CSF.

### Explain the difference between internal and external hydrocephalus.

**Internal hydrocephalus** is due to a block at the foramen of Monro, the aqueduct, or the foramen of Magendie and Luschka. **External hydrocephalus** could be due to a block at the foramen magnum or at the tentorial opening. It could also be due to diseases of the arachnoid mater or thrombosis of the dural sinuses. *Block at foramen magnum* prevents CSF from entering the spinal cord, thereby cutting off 20% of its absorptive surface. *Block at tentorial opening* prevents the passage of fluid from posterior fossa to supratentorial space, thereby occluding most of the absorptive surface.

### Explain the difference between communicating and non-communicating hydrocephalus.

In a **non-communicating hydrocephalus,** there is no communication between the CSF present in the ventricles and the spinal subarachnoid spaces. Hydrocephalus occurs due to the cutting off of 20% of the absorptive surface. In **communicating hydrocephalus**, the circulation of CSF is not obstructed. It occurs either due to excessive CSF formation (*hypersecretory hydrocephalus*) or reduced CSF absorption (*malabsorptive hydrocephalus*). The two may be differentiated clinically by the **phenolphthalein test** and the **Queckenstedt's tests** although both have been superceded by various types of **myeloencephalography**.

### Describe the phenolphthalein test.

The test involves injecting phenolphthalein into the lateral ventricle and looking for its appearance in urine. The possible outcome are shown in the flow chart below.

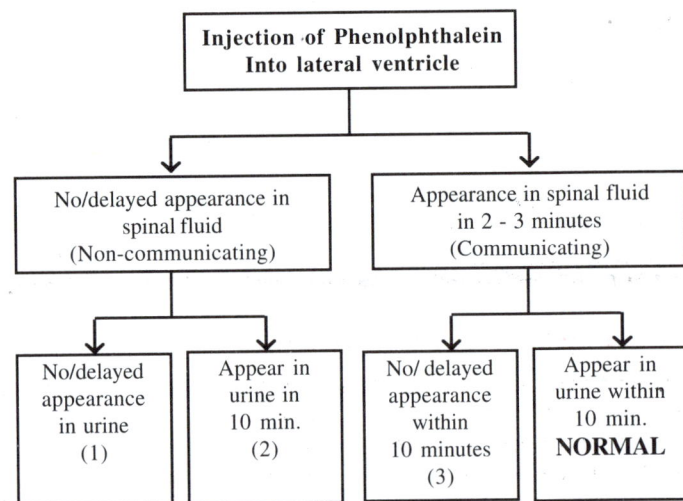

The results (1) – (3) are associated with the following conditions. (1) The CSF absorption through cerebral arachnoid is defective. Absorption through spinal arachnoid also not possible because the freshly formed CSF cannot flow out from the ventricles into the spinal subarachnoid space (hence the name non-communicating). (2) CSF absorption through cerebral arachnoid is normal. Hydrocephalus is due to the lack of CSF absorption through spinal arachnoid. (3) CSF absorption through cerebral and/or spinal arachnoid is defective.

### Describe the Queckenstedt's test.

It *is a clinical test for detecting non communicating* hydrocephalus. It is performed while doing a lumbar puncture by connecting the needle to a manometer. *Compression of one internal jugular vein causes a sudden rise in CSF pressure* followed by a sudden fall on release. Similar rise and fall occurs on coughing. *When there is a block, the rise and fall may be slow or absent.*

### Name the structures outside the blood-brain barrier.

The structures outside the blood-brain barrier are located mostly around the ventricles and therefore are called **circumventricular organs**. These areas are: (i) **posterior pituitary** and adjacent ventral part of median eminence of hypothalamus. (ii) **subfornical organ** where angiotensin II acts to increase water intake. (iii) **area postrema**, which initiates vomiting in response to toxic chemicals in plasma. (iv) **organum vasculosum of lamina terminalis (OVLT)**, which serves as an osmoreceptor. (v) The **pineal** and **anterior pituitary** also are outside blood-brain barrier but both are endocrine organs and not part of the brain.

### Name the factors that weaken the blood-brain barrier.

The blood-brain barrier is weak in **infancy.** Since blood-brain barrier is not properly developed in infancy, a high serum bilirubin level leads to accumulation of bilirubin in the brain causing kernicterus. The barrier is weakened by **brain tumor**. Hence, a radiolabelled amino acid that is injected into circulation gets localized in the tumor and not other parts of the brain. This is advantageous in diagnostic radiography. The barrier is also weakened in **inflammation**. Hence antibiotics like pencillin, which normally do not cross blood-brain barrier, can cross it during inflammation.

# 54

# Pulmonary Circulation

### What are the salient differences between systemic and pulmonary circulation?

Compared to the aorta, the pulmonary artery is much shorter, has a larger diameter and has about one-third its wall thickness. This is also true for pulmonary arteries and arterioles in relation to their systemic counterparts. Due to these characteristics, the pulmonary compliance is very high – about 7 mL/mm Hg. The pulmonary veins too, like systemic veins, are highly distensible.

The high distensibility of pulmonary artery enables them to offer a low resistance to blood flow from the right to the left ventricle. The distensibility of pulmonary circulation makes it **a low-pressure, high-capacitance system**.

### Why are bronchial vessels called physiological shunts?

Unlike the lung parenchyma which receives deoxygenated blood the bronchi receive oxygenated blood through bronchial arteries. Bronchial veins, instead of draining into the right atrium (which receives most of the deoxygenated blood), drain into the left atrium. The bronchial circulation therefore constitutes a **physiological shunt** – i.e., a channel that bypasses oxygenation in the lungs. *The other example of physiological shunt is the coronary vessels that drain into the left side of the heart.* These physiological shunts have two effects: they *reduce the $O_2$ saturation of arterial blood slightly*, and they *make the left ventricular output slightly greater* than the right ventricular output.

### How much is the normal pulmonary arterial pressure?

Pulmonary systolic pressure is 25 mm Hg, diastolic pressure is 8 mm Hg, mean pressure is 15 mm Hg and pulse pressure is 17 mm Hg.

### What is pulmonary wedge pressure?

The pulmonary wedge pressure gives *an approximate estimate of the pressure in the left atrium*, which is not easily accessible to catheters. It is measured by inserting a catheter through the right side of the heart and the pulmonary artery into one of the small branches of the pulmonary arteries and then pushing the catheter until it wedges tightly in the artery. The pressure so measured is called the **pulmonary wedge pressure**, and is about 5 mm Hg.

### How much is the pulmonary blood volume and what is its significance?

The blood volume of the lungs is approximately 600 mL, which is located mostly in the pulmonary arteries and veins. This volume of blood decreases when the intrathoracic pressure increases, e.g., during a Valsalva maneuver. Also, when there is loss of blood from the systemic circulation by hemorrhage, it can be partly compensated for by transfusion of blood from this pulmonary reservoir.

### What is the effect of gravity on pulmonary blood flow?

In the normal, upright person, the pulmonary arterial *pressure at the apex of the lung is about 15 mm Hg less* than the pulmonary arterial pressure at the level of the heart, and the *pressure at the base of the lungs is about 8 mm Hg greater*. There is a corresponding difference in regional blood flow, which forms the basis of three zones. In **Zone 1**, *no blood flows at all during any part of the cardiac cycle* because the local capillary pressure in that area of the lung never rises higher than the alveolar pressure during any phase of the cardiac cycle. *Zone 1 is present only under abnormal conditions*, e.g., in hypovolemia or in obstructive lung disorders. **Zone 2** has *intermittent blood flow*, occurring only during the peaks of pulmonary arterial pressure peaks. The zone extends from the apex down to a distance of 10 cm above the heart level. **Zone 3** has *continuous blood flow*, because the alveolar capillary pressure remains greater than alveolar pressure during the entire cardiac cycle. In the recumbent position, no part of the lung is more than a few centimeters above the level of the heart. Therefore, the entire lung, including the apex, becomes equivalent to zone 3, in recumbent position, receiving continuous blood flow.

### What is the effect of exercise on pulmonary blood flow?

During heavy exercise the average blood flow through the lungs increases as much as 4 to 7 fold. This extra flow is achieved in two ways: by *increasing the number of open capillaries*, and by *increasing the rate of flow through each capillary*. These two factors together decrease the pulmonary vascular resistance so much that the *pulmonary arterial pressure rises very little even during maximum exercise*. However, the rise in pressure is enough to *provide continuous blood flow to the apices*.

### When does pulmonary edema occur?

Pulmonary edema occurs in **left ventricular failure** when the high left atrial pressure is transmitted back to the pulmonary capillaries where the hydrostatic pressure rises. When the left atrial pressure rises to ~ 25 mm Hg, the capillary pressure is sufficiently high to produce pulmonary edema due to transudation of fluids across the capillary wall.

### What is the effect of sympathetic discharge on pulmonary circulation?

Stimulation of the sympathetic fibers causes a slight increase in resistance. However, the effect is insignificant and physiologically unimportant. More importantly, it *constricts the large pulmonary capacitance vessels, especially the veins.* The constriction produced is considerable and results in *transfusion of pulmonary blood into systemic circulation.*

### What are the functions of mechanoreceptors in the pulmonary circulation?

**Pulmonary baroreceptors** are present in the adventitia of the *pulmonary arteries.* These receptors detect rise in pulmonary arterial pressure and produce reflex *bradycardia* and *hypotension.* The afferent arc is through the vagus, and the efferent, through sympathetic fibers.

**Pulmonary volume receptors** are present at the junction of the pulmonary veins with the left atrium. When stimulated, they produce tachycardia. These vagal receptors could be the afferent limb of the Bainbridge reflex.

**Juxtapulmonary receptors** are present in the *alveolar interstitium, adjacent to the pulmonary capillaries.* It is triggered by microemboli in the small pulmonary vessels. It produces *bronchoconstriction* and *severe tachypnea.* Embolization of larger pulmonary vessels do not produce tachypnea because they do not stimulate the J-receptors. J-receptor stimulation also produces *hypotension* and *bradycardia.*

### What is the effect of hypoxia on pulmonary circulation?

Hypoxia induces **pulmonary vasoconstriction**. This is exactly opposite to what happens in systemic circulation where hypoxia produces vasodilatation. The physiological significance of this phenomenon is to *divert pulmonary blood flow from the alveoli that are poorly ventilated.* Acidosis and hypercapnia also produce pulmonary vasoconstriction, the functional significance of which is the same as in case of hypoxia.

### What is cor pulmonale?

**Chronic hypoxia** is associated with pulmonary vasoconstriction resulting in a marked increase in pulmonary arterial pressure (**pulmonary hypertension**). This imposes a heavy afterload on the right ventricle, leading to its hypertrophy and eventual failure which is called **cor pulmonale**. Pulmonary hypertension is *common in high altitude dwellers.*

# 55

# Cutaneous & Muscle Circulation

### How much is the normal cutaneous blood flow?

The oxygen and nutrient requirements of the skin are relatively small. *Cutaneous circulation is regulated not by its metabolic activity but by the requirements for maintenance of body temperature.* Depending on the amount of sweating, cutaneous blood flow varies from $\frac{1}{10}$th to 10 times the resting blood flow. Resting cutaneous blood flow is therefore *defined as the flow when a person is at thermal equilibrium with the environment*, i.e., at about 27°C. It is equal to 13 mL/min. per 100 g of skin tissue (i.e., 450 mL/min).

### Why is sweating called a prepotent reflex?

The increase in cutaneous blood flow in response to thermal challenge is a prepotent reflex. In shock, cutaneous vasoconstriction helps to divert blood to vital tissues. Yet, *if the temperature rises, the cutaneous blood flow increases regardless of the needs of vital tissues.* Maximal cutaneous blood flow that occurs on heat-exposure imposes a heavy circulatory load on the heart. It can lead to hypotension and shock.

### What is the role of counter-current exchanger in the skin?

In the limbs, the arteries supplying the extremities have accompanying veins (venae comites) which serve as a counter-current exchange mechanism to favor heat exchange. Thus, *heat conservation is enhanced in cold environment*, and *heat gain is minimized in warm environments.*

### Describe the triple response to cutaneous trauma.

A firm strong stroke across the skin using a blunt point evokes three sequential responses: the red reaction, flare and wheal. The **red reaction** is a red line that occurs along the line of the stroke. It occurs due to the dilatation of precapillary sphincters. The dilatation is not neurally mediated but caused by the histamine and bradykinin released from the injured skin. The **flare** is a warm, erythematous (red) area which develops surrounding the site of the red line. It occurs due to a dilatation of the arterioles, terminal arterioles and precapillary sphincters. The dilatation is mediated by the **axon reflex** in the cutaneous C fibers: the impulse is conducted from one branch of the nerve fiber to another (Fig. 55.1). The **wheal** is a swelling that develops along and around the line of the stroke. It is a direct consequence of capillary damage, which results in increased capillary permeability with consequent exudation of plasma. Some individuals have a striking triple response reactions so that anything drawn on the skin with a blunt point becomes conspicuous in minutes – a phenomenon called **dermatographia**.

### How much is the normal muscle blood flow?

The resting muscle blood flow is 3mL/100g/min. It can increase 20 times during strenuous exercise.

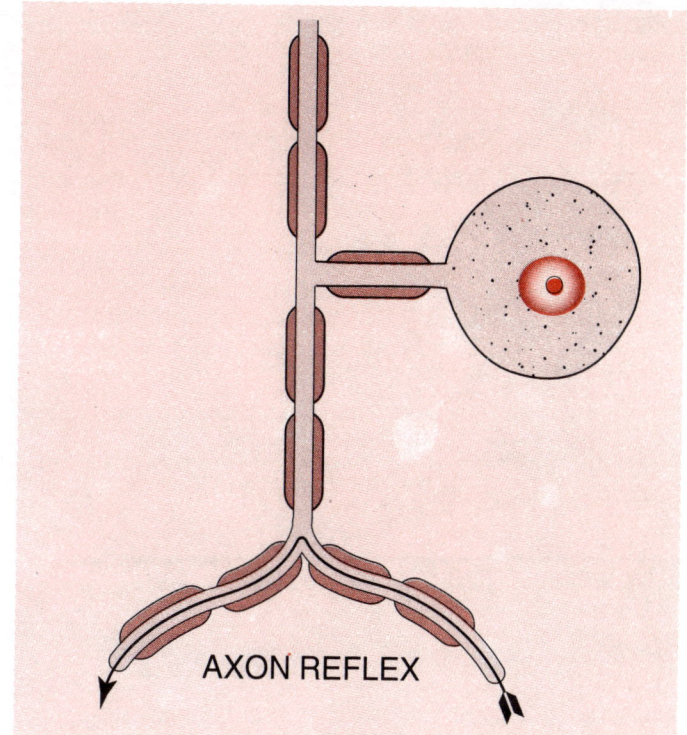

AXON REFLEX

**Fig. 55.1**

### What is the physiological significance of sympathetic vasodilator fibers?

Sympathetic vasodilator fibers are intermingled with other sympathetic fibers. They have acetylcholine and not norepinephrine as their neurotransmitter. The sympathetic vasodilator nerves are activated by *cortico-hypothalamic-reticulo-spinal pathways*, which are quite separate from the *vasomotor center-thoracolumbar spinal paths*. Yet, they are called sympathetic because they discharge only in emergencies. They are not influenced by the baroreceptor and chemoreceptor afferents and do not participate in the usual cardiovascular reflexes. Sympathetic vasodilator fibers are not important in providing improved nutritive flow to the muscles, either during or before exercise. The sympathetic vasodilator nerves *provide a safety valve that prevents dangerous increase in blood pressure before the onset of exercise.* Its mechanism is as follows.

Before exercise, even the thought of exercise brings about considerable sympathetic discharge, which causes widespread vasoconstriction in the muscle beds. As a result, the total peripheral resistance and blood pressure tends to rise to dangerous levels. At this time, the *discharge of the sympathetic vasodilator nerves lowers the blood pressure to safe levels.* It does so by dilating the A-V anastomotic channels in the muscle. Opening of these channels does not improve nutritive flow to the muscles. Once exercise commences, the precapillary sphincters are dilated by local metabolites and blood is diverted from the A-V channels to the muscle capillaries which now offer lesser resistance.

## Compare and contrast sympathetic vasoconstriction and vasodilator fibres.

### SIMILARITIES

Both are activated in emergency (fight or flight) situations.

Both affect blood pressure in general and muscle blood flow in particular.

### DIFFERENCES

| Sympathetic vasoconstrictor | Sympathetic vasodilator |
| --- | --- |
| Innervates nearly all circulatory beds. | Innervates only the blood vessels in skeletal muscles. |
| Reduces blood flow through the true capillary by contracting the pre capillary sphincter. | Increases blood flow through the capillary thoroughfare vessels, which connect the metarteriole with the venule, bypassing the sphincter. |
| Neurotransmitter is norepinephrine. | Neurotransmitter is acetylcholine. |
| Controlled directly by vasomotor center and indirectly by cortico-hypothalamic center. | Not under control of vasomotor center but is under direct cortico-hypothalamic control |
| Respond to baroreceptor and chemoreceptor afferents | Do not respond to baro-receptor and chemoreceptor afferents |
| Meant for increasing BP during exercise. | Meant for preventing rise in BP before exercise. |

# Splanchnic Circulation

### Define splanchnic circulation. How much is the normal splanchnic circulation?

The combined vascular beds of the *liver, spleen and the gut* are called the **splanchnic circulation**. The total splanchnic blood flow is ~ 1.5 L/min. If the entire gastrointestinal tract became simultaneously active, the splanchnic blood flow would have increased to ~4.0L. However, since during digestion and absorption, the gastrointestinal tract is sequentially activated, the maximum splanchnic circulation is about 3.0L/min.

### What is the villous countercurrent system?

The direction of the blood flow in the capillaries and venules in a villus is opposite to that in the main arteriole. This arrangement is a **countercurrent exchange system**. Its advantage is that it automatically *slows down the entrance of rapidly absorbed solutes* into the blood, so that the liver can handle them effectively. Its disadvantage is that it *reduces the supply of $O_2$ to the mucosal cells at the tip of the villus*. When intestinal blood flow is very low, the shunting of $O_2$ is exaggerated, which may cause extensive necrosis of the intestinal villi.

### Which are the two sources of hepatic blood flow? Which of the two provides more oxygen?

Nearly 70% of the $O_2$ used by the liver is derived from the **portal blood**. This is possible because the portal blood entering the liver is three times the volume of hepatic arterial blood entering the liver. Moreover, *portal blood is not markedly desaturated* because of the low $O_2$ demands of the other vascular beds. The remaining 30% of the $O_2$ is supplied by **arterial blood**.

### Why does ascites occur in congestive cardiac failure and in cirrhosis of liver?

Ascites occurs in **congestive heart failure** because the *elevated atrial pressure is transmitted backwards to the hepatic veins*. Rise in hepatic venous pressure is transmitted to the hepatic sinusoids, resulting in the pressure filtration of large amounts of fluids. Ascites occurs in **hepatic cirrhosis** because it leads to a *marked rise in hepatic vascular resistance*. The consequent increase in the portal venous system and the capillary hydrostatic pressure through the splanchnic circulation leads to extensive fluid transudation into the abdominal cavity.

### What are the consequences of portocaval anastomosis?

In portocaval anastomosis, the pressure rises substantially in the systemic veins that anastomose with the portal vein. For example, the esophageal veins may enlarge considerably to form **esophageal varices**. These varices may rupture and lead to severe, frequently fatal internal bleeding.

### What is the effect of sympathetic stimulation on hepatic blood flow?

The liver serves as a **blood reservoir**, storing about 400mL of blood in its sinusoids. The sympathetic nerves constrict the presinusoidal resistance vessels in the portal venous and hepatic arterial systems. More importantly, sympathetic stimulation causes a *marked reduction in the capacitance of the portal system* and helps to divert blood towards the heart.

# Cardiovascular Reflexes & Readjustments

### What is Valsalva maneuver?

A *forced expiration performed against a closed glottis* is called **Valsalva maneuver**. It is commonly performed during *straining at stools* and in the initial phase of *coughing*. It also occurs during straining at parturition.

### Describe the different phases of blood pressure changes during Valsalva maneuver.

Valsalva maneuver is associated with a *sharp rise in the intrathoracic pressure*. This results in a series of changes in cardiac output and arterial blood pressure, which can be described in four phases: In **phase 1**, the arterial pressure increases transiently as the increase in intrathoracic pressure *compresses the aorta*. **Phase 2** consists of a fall in the blood pressure which plateaus after several seconds owing to *reflex vasoconstriction* and heart-rate usually increases slightly. Its mechanism is as follows:

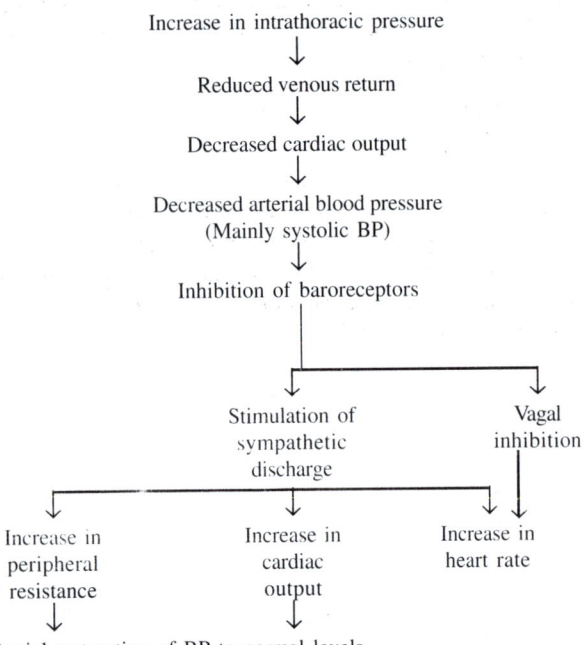

Partial restoration of BP to normal levels.

**Phase 3** occurs 1 – 2 seconds after release of the strain and consists of a transient fall in blood pressure. It is caused by a release of pressure compressing the aorta, i.e., *the reverse of the phenomenon in phase 1*. In **phase 4**, the systolic and mean blood pressures rise above the resting level within 10 seconds. The *blood pressure overshoot* is caused by the lingering effects of vasoconstriction induced by phase 2 and returns to resting values by 1-2 minutes after strain release. During the overshoot of the blood pressure, stimulation of the baroreceptor reflex causes a *decrease in heart rate* (Fig. 57.1).

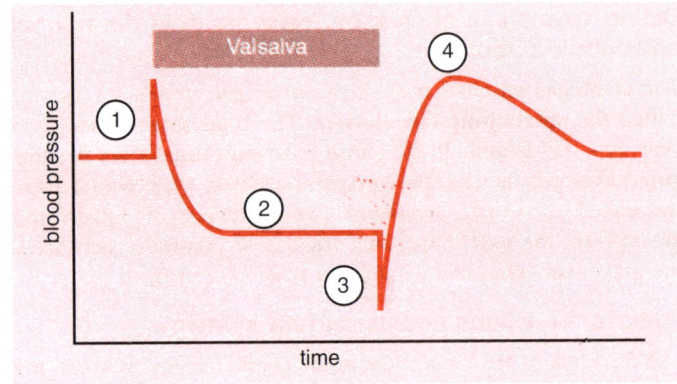

**Fig. 57.1**

### What is Valsalva ratio?

The Valsalva ratio is the *longest R-R interval* found after (within 20 beats of the end of the maneuver) to the shortest R-R interval during the Valsalva maneuver. The ratio indicates the *integrity of baroreceptor reflex* and is commonly employed in clinical practice.

### What is Müller's maneuver?

**Müller's maneuver** is *forced inspiration against closed glottis*. It can reduce the intrathoracic pressure to up to –80 mm Hg. It produces cardiovascular changes that are exactly opposite to those of Valsalva maneuver.

### What are the cardiovascular changes associated with a change of posture from lying to standing?

When the posture changes from the recumbent (lying) to the erect (standing) posture, the first change is a reduction in venous return due to venous pooling in the leg. This sets off a series of other changes. The changes during standing are summarized below.

| | |
|---|---|
| Central venous pressure | Slightly reduced |
| Total peripheral resistance | Increased |
| Stroke volume | Reduced |
| Heart rate | Increased |
| Cardiac output | Reduced. Reduction in cardiac output is less marked than the reduction in stroke volume due to the rise in heart rate. |
| Systolic blood pressure | Slightly reduced due to the fall in stroke volume |
| Diastolic blood pressure | Slightly elevated due to the rise in peripheral resistance |
| Pulse pressure | Reduced |
| Mean blood pressure | Nearly unchanged |

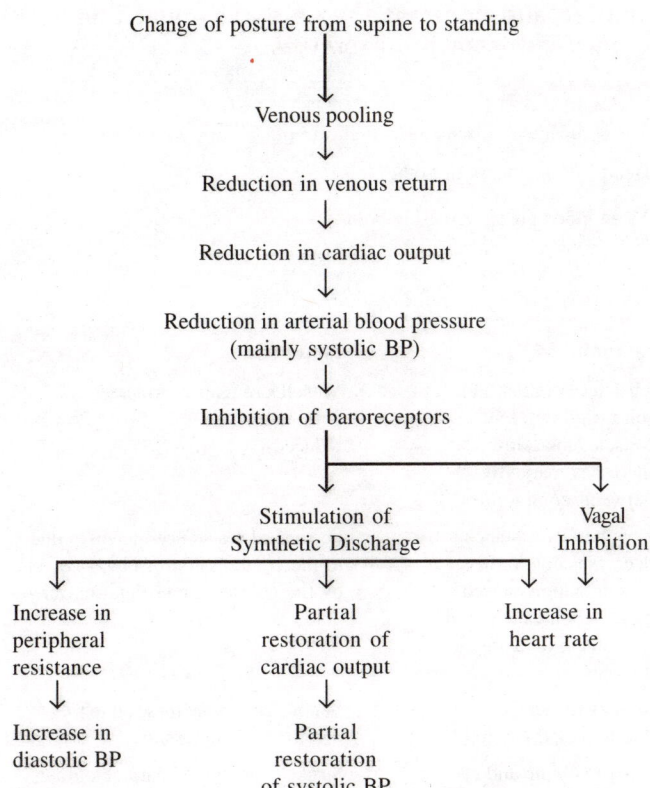

Change of posture from supine to standing

↓

Venous pooling

↓

Reduction in venous return

↓

Reduction in cardiac output

↓

Reduction in arterial blood pressure
(mainly systolic BP)

↓

Inhibition of baroreceptors

↓

Stimulation of Symthetic Discharge                    Vagal Inhibition

Increase in peripheral resistance    Partial restoration of cardiac output    Increase in heart rate

↓                                    ↓

Increase in diastolic BP             Partial restoration of systolic BP

### What is the effect of zero-gravity? When does it occur?

**Zero g** is *seen in orbiting satellites* where the gravitational forces are precisely counterbalanced by the centrifugal forces generated by the orbiting satellite. On earth, zero g is experienced *during free-fall*. The effects of zero g are the *same as those produced when the posture changes from the standing to lying*. This is because gravitational forces have significant consequences only when acting along the long axis of the body. In the recumbent posture, gravity is directed perpendicular to the long axis of the body and therefore, g effectively becomes zero.

### What is the effect of high-gravity? When does it occur?

**High g** is experienced when there is a higher than usual acceleration in the direction of earth's gravity. Very high g occurs *during the take off and landing of space rockets*. More commonly, a high g is experienced *when an airplane loops upward*, and during parachute jumping *when the parachute is suddenly opened out* after a period of free fall (the **opening shock load**). A feel of high g is obtained *in elevators (lifts) as it starts ascending or stops descending*. The effects of high g on circulation are primarily due to the inertia of blood in the blood vessels. When the body suddenly moves up, the blood fails to move quickly with it. As a result, there is a relative movement of blood downwards to the dependent portions of the body (venous pooling). The effect of high g are therefore the same as (though much more severe than) *those occurring during a change of posture from lying to standing*, i.e., changes occurring due to **excessive venous pooling**.

### What is the effect of negative-gravity? When does it occur?

**Negative g** is experienced when there is lower than usual

acceleration in the direction of earth's gravity. Low g occurs *when an airplane loops down*. A feel of negative g is obtained in *an elevator (lifts) as it stops ascending or starts descending*. The effects of high and low g on circulation are primarily due to the inertia of blood in the blood vessels. When the body suddenly moves down, the blood rushes up towards the brain. Negative g causes *a rise in cerebral arterial pressure, intense congestion of the head and neck vessels, ecchymoses around the eyes and severe throbbing head pain*. There is also a general increase in venous return leading to an increase in cardiac output. Most of the cardiac output however moves towards the upper parts of the body. *In spite of the great rise in cerebral arterial pressure, the vessels in the brain do not rupture*, because there is a corresponding increase in intracranial pressure which supports the walls of the blood vessels. In other words, the *CSF acts like a g-suit*. (see also Monro Kallie doctrine in Chapter 52).

### How does the antigravity suit work?

The antigravity suit or the **g-suit**, in its simplest form, is *a water-filled jacket* that is worn by astronauts. When there is a high positive g, there is tendency of venous pooling. Simultaneously, the water in the g-suit also rushes to the lower parts so that the pressure in the g-suit exactly matches *the pressure in the blood vessels. Thus, as g increases, the pressure in the g-suit parallels the blood pressure in the dependent parts of the body*, preventing venous pooling and edema.

### What is the role of sympathetic activity in exercise?

The sympathetic discharge has numerous important roles in exercise: (i) It *increases myocardial contractility* which makes the heart less dependent on heterometric mechanisms for increasing the cardiac output. (ii) It *increases the heart rate* which increases the cardiac output and at the same time, prevents an excessive increase in the end-diastolic volume. (iii) It causes contraction of the arteriolar smooth muscles, reducing arteriolar compliance. The *reduced arteriolar compliance* ensures that when cardiac output increases, the blood does not get 'stored' in distended arteries but moves forward into the tissues. (iv) It causes an *increase in pre-post capillary sphincter resistance ratio*. This reduces the capillary hydrostatic pressure and prevents an excessive transudation of fluid into tissue spaces. Excessive transudation losses would have caused hypovolemia. (v) It causes *venoconstriction*, thereby reducing venous compliance and accelerating the venous return.

### What are the cardiovascular changes associated with isotonic exercise?

Isometric exercise is characterized by a *marked dilatation of the capillary bed due to metabolic autoregulation*. This results in an increase in venous return and an increase in the cardiac output to 10 – 15 L, and even up to 25 L in champion athletes. Venous return is also aided by the respiratory pump, muscle pump and the *vis-a-fronte*. There is a *marginal rise in diastolic blood pressure – sometimes even a fall –* during isotonic exercise. This is because although the cardiac output rises manifold, there is a *marked fall in peripheral resistance*. The systolic blood pressure, which is comparatively less dependent on peripheral resistance and more dependent on stroke volume, shows a more marked rise. The *mean blood pressure and pulse pressure rise too.*

## What are the cardiovascular changes associated with isometric exercise?

In isometric exercise, the *muscle capillaries get squeezed by the contracting muscles and therefore there is a rise in peripheral resistance*. The *cardiac output decreases* due to both a high afterload (increased peripheral resistance) and a low preload (decreased venous return). The *diastolic blood pressure rises* due to the increased peripheral resistance but the *systolic pressure falls* due to a fall in stroke volume. The *mean blood pressure rises* but the *pulse pressure falls*. Such isometric exercises however cannot be sustained continuously for too long: they must be punctuated with periods of isotonic exercise.

## Compare and contrast the cardiovascular effects of isotonic and isometric exercises.

### SIMILARITIES

The sympathetic discharge is high in both.

Heart rate increases in both.

Mean blood pressure rises in both.

### DIFFERENCES

| Isotonic | Isometric |
|---|---|
| Muscles contract and relax rhythmically. Muscle blood flow increases markedly between contractions. | Muscles remain contracted continuously. Muscle blood flow is reduced. |
| Peripheral resistance decreases due to the vasodilatation caused by metabolites released from the exercising muscles. | Peripheral resistance increases due to the compression of blood vessels by the contracting skeletal muscles. |
| Venous return increases due to vasodilatation. | Venous return decreases due to capillary compression. |
| Stroke volume and cardiac output increase markedly due to increased preload (venous return) and reduced afterload (peripheral resistance). | Stroke volume and cardiac output do not increase much due to reduced preload (venous return) and increased afterload (peripheral resistance). |
| Diastolic blood pressure remains unchanged or falls due to reduced peripheral resistance. | Diastolic pressure rises (due to increased peripheral resistance). |
| Systolic blood pressure rises | Systolic blood pressure falls. |
| Pulse pressure increases markedly. | Pulse pressure does not change much. |

# 58

# Structure & Function of the Respiratory System

## How many times do the airways divide between the trachea and the alveolar sacs?

After passing through the nasal passages and pharynx where it is warmed and takes up water vapor, the inspired air passes down the trachea and through the bronchioles, respiratory bronchioles, and alveolar ducts to the alveoli. Between the trachea and the alveolar sacs, the airways divide **23 times**. The first **16 generations** of passages form the **conducting zone** of the airways that transports gas from and to the exterior. They are made up of bronchi, bronchioles, and terminal bronchioles. The remaining **7 generations** form the **transitional** and **respiratory zones** where

gas exchange occurs and are made up of respiratory bronchioles, alveolar ducts, and alveoli (Fig. 58.1). By definition, *bronchioles are airways with diameter less than 1 mm.*

## Which part of the airways offers maximum resistance to airflow, and why?

The multiple successive branching of the airways greatly increases the total cross-sectional area of the airways, from 2.5 $cm^2$ in the trachea to 12,000 $cm^2$ in the alveoli. Consequently, the resistance to airflow is much lower in the smaller airways, and *in health, most of the airways resistance is offered by the large airways.*

The trachea and bronchi have cartilage in their walls but relatively little smooth muscle. The walls of bronchioles and terminal bronchioles do not contain cartilage; instead, they contain more smooth muscle, of which the largest amount relative to the thickness of the wall is present in the terminal bronchioles. Hence, the diameter of smaller airways can change much more than that of the larger airways. *In obstructive lung diseases, it is the smaller airways that offer the bulk of the resistance.*

## What are the different types of cells lining the alveoli?

The alveoli are lined by two types of epithelial cells. **Type I cells** are flat cells with large cytoplasmic extensions and are the primary lining cells. **Type II cells (granular pneumocytes)** are thicker and contain numerous lamellar inclusion bodies. These cells secrete surfactant. The lungs also contain **pulmonary alveolar macrophages (PAM)** or the dust cells, lymphocytes, plasma cells, Clara cells (secretes a thin mucus), APUD (amine precursor uptake and decarboxylation) cells, and mast cells. The mast cells contain heparin, histamine, and various proteases that participate in allergic reactions.

## Compare and contrast coughing and sneezing.

**SIMILARITIES**

Both are concerned with the cleansing of the air passages by removing secretions or inhaled material.

Both are reflexes that have their centers in the medulla and efferent impulses of both the reflexes travel down vagus to the larynx / soft palate and by spinal nerves to diaphragm, abdominal and pelvic muscle that contract during cough / sneeze.

Both have the following sequence of: (i) a deep inspiration; (ii) trapping of air by shutting off its exit; (iii) initiation of expiratory effort, raising the intrathoracic pressure; (iv) augmentation of the pressure of the trapped air (the compressive stage); (v) sudden release of the trapped air at high pressure by opening up the exit passages (Fig. 58.2).

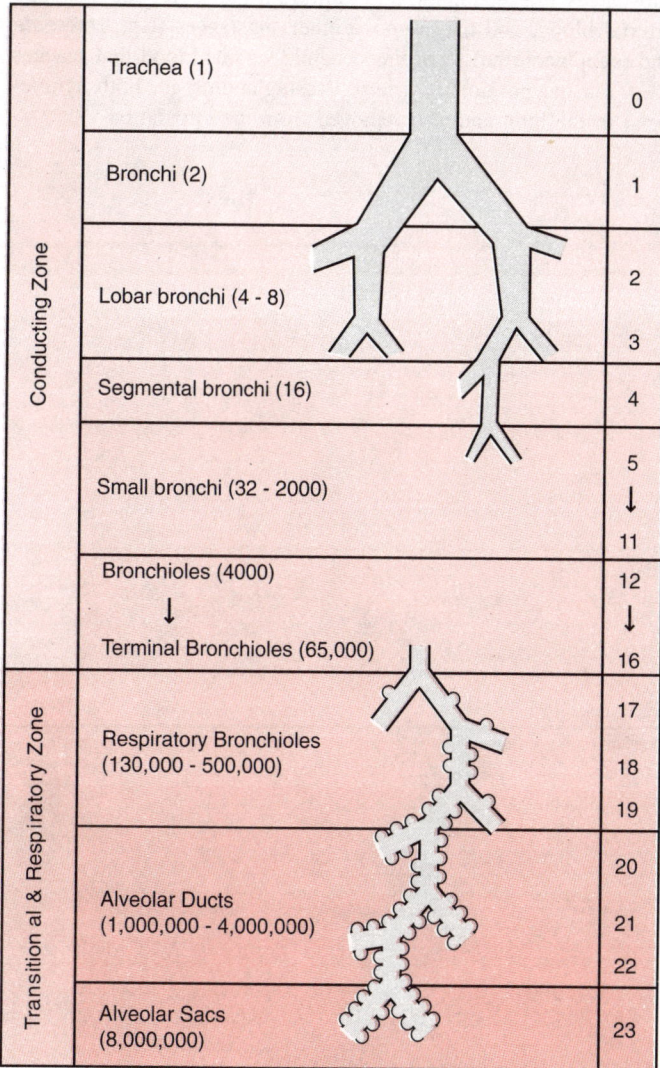

| | | |
|---|---|---|
| Conducting Zone | Trachea (1) | 0 |
| | Bronchi (2) | 1 |
| | Lobar bronchi (4 - 8) | 2 |
| | | 3 |
| | Segmental bronchi (16) | 4 |
| | Small bronchi (32 - 2000) | 5 ↓ 11 |
| | Bronchioles (4000) ↓ | 12 ↓ |
| | Terminal Bronchioles (65,000) | 16 |
| Transitional & Respiratory Zone | Respiratory Bronchioles (130,000 - 500,000) | 17 18 19 |
| | Alveolar Ducts (1,000,000 - 4,000,000) | 20 21 22 |
| | Alveolar Sacs (8,000,000) | 23 |

Fig. 58.1

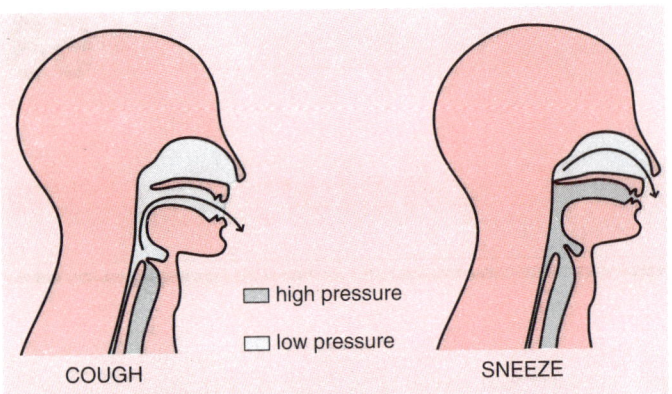

COUGH                               SNEEZE

☐ high pressure
☐ low pressure

**Fig. 58.2**

**DIFFERENCES**

| Cough | Sneeze |
| --- | --- |
| Stimulated by irritants in the tracheobronchial tree. | Stimulated by irritation of the nasal mucosa. |
| Impulses travel up via vagus and glossopharyngeal. | Impulses travel up via trigeminal. |
| Air is trapped behind the closed glottis by contraction of the laryngeal adductor muscles. | Air is trapped by shutting off the nasopharynx by raising of the soft palate and raising of the tongue to the hard palate. |
| Air is released by opening of the glottis. | Air is released by opening of the nasopharynx. |
| Can be reflex or voluntary. | Always reflex. |

### How do the cough originating in the upper and lower airways differ?

There are two types of cough, depending on the type of receptor stimulated. In the mucosa of large airways (larynx, trachea, bronchi), there are **mechanoreceptors** (rapidly adapting stretch receptors or irritant receptors sensitive to mechanical stimuli). They initiate a *forceful expiration without a preceding inspiration*. Absence of the preceding inspiration helps prevent aspiration of noxious material. Distal to the large airways up to the acinus, there are **chemical receptors**. When stimulated, these receptors *first initiate a deep inspiration and then a forceful expiration*.

### Enumerate the non-respiratory functions of the lung.

(1) They synthesize **surfactant**. (2) They contain a fibrinolytic system that lyses clots in the pulmonary vessels. (3) The lungs activate the physiologically inactive angiotensin I to angiotensin II in the pulmonary circulation. Large amounts of the **angiotensin-converting enzyme (ACE)** responsible for this activation are located on the surface of the endothelial cells of the pulmonary capillaries. ACE also inactivates bradykinin. (4) They release several substances like histamine and kallikrein that enter the systemic arterial blood, and they remove other substances (e.g., serotonin and norepinephrine) from the systemic venous blood that reaches them via the pulmonary artery. Prostaglandins are both synthesized in the lung and also removed from the circulation.

# 59

# Mechanics of Pulmonary Ventilation

### Name the muscles of inspiration.

The **diaphragm** and the **external intercostal muscles** maintain adequate ventilation at rest. Other muscles called **accessory muscles** of inspiration are required when greater inspiratory force is required as during exercise. These include the **quadratus lumborum** which serves a synergistic role with the diaphragm, acting as a stablizer, and the **scalenei** and the **sternocleidomastoid**.

### Name the muscles of expiration.

*Normal expiration occurs due to the passive recoil of the thoracic wall.* It does not require any muscle action. *Muscle action is required only during forced expiration* which is provided by the **internal intercostal muscle** and the **anterolateral abdominal muscles**.

### What are the different ways in which intrathoracic volume is changed?

During inspiration, all the three dimensions of the thoracic cavity expand, viz., the vertical (superoinferior) diameter, the anteroposterior diameter and the transverse diameter. There is a different mechanism for expansion in each direction. The **vertical diameter** increases when the diaphragm descends in the thoracic cavity. During quiet breathing, nearly 75% of this thoracic expansion occurs due **diaphragmatic descent** that ranges from 1.5cm (in eupnea) to 7.0 cm (in deep breathing). The **anteroposterior diameter** of the thorax increases during inspiration when the upper ribs ($2^{nd}$ to $6^{th}$ ribs), which normally slope obliquely downwards and forwards, swing upwards to a more horizontal position from their joints with the spine. This is called the **pump-handle movement**. The **transverse diameter** also increases during inspiration, but to a lesser degree. This occurs due to the movements of the lower ribs ($7^{th}$ to $10^{th}$ ribs) that swing outwards and upwards in inspiration. This is called the **bucket handle movement** (Fig. 59.1).

### What are Valsalva and Müller's maneuvers?

When forced expiration is performed against a closed glottis, it is called the **Valsalva's maneuver**. If this maneuver is performed simultaneously with contraction of abdominal muscles, it results in a sharp rise in intraabdominal pressure that helps in defecation and parturition. Conversely, forced inspiration against a closed glottis is called the **Müller's maneuver**.

### Why is pleural pressure subatmospheric?

At the end of quiet expiration, the thoracic pressure is –2.5 mm Hg. It is negative because at the end of quiet expiration, the lungs are trying to collapse to a smaller volume while the thorax is trying to expand to a larger volume. The *pleural pressure becomes more negative during inspiration* (Fig. 59.2).

### How is pleural pressure measured?

The intrapleural pressure is mostly inferred from **intraesophageal pressure** that is measured with an *intraesophageal balloon*. The intrapleural pressure can also be recorded by *inserting a needle into the intrapleural space*. A small air bubble is injected into the pleural space and the tip of the needle is kept in the bubble. This ensures that the tip of the needle does not get obliterated by the pleural membranes.

### Define compliance. What is the normal compliance of the lung and thorax?

**Lung compliance** (or stretchability) is defined as the change in lung volume for unit increase in pleural pressure. It is approximately 200mL / cm $H_2O$. **Thoracic compliance** is about the same as lung compliance, i.e., 200mL/cm $H_2O$. The combined compliance of lung plus thorax is given by the formula:

$$\frac{1}{\text{Total compliance}} = \frac{1}{\text{Lung compliance}} + \frac{1}{\text{Thoracic compliance}}$$

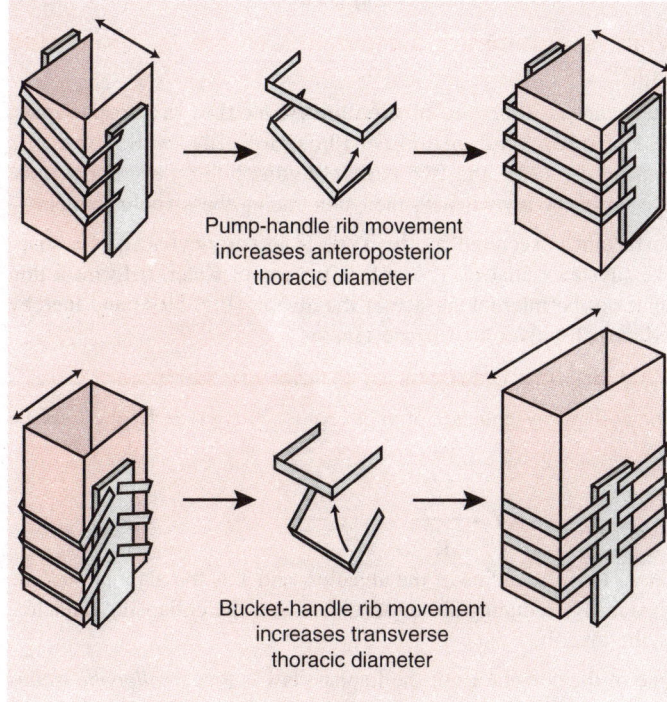

Pump-handle rib movement increases anteroposterior thoracic diameter

Bucket-handle rib movement increases transverse thoracic diameter

**Fig. 59.1**

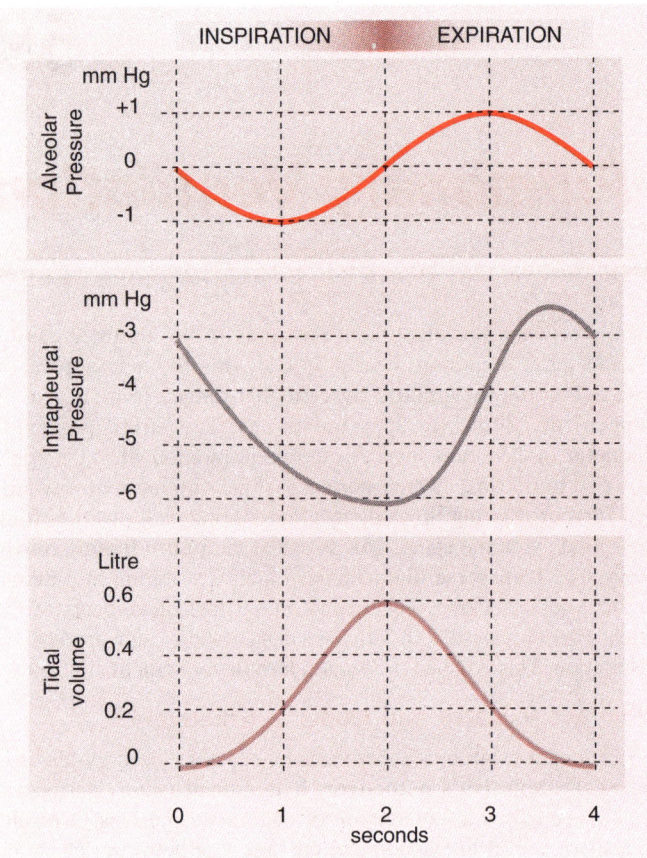

**Fig. 59.2**

The **combined compliance** of lung and thorax can therefore be calculated from the above formula to be about 100L/cm $H_2O$.

### What is specific lung compliance?

Specific compliance is lung compliance divided by the functional residual capacity (FRC) of the lung. The compliance of a large, healthy lung of an adult will be greater than the compliance of a small, healthy lung of a child. However, the specific lung compliance will be nearly equal in both. In other words, specific compliance is the *compliance of the lung tissue* and not of the lung as a whole.

### What is the difference between static and dynamic lung compliance?

For measurement of **static lung compliance**, adequate time must be allowed for lung volume to stabilize in response to a distending pressure. When adequate time is not allowed, what is measured is the **dynamic lung compliance**, as mostly done in clinics.

### How is lung compliance affected in emphysema?

In emphysema, the *static lung compliance increases* due to loss of elastic tissues but the *dynamic lung compliance decreases* due to dynamic airway compression.

### What are the conditions in which static lung compliance is reduced?

The compliance of the lung reduces in the recumbent position. This is due to the engorgement of the pulmonary vascular bed with blood that increases the overall stiffness of the lung tissue. Pathological conditions in which static lung compliance is decreased include fibrosis and pneumonia.

### What is hysteresis?

Measurement of compliance requires that the change of volume be recorded for unit change in pressure. The experimenter therefore has the liberty of making the measurements by either increasing or decreasing the pressure. Experimenters however noted that in case of the lungs, the compliance measured depended on whether measurements were made during its expansion or contraction. Thus, instead of getting a single compliance curve, experimenters obtained two curves – one for inspiration and the other for expiration. Together, the curves formed a loop called the **pressure-volume loop** (Fig. 59.3). This phenomenon is known as **hysteresis** (Gr. *hysterein* = to fall short, to lag behind). *Hysteresis occurs due to the presence of viscous (i.e., fluid) resistance* which is the resistance to movement offered by *surfactant* and *air*.

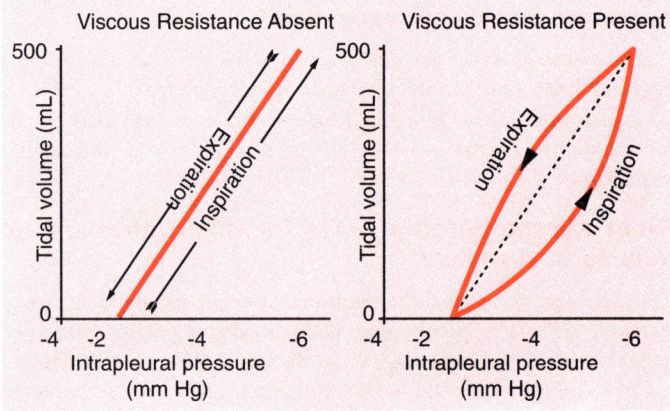

**Fig. 59.3**

### What is pulmonary surfactant? Where is it secreted from?

Surfactant is a mixture of **dipalmitoyl lecithin** (a phospholipid), other lipids, and proteins. Phospholipids, which have a *hydrophilic head* and two parallel hydrophobic *fatty acids tails*, line up in the alveoli with their tails facing the alveolar lumen.

Surfactant is secreted by the **Type-II pneumocytes**. It is a soap-like substance that lowers surface tension of water. It forms a thin layer on the internal surface of the alveoli (Fig. 59.4) and thereby reduces the alveolar surface tension.

### What are the functions of pulmonary surfactant?

The collapsing tendency of an alveolus (P) is given by the Laplace law:

$$P = \frac{2\,T}{R}$$

*where* R is the radius of the alveolus, and T is the alveolar surface tension. By reducing T, surfactant reduces the collapsing tendency of the alveoli.

One of the corrolaries of the Laplace law is that *smaller the radius of alveolus, greater is the collapsing tendency*. The alveoli in the lung are not uniform in size. Being interconnected, the smaller

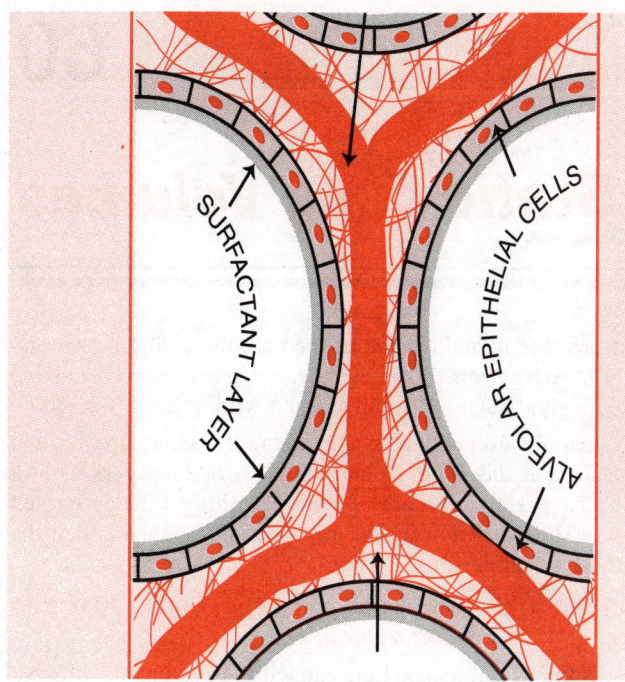

**Fig. 59.4**

alveoli would have emptied into the larger ones were it not for two factors: (i) Many of the alveoli share a common wall so that when one tends to collapse, it is prevented by the adjacent alveolus with which it shares a common wall, a phenomenon named **'interdependence'**. (ii) The total surfactant content of each alveolus is roughly the same. As a result, the smaller alveoli have a *greater concentration of surfactant molecules*, and therefore, a lower surface tension than the larger ones. According to Laplace law, the collapsing tendency is lesser when the surface tension is low. Hence, the difference in the surface tension in small and large alveoli effectively counterbalances the effect of difference in the radii.

### What happens when surfactant secretion is deficient?

Deficiency of surfactant occurs in *cigarette smokers* and in patients on *long-term 100% $O_2$ inhalation*. It is seen in *premature infants* not secreting adequate amounts of pulmonary surfactant (**infant respiratory distress syndrome** or the **hyaline membrane disease**). Deficiency of surfactant leads to collapse (**atelectesis**) of parts of the lung. It is possible that other cases of atelectesis, e.g., those occurring following bronchial or pulmonary artery obstruction, are also due to surfactant deficiency.

### What is work of breathing?

It is the work performed by the respiratory muscles in overcoming the elastic and viscous resistances offered by the chest wall, lungs and the airways. *During heavy breathing, the work of breathing can increase considerably.* It can be calculated graphically from the lung compliance curve (Fig. 59.5).

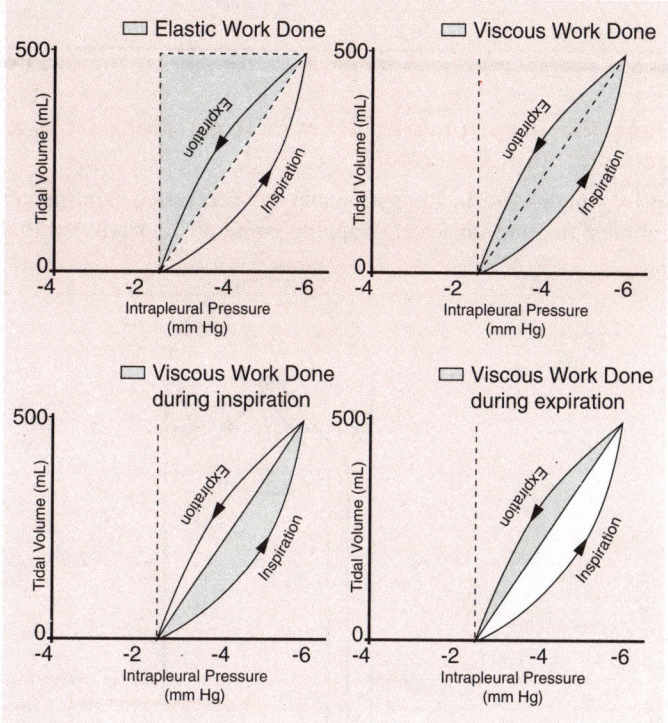

**Fig. 59.5**

# 60

# Static Lung Volumes

### Describe a spirometer. How is it different from a Benedict-Roth apparatus?

In its simplest form, the spirometer is an inverted light-metal cylinder floating on water, trapping some air under it. As the subject breathes in and out the trapped air, the cylinder rises and sinks. The movements of the cylinder are recorded on a moving drum through a system of a pulley and a writing lever (Fig. 60.1).

The system however involves rebreathing the same air over and over again and therefore, cannot be used for long periods at a stretch. To permit rebreathing, the breathing tube is passed through a soda-lime tower and the apparatus is then called the **Benedict-Roth apparatus** (Fig. 90.1).

### Enumerate the various lung volumes and capacities and give their normal values.

The terms **lung volumes** and **lung capacities** have slightly different meaning. *Capacities are made of one or more composite volumes* (Fig. 60.2). The **tidal volume (TV)** is the amount of air that moves into the lungs with a relaxed inspiration after a passive expiration. In other words, it is the amount of air that normally moves in or out of the lung with each breath. It is about 500mL. The **inspiratory reserve volume (IRV)** is the amount of air in excess of the tidal volume that can be inspired with a maximal inspiratory effort. It is about 2500 mL. The **expiratory reserve volume (ERV)** is the extra volume of air expelled after a passive expiration by a maximal expiratory effort. It is about 1000mL. The **inspiratory capacity (IC)** is the maximum amount of air that can be inspired after a passive expiration. It is about 3000mL. The **expiratory capacity (EC)** is the maximum amount of air that can be expired after a relaxed inspiration. It is about 1500 mL. The **vital capacity (VC)** is the maximum amount of air that can be inspired after a maximal expiration. It is about 4000mL.

$$IC = IRV + TV$$
$$EC = ERV + TV$$
$$VC = IRV + TV + ERV$$

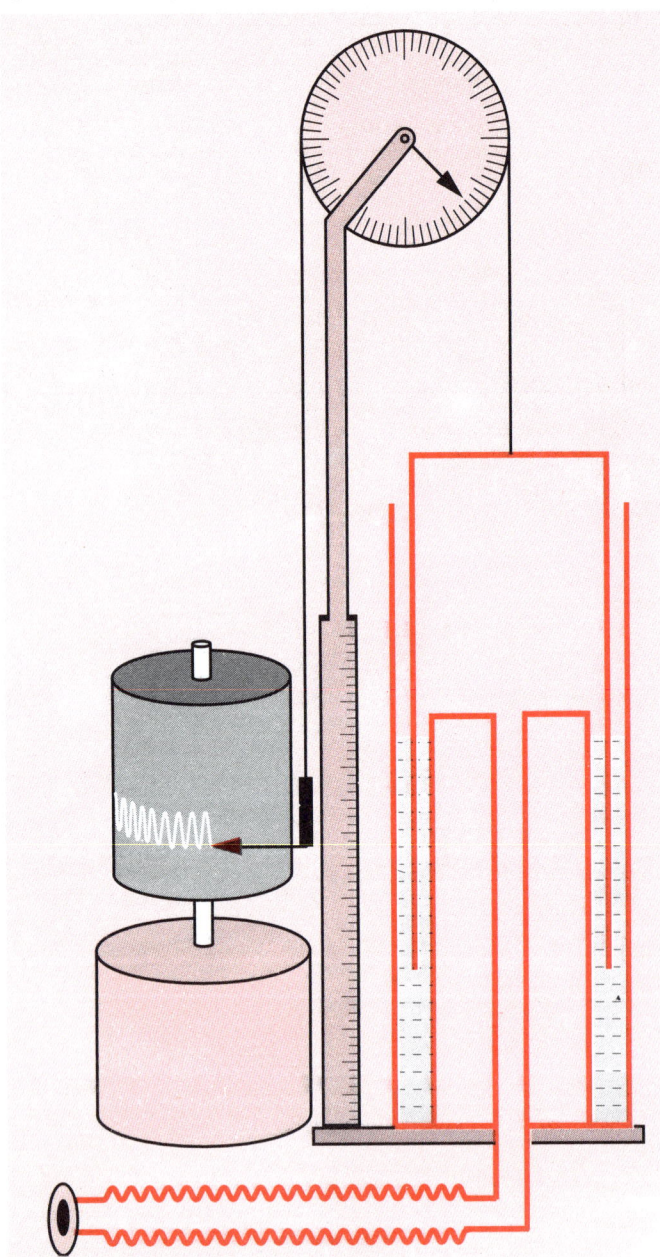

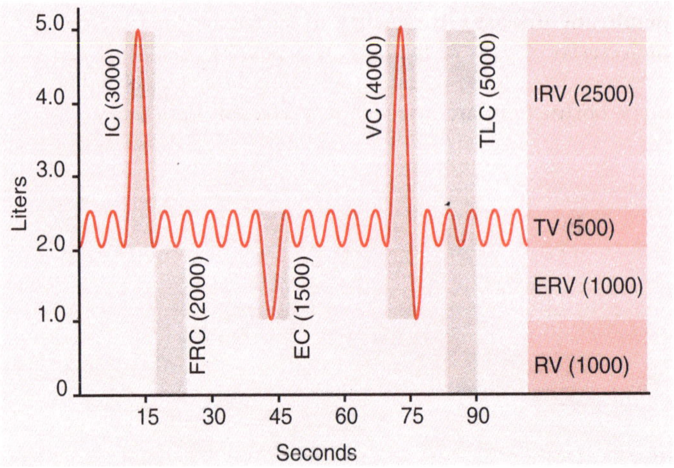

Fig. 60.1

Fig. 60.2

## Name the nonspirometric lung volumes and capacities.

Even after maximal expiration, a certain amount of air – called the **residual volume** – always remains in the lungs, which cannot be expelled in anyway. This amount cannot be estimated through spirometry and it requires special techniques to estimate it. The same is true for lung capacities that have residual volume as one of its components, like the **functional residual capacity** and the **total lung capacity**. **Residual volume (RV)** is the amount of air that remains in the lungs after maximal expiration. It is about 1000 mL. The **functional residual capacity (FRC)** is the amount of air that remains in the lungs after passive expiration. It is about 2000 mL. The **total lung capacity (TLC)** is the amount of air present in the lungs at the end of a maximal inspiration. It is about 5000 mL.

$$FRC = ERV + RV$$
$$TLC = IRV + TV + ERV + RV$$

## What is the physiological significance of FRC?

The FRC of about 2L represents the air that remains in the lung most of the time. Even after a forceful expiration, about 1L of air (the RV) remains in the lung. This has several advantages.

Because of the FRC, *$pO_2$ and $pCO_2$ do not fluctuate excessively*. Without the FRC, alveolar $pO_2$ would have risen to atmospheric levels (150 mm Hg) during inspiration, and reduced to nearly zero during expiration. However, because of the FRC, the $pO_2$ of the alveolar air remains fairly stable at ~ 100 mm Hg. In the same way, without FRC, the alveolar $pCO_2$ would have dropped to atmospheric levels (0.3 mmHg) during inspiration and to 0 mm Hg during expiration. In other words, the alveolar $pCO_2$ would have remained low throughout the breathing cycle. This *would have taken away the respiratory drive* that is provided mainly by $CO_2$. FRC helps to *dilute the effect of any toxic gases* that might be inhaled in small amounts. Without the FRC, the lungs would have collapsed totally at the end of each expiration. *Reexpansion of the lung from a totally collapsed state would have required tremendous breathing effort* in accordance with Laplace law. Moreover, the collapsed lung would have increased pulmonary vascular resistance and imposed a *heavy load on the left ventricle*.

## How is FRC measured?

Two methods are commonly employed for FRC estimation: the helium dilution technique (closed-circuit gas-dilution technique) and $N_2$-washout technique (open-circuit gas-dilution technique). A better but more expensive method is whole-body plethysmography. In the **closed circuit method**, the subject is given to rebreathe a known volume of gas mixture containing 80% oxygen and 20% helium (Fig. 60.3). As rebreathing progresses, the gas mixture gets diluted by the air inside the lungs and the helium concentration falls. The helium concentration stabilizes in about 5 minutes in normal individuals. The fall in helium concentration at equilibrium indicates the extent of dilution, which is proportional to the FRC.

*Example.*

A subject rebreathes into a 2L reservoir containing 20% helium and 80% oxygen. The total amount of helium in the reservoir is $2L \times 20/100 = 400mL$. After equilibrium, the helium concentration in the reservoir drops to 10%. Knowing that the total amount of helium was 400mL, it must have got distributed in $400mL \div 10/100 = 4000mL$ of gaseous space (the volume

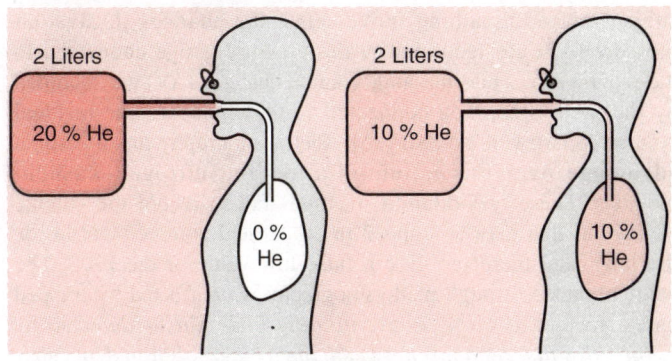

**Fig. 60.3**

of distribution). Since the volume of the reservoir is 2L, hence the remaining 2L of space must be the FRC.

In the **open circuit method**, the subject breathes in 100% oxygen and breathes it out into a large bag. Initially, the expired air contains a fairly large concentration of nitrogen. As the breathing continues, the concentration of nitrogen in the expired air decreases. The breathing is continued till the nitrogen concentration in the expired air is negligible. At this stage, it can be said that the nitrogen that was present in the lungs has been completely washed out. The product of the total volume of air collected (V) and the concentration of nitrogen (C) in it gives the total amount of nitrogen (Q) washed out of the lungs ($Q = C \times V$). Knowing that the concentration of nitrogen in the alveolar air was 80%, the FRC can be calculated using a similar formula $Q = 80\% \times FRC$.

*Example.*

A subject breathes in 40L of oxygen and the expired gas mixture has a nitrogen concentration of 5%. The total volume of nitrogen in the 40 liters of expired gas mixture (V) would be $40L \times 5\% = 2L$. Since the entire 2L of nitrogen must have been present in the lung at a concentration of 80%, the resting volume of the lung (FRC) must have been $2 \div 80/100 = 2.5L$.

In **plethysmography**, the subject sits in an air-tight chamber made of transparent plastic (the whole-body plethysmograph) and tries to breathe against a tube connected to pressure gauge. As the

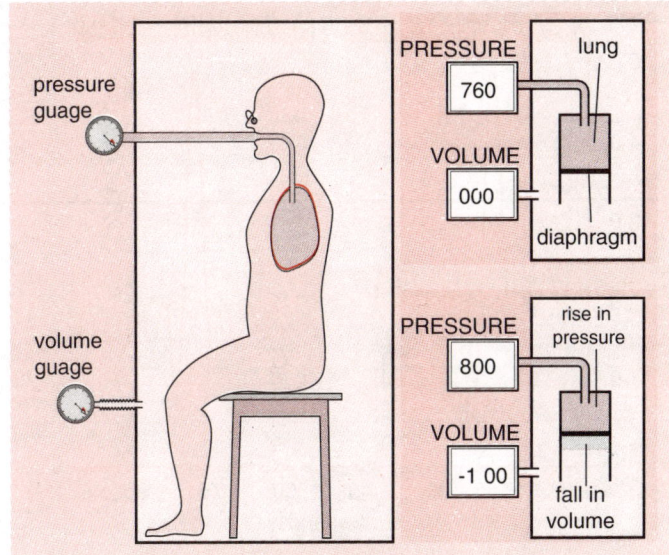

**Fig. 60.4**

subject makes breathing movements, the changes in alveolar pressure ($\Delta P$) are recorded by the pressure gauge connected to the mouthpiece while the lung volume changes ($\Delta V$) are recorded by the plethysmograph connected to the chamber. The residual volume V is given by $P \times \Delta V / \Delta P$. Plethysmography has a distinct advantage over the helium-dilution and nitrogen-washout methods. These 'gas-dilution' methods fail to record the volume of any gas that may be trapped in an isolated compartment inside the lung, and therefore give a false-low value of the FRC. The value obtained through plethysmography is unaffected by trapped gases. In fact, *a large, nonventilating bleb can be detected by noting the discrepancy between the values obtained by gas-dilution and plethysmography.*

### Example

While blowing into the pressure gauge, a subject records a rise in pressure from 760 to 800 mm Hg, i.e., a rise of 40 mm Hg. from Simultaneously, the plethysmograph records a decrease in volume by 100mL. The FRC of the subject can be calculated to be:

$$760 \times (100 \div 40)$$
$$= \quad 1900 \text{ mL}$$

## What are the physiological factors affecting lung volumes?

FRC denotes the *resting volume* of the lung. It is usually thought to be the volume at which the *collapsing force of the lung* balances the *expansive force of the thorax.* However, there is a third important factor: the *end-expiratory diaphragmatic tone.* If the diaphragm does not relax fully at the end of expiration, the FRC will remain somewhat high. This is true in most normal individuals. Hence, *during anesthesia, the FRC decreases by about 400 mL* due to the complete relaxation of the diaphragm.

Change in posture also affects FRC (Fig. 60.5). *During supine position, FRC decreases* by about 25% due to the pressure of the abdominal contents on the diaphragm and the restriction of thoracic cage movements by the bed or floor. Had it not been for the end-expiratory diaphragmatic tone, the reduction in FRC during supine position would have been greater.

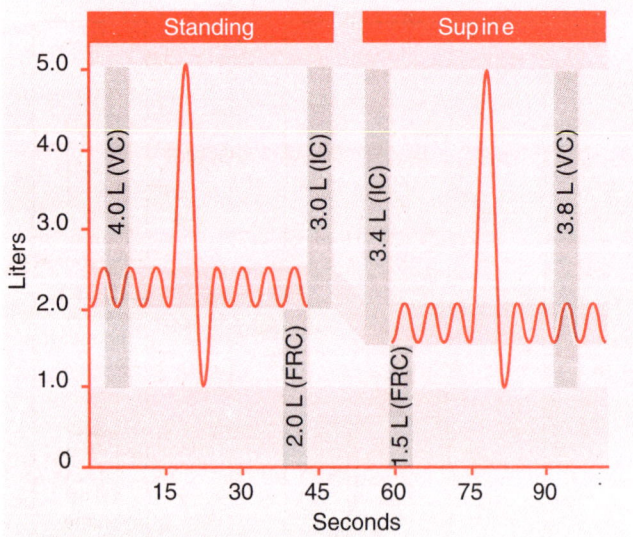

**Fig. 60.5**

In *supine position,* the vital capacity decreases mainly due to the increased venous return, which engorges the pulmonary vessels with blood and displaces an equal amount of air from the lung. However, the inspiratory capacity increases because while the FRC decreases by nearly 25% in the supine position, the VC decreases by only 5%.

FRC *increases with body height* and is slightly *more in males* than in females of same height. It is markedly *reduced in obesity,* and shows a slight *increase with age.*

The inspiratory capacity, and therefore the vital capacity are increased by *activities that strengthen the accessory muscles of inspiration* like swimming and rowing.

*Obesity* is also associated with a reduction in FRC and ERV and a compensatory increase in IC. The RV is not reduced. The reduction in FRC is due to reduced thoracic compliance caused by the weight added to the chest wall. TLC and VC do not change much. Thus, on the whole, the changes associated with obesity are similar to the changes associated with supine position.

In *pregnancy,* the RV is reduced due to the gravid uterus pushing the diaphragm up. However, the IC increases due to a compensatory increase in the rib excursions. Hence, the VC and TLC remain unchanged (Fig. 60.6).

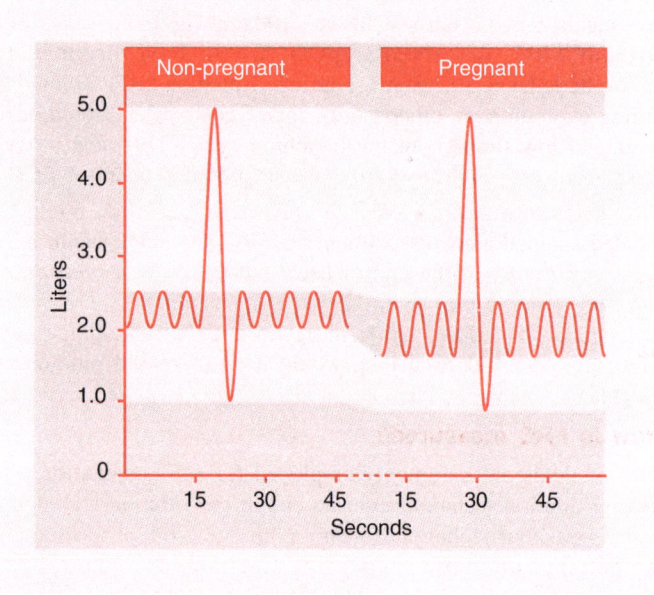

**Fig. 60.6**

Pregnancy is also associated with an increase in the respiratory rate and a greater increase in the tidal volume so that there is 70% increase in the respiratory minute volume. These ventilatory changes are caused by the hormone progesterone, which increases greatly in pregnancy.

# 61

# Dynamic Lung Volumes

## What are forced expiratory volumes? How are they measured?

**Forced expiratory volume** (also called **timed vital capacity**) is a general term for the *volume of air that is expired forcefully in a specified time interval*. It can be measured with a spirometer. The subject is initally asked to breathe normally into a spirometer while the spirogram is recorded on a drum moving at low speed (about 1mm/s). Thereafter, the subject breathes in maximally, holds his breath as the drum speed is increased (to about 20mm/s), and then expires maximally as fast as possible. The graph thus obtained (Fig. 61.1) is almost identical to a typical spirogram (Fig. 60.2) except that a small part of it has been stretched out in time.

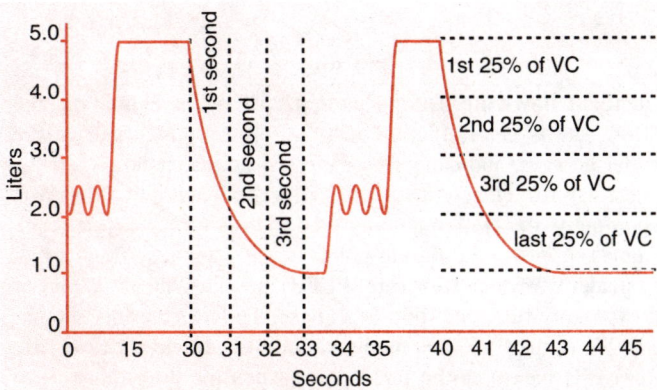

**Fig. 61.2**

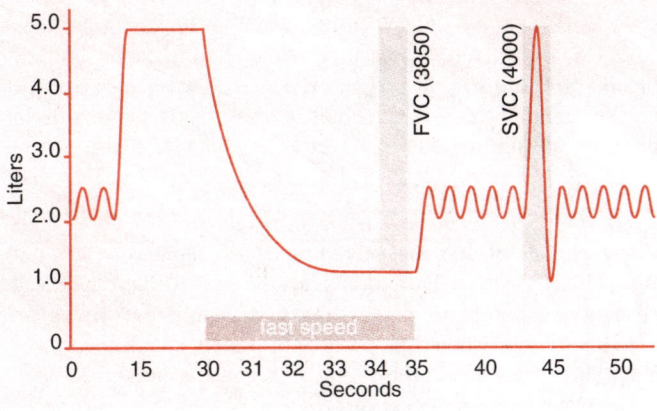

**Fig. 61.1**

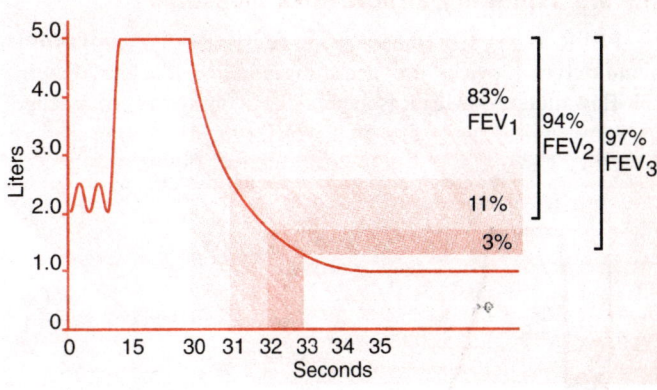

**Fig. 61.3**

The graph permits the measurement of all the sprometric volumes and capacities. Numerous specific indices can be defined based on the time interval in which the expired volume is measured. However, the most commonly measured index is the $FEV_1$. It is the *maximal volume of air which the subject can breathe out in the first second of a forced expiration*. The other forced expiratory volumes are $FEV_2$ and $FEV_3$.

$FEV_1$ becomes more meaningful when it is expressed as a percentage of the FVC. The *$FEV_1$/ FVC ratio is the cornerstone of the diagnosis of obstructive airway disease*. Normally, $FEV_1$/FVC is 83%, $FEV_2$/FVC is 94% and $FEV_3$/FVC is 97% (Fig. 61.3).

## What is the difference between slow and fast vital capacities?

The *vital capacity recorded during forceful expiration is lesser than the vital capacity recorded when it is not forceful*. Hence, the former is called **forced vital capacity (FVC)** to distinguish it from the latter which is called the **slow vital capacity (SVC)**.

## What is forced expiratory time?

The time taken for completing the expiration forcefully (approximately 4 seconds) is called **forced expiratory time (FET)**. Although not a very precise index, it provides a useful bedside test to the clinician. The forced expiration is heard by auscultating (hearing through the stethoscope) the lungs and is timed using the wrist watch. *When FET exceeds 4 seconds, airway obstruction is suspected* and when it exceeds 6 seconds, the clinician is almost sure.

## What are expiratory airflow rates? What is their significance?

For measurement of expiratory airflow rates, the entire volume of expired air is segmented into four quarters (Fig. 61.2). The indices obtained are called **expiratory airflow rates.** During the first 25% of the expiration, the airflow rate is determined almost entirely by the strength of the expiratory muscles. Hence, it is called **effort**

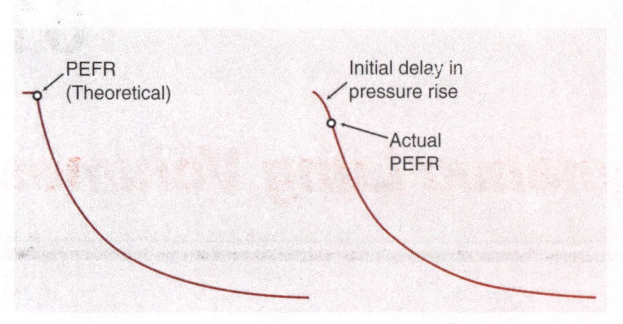

**Fig. 61.4**

**dependent flow-rate**. During the last 25% of the expiration, the airflow rate is determined almost entirely by the caliber of the smaller airways, and cannot be increased no matter how hard the subject expires. Hence, it is called **effort-independent flow-rate**. Accordingly, the two commonly used indices of airflow rates are designed to measure different points of the expiratory flow curve. The **peak expiratory flow rate (PEFR)** measures the initial part of the expiratory flow rate (Fig. 61.4) when the lungs are full to more than 75% of the FVC, and the **maximal mid-expiratory flow rate (MMEFR)** measures the middle part when the lungs are full to about 50% of the FVC.

## How are expiratory airflow rates measured?

The PEFR is mostly measured directly with **respiratory anemometers** (devices for measuring airflow) like the **Wright peak-flow meter**. MMEFR is measured by considering the average flow between 75% and 25% of the FVC (Fig. 61.5). Hence, it is also called **FEF$_{25-75\%}$** (FEF = forced expiratory flow).

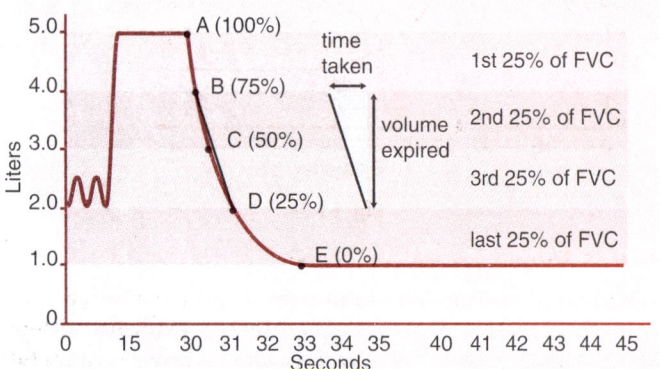

**Fig. 61.5**

## How much is the normal PEFR?

PEFR ranges from *5-15L/s in males* and *2.5-10L/s in females*. Much higher flow rates are recordable during cough. Hence it is important that the subject does not 'cough' into the mouthpiece.

## What are the advantages and disadvantages of recording PEFR?

Since PEFR measures the initial part of expiration, it reflects mainly the caliber of the *bronchi and larger bronchioles*. Hence, the test is widely used to monitor patients of asthma who have variable degrees of bronchoconstriction. Being effort-dependent, it may

be *reduced if the respiratory muscles are weak*. For the same reason, it is also *low if the TLC is reduced* (i.e., restrictive disorder) since at low lung volumes, expiratory force produced is lesser. Measuring PEFR alone is therefore a poor substitute for a complete spirometry. Its only advantage is that it can be measured using small and handy instrument and is therefore used for monitoring airway obstruction for large health surveys or when a spirometer is not available.

## How much is the normal respiratory minute volume? How is it measured?

Respiratory minute volume is the amount of air expired over a period of 1 minute when the subject is breathing normally. It is also called **pulmonary ventilation**.

Respiratory minute volume = Tidal volume × Respiratory rate

It can be measured simply by asking the subject to breathe in through nose and expire the air into a large bag (the **Douglas bag**) for 1 minute and then measuring the volume of air collected. The *normal respiratory minute volume is 6L*.

## What is the normal maximum breathing capacity? What is the use of measuring it?

Maximum breathing capacity (MBC) is the maximum volume of air which the subject can expire in 1 minute *when breathing as deeply and as rapidly as possible*. Ideally, maximum breathing capacity is attained, and therefore measured, either during exercise or by rebreathing into a bag so that the $CO_2$ is not washed out of the lungs. In actual practice, what is mostly measured is the **maximum voluntary ventilation (MVV)** which is less than the MBC.

For determination of MVV, the subject is asked to breathe in and out of a spirometer *as fast and as deeply as possible* for 15 seconds (Longer periods of maximal breathing causes faintness). It is left to the subject to strike the right balance between tidal volume and respiratory rate so as to achieve maximal ventilation. However, the breathing rate should be preferably greater than 80/min. The amount of air breathed in (or out) in 15 seconds is multiplied by 4, and the results are expressed in L/min.

The *normal MVV is 125 ± 25L/min.* in young males. Before the introduction of FEV$_1$, *MVV used to be the major dynamic spirometric test used for diagnosis of airway obstruction*. The MVV is less in such patients. However, *the test is exhausting and causes faintness*. It is affected by the motivation and endurance of the subject. Other factors affecting it are the compliance of the lung and thorax and the strength of respiratory muscles. *After the advent of FEV$_1$, MVV is left with very little utility*.

## Define breathing reserve and dyspneic index.

The difference between MVV and RMV is called the **breathing reserve (BR)**. The breathing reserve expressed as a fraction of the MVV is called the **dyspneic index** because a reduction of the dyspneic index below 60% is associated with dyspnea. Current medical opinion does not attach any significance to these indices.

$$\text{Breathing reserve} = \text{MVV} - \text{RMV}$$

$$\text{Dyspneic index} = \frac{\text{MVV} - \text{RMV}}{\text{MVV}} \times 100$$

# 62

# Alveolar Ventilation, Perfusion & Gaseous Exchange

## What is anatomic dead space? How is it measured?

During quiet breathing, about 500 mL of air in inspired and expired (the tidal volume). Not all the air that is breathed in enters the alveoli. *About 150 mL of inspired air remains in the upper airways, trachea and bronchi*, and therefore *do not participate in gaseous diffusion*. This is called the **anatomic dead space**. The anatomic dead space can be measured by the **single-breath** $N_2$ method, which is as follows. At the end of a quiet expiration, the subject takes in a deep breath of pure $O_2$ and breathes it out slowly and steadily. The exhaled air is instantaneously monitored for its $N_2$ content. The initial volume of air which is entirely $N_2$ free gives the anatomic dead space. The air exhaled thereafter, which comes from the alveoli, has a higher concentration of nitrogen (Fig. 62.1).

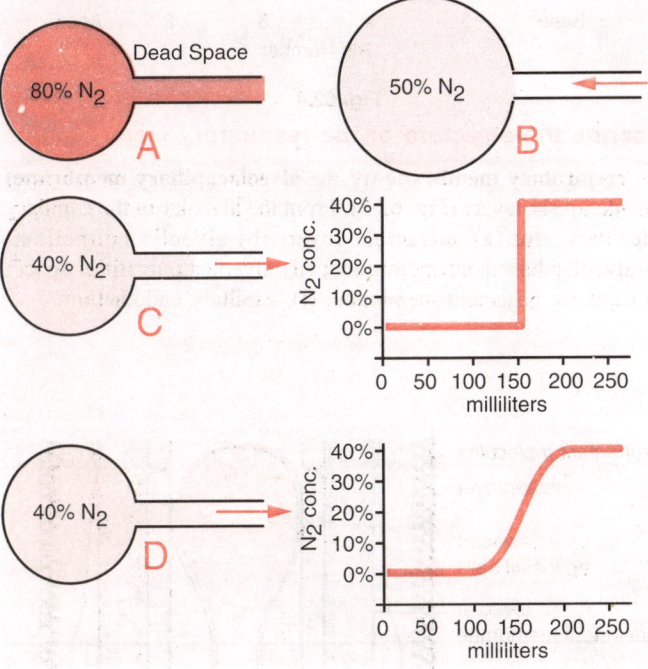

**Fig. 62.1**

## What is physiologic dead space? How is it measured?

Normally, about 350 mL enters the alveoli with each breath. Not all the air that enters the alveoli participates in alveolar gas exchange. This is because the alveolus might not be getting adequate blood supply, or its walls might not permit adequate diffusion. Such spaces in the alveoli are called **alveolar dead space**. The sum of anatomic dead space and alveolar dead space is called the **physiological dead space**. Hence, the physiological dead space is

the volume of inspired air, either in the airways or in the alveoli, that does not participate in gaseous exchange. The physiological dead space (PDS) can be calculated using the **Bohr equation**:

$$P_{CO_2\,[exp]} \times TV = P_{CO_2\,[art]} \times (TV - PDS) + P_{CO_2\,[insp]} \times PDS$$

*where:*

| | | |
|---|---|---|
| $P_{CO_2\,[exp]}$ | *is* | $P_{CO_2}$ in expired air |
| $P_{CO_2\,[art]}$ | *is* | $P_{CO_2}$ in arterial blood |
| $P_{CO_2\,[insp]}$ | *is* | $P_{CO_2}$ in inspired air |
| TV | *is* | Tidal volume |

Ignoring $P_{CO_2\,[insp]}$, the formula reduces to

$$P_{CO_2\,[exp]} \times TV = P_{CO_2\,[art]} \times (TV - PDS)$$

*Example*

| | | |
|---|---|---|
| $P_{CO_2\,[exp]}$ | = | 28 mm Hg |
| $P_{CO_2\,[art]}$ | = | 40 mm Hg |
| TV | = | 500 mL |
| $28 \times 500$ | = | $40 \times (500 - PDS)$ |
| | = | 150 mL |

## How is alveolar ventilation calculated?

Alveolar ventilation is defined as amount of inspired air entering the alveoli per minute during normal breathing. It is given by the formula:

| | | |
|---|---|---|
| Alveolar ventilation | = | (tidal volume – anat. dead space) × respiratory rate |
| | = | (500 mL – 150 mL) × 14/min |
| | = | 4900 mL /min |
| | = | 5 L/min (approximately) |

## What is the effect of gravity on alveolar air ventilation?

Gravity reduces the ventilation of the apical alveoli, i.e., the alveoli that are nearer to the apex of the lungs. The reason is two-fold: (a) gravity reduces the compliance of the apical alveoli, and (b) gravity increases the pleural pressure near the base of the lungs. In the erect posture, the *apical alveoli are larger but poorly ventilated* while the basal alveoli are smaller but better ventilated. This is because the weight of the lungs stretches the apical alveoli to nearly their maximum size, leaving little room for further expansion during inspiration (Fig. 62.2). In other words, apical alveoli have lower compliance. *Although apical alveoli are poorly ventilated, the $P_{O_2}$ of apical alveoli is higher*. This is because of the effect of gravity on alveolar perfusion.

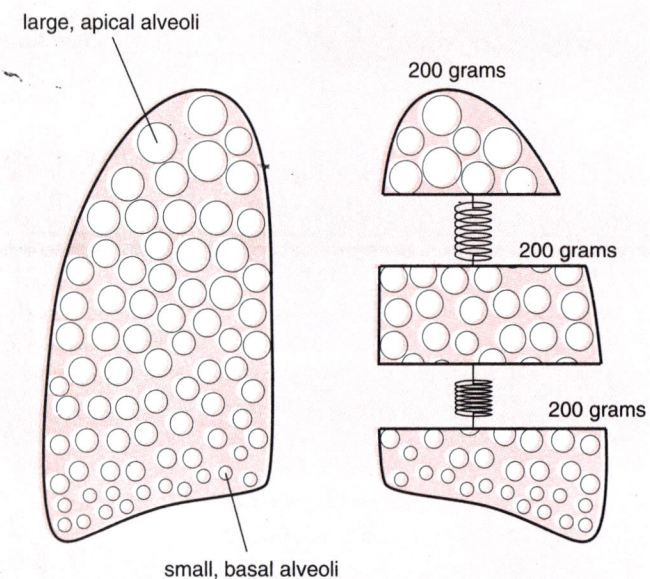

**Fig. 62.2**

### What is the effect of gravity on alveolar perfusion?

In the erect posture, the basal alveoli are much better perfused than the apical alveoli. The composition of air in the well-perfused basal alveoli therefore tends to approximate with that of pulmonary arterial blood, i.e., having high $P_{CO_2}$ and low $P_{O_2}$. Conversely, the alveolar air composition of the poorly perfused apical alveoli approximates more with that of inspired air, i.e., it has low $P_{CO_2}$ and high $P_{O_2}$ (Fig. 62.3). The high $P_{O_2}$ in apical alveoli is the reason for the vulnerability of apical areas of the lungs to infection by *Mycobacterium tuberculosis*.

### What is ventilation-perfusion ratio?

Considering that the cardiac output is 5.0L/min and alveolar ventilation too is about 5.0L/min, the overall ventilation: perfusion (V/Q) ratio is 1:1. Ideally, therefore, each alveolus should have a V/Q ratio of 1:1. However, that is not so even in the normal lungs.

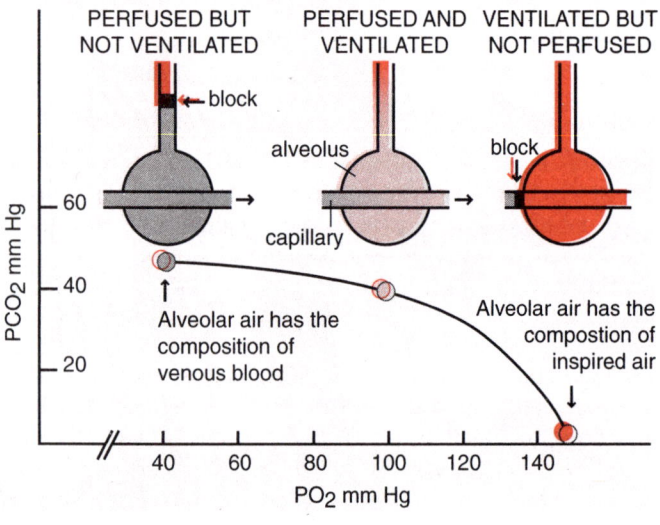

**Fig. 62.3**

The *apical alveoli are both underventilated and underperfused* while the *basal alveoli are both overventilated and overperfused* (Fig. 62.4). However, gravity affects perfusion much more than it affects ventilation. Hence, *apical alveoli are more underperfused than underventilated* (V/Q = 3) while the *basal alveoli are more overperfused than overventilated* (V/Q = 0.6). These regional inequities in ventilation and perfusion get exaggerated in diseases, resulting in gross impairment of alveolar gas exchange with consequent hypoxic hypoxia.

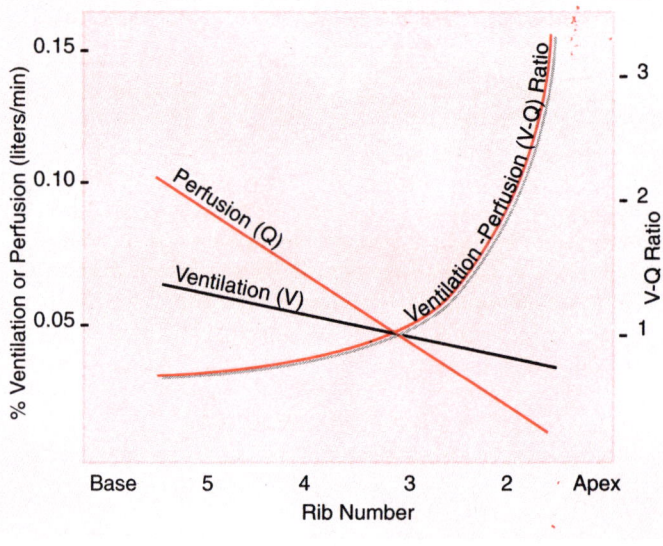

**Fig. 62.4**

### Describe the structure of the respiratory membrane.

The **respiratory membrane** (or the **alveolocapillary membrane**) is made up six layers (Fig. 62.5). From the alveolar to the capillary side, they are: (a) surfactant layer; (b) alveolar epithelium; (c) alveolar basement membrane; (d) alveolar interstitial space; (e) capillary basement membrane; (f). capillary endothelium.

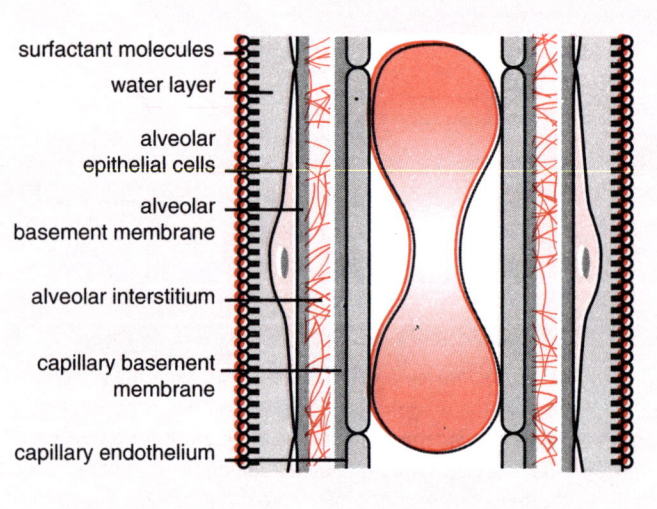

**Fig. 62.5**

It is ~0.5μ thick, and its total surface area in the two lungs equals ~100m². The gases have to pass through these layers while diffusing from the alveoli to pulmonary blood.

### Define the diffusion capacity of the lung.

The **diffusion capacity** of the lung for a given gas is defined as *the volume of gas diffusing across the respiratory membrane in 1 minute when the pressure gradient is 1 mm Hg*. It is given by the formula:

$$D_L = K \times \frac{A}{D} \times \frac{S}{\sqrt{W}}$$

*where*

A is the surface area of the respiratory membrane
D is the thickness of the respiratory membrane
S is the solubility of the gas in the respiratory membrane
W is the molecular weight of the gas.

$S \div \sqrt{W}$ is also called the **diffusion coefficient** of the gas. Other things remaining constant, gases diffuse through the respiratory membrane in proportion to their diffusion coefficients.

### How is the diffusion capacity for oxygen measured?

The diffusion capacity for $O_2$ is rarely measured directly because it involves measurement of $P_{CO_2}$ in pulmonary venous blood, which is very difficult. Instead, it is calculated from the diffusion capacity for carbon monoxide (CO), which has the advantage that once in blood, it reacts with hemoglobin to form carboxyhemoglobin. Hence, CO has a *negligible partial pressure in pulmonary venous blood*. The diffusion capacity measured for CO at rest is about 17 mL/min/mm Hg. Since the diffusion coefficient of $O_2$ is 1.23 times greater than that of CO, the diffusion capacity for $O_2$ can be calculated to be approximately 20 mL / min / mm Hg.

### How is diffusion capacity affected by exercise?

The diffusion capacity *increases up to threefold* during exercise because of capillary dilation and an increase in the number of active capillaries.

# 63

# Transport of Gases in Blood

### What is the normal alveolar air composition?

The alveolar $pO_2$ is 100mmHg and $P_{CO_2}$ is 40 mm Hg. Aqueous tension is 47 mm Hg (Fig. 63.1).

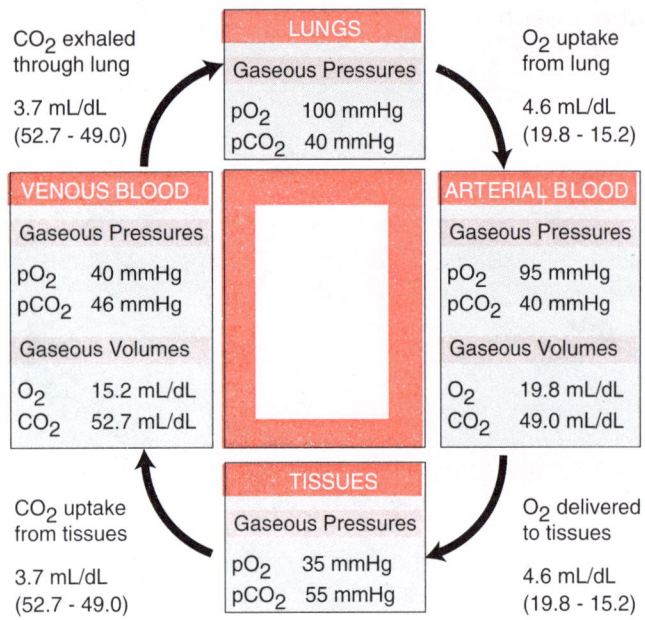

**Fig. 63.1**

### What are the different forms in which $O_2$ is carried in blood?

Oxygen is carried in blood, either in **dissolved form**, or as **oxyhemoglobin**.

### How much oxygen is carried in plasma?

The amount of $O_2$ normally transported in plasma is only about 1.5% of the total amount transported. The volume of oxygen (ml/ 100 ml of blood) that is dissolved in plasma is directly proportional to the $pO_2$ and is given by the formula: $0.003 \times pO_2$ (Fig. 63.2).

### How much oxygen is carried in hemoglobin?

Hemoglobin carries the bulk of the $O_2$ under normal circumstances. When 100% saturated:

*   1 gram of hemoglobin can carry a maximum of **1.34 ml of oxygen**.
*   100 mL of blood with 15 g/100mL of hemoglobin contain **20.1 mL of oxygen**.

The amount of oxygen carried is actually higher (1.39 mL) for pure

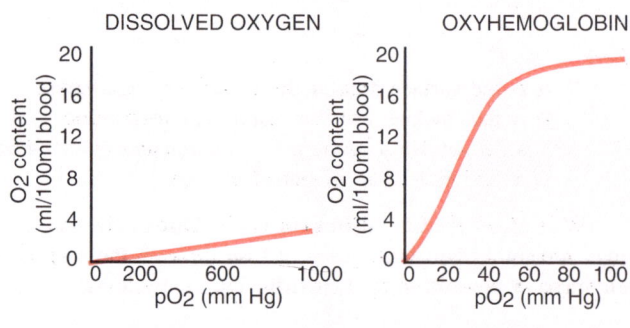

**Fig. 63.2**

hemoglobin-A. However in blood, a small amount of hemoglobin always remains in inactive form and hence, the clinically measured values are lower.

### How much oxygen is delivered to the tissues?

100ml of arterial blood contains 19.8ml of $O_2$ while venous blood contains 15.2 ml of $O_2$. Therefore the amount of $O_2$ delivered by 100ml of blood is 4.6ml (i.e., 19.8 - 15.2). For 5L of blood, this translates to 230mL of $O_2$.

| $O_2$ content of 100 ml of blood | | |
|---|---|---|
| | *Arterial* | *Venous* |
| | *($pO_2$=95 mm Hg)* | *($pO_2$=40 mm Hg)* |
| *Hemoglobin-bound* | 19.5 | 15.08 |
| *Dissolved* | 0.29 | 0.12 |
| *Total* | 19.8 | 15.2 |

### What is the $O_2$ dissociation curve?

The amount of oxyhemoglobin formed is proportional to the partial pressure of oxygen. By plotting the amount of oxyhemoglobin against the $pO_2$, the **oxygen dissociation curve** is obtained. The curve is not straight (as in case of dissolved $O_2$) but **sigmoid**. The amount of oxyhemoglobin is often expressed as **percentage saturation**, i.e., the percentage of total hemoglobin that gets oxygenated (Fig. 63.3).

### What are the factors causing a shift in the $O_2$ dissociation curve?

Factor causing right-shift (Fig. 63.3) are (i) increased $P_{CO_2}$; (ii) decreased (acidic) pH; (iii) increase in temperature; and (iv) increase in the DPG content of RBC.

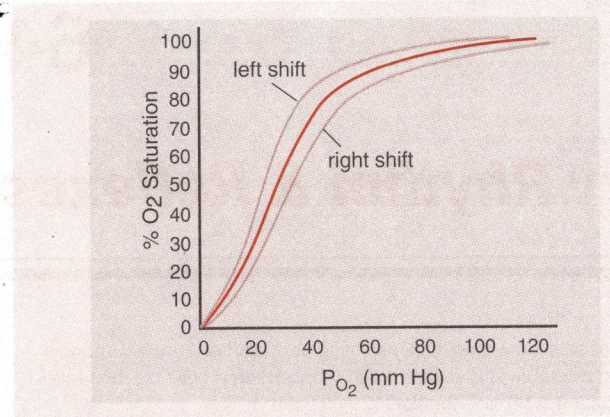

**Fig. 63.3**

## What is Bohr effect?

The right-shift in $O_2$ dissociation curve that is brought about by $H^+$, and therefore, by increased $P_{CO_2}$ or decreased pH is known as the Bohr effect.

## What are the different forms in which $CO_2$ is transported in blood?

$CO_2$ is transported in the blood in 3 forms: as **bicarbonate**, as **carbamino hemoglobin** and as **dissolved $CO_2$**. In carbamino hemoglobin, $CO_2$ binds to the terminal $NH_2$ groups of valine of $\alpha$ and $\beta$ chains. The volume of dissolved $CO_2$ (ml/100 ml) is 6% of $CO_2$.

## What is chloride shift?

RBCs contain the enzyme carbonic anhydrase that catalyzes the following reaction:

$$CO_2 + H_2O = HCO_3^- + H^+$$

Hence, when $CO_2$ diffuses into the RBC, it reacts chemically with water to generate $HCO_3^-$. The $H^+$ are mopped up by hemoglobin which is an excellent buffer. This enables the reaction to proceed in the forward direction. The $HCO_3^-$ ions generated diffuse out into the plasma in exchange for $Cl^-$ ions which diffuse in simultaneously. The *movement of chlorides into the RBC is called* **chloride shift**. The above events result in an increase in the total number of ions inside the RBC, which increases its osmolarity. As a result, water enters the RBC through osmosis. Hence, RBCs carrying $CO_2$ in bicarbonate form will be somewhat larger than normal. This is manifest in the *slightly higher (~ 3%) PCV of venous blood*.

## How much $CO_2$ is brought back from the tissues?

100 ml of venous blood carries 53 ml of $CO_2$ while the same volume of arterial blood carries 49 ml $CO_2$. Thus 100 ml of blood takes away 4 ml of $CO_2$ (53 ml – 49 ml) from the tissues. Therefore 5 L blood takes away 200 mL of $CO_2$ from the tissues each minute.

| $CO_2$ content of 100 ml of blood | | | | |
|---|---|---|---|---|
| | **Arterial blood** | **%** | **Venous blood** | **%** |
| $HCO_3^-$ | 43.8 ml | 90 | 46.3 ml | 88 |
| Carbamino Hb | 2.6 ml | 5 | 3.4 ml | 6 |
| Dissolved | 2.6 ml | 5 | 3.0 ml | 6 |
| Total | 49.0 ml | 100 | 52.7 ml | 100 |

## What are the factors causing a shift in the $CO_2$ dissociation curve?

The $CO_2$ dissociation curve is shifted to the right by $O_2$ and DPG.

## What is Haldane (CDH) effect?

Haldane effect is the right-shift in $CO_2$ dissociation curve that is brought about by a rise in $P_{O_2}$.

## How does the $O_2$ dissociation curve of myoglobin compare with that of hemoglobin?

Myoglobin is an iron-containing pigment that is similar to hemoglobin except that it *contains only one polypeptide chain* instead of four. It binds to one molecule of $O_2$. Its dissociation curve is a rectangular hyperbola and lies well to the left of the $O_2$ dissociation curve of hemoglobin. Its *left-shifted curve* makes it specially suitable for taking up $O_2$ at low $pO_2$. It *does not show the Bohr effect* which if present would be disadvantageous to its very purpose.

## Compare and contrast Bohr and Haldane effects.

**SIMILARITIES**

Both relate to the factors affecting transport of blood gases.

Both are ultimately due to the fact that deoxyhemoglobin binds $H^+$ more actively.

**DIFFERENCES**

| Bohr effect | Haldane effect |
|---|---|
| It is the effect of $H^+$ and $CO_2$ on the $O_2$ dissociation curve | It is the effect of $O_2$ on the $CO_2$ dissociation curve |
| Due to Bohr effect, blood takes up more $O_2$ in lungs and gives off more $O_2$ to the tissues | Due to Haldane effect blood takes up more $CO_2$ in tissues and give off more $CO_2$ in lungs |

# 64

# Neural Bases of Respiratory Rhythm & Reflexes

## Describe the classical theory of neural control of respiration.

According to the classical theory, the respiratory rhythm is controlled by four centers (Fig. 64.1). (i) the **inspiratory center** having a pacemaker activity, enabling it to initiate inspiration; (ii) the **expiratory center** which terminates the inspiratory activity; (iii) the **apneustic center** which accentuates inspiration by stimulating the inspiratory center; and (iv) the **pneumotaxic center** which promotes expiration by stimulating the expiratory center and also, by inhibiting the apneustic center. In addition, vagal afferents from the stretch receptors in the lungs inhibit the apneustic center once the lung expansion exceeds 800 mL.

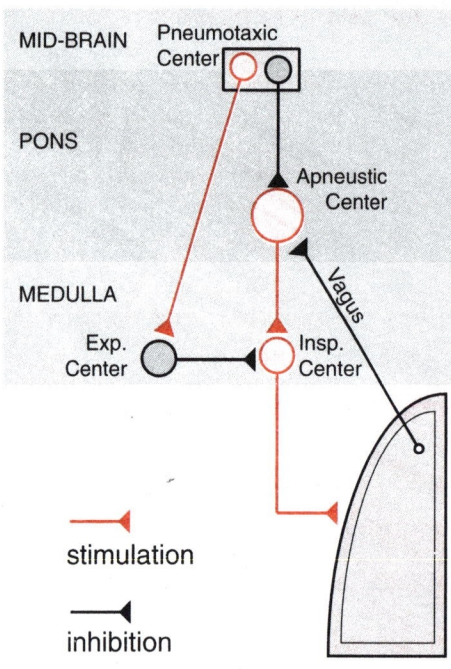

**Fig. 64.1**

## Describe the classical experiments related to the neural control of respiration.

| Experimental observation | Classical interpretation |
|---|---|
| Respiration ceases if the brainstem is transected below the calamus scriptorius (lower border of the fourth ventricle) but is maintained if sectioned at the upper border of the medulla. | 'Centers' or 'neurons' driving the respiration lie between these two levels. |
| Stimulation of ventral regions of the medial medulla stimulates inspiration whereas stimulation of dorsal regions of medial medulla stimulates expiration. | The stimulated areas are the 'inspiratory' and the 'expiratory' centers. |
| Stimulation of the lateral-most part of the lower pons produced apneustic breathing | The area contains the 'apneustic' center'. |
| Hering (1968) and Breuer (1868) observed that vagotomy produced deep and slow breathing in anaesthetized dogs. | Afferent vagal impulses normally inhibit the apneustic center. |
| Mid-pontine section produced deep, slow breathing while mid-collicular section did not alter the breathing pattern | A 'pneumotaxic center' lies between these two levels. It inhibits the apneustic center and stimulates the expiratory center. |
| Mid-pontine section together with vagotomy produces apneustic breathing in (and only in) an anaesthetized animal. | The apneustic center is totally disinhibited. |

## What is the present concept of neural regulation of respiration?

The neurons with respiratory discharge patterns are organized in three main aggregates of neurons: (i) one is located dorsomedially in medulla in the region of the nuclear complex of the tractus solitarius (NTS). This group is known as the **dorsal respiratory group** (DRG). (ii) The second group of respiratory neurons constitutes a longitudinal column of neurons in a more ventral and lateral region of the medulla oblongata, extending from its rostral to its caudal border. They are called the **ventral respiratory group** (VRG). (iii) A group of pacemaker neurons in the **pre-Bottzinger** complex in the medulla generates the rhythm and pattern of breathing.

## What is apneustic breathing?

Apneustic breathing is the pattern of breathing that is punctuated by **apneusis** (stopping of breathing) at inspiration. Apneustic breathing is characterized by *prolonged deep inspiration separated by periods of brief expiration*.

## How does the vagus affect breathing?

Vagus carries the afferents of the Hering-Breuer reflex. Vagal stimulation therefore tends to trigger expiration. Vagotomy in anesthetized dogs produce **deep slow breathing**. Vagotomy in anesthetized dogs with mid-pontine section produces **apneustic breathing**.

## What is Hering-Breuer inflation reflex?

In the **Hering-Breuer inflation reflex**, inflation of the lung to a volume greater than 800 mL initiates *reflex expiration*. It is triggered by *slow-adapting* **stretch receptors** located in the smooth muscle of the bronchial wall, especially at points of bronchial branching. Thus, the reflex tends to limit the tidal volume while increasing the respiratory frequency. The reflex also results in *bronchodilatation*. It seems that the physiological role of the Hering-Breuer reflex is to adjust the tidal volume and respiratory rate under different conditions of lung compliance and airway resistance.

## Enumerate the various afferents that influence breathing.

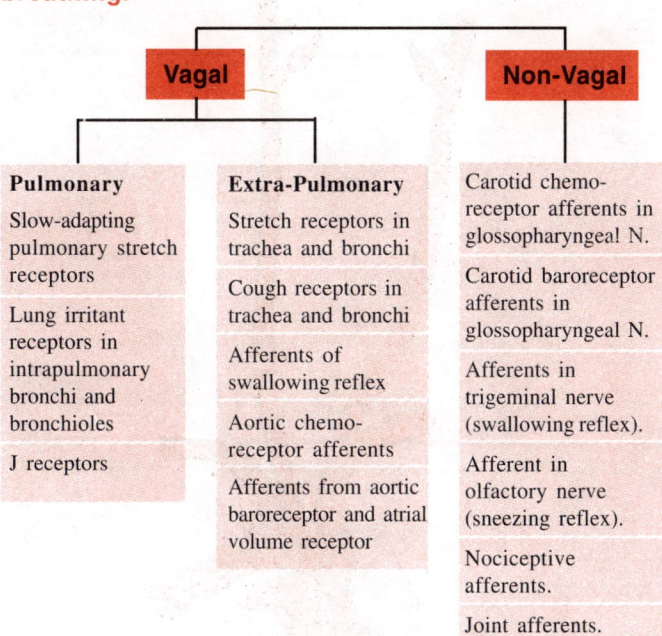

| Pulmonary | Extra-Pulmonary | |
|---|---|---|
| Slow-adapting pulmonary stretch receptors | Stretch receptors in trachea and bronchi | Carotid chemo-receptor afferents in glossopharyngeal N. |
| Lung irritant receptors in intrapulmonary bronchi and bronchioles | Cough receptors in trachea and bronchi | Carotid baroreceptor afferents in glossopharyngeal N. |
| | Afferents of swallowing reflex | Afferents in trigeminal nerve (swallowing reflex). |
| J receptors | Aortic chemo-receptor afferents | Afferent in olfactory nerve (sneezing reflex). |
| | Afferents from aortic baroreceptor and atrial volume receptor | Nociceptive afferents. |
| | | Joint afferents. |

## What is Hering-Breuer deflation reflex?

Large deflations of the lung distort the bronchial epithelium. The *reflex hyperpnea in response to deflation* is called the **Hering-Breuer deflation reflex** and is seen pneumothorax and lung collapse (atelectasis). The reflex may also be responsible for the sighs or yawning in response to the increase in compliance that occurs periodically due to the collapse of the smaller alveoli. The reflex helps in opening up the collapsed alveoli again.

## What are J-receptors?

J-receptors are present in the alveolar wall, adjacent to pulmonary capillaries. These **juxtapulmonary receptors** were discovered by AS Paintal and were found to be stimulated by an *increase in the alveolar interstitial fluid. Irritant gases* too stimulate J-receptors, which could be a direct effect or due to increase in the alveolar interstitial fluid.

Stimulation of the J receptors reflexly brings about several effects including a *strong and prolonged expiration, broncho-constriction,* and *contraction of the laryngeal adductors, hypotension* and *bradycardia.* It also causes *inhibition of the myotatic stretch reflex.*

## What is the J-reflex?

It is a protective reflex in which inhibition stimulation of the J-receptors causes inhibition of the stretch receptors of skeletal muscles. J-reflex is triggered by strenuous exercise due to interstitial edema. The reflex in turn terminates the exercise by inhibition of the stretch reflex.

In the 1984 Bhopal gas tragedy, methyl isocyanide (MIC) was found to cause paralysis of skeletal muscles for no apparent reasons. Paintal argued that the highly irritant MIC gas had caused interstitial edema and stimulated the J-reflex, which caused paralysis by inhibiting the muscle stretch reflex.

# 65

# Chemical Control of Breathing

## Where are the various central and peripheral chemoreceptors located?

**Central chemoreceptors** (Fig. 65.1) are located within the central nervous system. Central chemoreceptors are *located on the ventral surface of the medulla oblongata* and are therefore also called medullary chemoreceptors. (The central chemoreceptors are not the same as the respiratory neurons that are located deeper inside the medulla and generate the respiratory rhythm.)

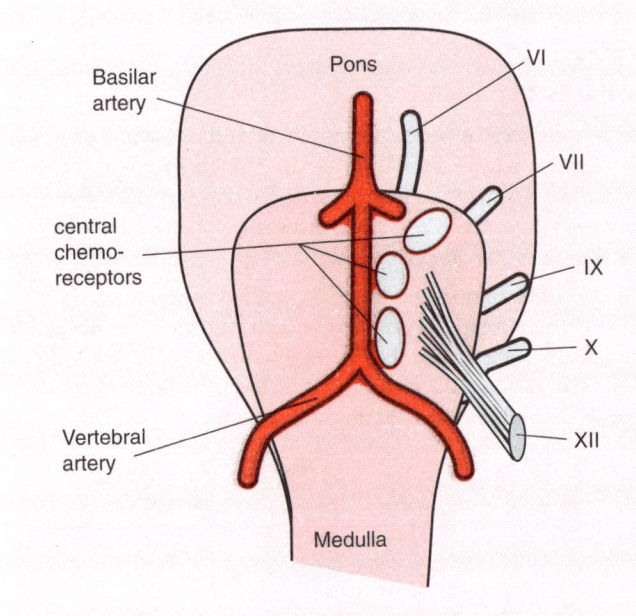

**Fig. 65.1**

**Peripheral chemoreceptors** (Fig. 65.2) are attached to the peripheral nervous system. The **carotid bodies** are located near the carotid bifurcation on each side. The **aortic bodies**, two or more in number, are located near the arch of the aorta.

## Briefly describe the structure of the carotid bodies.

Each carotid and aortic body is made of two types of cells, type I and type II cells (Fig. 65.3). The **type I** or **glomus cells** contain dopamine that is released in response to hypoxia. The cells are in close contiguity with afferent nerve endings bearing dopamine ($D_2$) receptors. The **type II cells** are glia-like supporting cells.

## What is the type and course of the carotid body afferents?

Afferents neurons innervating the carotid bodies are thinly myelinated A$\delta$ fibers. They ascend to the medulla via the carotid

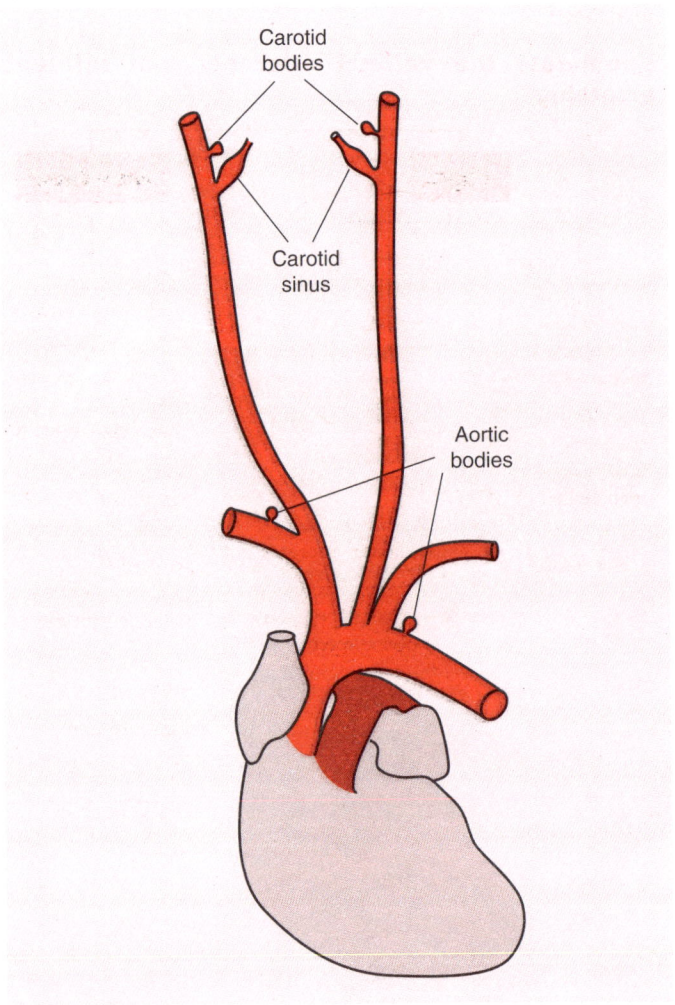

**Fig. 65.2**

sinus and glossopharyngeal nerves. Fibers from the aortic bodies ascend in the vagi.

## How do the chemoreceptors regulate breathing?

The peripheral and central chemoreceptors work in unison to *bring about increased ventilation* in response to (i) a rise in arterial $P_{CO_2}$ (ii) a rise in arterial $H^+$ concentration, or (iii) a fall in arterial $P_{O_2}$ below 60 mmHg. Of the three, *hypercapnia provides the strongest respiratory drive*.

## What are the differences between central and peripheral chemoreceptors?

Peripheral chemoreceptors are stimulated by a *low $P_{O_2}$* and *high*

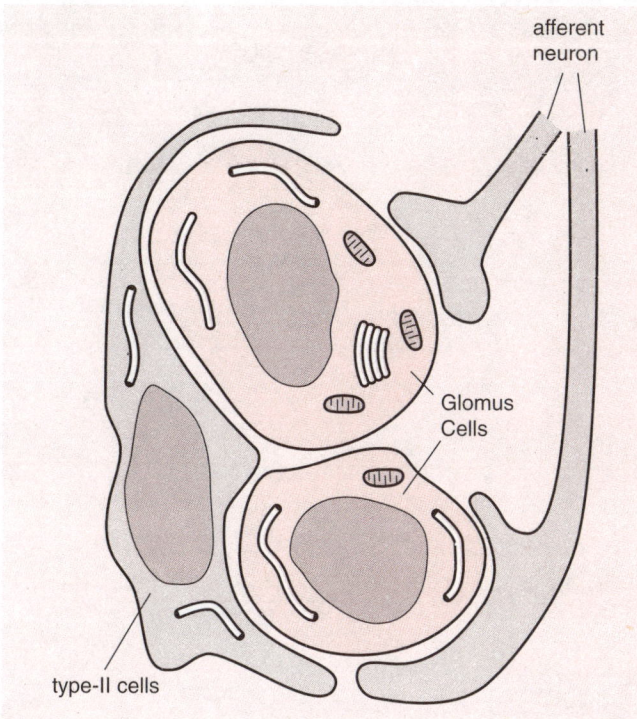

**Fig. 65.3**

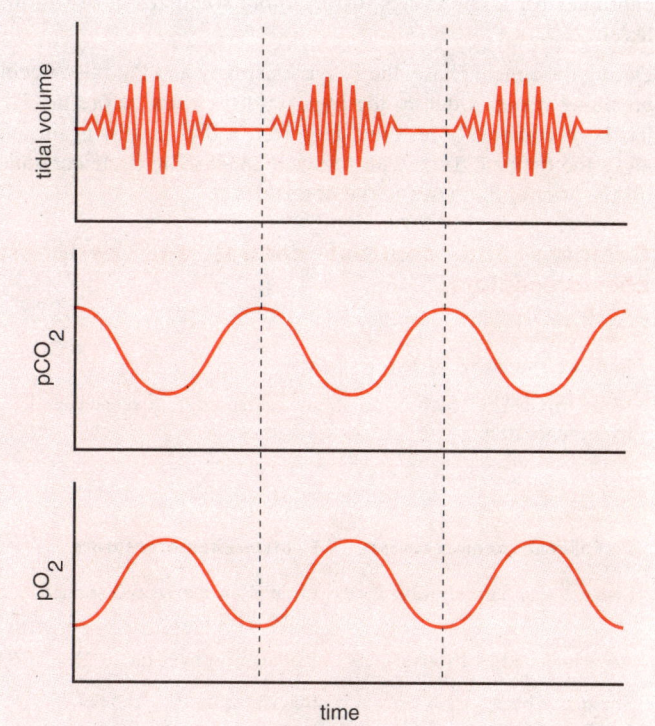

**Fig. 65.4**

$P_{CO_2}$ in the arterial blood perfusing it. Central chemoreceptors are stimulated by a *fall in the pH* of the CSF and the pH of the interstitial fluid of the brain. High $P_{CO_2}$ decreases the pH of CSF and cerebral interstitial fluid, and thereby stimulates the central chemoreceptors. *Central chemoreceptors are not stimulated by hypoxia*; rather, like any other cell, they are depressed by hypoxia.

### Describe the common causes of respiratory acidosis and alkalosis.

The causes of respiratory acidosis and alkalosis are the same as those of hypercapnia and hypocapnia respectively (see Chapter 66).

### Describe the respiratory regulation of pH.

The lungs can compensate for both acidosis and alkalosis that are of non-respiratory, i.e., metabolic origin. In *metabolic acidosis*, the high $P_{CO_2}$ stimulates hyperventilation causing $CO_2$ washout. As a result, the $P_{CO_2}$ decreases and the pH is restored to near normal levels. For example, in diabetic ketoacidosis, there is pronounced respiratory stimulation (Kussmaul breathing). The hyperventilation decreases alveolar $P_{CO_2}$ ("blows off $CO_2$") and thus produces a compensatory rise in pH. In *metabolic alkalosis*, the low $P_{CO_2}$ levels depress ventilation resulting in $CO_2$ retention. As a result, the $P_{CO_2}$ and the pH are restored to near normal levels. For example, excessive vomiting with loss of HCl from the body results in metabolic alkalosis. The alkalosis depresses ventilation and the arterial $P_{CO_2}$ rises, lowering the pH toward normal.

### What is Cheyne-Stokes breathing? What are its causes?

Cheyne-Stokes breathing (**periodic breathing**) is characterized by a *regular waxing and waning of ventilation at a constant frequency, punctuated by periods of apnea* (Fig. 65.4). The arterial $P_{O_2}$ and $P_{CO_2}$ fluctuate during each cycle of Cheyne-Stokes

breathing. The $P_{O_2}$ is lowest and the $P_{CO_2}$ highest at the end of the apnea. Cheyne Stokes breathing tends to occur (i) when circulation time is prolonged, as in shock; (ii) in premature infants; (iii) in old age (iv) in NREM sleep stages 1 and 2; (v) following consumption of sedative drugs; (vi) in hypoxia and (vii) when FRC of the lungs is reduced.

### What is Biot's breathing?

Also called **ataxic breathing**, this is a pattern of *slow and irregular respiration* (Fig. 65.5). It indicates a disruption of the normal medullary rhythmicity of respiration. The ventilatory response to $CO_2$ and $O_2$ is usually impaired. This type of breathing is seen in a wide variety of medullary disorders, including head injury, meningitis and medullary compressions like pontine hematomas or cerebellopontine herniation. It is commonest with *central medullary lesions*.

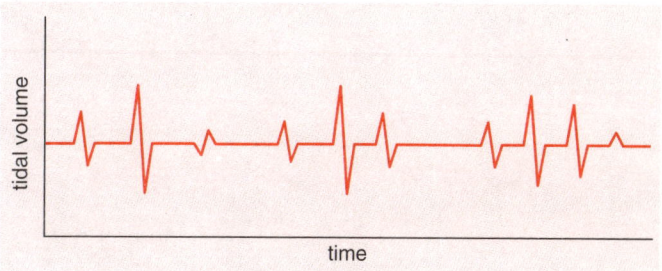

**Fig. 65.5**

### Why is hyperventilation followed by periodic breathing?

When a subject hyperventilates till there is a feeling of faintness (about 1 - 2 minutes), it is followed by a period of apnea. There is a slow recovery from apnea. However, after a few breaths, apnea follows again (**post-hyperventilation periodic breathing**). This continues for a few cycles till breathing stabilizes at the normal level.

During the apneic phase, the $P_{CO_2}$ rises slowly and $P_{O_2}$ falls. Feeble breathing resumes due to the hypoxic drive even before the $P_{CO_2}$ has been completely restored. However, a few breaths again take away the hypoxic drive with resultant apnea. The cycle continues till the arterial $P_{CO_2}$ rises to the normal level.

## Compare and contrast central and peripheral chemoreceptors.

**SIMILARITIES**

Both are stimulated by hypercapnia.

When stimulated, both bring about similar efferent responses, i.e. hyperventilation.

**DIFFERENCES**

| Peripheral chemoreceptors | Central chemoreceptors |
| --- | --- |
| Located near carotid bifurcation | Located on the ventral surface of the medulla. |
| Are stimulated by hypoxia | Inhibited by hypoxia |
| Stimulated by $P_{CO_2}$, pH and $P_{O_2}$ *of blood* | Stimulated by $P_{CO_2}$ and pH *of CSF and cerebral intestitial fluid* |

# 66

# Respiratory Disequilibria

## Define the four types of hypoxia, giving examples.

Hypoxia is $O_2$ deficiency at the tissue level. There are four types of hypoxia: (i) **hypoxic hypoxia**, in which the $P_{O_2}$ of the arterial blood is reduced, as in *high-altitude hypoxia*; (ii) **anemic hypoxia**, in which the arterial $P_{O_2}$ is normal but the amount of hemoglobin available to carry $O_2$ is reduced, as in *severe anemia, carbonmonoxide poisoning* and *methemoglobinemia*; (iii) **stagnant hypoxia**, in which the blood flow to a tissue is so low that adequate $O_2$ is not delivered to it despite a normal $P_{O_2}$ and hemoglobin concentration, as in *circulatory shock* and *congestive heart failure*; and (iv) **histotoxic hypoxia**, in which the amount of $O_2$ delivered to a tissue is adequate but, because of the action of a toxic agent, the tissue cells cannot make use of the $O_2$ supplied to them. An example is *cyanide poisoning*, which inhibits cytochrome oxidase.

## What are the causes of hypoxic hypoxia?

Hypoxic hypoxia is the most common form of hypoxia seen clinically. The causes of hypoxic hypoxia are: (i) *Reduced $P_{O_2}$* of atmospheric air as at high altitudes (high-altitude hypoxia); (ii) *Reduced ventilation* due to restrictive or obstructive lung disorders; (iii) *Reduced diffusion capacity* of $O_2$ across the respiratory membrane. This commonly occurs when there is a marked reduction in the area of the respiratory membrane, as in emphysema. (iv) *Shunting of blood*, bypassing the ventilated alveoli. This is commonly due to ventilation-perfusion mismatch within the lung. It also occurs when there is a right-to-left shunt in the heart, i.e., deoxygenated blood from the right side of the heart bypasses the lung to get access to the left ventricle. This is seen in congenital heart diseases like Fallot's tetralogy.

## Explain the pathophysiology of carbon monoxide poisoning.

Carbon monoxide poisoning results in the formation of **carboxyhemoglobin (COHb)**, which *reduces the amount of Hb available for $O_2$ transport*. CO has a very high affinity for hemoglobin and once bound, is difficult to dislodge from hemoglobin. Moreover, the *COHb shifts the $O_2$ dissociation curve of the remaining Hb to the left*, decreasing the amount of $O_2$ that can be released. Hence, inactivation of Hb by carbon monoxide poisoning is worse than having a reduced Hb concentration. The **cherry-red color** of COHb visible through skin and mucous membranes can be confused with cyanosis. Death results due to hypoxic brain damage. Management of CO poisoning includes termination of exposure to CO and $O_2$ therapy (hyperbaric $O_2$ if required)

## What is methemoglobinemia?

Methemoglobin is denatured hemoglobin in which the heme $Fe^{2+}$ is oxidized to the $Fe^{3+}$. Presence of methemoglobin in blood is called methemoglobinemia.

## Outline the treatment of cyanide poisoning.

The general treatment for histotoxic hypoxia is **hyperbaric oxygen therapy**. Specific treatment for cyanide poisoning includes **nitrites or methylene blue**, which act by forming methemoglobin from hemoglobin. **Methemoglobin** then detoxifies cyanide by converting it to **cyanmethemoglobin**. However, overenthusiastic treatment with nitrites can cause anemic hypoxia by forming too much methemoglobin.

## What are the clinical features of hypoxia?

Hypoxia is usually associated with (i) hyperventilation; (ii) cyanosis; (iii) circulatory changes; and (iv) cerebral symptoms.

**Hyperventilation** occurs only when the central chemoreceptors are stimulated by low $P_{O_2}$. Hence, it is present in hypoxic hypoxia. It also occurs in histotoxic hypoxia if the chemoreceptor cells get poisoned. However, it is not seen in anemic hypoxia so long as the arterial $P_{O_2}$ remains normal. It is also *not seen in stagnant hypoxia* either, because the blood supply to the carotid bodies is extremely high and the glomus cells rarely if ever suffer from $O_2$ deficiency so long as the blood $P_{O_2}$ is normal.

**Cyanosis** is a bluish discoloration of skin and mucous membrane. It is seen when the deoxyhemoglobin concentration in blood exceeds 5g/dL. There are two types of cyanosis: peripheral and central. **Peripheral cyanosis** is seen in the nail beds and is suggestive of *stagnant hypoxia*. **Central cyanosis** is seen in the mucous membranes of the tongue-tip and lips and in the earlobes where the skin is thin. These areas receive a good blood supply and become cyanotic only if the $O_2$ saturation of blood is low, as in *hypoxic hypoxia*. Cyanosis *does not occur in anemic hypoxia*. In fact, it cannot occur in severe anemia if the Hb concentration is 5g/dL or less. Cyanosis *does not occur in histotoxic hypoxia* either, because the $O_2$ saturation of Hb is normal.

**Circulatory changes** occur due to the *peripheral vasodilatation* caused by tissue hypoxia. A fall in peripheral resistance increases the venous return and the cardiac output. *Increased cardiac output* causes turbulent blood flow near the heart valves, resulting in *soft systolic murmurs* that are characteristic of hyperdynamic circulation. The patient also complains of *palpitation*.

**Cerebral symptoms** are prominent in hypoxic and anemic hypoxia. They *resemble alcohol toxicity*: impaired judgment, drowsiness, dulled pain sensibility, excitement, disorientation and headache.

Other symptoms include nausea, vomiting, tachycardia and hypertension.

### What are the indications and contraindications of oxygen therapy?

An $O_2$-rich gas mixture helps in increasing the blood $P_{O_2}$. Hence, it is *useful in most types of hypoxic hypoxia* and is commonly used in chronic obstructive pulmonary diseases. For the same reason, it is of little use in those types of hypoxia (stagnant, anemic, and histotoxic) in which reduction in blood $P_{O_2}$ is not the primary problem. Breathing $O_2$ is also *useless in hypoxic hypoxia if it is due to ventilation-perfusion mismatch* i.e., deoxygenated blood bypasses the well-ventilated alveoli. Caution is required while giving $O_2$ therapy to *patients with severe pulmonary failure and high $P_{CO_2}$*. The central chemoreceptors in these patients are inhibited by hypercapnia, and the breathing is driven by hypoxia through the peripheral chemoreceptors. Oxygen therapy may produce apnea by taking away this hypoxic drive.

### What are the indications of hyperbaric oxygen therapy?

The advantage of hyperbaric $O_2$ is that it raises the amount of $O_2$ dissolved in plasma and therefore, is unaffected by the hemoglobin concentration. It is useful in the treatment of (i) carbon monoxide poisoning; (ii) decompression sickness and air embolism; (iii) severe anemia; (iv) wounds with poor blood supply.

### What are the clinical features of oxygen toxicity?

100% $O_2$ has toxic effects due to the production of the **superoxide anion** (a free radical), and hydrogen peroxide. When administered for 8 hours or more, there is *irritation of the airways*. Administered chronically, infants may develop *bronchopulmonary dysplasia* (characterized by lung cysts and opacities) and *retrolental fibroplasia*, (formation of opaque vascular tissue in the eyes, which can lead to serious visual detects). Hyperbaric 100% $O_2$ at higher pressures produces, in addition to airway irritation, *nervous symptoms* like muscle twitching, tinnitus, convulsions, and coma.

### What are the causes of hypercapnia?

An increase in $CO_2$ production rarely produces hypercapnia because it is promptly *washed out* by the resulting hyperventilation. The $P_{CO_2}$ does not rise even when there is considerable reduction in the diffusion capacity of the lung, as in pulmonary fibrosis. This is because $CO_2$ is lipid soluble and promptly diffuses out across the respiratory membrane. Hence, hypercapnia occurs essentially in: (i) *Reduction of pulmonary ventilation*, as occurs in all *restrictive lung disorders*; or due to respiratory depression following drugs and cerebral diseases. (ii) *Reduction of effective alveolar ventilation* as occurs due to *ventilation-perfusion mismatch*. This is commonly seen in chronic obstructive pulmonary disease (COPD). (iii) Hypercapnia can also occur as a compensatory response to *metabolic alkalosis*.

### What are the clinical features of hypercapnia?

Hypercapnia is associated with **respiratory acidosis**, since any increase in $CO_2$ will promptly generate excess $H^+$ through the following reaction:

$$H_2O + CO_2 \xrightarrow{\text{Carbonic Anhydrase}} H_2CO_3 \longrightarrow H^+ + HCO_3^-$$

Hypercapnia stimulates respiration, leading to **hyperpnea**. However, the pulmonary ventilation does not improve if there is restrictive lung disorder, which is often the cause of the hypercapnia. Retention of large amounts of $CO_2$ produces **$CO_2$ narcosis**, which is characterized by *symptoms of CNS depression:* confusion, diminished sensory acuity, and coma with respiratory depression and death.

### What are the causes of hypocapnia?

Hypocapnia occurs due to hyperventilation. It is seen in the following conditions: (i) *hypoxic conditions* that are not due to restrictive lung disorders, e.g., high altitude hypoxia or diseases impairing alveolar diffusion of gases; (ii) *metabolic acidosis*, as a compensatory response; (iii) *compulsive hyperventilation* due to hysteria; (iv) excessive stimulation of respiratory center due to *fever, anxiety, cerebral tumors* or in *pregnancy*; (v) over-enthusiastic *artificial ventilation;* (vi) *excessive exercise*.

### What are the clinical features of hypocapnia?

Hypocapnia results in **respiratory alkalosis**, since any decrease in $CO_2$ drives the following reaction in the backward direction, resulting in a decrease in $H^+$ concentration:

$$H_2O + CO_2 \xleftarrow{\text{Carbonic Anhydrase}} H_2CO_3 \longleftarrow H^+ + HCO_3^-$$

Hypocapnia produces *faintness* and *parasthesias* due to reduction of cerebral blood flow. The associated respiratory alkalosis results in a lowering of ionized $Ca^{2+}$ in plasma and the appearance of symptoms of **tetany** (carpopedal spasm, a positive Chvostek sign etc.)

### What is asphyxia?

Asphyxia is the simultaneous development of *acute hypercapnia and hypoxia* and commonly occurs due to airway obstruction as occurs in *choking* or *drowning*. It is associated with: (i) violent respiratory efforts; (ii) acidosis; (iii) increased catecholamine secretion, which causes high blood pressure and heart rate, and also predisposes the hypoxic myocardium to *ventricular fibrillation*. Eventually the respiratory efforts cease, the blood pressure falls, and cardiac arrest occurs in 4-5 minutes.

### How does death occur in drowning?

Only 10% of deaths in drowning occur due to **asphyxia**. The asphyxia occurs initially due to breath holding and after breaking breath, due to the laryngospasm triggered by the cold water. The lungs remain dry in these deaths. In others, the lungs are flooded with water. *Fresh water drowning* causes **plasma dilution** and **intravascular hemolysis**. *Drowning in the hypertonic seawater* results in **hypovolemia**. If timely rescued and resuscitated, these circulatory effects has to be taken care of.

# Compare and contrast the 4 different types of hypoxia.

## SIMILARITIES

All of them are associated with oxygen deficiency at the tissue level.

## DIFFERENCES

| | Hypoxic hypoxia | Anemia hypoxia | Stagment hypoxia | Histotoxic hypoxia |
|---|---|---|---|---|
| Cause | Reduced oxygenation of blood, e.g. in high attitude or restrictive lung disorder | Reduced $O_2$ carrying capacity of blood | Reduced rate of oxygen delivery (reduced blood flow) to tissues, e.g. in shock | Impaired oxygen utilization, e.g. in cyanide poisoning |
| Arterial $PO_2$ | Reduced | Normal | Normal | Normal |
| Hyperventilation | Present | In severe anemia only | In severe cases only | Present only if carotid bodies get poisoned. |
| Cyanosis | Central cyanosis | Absent | Peripheral cyanosis | Absent |
| Cerebral symptoms | Prominent | Prominent | Present | May be present |

# 67

# High & Low Pressure Breathing

## What is high-pressure breathing and what are the problems associated with it?

High-pressure breathing is breathing compressed air. The problems associated with it are due to (i) the toxic effects of gases at high partial pressure e.g., oxygen toxicity, nitrogen narcosis and high pressure nervous symptoms (HPNS); and (ii) increased work of breathing associated with moving compressed gases in and out of the lungs. (a) **Oxygen toxicity** occurs with 100% $O_2$ at high pressures. It produces *nervous symptoms* like muscle twitching, tinnitus, convulsions, and coma. This is in addition to *airway irritation* which occurs even on breathing 100% $O_2$ at atmospheric pressure. (b) **Nitrogen narcosis** is also known as **rapture of the deep**. At pressures of 4 – 5 atmospheres (i.e., at depths of 30 - 40 m in the ocean), 80% $N_2$ produces euphoria. At greater pressures, the symptoms resemble alcohol intoxication. Manual dexterity is maintained, but *intellectual functions are impaired.* (c) **High-pressure nervous syndrome** or **HPNS** develops with inert gases in the atmosphere like helium, neon, argon, krypton and xenon. All these gases, when at high pressure, have a *non-specific anesthetic effect.* Their anesthetic activity parallels their lipid solubility, and the anesthesia may be due to an action on nerve cell membranes. HPNS is characterized by tremors and drowsiness. Unlike nitrogen narcosis, intellectual functions are not severely affected but *manual dexterity is impaired.*

## What are the problems associated with rapid decrease in pressure?

Rapid decrease in pressure causes **decompression sickness (Caisson disease)**. It occurs on rapid ascent by divers, usually due to a panic reaction to trouble. It is also seen when an unpressurized airplane rapidly gains in height. In **explosive decompression**, as occurs when an airplane flying at a great height gets suddenly depressurized, there is fatal air embolism. Less severe decompression sickness is characterized by bends, chokes and strokes. **Bends** are intense joint pains that occur when gas bubbles form in tissues. There is associated parasthesia and itching. **Chokes** are a choking sensation or dyspnea that occurs due to gas bubbles in pulmonary capillaries. **Strokes** – cerebral or coronary – occur due to gas bubbles in cerebral or coronary microcirculation.

## What is the pathophysiology of decompression sickness?

Decompression sickness occurs only when breathing pressurized air. As a diver breathing 80% $N_2$, ascends from a dive, the elevated alveolar $P_{N_2}$ falls, and with it, the $P_{N_2}$ of the blood and arterial fluids also fall. When the partial pressure of $N_2$ decreases, it is unable to keep in solution the large volumes of $N_2$ that was dissolved at a much higher pressure. The $N_2$ thus bubbles rapidly out of solution from blood. If the $P_{N_2}$ falls slowly, then the $N_2$ that comes out of solution is exhaled before it can form bubbles. This is called **slow decompression**. However, during rapid ascent through water, the decompression is fast and bubbles form in the tissues and blood, causing **decompression sickness.**

## How is decompression sickness treated?

Treatment of this disease is prompt **recompression** in a pressure chamber, followed by **slow decompression**. Recompression is frequently lifesaving. Recovery is often complete, but there may be residual neurological signs as a result of irreversible damage to the nervous system.

## What are the problems associated with ascent to high altitude?

The atmospheric pressure decreases at higher altitudes. If a person ascends to high altitude without carrying oxygen, then the following bodily events will occur:

| | |
|---|---|
| 3000 m | Hyperventilation starts (Alveolar $pO_2$ = 60mm Hg.) |
| 4000 m | Hypoxic symptoms appear; |
| 5000 m | Hypoxic symptoms become severe; |
| 6000 m | Consciousness is lost. |

It is possible for a person to climb higher up if he carries 100% $O_2$. However, if the $O_2$-cylinder is not pressurized so as to provide $O_2$ at 760 mm Hg, then the $P_{O_2}$ will still fall as the ambient (surrounding) pressure decreases. Thus, the atmospheric pressure of 187 mm Hg (at ~ 10,000m altitude) is the lowest barometric pressure at which the normal alveolar $pO_2$ of 100 mm Hg is possible even when breathing 100% oxygen. The following events occur in treating unpressurized 100% $O_2$.

| | |
|---|---|
| 10,000 m | Body at the brink of hypoxia ($P_{Atm}$ = 187 mm Hg; alveolar $pO_2$ = 100mm Hg); |
| 14,000m | Consciousness is lost. |
| 20,000m | At this height, the atmospheric pressure falls below 47 mm Hg, and blood will begin to boil. This is entirely a theoretical proposition because a person trying to climb to this height without pressured air will die long before his/her blood boils. |

## What are the clinical features of acute mountain sickness? How is it treated?

When unacclimatized individuals first arrive at a high altitude, they develop transient **mountain sickness**. This syndrome develops 8-24 hours after arrival at altitude and lasts 4-8 days. It is characterized by (i) hyperventilation, which is transient; (ii) cerebral edema; (iii) pulmonary edema. Treatment includes, rest, $O_2$ therapy and $Ca^{2+}$ channel-blocking drug nifedipine, which lowers pulmonary arterial pressure.

## What are the physiological changes associated with acclimatization?

The physiological changes associated with acclimatization include: (i) barrel chest and persistent hyperventilation; (ii) increased diffusion capacity of lungs; (iii) Increased cardiac output; (iv) polycythemia produced by increased erythropoietin secretion; (v) right-shift of $O_2$ dissociation curve; (vi) increased tissue capillary density; (vii) increase in myoglobin; (ix) larger lumber of mitochondria in cells; (x) increase in the tissue content of cytochrome oxidase.

## Explain why acclimatized persons are able to hyperventilate indefinitely while unacclimatized persons are unable to do so.

Unacclimatized individuals are unable to keep up the hyperventilation due to the effects of $CO_2$ washout. The $CO_2$ washout not only takes away the respiratory drive but also causes faintness due to the cerebral vasoconstriction associated with hypocapneic alkalosis. Persons acclimatized to high altitudes are however able to hyperventilate unabated, even when their alveolar and arterial $pCO_2$ is low due to $CO_2$ washout. This is because an *acclimatized person has a normal arterial pH* due to renal compensatory mechanisms. This ensures that their peripheral chemoreceptors are adequately driven. More importantly, *acclimatized persons are able to maintain a slightly acidic CSF pH*. This is made possible by a $HCO_3^-$ pump located at the blood-brain barrier, which pumps out $HCO_3^-$. The acidic CSF helps maintain adequate respiratory drive of the central chemoreceptors. It also prevents cerebral vasoconstriction and faintness.

# 68

# Respiratory Medicine

## What is hemoptysis?

It is defined as the expectoration of blood from the respiratory tract. It can occur with airway disease (e.g. chronic bronchitis) or parenchymal disease (e.g. tuberculosis, pneumonia). Hemoptysis can also result from cardiovascular disease (e.g. acute left ventricular failure).

## What is dyspnea?

Dyspnea or breathlessness is the unpleasant awareness of breathing effort. According to the theory of **length-tension inappropriateness**, there is a constant subconscious comparison between ventilation required and ventilation achieved and between muscle tension exerted and change in muscle length achieved. Dyspnea occurs when these inappropriateness reach a certain threshold.

## What is orthopnea?

Any patient who is severely dyspneic tends to sit up and bend forwards as dyspnea is worst in supine position (**orthopnea**). Although classically orthopnea is thought to suggest left ventricular failure it is also seen in purely respiratory disorders with severe breathlessness such as asthma and COPD. In supine position the abdominal contents tend to press on the diaphragm and causes dyspnea. Sitting up takes this load off the diaphragm and relieves dyspnea.

## What are wheeze and ronchi?

Wheeze is a high-pitched (~ 400 Hz) continuous 'whistling' sound more than 250ms in duration. **Rhonchi** are similar lung sounds with a lower frequency (~ 200 Hz). Wheeze is produced when air flows through narrowed airways (as in asthma), setting up oscillations in the airway walls. Wheeze is of higher pitch during expiration when the airways become narrower.

## What is clubbing?

The normal angle between the nail and the distal skin over the nail bed is lost over fingers and toes in certain respiratory (and non respiratory conditions). This is called **clubbing**. In more advanced clubbing, the terminal phalanx looks swollen like a drumstick. Severe clubbing is sometimes associated with **hypertrophic osteoarthropathy**, i.e., swelling, pain and oedema of the ankle and wrist joint and subperiosteal calcification of distal long bones near these joints.

Clubbing from respiratory causes is seen in conditions associated with *hypoxemia, suppuration* (pus-formation) or *malignancies*. Hypertrophic osteoarthropathy is most commonly seen with bronchial carcinoma.

## Describe some abnormal shapes of the thoracic cage.

Abnormal shape of the thorax include **pectus excavatum** or funnel chest (depression of sternum with anterior protrusion of ribs), **pectus** carinatum or pigeon chest (sternum protrudes anteriorly) and **kyphoscoliosis**. In **barrel chest,** the anteroposterior diameter of the chest is increased. It is seen in COPD but is also seen in the elderly.

## What is vocal fremitus?

Vocal fremitus is the assessment of conducted vibrations to chest wall during speech. It is assessed by placing ulnar border of hand on intercostal spaces while the patient is asked to repeat numbers like nine-nine-nine. Increase in vocal fremitus indicates increased density of lungs (as in consolidation or atelectasis) allowing better transmission of voice sounds from the airways to the chest wall. Increased fat on chest wall (obesity), presence of air (pneumothorax) or fluid (pleural effusion) in the pleural cavity and hyperinflated lung decrease vocal fremitus.

## What is percussion? What is its clinical significance?

The term 'percussion' means 'hitting one body against another'. To a clinician, the word means 'striking or tapping of the chest with the fingertips so as to determine from the sound produced the condition of internal organs'. When the finger (called the **plexor finger**) strikes the chest wall, the chest wall tends to vibrate as a resonant cavity, which is partially damped by the thoracic contents.

If the underlying lung is replaced by air as in pneumothorax, the sound is of greater amplitude and duration and is called **tympanic**. If the underlying lung alveolar air is replaced by fluid in the pleural cavity or by exudative fluid in the alveolar space as in pneumonia, the sound has low amplitude and short duration and is called dull.

## What are adventitious sounds?

Normally, the only sounds heard on auscultation (i.e., listening with the aid of a stethoscope) of the lungs are the **normal breath sounds**. Any other sound (wheeze, crackles, pleural rub) is called **adventitious sound** and mostly (but not always) suggests some disease process.

## What are the differences between vesicular and bronchial breath sounds?

| Vesicular | Bronchial |
| --- | --- |
| Has a soft, low-pitched 'rustling' quality. | Harsh and high-pitched. Has a hollow, 'tubular' quality. |
| Expiratory sound much softer than the inspiratory sound. | The expiratory sound is harsher than the inspiratory sound. |

| | |
|---|---|
| Duration of expiratory sound is twice that of inspiration. | Duration of inspiratory sound is equal to that of expiratory sound. |
| There is no gap between the inspiratory and expiratory sounds. | There is a definite gap between the inspiratory and expiratory sounds. |
| The inspiratory sound originates within the lungs while the expiration-phase sound comes partly from the upper airways. | It is generated in upper airways. |
| Normally heard on the chest wall over the lungs. | Normally not transmitted to the chest wall. When present, signifies consolidation of lungs. |

## What are crackles?

Crackles are short 'clicking' sounds heard on auscultation over the chest with a variety of pulmonary disease (pneumonia, bronchiectesis) as also congestive cardiac failure. **Early inspiratory crackles** are produced in the more proximal and larger airways. **Late inspiratory crackles** on the other hand are produced in peripheral airways and are best heard in the dependent regions of these areas. **Fine crackles** (earlier called **crepitations**) have high pitch and are shorter in duration. **Coarse crackles** (earlier called **rales**) have lower pitch, longer duration and are louder.

## What is pleural rub?

It is a coarse, low-pitched sound generated by rubbing of pleural surfaces when they become rough due to inflammation. It is usually audible both during inspiration and expiration, usually near peak lung volumes (later part of inspiration and early part of expiration).

## What is the role of PFT in clinical setting?

In the clinics, PFT is done for (i) confirmation of clinical diagnosis; (ii) exclusion of a diagnosis; (iii) early diagnosis of diseases; (iv) planning of further investigations; (v) objective assessment of severity of disease; (vi) monitoring response to treatment; (vii) evaluation of fitness for surgery or sports / flight fitness.

## Which are the commonly used parameters in PFT?

The most commonly used **spirometric parameters** are (i) Forced vital capacity (FVC); (ii) Forced expiratory volume during the first second ($FEV_1$) (iii) Ratio of $FEV_1$ and FVC ($FEV_1\%$); (iv) Flow rates at low volume, i.e., $FEF_{50}$, $FEF_{25}$, $FEF_{25-75}$ etc; (v) Peak expiratory flow rate (PEFR). Less commonly used spirometric parameters are (vi) Slow vital capacity (SVC); (vii) Expiratory reserve volume (ERV); (viii) Maximum voluntary ventilation (MVV). **Non-spirometric parameters** recorded in PFT include functional residual capacity (FRC) and diffusion capacity.

## How is an obstructive lung disorder differentiated from a restrictive lung disorder?

| Obstructive | Restrictive |
|---|---|
| TLC normal. VC mostly normal but may be reduced at the expense of increased FRC due to 'air-trapping' | TLC and VC always reduced. |
| $FEV_1$/FVC normal | $FEV_1$/FVC reduced |
| Examples are asthma, chronic bronchitis and emphysema (COPD) | Examples are pneumothorax, pleural effusion, and atelectasis. Also occurs in kyphoscoliosis, and neuromuscular disorders. |

## What is COPD?

The term **chronic obstructive pulmonary disease (COPD)** includes both chronic bronchitis and emphysema. Most patients with these diseases have airway obstruction. Two hallmark of COPD are *chronic cough with hypersecretion of mucus* and *progressive persistent airflow obstruction*. In **chronic bronchitis,** persistent cough and mucus hypersecretion result from *bronchial gland enlargement* in the airways. The smaller peripheral bronchi are thickened and distorted by scar tissue and result in increased airflow resistance.

In **emphysema** there is abnormal enlargement of airspaces distal to terminal bronchioles accompanied by destruction of their walls. The destruction of elastic tissues in the airway walls makes them susceptible to *dynamic airway compression*, resulting in airway obstruction.

## What is bronchial asthma?

Asthma is characterized by airway narrowing due to smooth muscle constriction, mucosal edema and mucous plugging. Characteristic feature of this airway narrowing is its variability with time (spontaneously) on exposure to triggering factors (allergens, cold air, exercise etc.) or bronchodilators.

# 69

# Structure & Functions of the Kidney

## Enumerate the functions of the kidney.

The main function of the kidney is **homeostasis**, i.e. the maintenance of the **milieu interior** (internal environment). In doing so, the kidney has to deal effectively with: (1) *Products of protein metabolism*. These include substances like urea, uric acid, $SO_4^{2-}$, $PO_4^{3-}$, creatinine, and several other substances that must be effectively eliminated from the body. Metabolism of carbohydrates and fats produce only water and $CO_2$ and therefore, does not load the kidney with metabolites. Hence in kidney dysfunctions, only protein restriction is advised. (2) Water, $Na^+$, and $K^+$ which must be dealt with according to whether there is a surplus or deficit in the body. Thereby, it *regulates water and electrolyte balance*, and also, the blood and ECF volume. (3) $HCO_3^-$ ions and buffer mechanisms of the body. Along with the respiratory system, the kidney thereby *regulates the acid-base balance*. The kidney plays a relatively minor part in the homeostasis of certain other substances like $Ca^{2+}$, $Mg^{2+}$ and glucose that are regulated primarily through hormones.

Other functions of the kidney include: (4) *long-term maintenance of blood pressure*; chronic renal disorders are invariably associated with hypertension; (5) *intermediate-term regulation of blood pressure* (renin secretion); (6) *Regulation of erythropoiesis*. The kidney secretes erythropoietin. Reduced kidney mass, as occurs in chronic renal failure, is associated with normocytic, normochromic anemia; (7) *regulation of $Ca^{2+}$/bone metabolism*. The kidney activates vitamin D precursor 25-hydroxycholecalciferol to 1,25 dihydroxycholecalciferol. Chronic renal disorders are associated with renal osteodystrophy; (8) *Synthesis of metabolic substrate* like L-arginine. L-arginine is the precursor for nitric oxide (NO), a mediator for several functions including an 'anti-atherosclerotic' effect; (9) Under exceptional conditions, the kidneys can contribute significantly to the body's *gluconeogenetic capability*.

## Briefly describe the internal structure of the kidney.

A longitudinal section of the kidney shows two distinct zones: the outer cortex and the inner medulla. The **medulla** comprises the renal pyramids, 4 to 14 in number, separated by the cortical columns of Bertin. The **pyramid** shows radial striations on it that are due to the straight portions of the nephrons. The apex of the pyramid is called the **papilla**. The tip of the papilla has pores, which are the openings of the collecting ducts into the **minor calyx**. The minor calyces join together to **major calyces**, which in turn drain in to the pelvis. The **pelvis** narrows down to continue as the ureter that drains into the bladder.

The medulla can be subdivided into: an *outer medulla* that is further subdivided into the outer strip, and the inner strip, and an *inner medulla*, also called the papillary zone.

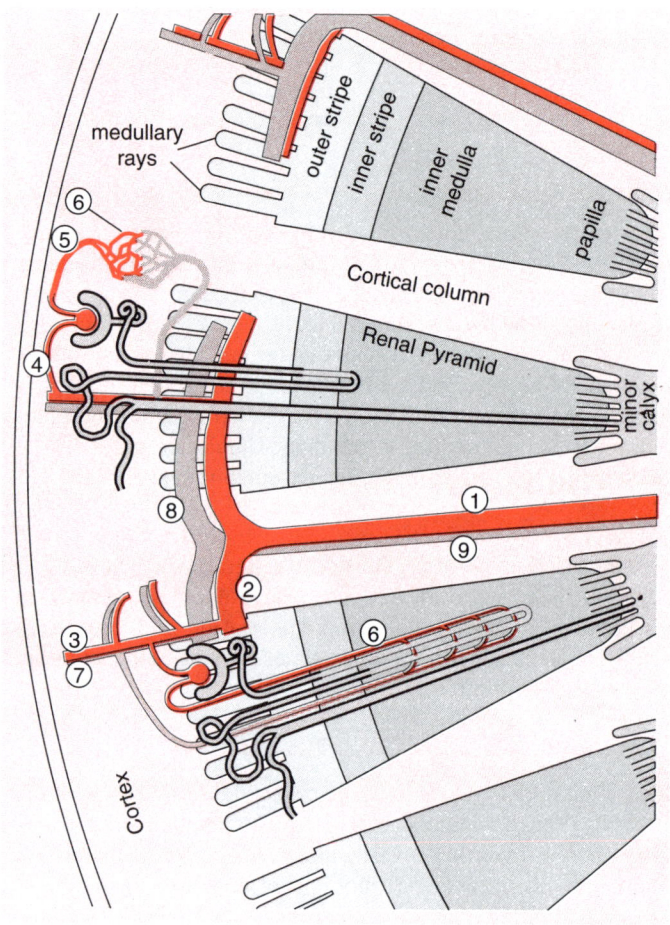

**Fig. 69.1**

## Briefly describe the blood vessels of the kidney.

The renal artery enters the hilus and gives rise to **segmental arteries**. The segmental arteries provide the **lobar arteries** to each renal pyramid. The lobar arteries divide into two **interlobular arteries** just before entering the substance of the kidney, and run in the cortical columns. The **interlobar arteries** dichotomize into the arcuate arteries at the corticomedullary junction and run parallel to the surface of the kidney. The **arcuate arteries** give off the cortical radial arteries (formerly called inter-lobular arteries), which ascend radially towards the cortex. The **cortical radial arteries** give off the afferent arterioles. The **afferent arterioles** ramify into a tuft of capillaries – the **glomerulus** – inside the Bowman's capsule. Glomerular capillaries reunite to form the **efferent arteriole**. In cortical nephrons, the efferent arterioles have a small caliber and ramify to form the dense **peritubular capillary network**.

The efferent arterioles drain into **stellate veins**, which in turn drain into **interlobular veins** (Fig. 69.1).

### What is the vasa recta?

In juxtamedullary nephrons, the efferent arterioles are larger than those in the cortical nephrons. They branch into long and straight capillaries called the **vasa recta**. The vasa recta follow the course of the loop of Henle. The descending and ascending limbs of the vasa recta run close together which facilitates counter-current exchange. Between the descending and ascending limbs are present the peritubular capillary network of the medulla which is less dense than the cortical network.

### Why is the blood flow through the vasa recta slow?

The factors responsible for the low inner medullary blood flow are to be found in the **Poiseuille-Hagen formula**. These are: (i) The long length of the vasa recta (vascular resistance is proportional to the length of the vessel); (ii) The sharp rise in the viscosity of blood in the inner medulla due to the loss of large amounts of water into the hyperosmolar interstitium; (iii) The capillary hydrostatic pressure is lower in the vasa recta because the efferent arterioles of the juxtamedullary nephrons have smaller diameter.

### What is the relative blood supply of the different parts of the kidney?

90% of the RBF goes to the renal cortex, 9% goes to the outer medulla and 1% goes to the inner medulla.

### Which metabolic process in the kidney accounts for its high $O_2$ consumption?

The $O_2$ consumption per 100g of renal tissue (5 ml/min.) is fairly high and next only to that of the heart (8 ml/min). Renal $O_2$ is determined mainly by the amount of **Na⁺ reabsorption**.

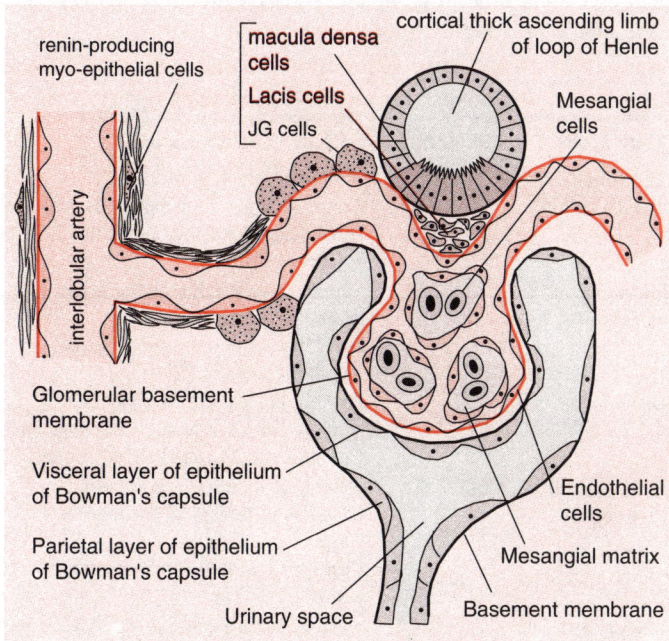

**Fig. 69.2**

### What are the components of the glomerular membrane?

The glomerular membrane (or filtration barrier) (Fig. 69.2) comprises: (i) **Capillary endothelium**. The endothelium is fenestrated. The fenestrae are 50 to 100 nm wide; (ii) **Basement membrane**. It is composed of glycoproteins and mucopolysaccharides, but no cells. It contains hydrated channels approximately 6 nm wide. These channels account for the *selectivity of the glomerular membrane*; (iii) **Bowman's visceral epithelium** (made of podocytes). The podocytes are separated by slits that are approximately 25 nm wide.

### What are the components of the juxtaglomerular apparatus?

The juxtaglomerular apparatus is *located at the angle of the afferent and efferent arterioles* where they come in contact with the *cortical part of the thick ascending limb* (CTAL) (Fig. 69.3). It comprises the macula densa, the juxtaglomerular (JG) cells and the Lacis cells. (i) The **macula densa** are specialized cells of the distal tubule where it comes in contact with the afferent arteriole. (ii) The **juxtaglomerular cells** are modified smooth muscle cells in the scala media of the terminal part of the afferent arterioles. They secrete renin. (iii) The Lacis cells (**extra glomerular mesangial cells**) are also derived from smooth muscle cells. They are present in the angular interspace between the glomerulus and the diverging afferent and efferent arterioles.

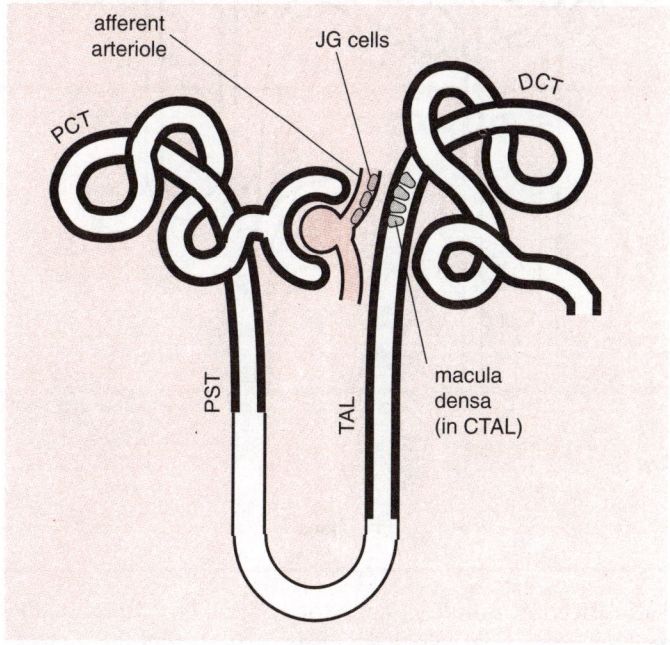

**Fig. 69.3**

### What are the various functionally distinct parts of the renal tubule?

The tubule can be subdivided into four parts: proximal tubule, thin segment, distal tubule and collecting duct (Fig. 69.4). The **proximal tubule** is the longest part of the nephron. It is further subdivided into: (i) the *proximal convoluted tubule (PCT)* located in the cortex and, (ii) the *proximal straight tubule (PST)* located in the medullary rays and the outer stripe of the medulla.

The intermediate tubule or the **thin segment** is divided into: (i) the *descending thin segment (DTS)* which traverses the inner stripe and extends deep into the inner medulla and (ii) the *ascending thin segment (ATS)*. In *juxtamedullary nephrons*, the DTS loops around as the ATS to reach the junction of the outer and inner medulla. In *cortical nephrons*, there is no ATS. The DTS is continuous at the bend of the loop with the distal tubule. The **distal tubule** is divided into: (i) the *distal straight tubule (DST)*, more commonly known as the *thick ascending limb (TAL)*, which extends across the outer medulla. The TAL is further subdivided into the *medullary thick ascending limb (MTAL)* and the *cortical thick ascending limb (CTAL)* (ii) the *distal convoluted tubule (DCT)* lying in the cortex. It is connected by a short *connecting tubule (CNT)* to the *collecting duct (CD)*. The PST, this segment and TAL together constitute the loop of Henle. The PST, thin segment and TAL together constitute the loop of Henle.

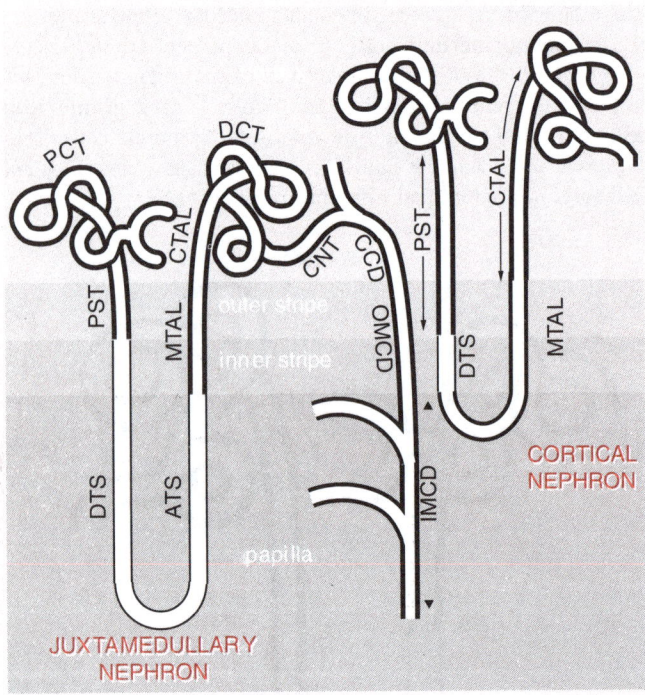

**Fig. 69.4**

The **collecting tubule** is not, strictly speaking, a part of the nephron since embryologically, it is derived from the ureteric bud. It consists of: (i) *Connecting tubule (CNT)*, which lies entirely in the cortex. In this segment, several tubules coalesce to form the collecting duct. (ii) *Collecting duct (CD)* runs through the cortex, medulla and the papilla, finally opening at the tip of the papilla. Accordingly, it is subdivided into: (i) the *cortical collecting duct (CCD)*; (ii) the *outer medullary collecting duct (OMCD)* and (iii) the *inner medullary collecting duct (IMCD)* or the papillary collecting duct. In the IMCD region, several collecting ducts coalesce together before finally opening at the tip of the renal papilla.

## What are the differences between cortical and juxtamedullary nephrons?

| Cortical Nephrons | Juxtamedullary Nephrons |
|---|---|
| Constitute 85% of the nephrons | Constitute 15% of the nephrons |
| Bowman's capsules are located in the outer and middle regions of the cortex | Bowman's capsules are located near the corticomedullary junction |
| Glomeruli of cortical nephrons are smaller than those of juxtaglomerular nephrons | Glomeruli of juxtaglomerular nephrons are about 20% larger than those of superficial glomeruli. |
| Efferent arterioles have larger diameter and break up again into the peritubular capillary network. | Efferent arterioles have smaller diameter and continue as the descending vasa recta. |
| Thin segment is short and confined to the inner stripe of the outer medulla; forms a part of the descending limb of the loop of Henle | Thin segment is long; forms a part of both the descending and ascending limb |
| Loop of Henle lies in the medullary *rays*. Hairpin bend located at the junction of the outer and inner medulla | Loop of Henle lies in the medulla. Hairpin bend located deep inside the inner medulla (papillary zone). |
| The thin segments are poorly permeable to $Na^+$ and urea. | The thin segments are highly permeable to water and urea. |
| Important for the reabsorption of tubular fluid and electrolytes. | Important for the production of medullary hyperosmolarity. |

## What is transepithelial potential difference?

An electrical potential is recordable from the lumen of the tubules. Different segments of the tubular lumen have different electrical potentials. Some of these are of importance in the tubular transport of certain ions. The potential in the proximal tubule is very slight (-2mV in the convoluted part, +2mV in the straight part). In the thick ascending limb, it is lumen positive (+6 to +10 mV). In the distal tubule, it is highly lumen negative (-70 mV).

## Names the different types of cells present in a nephron segment and mention their characteristics.

| Cell type | Present in | Salient characteristics |
|---|---|---|
| Proximal tubular cell | PCT PST | Prominent brush border. Features suggest high metabolic activity. Have leaky tight junctions with adjacent cells. |
| Intermediate tubule cell | DTS ATS | Squamous type (all other cells are cuboidal). No features suggesting significant metabolic activity. |
| Distal tubule cell | TAL DCT | Has the highest $Na^+$-$K^+$ ATPase activity compared to any other segment. Contains the Tamm-Horsfall protein. |
| Principal cell (light cells) | CD | Have microtubules with water channels in the apical cytoplasm. Responsive to ADH. Concerned with $Na^+$ reabsorption and $K^+$ secretion. |
| Intercalated cell (dark cells) | CD | Have high carbonic anhydrase activity. Concerned with $K^+$ and $Cl^-$ reabsorption and $H^+$ secretion. |

# 70

# Glomerular Filtration & Tubular Reabsorption

## What are the Starling forces operating at the glomerular capillaries?

The Starling forces, viz., the hydrostatic and colloid osmotic pressures in the glomerular capillary and the Bowman's capsule are given below:

| Glomerular capillaries | | | | |
|---|---|---|---|---|
| ← afferent arteriolar end | | | efferent arteriolar end → | |
| P=45 | π=25 | glomerular capillary | P=45 | π=35 |
| P=10 | π=0 | Bowman's capsule | P=10 | π=0 |

The Starling forces results in the following filtrative and reabsorptive pressures (*mm Hg*) at the afferent and efferent arteriolar ends:

| AFFERENT ARTERIOLAR END | |
|---|---|
| Capillary hydrostatic pressure *(which pushes out fluid)* | 45 |
| Capsular oncotic pressure *(which pulls out fluid)* | 0 |
| **Total OUTward force** | **45** |
| Plasma oncotic pressure *(which pulls in fluid)* | 25 |
| Capsular hydrostatic pressure *(which pushes in fluid)* | 10 |
| **Total INward force** | **35** |
| EFFERENT ARTERIOLAR END | |
| Capillary hydrostatic pressure *(which pushes out fluid)* | 45 |
| Capsular oncotic pressure *(which pulls out fluid)* | 0 |
| **Total OUTward force** | **45** |
| Plasma oncotic pressure *(which pulls in fluid)* | 35 |
| Capsular hydrostatic pressure *(which pushes in fluid)* | 10 |
| **Total INward force** | **45** |

Hence, fluid is filtered out from the arteriolar side of the glomerular capillaries under a net outward pressure of 10 mm Hg.

| AFFERENT ARTERIOLAR END | |
|---|---|
| Total OUTward force | 45 |
| Total INward force | 35 |
| **NET force is OUWARD** | **10** |
| EFFERENT ARTERIOLAR END | |
| Total OUTward force | 45 |
| Total INward force | 45 |
| **NET force is ZERO** | **0** |

## What are the salient differences between glomerular capillary circulation and systemic capillary circulation?

The Starling forces that operate at the glomerular capillary level are the same as in systemic capillaries but are different in magnitude. The salient differences are: (i) there is no drop in hydrostatic pressure along the glomerular capillaries despite the filtering out of fluids; (ii) there is considerable rise in plasma oncotic pressure along the glomerular capillaries; (iii) the oncotic pressure of the glomerular filtrate is zero; (iv) the capsular hydrostatic pressure is higher than that in the tissue interstitial fluid; and (v) the Starling forces equilibrate towards the efferent arteriolar end of the glomerular capillaries.

## What are the factors affecting the glomerular filtration of solutes?

The **glomerular filtration barrier** for solutes resides at the glomerular basement membrane (GBM). The concentration ratio of a substance in the Bowman's space and plasma is called its **glomerular sieving coefficient** (θ). The barrier explains the following observations: (i) Molecules less than 4 nm are freely filtered while molecules larger than 8 nm are excluded from the glomerular filtrate. (ii) The basement membrane contains negatively charged proteoglycans. Hence, *negatively charged molecules have greater difficulty passing through it*. This explains why *albumin, which is about 7 nm is totally excluded from the filtrate.* (iii) Loss of the negative charge on the basement membrane even *without any structural damage to the membrane* is enough to produce albuminuria. (iv) For comparable effective radii, flexibly coiled molecules (like dextran) pass more readily than molecules which behave like rigid spheres. (v) As a consequence of the impermeable proteins and the resultant Donnan effect, there is a slight (5%) excess of anions in the glomerular filtrate.

## What are the factors affecting the glomerular filtration of fluids?

The primary factors controlling the GFR are the Starling forces, the filtration coefficient and the surface area of the glomerular capillary membrane.

$$GFR = K_f [P_G - P_B) - (\pi_G - \pi_B)]$$

**$K_f$** is the **filtration coefficient**.

The effective surface area of the glomerular membrane is regulated physiologically by the mesangial cells that are contractile and can effectively constrict adjacent capillaries. *Secondary factors* affecting glomerular filtration are: (i) increased systemic blood pressure (which increases the capillary hydrostatic pressure thereby increasing GFR). (ii) increase in renal blood flow (which reduces the rise in colloid osmotic pressure along the glomerular capillary, thereby increasing glomerular filtration). (iii) ureteric obstruction or renal edema (which augments the hydrostatic pressure in the Bowman's capsule, thereby decreasing GFR). (iv) dehydration (which increases the plasma oncotic pressure) and hypoproteinemia (which decreases the plasma oncotic pressure, thereby decreasing and increasing the GFR respectively). (v) the numerous pathological conditions which affect the permeability and effective surface area of the GBM.

### What is autoregulation? What are the theories of autoregulation of GFR?

The GFR is normally well *autoregulated in the range of 70 to 180 mm Hg of systemic pressure* (Fig. 70.1). However, this autoregulation can be over-ridden by renal nerves. There are two hypotheses for explaining the autoregulation of GFR: the myogenic hypothesis, and the tubuloglomerular feedback (TGF) hypothesis.

The **myogenic hypothesis** of autoregulation suggests that the afferent arterioles constrict in response to augmented blood pressure. Arteriolar constriction restores GFR to normal levels. Possibly, stretch leads to the opening of $Ca^{2+}$ channels on the smooth muscle cell membrane, resulting in a $Ca^{2+}$ influx that causes contraction of arteriolar smooth muscles. According to the **tubuloglomerular feedback (TGF) hypothesis**, any increase in GFR results in increased delivery of NaCl to the distal tubule. The concentration of $Cl^-$ is sensed by the macula densa and signaled to the afferent arteriole (Fig. 69.3). Infusion of $Na^+$ salts other than NaCl does not produce TGF. The signal is transmitted probably by some adenosine or eicosanoid compound that results in vasoconstriction of afferent arteriole by opening up $Ca^{2+}$ channels of the smooth muscles.

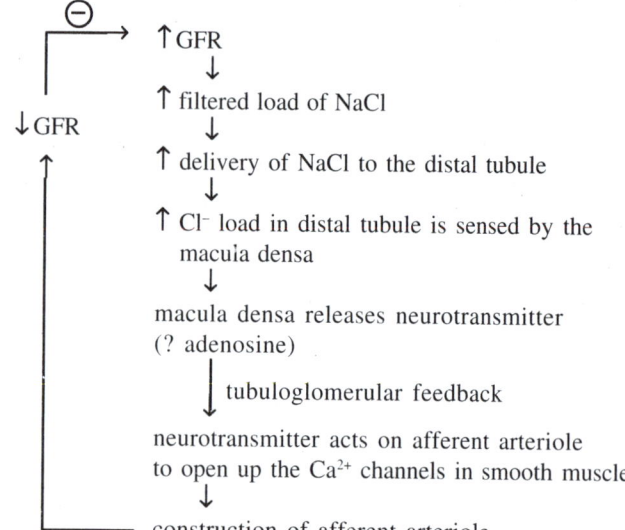

### What are the differences between obligatory and facultative water reabsorption?

85% of the water is always reabsorbed, irrespective of the body water balance. This reabsorption is called is **obligatory** (must occur). About 65% of the obligatory reabsorption occurs in the proximal tubules. Another 20% of the obligatory reabsorption occurs in the distal tubules. The remaining 15% of the water may or may not be reabsorbed depending on the body water balance. It is called

**facultative** reabsorption (optional). The facultative reabsorption occurs from the collecting tubule as it courses through the renal medulla. It is *under control of the antidiuretic hormone (ADH)* which controls the permeability of the collecting tubule to water. The renal medulla has a very high osmolarity and would normally extract water from the collecting tubules. In the presence of ADH, the collecting tubule epithelium is permeable to water, which is reabsorbed, in large amounts. However, in the absence of ADH, the collecting tubule is impermeable and no water is reabsorbed.

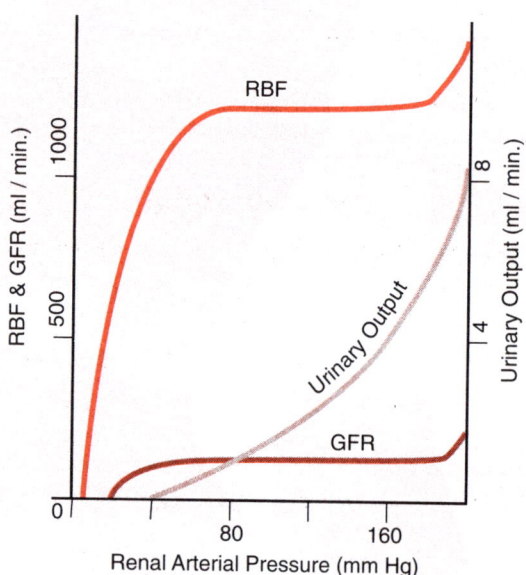

**Fig. 70.1**

### Enumerate the effects of renal sympathetic discharge to the kidneys.

Renal sympathetic discharge results in *salt and water retention* in the body due to (i) Decreased urinary output due to decreased GFR and increased tubular water reabsorption; (ii) Decreased urinary $Na^+$ excretion due to increased tubular reabsorption of $Na^+$; and (iii) Increased thirst and water intake (due to angiotensin II production). The mechanisms are as follows:

Sympathetic discharge causes (1) **afferent arteriolar vasoconstriction** that decreases RBF and GFR. The result is a decrease in urinary output with consequent water retention; (2) **efferent arteriolar vasoconstriction** resulting in a decrease in peritubular capillary pressure. The decreased peritubular capillary pressure increases tubular water reabsorption and decreases UO, producing water retention. (3) **renin-degranulation** and activation of angiotensin. The angiotensin II has 3 important effects: (a) it constricts the efferent arterioles and to a lesser degree, the afferent arterioles too. Hence, it decreases RBF, and to a lesser degree, the GFR too. Consequently, UO decreases leading to water retention. (b) it stimulates aldosterone secretion from the adrenals, resulting in increased retention of $Na^+$ and water in the body. (c) It stimulates the thirst center located in the SFO and OVLT and promotes water intake.

*At moderate stimulation rates*, sympathetic nerve stimulation causes more vasoconstriction in the efferent arteriole than in the afferent arteriole, resulting in a moderate decrease in renal blood flow, but little change in the glomerular filtration rate. *At higher stimulation rates*, sympathetic nerve stimulation causes vasoconstriction predominantly at the afferent arterioles, resulting in a marked decrease in renal blood flow and a marked decrease in the glomerular filtration rate.

## Compare and contrast the starling forces in systemic and glomerular capillaries.

### SIMILARITIES

In both, there is a net filtration of fluid, which is reduced by sympathetic stimulation.

In both, the main force for filtration is provided by the capillary hydrostatic pressure.

### DIFFERENCES

| Systemic capillaries | Glomerular capillaries |
| --- | --- |
| The net filtration pressure is only 2 mm Hg | The net filtration pressure is 10 mm Hg |
| The amount of fluid filtered is small (15 ml/min) | The amount of fluid filtered is large (125 ml/min) |
| There is a marked drop in hydro-static pressure along the capillary | There is very little drop in hydrostatic pressure along the capillary |
| There is no change in the plasma colloid oncotic pressure along the capillary | There is marked increase in plasma colloid oncotic pressure along the capillary |
| There is fluid reabsorption at the venous end of the capillary | Fluid reabsorption occurs in the peritubular capillaries |

# Renal Handling of Sodium & Diuretic Mechanisms

### Enumerate the different mechanisms of Na⁺ reabsorption in the different parts of the tubule.

About 50% of the filtered load of Na⁺ is actively reabsorbed in the PCT, and another 10% of the filtered Na⁺ load is passively reabsorbed in the PST. In the TAL, another 30% of Na⁺ is actively reabsorbed. In the DCT and CNT, about 7% of the tubular Na⁺ load is reabsorbed. The reabsorption is increased by aldosterone. In the collecting duct (CCD, OMCD and IMCD) about 3% of the Na⁺-load is actively reabsorbed (Fig. 71.1). These segments are responsive to aldosterone which increase the reabsorption of Na⁺.

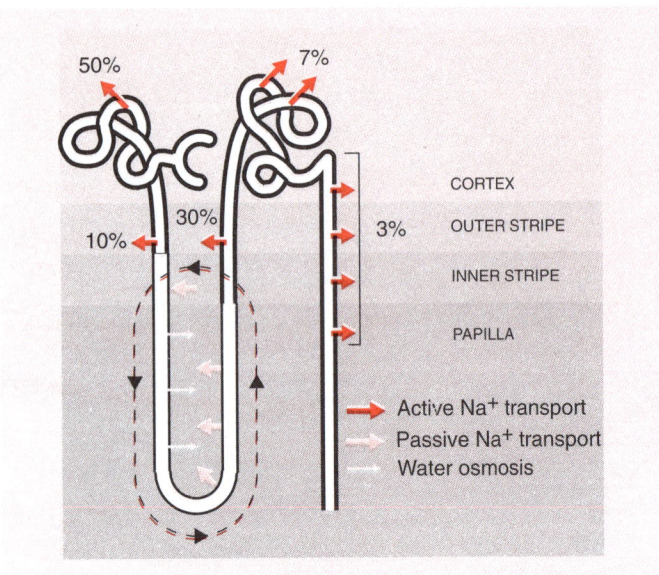

**Fig. 71.1**

The Na⁺ which is actively pumped out from the TAL into the outer medullary interstitium mostly enters the outer medullary DTS. This results in **recycling of Na⁺** in the long loops of the juxtamedullary nephrons. The recycling causes accumulation of Na⁺ in the interstitium of the renal medulla.

### What are the mechanisms of Na⁺ reabsorption?

Almost all renal tubular cells (except the intercalated cells) reabsorb Na⁺ actively. The reabsorption is driven by the Na⁺-K⁺ pump located on the basolateral membrane which pumps Na⁺ into the paracellular spaces and lowers the intracellular Na⁺ concentration. However, the mechanisms of Na⁺ transport across the apical membrane differ in the different segments of the tubule (Table 71.1). These mechanisms are: (A) Unitransport of Na⁺ (B) Na⁺ cotransport with non-Cl⁻, non-H⁺ substrates; (C) Na⁺-H⁺ exchange, usually

with a parallel Cl⁻-HCO₃⁻ (D) Na⁺/K⁺-2Cl⁻ cotransport; (E) Na⁺-Cl⁻ cotransport; (F) Chloride-driven Na⁺ transport (Fig. 71.2).

| Table 71.1 | |
|---|---|
| **Tubular segment** | **Transport mechanism** |
| PCT | A, B, C |
| PST | A, F |
| TAL | D |
| DCT | E |
| CNT | |
| CCD | |
| OMCD | A, C |
| IMCD | |

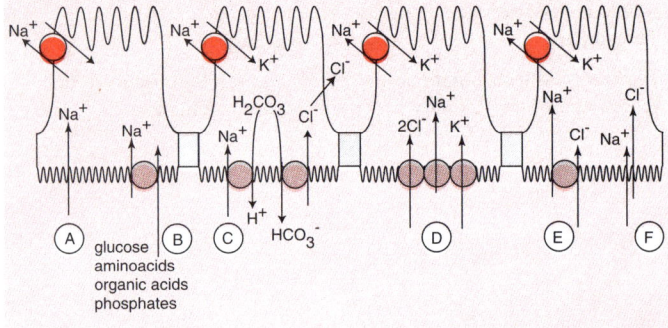

**Fig. 71.2**

### What are the factors affecting Na⁺ reabsorption?

(1) Na⁺ reabsorption *in proximal tubule* is *load-dependent* and shows **glomerulotubular balance**. It means that greater the amount of Na⁺ filtered, greater is its reabsorption. However, despite glomerulotubular balance, a rise in GFR increases the urinary excretion of Na⁺. Na⁺ reabsorption *in distal nephron* too is *load dependent* and therefore is proportional to the Na⁺ load reaching there. Thus, when proximal tubular Na⁺ reabsorption decreases, distal tubular Na⁺ load increases, and the Na⁺ reabsorption increases to compensate. Hence, **Na⁺ delivery to the distal tubules** is an important controller of distal tubular Na⁺ reabsorption. (2) Increase in **ECF volume** reduces water reabsorption from the proximal tubules due to alteration in the Starling forces. Concomitantly, there is also a reduction in Na⁺ reabsorption from the proximal tubules. (3) Most **diuretics** inhibit Na⁺ reabsorption by inhibiting apical Na⁺ transport. Osmotic diuretics reduce water reabsorption with concomitant reduction in Na⁺ reabsorption. **Aldosterone** acts on the distal tubules to stimulate the basolateral Na⁺/K⁺-ATPase and the apical Na⁺ unitransport.

## What are diuretics? Enumerate the diuretics acting on different parts of the tubule.

Diuretics are *drugs that increase the rate of urine flow*. They are used to adjust the volume and/or composition of body fluids in conditions like hypertension and edema. The diuresis produced is almost always secondary to natriuresis (increased $Na^+$ losses in urine). Most diuretics have undesirable side effects like hypokalemia and pH disturbances. Diuretics act on specific nephron segments and inhibit specific $Na^+$ transport mechanisms.

### Table 71.2

| Diuretic | Segment & mechanism |
|---|---|
| CA inhibitors | Inhibits $Na^+$-$H^+$ antiport in PCT |
| Loop diuretics | Inhibits $Na^+$-$K^+$-$2Cl^-$ cotransport in TAL |
| Thiazides | Inhibits $Na^+$-$Cl^-$ cotransport in DCT |
| Aldosterone antagonists | Inhibits unitransport of $Na^+$ in collecting duct |
| $Na^+$ channel inhibitors | Inhibits unitransport of $Na^+$ in collecting duct |

## Which type of diuretic has the maximum efficacy?

Diuretics acting on the proximal tubule have limited efficacy since the TAL, which has a great reabsorptive capacity compensates for any decrease in $Na^+$ and $H_2O$ reabsorption that might occur in the proximal tubule. Diuretics acting on sites distal to the TAL also have limited efficacy because only a small part of the filtered solute load and fluid reaches that part of the tubule. Diuretics acting on the TAL are called **loop diuretics** or **high ceiling diuretics**. They are the most efficacious of all diuretics. They abolish the urine concentrating ability of the nephron.

## What are osmotic diuretics? How do they act?

Commonly used osmotic diuretics are *glycerin*, *mannitol* and *urea*. Being non-reabsorbable, they 'hold water' in the tubule. They are most effective in the proximal tubule where normally, the maximum amount of water is reabsorbed. The water retained in tubule dilutes the tubular concentration of $Na^+$ and other electrolytes, thereby, reducing their reabsorption too. Hence, *osmotic diuretics increase the urinary excretion of nearly all electrolytes* including $Na^+$, $K^+$ (kaliuresis), $Cl^-$, $HCO_3^-$ (resulting in acidosis), $Ca^{2+}$, $Mg^{2+}$ and $PO_4^3$.

Presence of more glucose in the tubules than can be reabsorbed results in glycosuria. The unabsorbed glucose in the tubule holds water and acts as an osmotic diuretic. This is called **glycosuric osmotic diuresis**, and is seen in diabetes mellitus.

## Compare and contrast osmotic diuresis and water diuresis.

### SIMILARITIES

Both increase the rate of urine flow.

Both are associated with increased urinary excretion of electrolytes.

### DIFFERENCES

| Osmotic diuresis | Water diuresis |
|---|---|
| Induced by substances like glycerin, mannitol and urea | Induced by ingestion of large amounts of water |
| Acts by osmotically extracting body water into the tubule. | Acts by increasing body water, and excretion of excess body water |
| Stimulates ADH secretion (by causing plasma volume contraction) | Inhibits ADH secretion (by causing plasma volume expansion) |

# 72

# Renal Regulation of Urine Volume & Osmolarity

### How does the osmolarity of the filtrate change as it flows down the tubule?

In the *proximal tubules*, solutes and water are reabsorbed in isoosmolar proportions. Hence, the tubular fluid remains isoosmotic (~ 300 mOsm/L) to body fluids till the end of the proximal tubule. As the *thin segment descends* into the deeper parts of the renal medulla, the tubular fluid in it becomes progressively hyperosmolar (up to 1200 mOsm/L). This happens because the interstitium of the renal medulla is extremely hyperosmolar. As a result, water moves out of the tubular fluid into the hyperosmolar medulla. As the *thin segment ascends* back from the hyperosmotic medulla, the tubular fluid in it again becomes nearly isoosmolar. The thin ascending limb is impermeable to water. Hence, the osmolarity changes occur due to the diffusion of Na⁺ from the tubular fluid into the interstitium of the outer medulla that has relatively lower osmolarity.

In the *thick ascending limb* (TAL) of the distal tubule, *the urine becomes hypoosmolar for the first, and the only time.* This is because the TAL cells actively pump out Na⁺ from the tubular fluid into the interstitium. Water cannot follow since the distal tubule is impermeable to water. As a result, the osmolarity of the tubular fluid becomes ~ 200 mOsm lower than the adjacent

interstitium. The minimum possible osmolarity of the tubular fluid is ~ 100 mOsm / L (i.e. 300 minus 200) (Fig. 72.1).

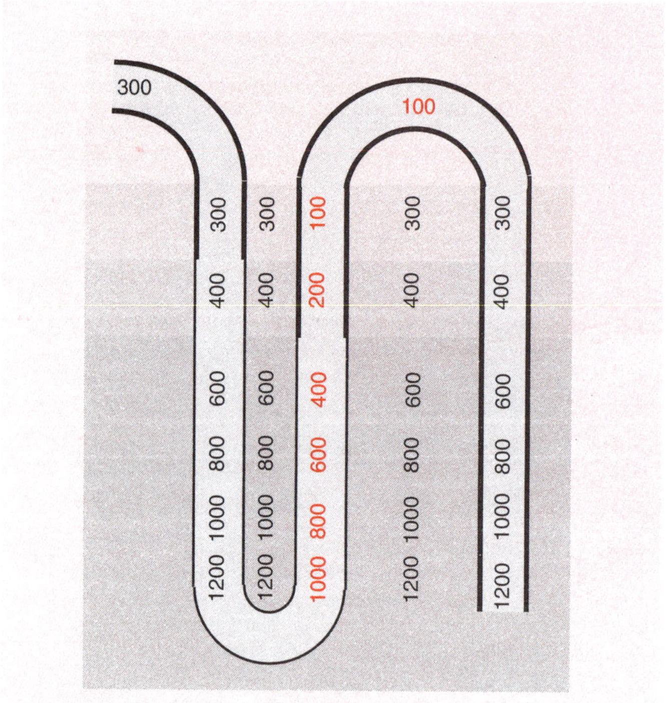

The permeability of the *collecting duct* to water is variable. In the presence of the antidiuretic hormone (ADH), it is highly permeable to water. In the absence of ADH, it is impermeable to water. Accordingly, as the collecting tubule descends through the hyperosmolar medulla, the osmolarity of the tubular fluid can change either way: (i) In the absence of ADH, the osmolarity of the tubular fluid remains unchanged. The urine finally formed will be hypoosmolar. (ii) In the presence of ADH, the osmolarity of the tubular fluid tends to equal that of the inner medulla. The urine formed is therefore hyperosmolar. Thus, it is in the collecting tubule, that the *urine becomes hyperosmolar for the second, and the last time.* (It becomes hyperosmolar for the first time in the thin segment). The maximum possible osmolarity of the tubular fluid is ~ 1200 mOsm/L (i.e. equal to the osmolarity in the innermost medulla) Thus, urine is always diluted in the distal tubule. However, its reconcentration in the collecting tubule is optional.

### What is the difference between the counter-current multiplier and counter-current exchanger mechanisms?

The interstitial fluid in the renal cortex has the same osmolarity as that of the plasma i.e., 290 mOsm/L. In the renal medulla however, it is much higher, more so in the inner medulla where it is ~ 1200 mOsm/L. This hyperosmolarity is generated by a mechanism called the **counter-current multiplier system** *that operates in the loop of Henle.* Since the vasa recta carries blood through the medulla, the solutes in the hyperosmolar zone would be expected to diffuse into blood and thus get 'washed away' from the medulla. This however does not happen due to the **counter-current exchanger system** *that operates in the vasa recta.*

### Briefly explain the mechanism of the counter-current multiplier system.

The development of medullary hyperosmolarity through counter-current multiplier can be understood in five steps (Fig. 72.2): (A) Initially, the tubular fluid and the renal interstitium has uniform osmolarity of 290 mOsm/L. (B) The thick ascending limb (TAL) of the loop of Henle pumps out Na⁺ ions (along with Cl⁻ and HCO₃⁻) into the adjacent areas of medullary interstitium. Since the TAL is impermeable to water, the osmolarity of the medullary interstitium rises and that of the tubular fluid in the TAL decreases. The difference in osmolarity between the interstitium and the tubular fluid is around 200 mOsm, which is limited by the power of the Na⁺-K⁺ pump. Establishment of this osmotic gradient is called the

**Fig. 72.1**

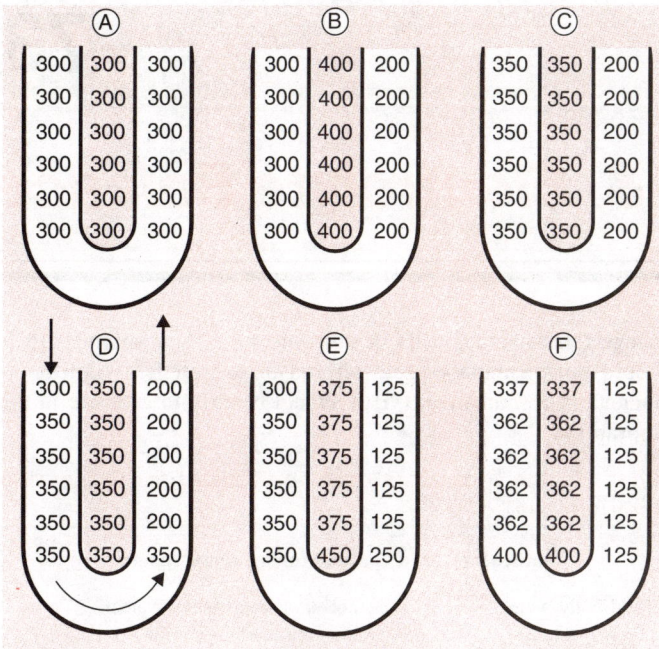

**Fig. 72.2**

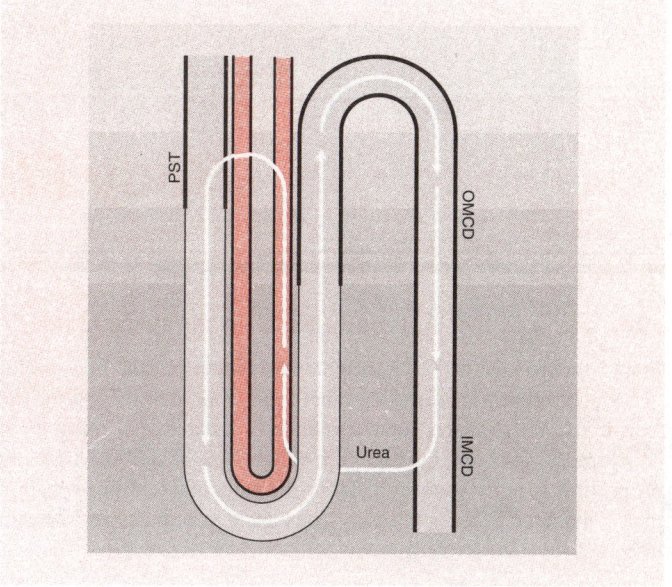

**Fig. 72.3**

**single-effect**. (C) The portion of the DTS that is located in the outer medulla is moderately permeable to Na⁺. The Na⁺ in the adjacent interstitium therefore diffuses into the tubular fluid in the DTS and equilibrates with the hyperosmolar medullary interstitium around it. (D) Fresh isoosmolar filtrate (~ 300 mOsm/L) trickles down into the descending loop and pushes some of the hyperosmolar fluid into the ascending limb round the bend. (E) As the cycle of above steps are repeated several times over, the tubular fluid and the medullary interstitium in the deeper regions of the medulla become more and more hyperosmolar.

In short, it can be said that *Na⁺ gets trapped in the loop of Henle*: it leaves the thick ascending segment only to reenter the descending segment. Since filtered Na⁺ ions enter the loop continuously and get trapped there, its concentration in the loop increases.

### What is the role of urea in the countercurrent multiplier system?

The distal and collecting tubules are *impermeable to urea*. Therefore, as water is reabsorbed from these segments, *urea gets more and more concentrated within the collecting duct*. When the luminal fluid finally reaches the urea-permeable terminal IMCD, the intraluminal urea concentration is very high, and the urea is rapidly reabsorbed into the interstitium. From the medullary interstitium, most of the urea enters the vasa recta, and is carried upwards towards the renal cortex by the ascending vasa recta. From there, urea diffuses out to reenter the renal tubule at PST of cortical nephrons. Thus, the urea is carried back to the IMCD from where it diffuses out again, resulting in a constant *recycling* (Fig. 72.3).

The recycling of urea and its continuous efflux from IMCD results in high concentration of urea in the inner medullary interstitium. Thus, while the hyperosmolarity of the outer medullary interstitium is largely due to high concentration of Na⁺ alone, the *hyperosmolarity of the inner medullary interstitium is due to high concentrations of both Na⁺ and urea*.

### Briefly explain the mechanism of the counter-current exchanger system.

As the vasa recta passes through the hyperosmolar medulla, the blood in the vasa recta equilibrates with the surrounding interstitial fluid and becomes more and more hyperosmolar. As the vasa recta loops around and exits the medulla, the blood in it once again equilibrates with the interstitium around it which now has lesser osmolarity than in the deeper regions of the medulla. Consequently, by the time the vasa recta leaves the medulla, the blood in it is only slightly hyperosmolar than when it had entered the medulla. In other words, the electrolytes in the medulla that make it hyperosmolar are not washed away by the blood flowing through the medulla. The slow rate of blood flow through the vasa recta is yet another factor which ensures that very little electrolytes are washed away from the renal medulla (Fig. 72.4).

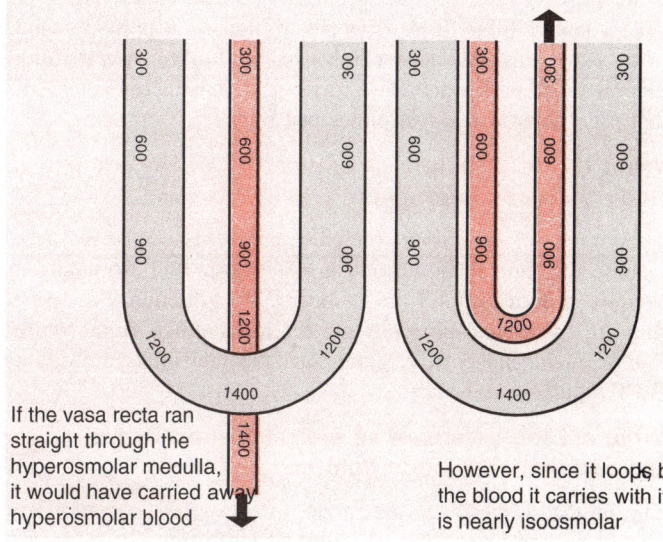

If the vasa recta ran straight through the hyperosmolar medulla, it would have carried away hyperosmolar blood

However, since it loops t the blood it carries with i is nearly isoosmolar

**Fig. 72.4**

# 73

# Body Fluid & Electrolyte Balance

## How much is the total body water in an average man ?

In an average man of 72 kg weight, the volume of total body water (TBW) is approximately 44L. The TBW constitutes 72 % of the lean body mass. Males have a relatively greater lean body mass compared to females of equivalent weight, and therefore, a greater proportion of body water too. Thus, the percentage of body weight that is made of water is 62% in males, 52% in females and 72% in infants.

## What are the various body fluid compartments?

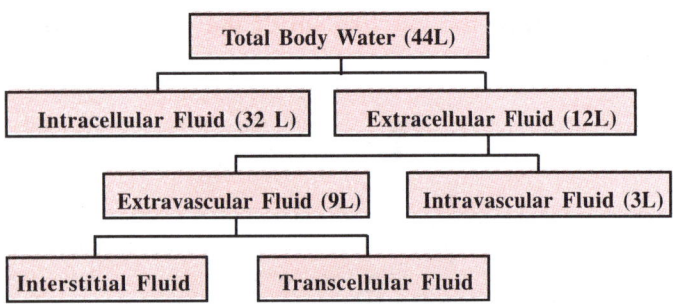

Extracellular fluid (ECF) is present outside the cells. Of the 12 L of ECF, 3L is present inside the blood vessels as plasma (the **intra-vascular fluid**) while the remaining is present around the cells (**interstitial fluid**) and is separated from the intravascular fluid only by the walls of the blood vessels. Some of the extracellular fluid however is present in specialized compartments. These are called **transcellular fluid**. Examples of transcellular fluid include urine in the urinary tract, cerebrospinal fluid, synovial fluids, pleural fluid, pericardial fluid, peritoneal fluid, intraocular fluid and secretions in the gastrointestinal tract.

## What is the principle of estimation of the volume of body fluid compartments?

The volume of the various body compartments can be measured by injecting into them an indicator substance and estimating its **volume of distribution** from the degree of its dilution. Two spaces that are calculated *indirectly* are the intracellular fluid volume (TBW volume *minus* ECF volume) and the interstitial fluid volume (ECF volume *minus* plasma volume).

## What are the criteria of an indicator substance used for the estimation of body fluid compartments?

The indicator substance used must fulfill certain criteria: (i) It should be non-toxic; (ii) It should get uniformly diluted by the fluid in the compartment; (iii) It should remain confined to the compartment whose volume is to be measured; (iv) It should not

change (pharmacologically or otherwise) the fluid volume; (v) It should not be metabolized, altered or excreted in significant amounts in a short time; (vi) It should be easy to estimate in the laboratory.

## What are the indicators commonly used for measuring body spaces?

| Indicators used for measuring body spaces | |
|---|---|
| Total body water (TBW) Volume | Deuterium oxide (heavy water), tritium oxide, aminopyrine |
| Extracellular fluid (ECF) volume | Sodium thiosulfate, sucrose, inulin, mannitol |
| Intravascular space | Evans Blue (T-1824), $^{131}I_2$ (these bind to plasma albumin, and therefore cannot escape from the blood vessels) |

## Which are the predominantly extracellular and intracellular ions?

The normal osmolarity of (extracellular) body fluids is 290 mOsm/L. The predominantly intracellular ions are $K^+$, $Mg^{2+}$ and $PO_4^{3-}$ while the predominantly extracellular ions are $Na^+$, $Ca^{2+}$ and $Cl^-$.

## Name the main contributors to body osmolarity.

The *major contributors* to the body osmolarity are $Na^+$ and $Cl^-$. The important contributors to body osmolarity are:

| Constituent | Concentration |
|---|---|
| $Na^+$ | 135-145 mEq/L |
| $Cl^-$ | 90-110 mEq/L |
| $HCO_3^-$ | 25 mEq/l |
| $K^+$ | 3.5-5.0 mEq/L |
| Glucose | 60-100 mg/dL (3.4-5.6 mEq/dL) |
| Urea | 10-20mg/dL (3.6-7.1 mEq/dL) |

## How is the total body osmolarity calculated?

The total body osmolarity can be approximately calculated from either of the following formulas. The square brackets indicate concentration in mEq/L.

$$2 \times [Na^+] + [glucose] + [urea]$$

A more accurate formula is:

$$[Na^+] + [Cl^-] + [HCO_3^-] + [K^+] + [glucose] + [Urea] + 10$$

## Briefly outline the balance of gains and losses of body water.

| Daily water gains | |
|---|---|
| Water ingested as fluids | = 1 L |
| Water contained in ingested food | = 1 L |
| Water obtained through metabolism of food | = 500 ml |
| **Total** | **= 2.5 L** |
| **Daily water losses** | |
| Water lost in urine | = 1.5 L |
| Water lost through insensible perspiration | = 800 ml |
| Water lost through sweating | = 100 ml |
| Water lost through feces | = 100 ml |
| **Total** | **= 2.5 L** |

## How much fluid is lost in gastrointestinal secretions? What is its significance?

Nearly 7 liters of secretions enter the gastrointestinal tract daily but these are mostly reabsorbed back into the blood. However, when there is a gastrointestinal obstruction, large volumes of secretions accumulate in the GIT. These accumulated secretions represent losses of fluid and electrolytes from the body.

| Secretion | Volume |
|---|---|
| Saliva | 1000 |
| Gastric juices | 2000 |
| Bile | 500 |
| Pancreatic juice | 500 |
| Succus entericus | 3000 |

## Briefly outline the balance of gains and losses of body sodium.

About 100 to 400 mmol of $Na^+$ is lost daily, mostly in urine, but also in sweat and feces. The same amount is replenished daily through dietary intake.

## What are the mechanisms of regulation of body fluid and electrolyte balance?

Derangements of fluid and electrolyte balance result directly or indirectly in changes in *blood volume* and / or changes in *colloid osmotic pressure (oncotic pressure)*. These changes set off a series of circulatory *readjustments* and neurohormonal and behavioral *reflexes*, ultimately leading to the restoration of normal fluid and electrolyte composition of body.

**Readjustments** are brought about by any change in the volume and oncotic pressure of the body fluids that leads to changes in the Starling forces operating at the renal glomeruli and renal tubules. The end result is a readjustment of glomerular filtration and tubular reabsorption so that the normal volume and oncotic pressure is restored.

Starling mechanisms affect tubular reabsorption mainly in the proximal tubule where high amounts of $H_2O$ and $Na^+$ are

reabsorbed. Hence, these mechanisms are more suited for *large-scale adjustments in fluid and electrolyte balance*. It works as follows:

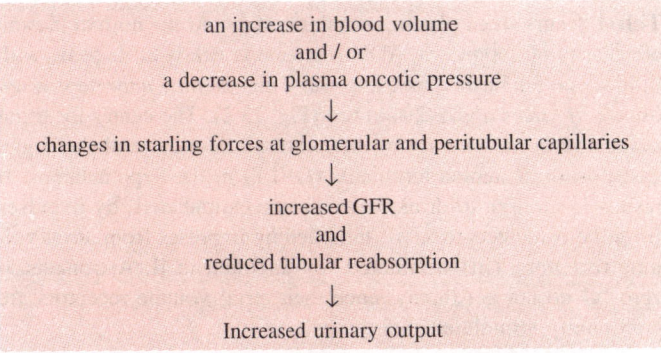

an increase in blood volume
and / or
a decrease in plasma oncotic pressure
↓
changes in starling forces at glomerular and peritubular capillaries
↓
increased GFR
and
reduced tubular reabsorption
↓
Increased urinary output

**Reflexes** are triggered by any change in the volume and electrolyte composition of the body that is sensed by **volume receptors** and **osmoreceptors** respectively. These receptors reflexly trigger neural, hormonal and behavioral mechanisms, which bring about a correction of the original disturbance (see flow chart).

## What are the various effector mechanisms involved in the reflex regulation of body fluid and electrolyte balance?

The effector mechanisms include: (i) *Neural:* sympathetic discharge; (ii) *Hormonal:* ADH and aldosterone secretion; (iii) *Behavioral:* thirst and salt craving.

**Sympathetic discharge** to the kidneys is stimulated by hypovolemia (due to reduced stimulation of atrial volume receptors). It brings about retention of $Na^+$ and water.

**ADH** is secreted largely by the neurons of the suprachiasmatic nuclei, and also by the paraventricular nuclei in the hypothalamus (Fig. 73.1). ADH secretion is stimulated by inputs both from osmoreceptors as well as volume receptors. ADH promotes water reabsorption from the collecting duct and makes it iso- or hypertonic as required.

**Aldosterone** secretion is stimulated by: (i) circulating angiotensin II formed as a result of sympathetic activation (the main stimulus); (ii) rise in plasma $K^+$. (iii) fall in plasma $Na^+$ osmolarity (a weak stimulus). Aldosterone promotes reabsorption of $Na^+$ from the DCT.

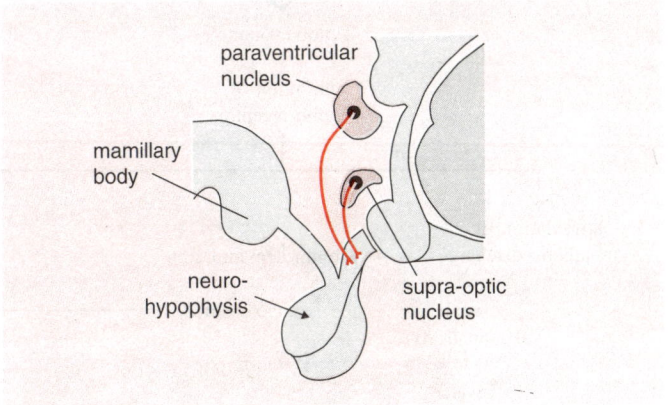

**Fig. 73.1**

Both ADH and aldosterone operate in the distal tubule where the amount of $H_2O$ and $Na^+$ reabsorbed are much lesser than in the proximal tubule. Hence, these mechanisms, unlike the 'readjustments' are more suited for *fine adjustments in fluid and electrolyte balance*.

**Thirst** occurs when plasma osmolarity rises. At the normal plasma osmolarity of 290mOsm, ADH secretion is nearly at its peak, with little scope for further rise. It is thirst that is *most important when osmolarity rises above 290mOsm* (Fig. 73.2). The center for thirst is located *in the vicinity of* the subfornical organ and the organ vasculosum of lamina terminalis (OVLT) in the hypothalamus. It results in an urge to drink water. It is (i) stimulated by impulses from the osmoreceptors; (ii) inhibited by impulses from atrial volume receptors. (iii) stimulated by angiotensin II. Astronauts at zero 'g' do not get thirsty since their atrial volume receptors are continually stimulated.

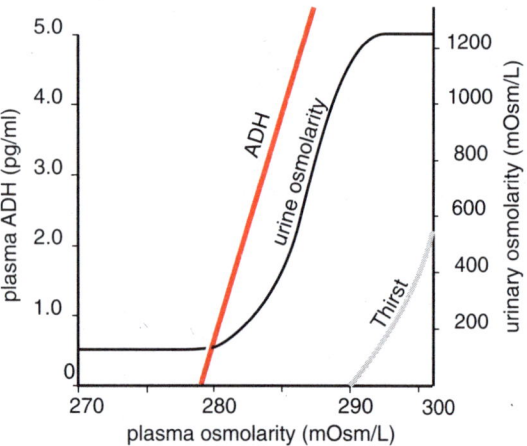

**Fig. 73.2**

**Salt craving** is the intense desire for excessive consumption of NaCl evoked by a decrease in the plasma Na$^+$ concentration. The changes in plasma Na$^+$ concentration is sensed by *receptors probably located in the amygdala*.

## What are the various receptors involved in the regulation of body fluid and electrolyte balance?

The receptors involved in the regulation of body fluid and electrolyte balance are the osmoreceptors and the volume receptors. The **osmoreceptors** are located in the anterior hypothalamus, *near* but *distinct from* the supraoptic nuclei. They respond to *as little as 1%* changes in the osmolarity by firing rapidly. Impulses from the osmoreceptors reach the thirst center and the ADH center. The osmoreceptors *do not respond to hypertonic solutions of urea or glucose* (which easily enter the osmoreceptor cells). That is significant because if it did, a rise in plasma urea concentration would have decreased the urinary output (by stimulating ADH) and thereby, hampered the excretion of urea.

The **volume receptors** are *located in the right atria*. When the blood volume increases, the venous return to the right atrium, and with it, the right atrial pressure increase. The change in the right atrial pressure is sensed by the atrial volume receptors. Increased venous filling increases the firing rate of the volume receptors. Impulses from the volume receptors *travel through the vagus nerve* and reach the medulla where they *inhibit the pressor area* of the **vasomotor center** and thereby *suppress the sympathetic discharge*. Conversely, a decrease in the blood volume would increase the sympathetic discharge. The afferents from the atrial volume receptors also reach the **thirst center**. The blood volume must change by *as much as 10%* before any change in the sympathetic discharge or thirst is evoked.

Volume receptors are *less sensitive* than osmoreceptors. But, volume receptors, once stimulated, bring about *much stronger* effects than osmoreceptors. This is apparent when a decreased plasma volume coexists with a decreased osmolarity. Water is retained (by stimulation of thirst and ADH) to restore the volume at the expense of decreasing the osmolarity further. Hence the axiom: *volume overrides tonicity*.

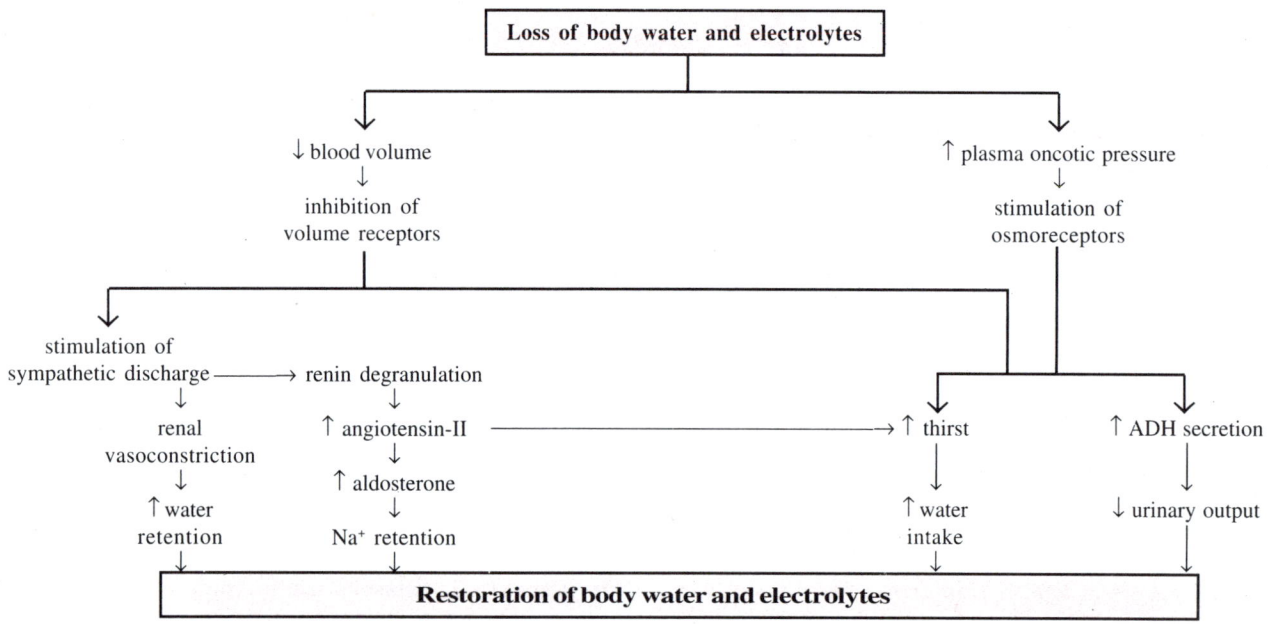

# 74

# Renal Handling of Hydrogen Ions & Acid-Base Balance

## Briefly describe the site and mechanism of H⁺ secretion.

Hydrogen ions are secreted into the tubule in most parts of the nephron: in the PCT, PST, TAL, CCD, OMCD and IMCD. Very little amounts of H⁺ are secreted in the DCT. In the collecting duct segments, H⁺ is secreted by the intercalated cells only (and *not* by the principal cells) (Fig. 74.1).

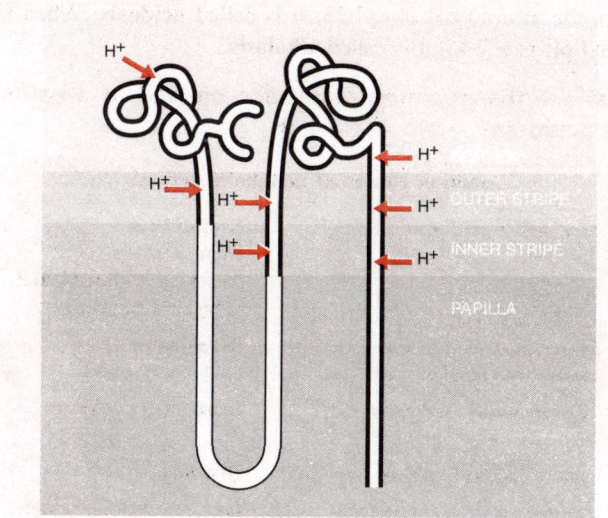

**Fig. 74.1**

The H⁺ are produced in the tubular cell by the following reaction:

$$H_2O + CO_2 \xrightarrow{\text{Carbonic Anhydrase}} H_2CO_3 \longrightarrow H^+ + HCO_3^-$$

The H⁺ is secreted into the tubules by **H⁺–Na⁺ antiport**, **H⁺-K⁺ antiport**, or **proton pump** (primary active H⁺ transport). The $HCO_3^-$ leaves the basolateral membrane through a **$HCO_3^-$ - Cl⁻ antiporter**. The H⁺ are mopped by the $HCO_3^-$, $HPO_4^{2-}$, and $NH_3$ buffers present in the tubular fluid (Fig. 74.2).

## What are the different types of blood buffers?

**Hemoglobin** is the largest contributor to the buffering capacity of blood. The $NH_2$ groups on intermediate histidine residues of the hemoglobin provide most of the buffering action. **Plasma proteins** are the next largest contributors to the buffering capacity. They also owe their buffering action to their $NH_2$ residues. **Bicarbonates** are the most *important* buffers in blood. This is because the components of this buffer system can be regulated by the body.

$$H^+ + HCO_3^- \xrightarrow{\text{Carbonic Anhydrase}} H_2O + CO_2$$

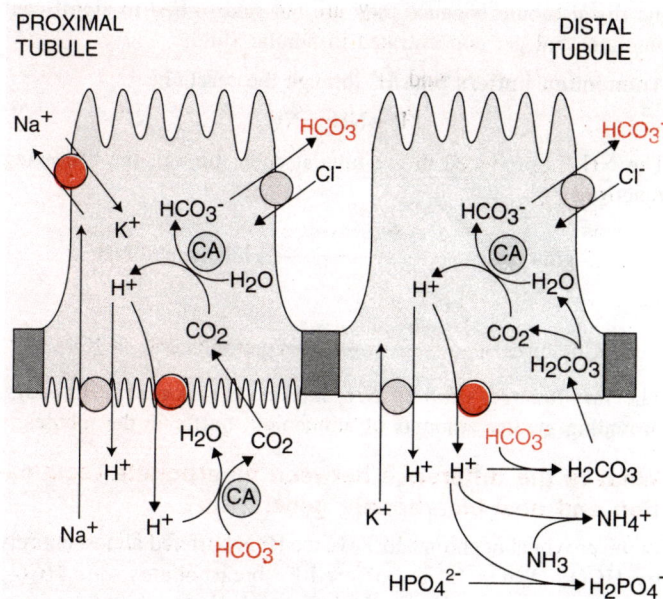

**Fig. 74.2**

The $HCO_3^-$ *concentration is regulated by the kidney* while the $P_{CO_2}$ *is regulated by adjusting the ventilation.* The pK of the bicarbonate buffer system is 6.1. Yet, it is a very effective buffer because $CO_2$ escapes from the field of reaction, preventing the backward reaction.

**Phosphates** are the predominant intracellular buffers in the body.

$$H^+ + HPO_4^{2-} = H_2PO_4^-$$

In blood, their concentration is small and therefore, they are not very important as blood buffer.

## What is the role of urinary buffers?

In the proximal as well as the distal tubule, the H⁺ secreted tend to *leak back* through the tight junctions into the intercellular spaces. The leakage is more in the proximal tubular cells where the 'tight junctions' are 'leaky'. Also, higher the tubular concentration of H⁺, greater is the leakage. *To reduce this backward leakage,* the presence of buffers in the renal tubules (the urinary buffers) is essential.

## Name the different types of urinary buffers.

**Bicarbonate buffers** mop up H⁺ to form $H_2CO_3$, which dissociates in the presence of carbonic anhydrase to form $CO_2$ and $H_2O$.

$$H^+ + HCO_3^- \xrightarrow{\text{Carbonic Anhydrase}} H_2O + CO_2$$

The carbonic anhydrase is present on the brush border of the proximal tubules and in the TAL. It is absent in the apical membrane of distal tubular cells. Consequently, the carbonic acid remains undissociated in the distal tubule and is excreted as such.

**Phosphate buffers** comprise a mixture of monobasic and dibasic phosphates. The monobasic phosphate binds H+ forming dibasic phosphates.

$$H^+ + HPO_4^{2-} = H_2PO_4^-$$

Phosphates are quite effective as urinary buffers, especially in the distal tubule because they are not reabsorbed in significant amounts and get concentrated in tubular fluid.

**Ammonium buffers** bind H+ through the reaction:

$$H^+ + NH_3 = NH_4^+$$

The $NH_3$ is produced in the tubular cells through the following reactions:

$$\text{glutamine} \xrightarrow{\text{glutaminase}} \text{glutamate} + NH_3$$

$$\text{glutamate} \xrightarrow[\text{dehydrogenase}]{\text{glutamate } \alpha} \alpha\text{-ketoglutarate} + NH_3$$

The *tubular secretion of $NH_3$ increases in chronic acidosis*, providing greater amounts of ammonium buffer in the tubules.

### What is the difference between bicarbonate reclamation and new bicarbonate generation?

In the proximal nephron and TAL, the H+ is buffered almost entirely by $HCO_3^-$. When H+ is buffered by bicarbonates, *one $HCO_3^-$ appears in the peritubular fluid for each $HCO_3^-$ that disappears from the tubular fluid*. This is called **$HCO_3^-$ reclamation**, or less appropriately, **$HCO_3^-$ reabsorption**. The PCT reclaims 80% of the filtered load of bicarbonate. Another 15% of the filtered bicarbonate load is reclaimed in the TAL. In the distal nephrons, only 5% of the filtered load of $HCO_3^-$ is available for buffering H+. This amount of $HCO_3^-$ is *completely reclaimed*.

*After all the tubular $HCO_3^-$ is completely reclaimed, the remaining H+ is mopped up by buffers other than $HCO_3^-$, like $HPO_4^{2-}$. In such a situation, the appearance of $HCO_3^-$ ions in peritubular fluid is not associated with the disappearance of $HCO_3^-$ ions from tubular fluid.* Hence, the $HCO_3^-$ that appears in the peritubular fluid represents a **new $HCO_3^-$ generation**.

### What is the normal body pH?

The arterial plasma pH is 7.40 (7.35 to 7.45), mixed venous plasma pH is 7.28 and intracellular fluid pH 6.90.

### What are the factors that routinely threaten the constancy of pH in the body?

The constancy of pH is threatened mainly by the *continuous production of acids* in the body. Each day, the amount of acid produced by the body ranges from 0.3 mEq/L to 1.0 mEq/L. The acids routinely produced in the body are either volatile or non-volatile. **Carbonic acid** is called *volatile* since it normally dissociates into carbon dioxide and eliminated by the lung. *Non-volatile acids* are also called fixed acids, e.g., **sulfuric** and **phosphoric acids**. Sulfuric acid is an end product of the sulfur-containing aminoacids methionine and cystine, while phosphoric acid is formed in the metabolism of phospholipids, nucleic acids, phosphoproteins and phosphoglycerides. Non-volatile acids also include organic acids like **lactic acid, acetoacetic acid, and β-hydroxy butyric acid**. These are however normally oxidized to $CO_2$ and water, but appear in blood following incomplete combustion of carbohydrates and fats. **Uric acid** is formed through the metabolism of nucleoproteins.

The body pH is also affected by *consumption of acid/alkali* or potentially acidic/alkaline substances in the diet (acidic, e.g., lysine; alkaline e.g. citrates). Occasionally, *acids are lost from the body* in large amounts, e.g., in **vomiting**. There is then an *alkali load* instead of the usual acid load on the body. Similarly, in **diarrhea**, alkalis are lost from the body, resulting in the increase in the acid load on the body.

### At what pH is it called acidosis or alkalosis?

When the arterial pH is < 7.35, it is called **acidosis**. When the arterial pH is > 7.45, it is called **alkalosis**.

### What are the common metabolic causes of alkalosis and acidosis?

| Common causes of metabolic acidosis | |
|---|---|
| I. *Increased acid production* | Ketoacidosis Lactic acidosis poisoning with methanol, salicylates (aspirin) etc. |
| II. *Decreased filtration of acids into tubules* | Renal failure |
| III. *Decreased H+ secretion by tubules* | Renal tubular acidosis |
| IV. *Excess alkali loss from body* | Diarrhea |
| V. *Increased acid consumption* | Intake of $NH_4Cl$, lysine |

Rise in H+ is associated with a rise in either Cl- (the *hyperchloremic variety* of metabolic acidosis like types III, IV & V above) or anions like lactate, acetoacetate etc. (types I & II) the *high-anion gap variety.*

| Common causes of metabolic alkalosis | |
|---|---|
| I. *Loss of acids &/or NaCl* | Vomiting, diuretic therapy |
| II. *Increased tubular H+ secretion* | Hyperaldosteronism Cushing's syndrome Severe K+ depletion |
| III. *Increased intake of alkali* | Milk-alkali syndrome |

### What is the plasma anion gap and how is it useful?

The estimation of the plasma anion gap provides a quick laboratory method to distinguish hyperchloremic and the non-hyperchloremic types of metabolic acidosis. The cations in the extracellular fluid almost entirely comprise Na+ (The concentrations of K+, $Ca^{2+}$ and $Mg^{2+}$ in the ECF are negligible in comparison.) The anions on the other hand are of two types: (i) those which are routinely estimated in clinical practice, i.e. $HCO_3^-$ and Cl-, and (ii) those which are not e.g. albumin, phosphates, sulfates and several other organic acids. The **anion gap** refers to the difference between plasma $Na^+$ concentration, and the sum of plasma $HCO_3^-$ and $Cl^-$ concentrations. Its *normal value* is $12 \pm 2$ mEq/L.

**Plasma anion gap = plasma $Na^+$ – (plasma $HCO_3^-$ + plasma $Cl^-$)**

It therefore gives an indirect measure of the anions other than $HCO_3^-$ and Cl-, viz., albumin, phosphates, sulfates and other organic acids. *Plasma albumin accounts for most of the anion gap.* Although each of these can be estimated separately and precisely, the anion gap is a quick estimate of all these anions taken together.

*In types I and II metabolic acidosis, the anion gap increases* due the accumulation in plasma of the anions of various acids such as acetoacetic acid or lactic acid. In renal failure, the anion gap increases because sulfates, phosphates and organic acid anions are not excreted efficiently. However, *in types III, IV and V, the anion gap is unchanged.*

### Briefly explain the regulation of acid-base balance

In **metabolic acidosis**, due to the presence of excessive $H^+$, the $HCO_3^-$ decreases (they are consumed) and $P_{CO_2}$ increases (it is generated).

$$H^+ + HCO_3^- = H_2O + CO_2$$

**Respiratory acidosis** on the other hand is due to increased $P_{CO_2}$. It results in the production of $H^+$ (which accounts for the acidosis) and $HCO_3^-$.

$$H_2O + CO_2 = H^+ + HCO_3^-$$

*In either case, the $P_{CO_2}$ is high in acidosis. The high $P_{CO_2}$ results in increased tubular secretion of $H^+$.* The $H^+$ secreted binds to tubular $HCO_3^-$ resulting in *increased $HCO_3^-$ reclamation.* However, in metabolic acidosis, the plasma $HCO_3^-$ is low and hence, the filtered load of $HCO_3^-$ in the tubules too is low. Hence, there is not much tubular $HCO_3^-$ available to be reclaimed. However, in acidosis, there is also increased renal **ammoniagenesis**. This increases the amount of ammonia buffer available in the tubule for buffering the augmented $H^+$ secretion in acidosis and results in *new $HCO_3^-$ generation.* Thus, *without increased renal ammoniagenesis, correction of metabolic acidosis is not possible.*

In **metabolic alkalosis**, $HCO_3^-$ is raised and the $P_{CO_2}$ gets reduced due to presence of excess hydroxyl ions.

$$OH^- + CO_2 = HCO_3^-$$

In **respiratory alkalosis**, the $P_{CO_2}$ is reduced due to excessive ventilation ($CO_2$ wash-out) and $HCO_3^-$ decreases as the equilibrium shifts to the left. *In either case, $P_{CO_2}$ is low in alkalosis.* Consequently, the tubular secretion of $H^+$ decreases and so does the amount of $HCO_3^-$ reclamation. If the plasma $HCO_3^-$ is high (as in metabolic alkalosis), large amounts of it are filtered into the tubules and go unabsorbed due to the reduction of $H^+$ secretion. As a result, plasma $HCO_3^-$ decreases, and the pH rises towards normal.

# Renal Handling of Potassium Ions & Potassium Balance

## How are potassium ions handled by the tubules?

In the *proximal tubule*, a large amount of K$^+$ is reabsorbed, mainly through bulk flow but partly through active transport. In the *distal tubule*, large amounts of K$^+$ are secreted into the tubule.

## Name some factors affecting K$^+$ handling by the tubules?

**Aldosterone** increases K$^+$ secretion because. (i) it stimulates Na$^+$-K$^+$ ATPase. (ii) it makes the lumen more negative by increasing Na$^+$ reabsorption and (iii) it increases the permeability of apical membrane to K$^+$. Aldosterone-mediated changes in K$^+$ secretion are important for acute response to external K$^+$ imbalances. **Acidosis** *decreases K$^+$ secretion by the principal cells.*

## What is the difference between external and internal balance of K$^+$.

**External K$^+$ balance** refers to the constancy of the total body K$^+$ that can be maintained only if the *net amount* of K$^+$ gained or lost by the body from the external environment is zero. In other words, the *daily intestinal absorption of K$^+$ must be equal to its daily urinary excretion*. **Internal K$^+$ balance** refers to the constancy of the distribution of K$^+$ in the intracellular and extracellular compartments. Acute changes in plasma K$^+$ results within minutes in a rapid redistribution of K$^+$ between the ECF and ICF.

## What are the two main determinants of external K$^+$ balance?

The two main determinants of external potassium balance are (i) dietary intake and intestinal absorption of potassium, and (ii) urinary excretion of potassium. The average dietary intake of potassium is approximately 100 mEq/day (~ 5g/day). Normally, 90% of ingested potassium is absorbed and the remaining 10% appears in the stool. The kidneys must excrete the 90 mEq each day for maintaining zero K$^+$ balance.

## Briefly outline the regulation of external K$^+$ balance.

Any change in the body K$^+$ balance triggers an acute and a chronic response. In the **acute response**, an increase in plasma K$^+$ stimulates *aldosterone* secretion. Aldosterone in turn acts on the distal nephron and increases K$^+$ excretion in 1 – 2 hours. The **chronic response** is *aldosterone-independent.* An increase in plasma K$^+$ inhibits the apical K$^+$-H$^+$-ATPase in the intercalated cells of the collecting duct and thereby increases K$^+$ secretion, restoring normal plasma K$^+$ levels. Conversely, K$^+$ deprivation stimulates K$^+$-H$^+$-ATPase.

## Enumerate the common causes of hypokalemia and hyperkalemia.

| Causes of hypokalemia | Causes of hyperkalemia |
|---|---|
| Decreased dietary intake | Excessive dietary intake Tissue damage (muscle crush, hemolysis, internal bleeding) |
| Metabolic alkalosis Renal tubular acidosis | Metabolic acidosis |
| Hyperaldosteronism Cushing's disease | Hypoaldosteronism Addison's disease |
| Diuretics | Potassium-sparing diuretics |
| Renal Failure (ARF, CRF) | |

## Enumerate the clinical features of hypokalemia and hyperkalemia.

**Neuromuscular symptoms** are prominent in hypokalemia. It ranges from muscle weakness to total paralysis. **Cardiac symptoms** are more prominent in hyperkalemia, usually resulting in cardiac arrhythmias. Nonetheless, the ECG signs are present in both hypokalemia and hyperkalemia (Fig. 75.1). *Hypokalemic ECG changes* include depression of ST segment, flattening or inversion of T wave and prominence of U wave. *Hyperkalemic ECG changes* include tall T waves, broad QRS complexes and prolongation of PR interval. **GIT symptoms** in hypokalemia include abdominal distension due to paralytic ileus (absence of intestinal peristalsis).

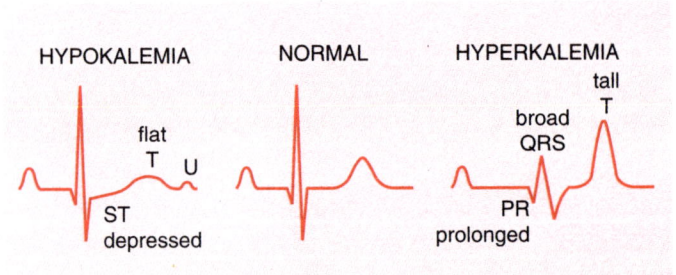

**Fig. 75.1**

# *Renal Handling of Miscellaneous Substances*

## Outline the mechanism of tubular reabsorption of glucose.

Glucose is freely filtered into the glomerular filtrate. It is completely reabsorbed in the proximal tubule. Glucose is reabsorbed by secondary active transport (Fig. 76.1). At the apical membrane, there is a **carrier-mediated Na⁺- glucose cotransport**. The carrier is called sodium-dependent glucose transporter (**SGLT**).

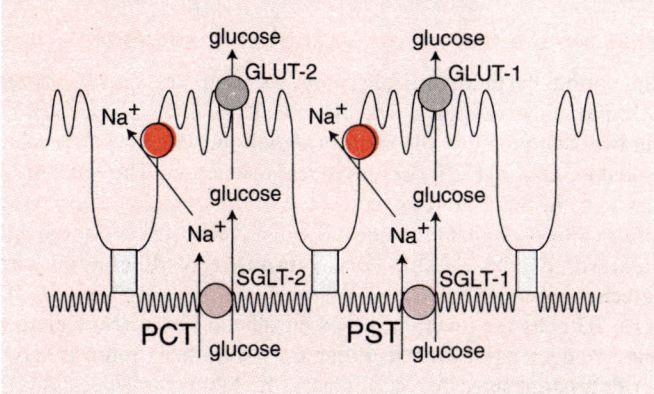

**Fig. 76.1**

The glucose that enters the cell through the apical membrane diffuses out of the basolateral membrane through facilitated diffusion. The carrier for facilitated diffusion across the apical membrane is called **glucose transporter** (**GLUT**), which belongs to a different family of glucose transporter than SGLT (Fig. 76.1).

## How are aminoacids and peptides handled by the renal tubules?

Aminoacids are normally completely reabsorbed in the proximal tubule. They are transported across the apical border of proximal cells by secondary active transport. There are different symports for neutral, basic and acidic aminoacids and iminoacids. Cystine and methionine seem to possess specific carriers.

Peptides and small proteins that do enter the tubules get endocytosed through the apical membrane of the proximal cells. Inside the cell, they are cleaved into the constituent aminoacids, which then diffuse out of the basolateral membranes.

## How are organic acids and bases handled by the renal tubules?

In the non-ionized form, organic acids and bases are sufficiently lipid-soluble to quickly diffuse across the tubular epithelium. In the ionized form however, organic ions and bases have separate transport systems. For example, PAH is transported by a **PAH-anion antiport** working together with a **Na⁺-anion symporter**. The

anion is a dicarboxylate or a tricarboxylate. The entire transport mechanism is non-electrogenic.

These transport systems are non-specific: e.g., one anion transporter can transport several endogenous (bile salts, hippurate, urate) and exogenous (PAH, penicillin, probenecid, aspirin) substances. There is competition among substances sharing the same transport system for elimination. For example, **probenecid** *inhibits the tubular secretion of penicillin.*

*Passive diffusion is speedier than transport of the ionized forms.* Many drugs and drug metabolites are weak acids or bases that are predominantly non-ionized and quickly diffuse into the tubules.

## What is the therapeutic use of alkalization of urine?

Alkalization of the urine ionizes the drug in the tubular fluid, resulting in a reduction of the non-ionized form of the drug in the tubular fluid. This increases its concentration gradient, which favors its passive diffusion from blood into the tubules. This process is known as **non-ionic diffusion and diffusion trapping**. Alkalization of urine is employed for achieving high urinary concentration of antibiotics during the treatment of urinary infections (Fig. 76.2).

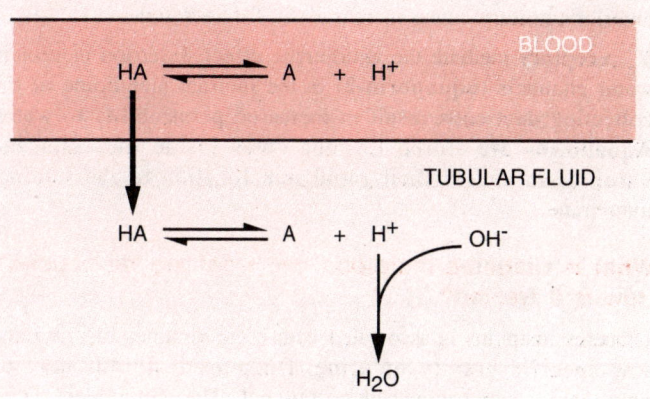

**Fig. 76.2**

## How is urea handled by the renal tubules?

Urea is filtered freely into the glomerular filtrate. About 50% of the filtered urea is reabsorbed passively in the proximal tubule. In the thin segment, urea, which is present in high concentration in the renal medulla, diffuses into the tubular lumen (**tubular secretion**). The distal tubule is mostly *impermeable to urea*. In the terminal part of the collecting duct (IMCD), however, large amounts of urea are reabsorbed. The reabsorption employs a specialized **urea transport protein**.

# Hormones acting on the Kidney

### Where is ADH secreted from?

**Antidiuretic hormone (ADH)** or **arginine vasopressin (AVP)** is a neurohormone, i.e. a hormone secreted into circulation by nerve cells. The precursor of AVP is *pre-pro-pressophysin*, which is synthesized in the cell bodies of the neurons in the **supraoptic** and **paraventricular nuclei**. Pre-pro-pressophysin is cleaved in the endoplasmic reticulum to form AVP and packaged into secretory granules (called **Herring bodies**) in the Golgi apparatus. The Herring bodies are transported down the axons by axoplasmic flow to their the endings in the **posterior pituitary**. When stimulated by inputs from the osmoreceptors and volume receptors, AVP-secreting neurons fire off action potentials. The action potentials reaching the neural endings trigger release of hormone from them by $Ca^{2+}$-dependent exocytosis.

### Briefly enumerate the actions of ADH and the receptors mediating them.

There are 2 types of AVP receptors: **$V_1$ receptors** have various effects depending on their location: (i) $V_{1a}$ receptors mediate smooth muscle contraction; (ii) $V_{1a}$ receptors in area postrema. Decrease the cardiac output. (iii) $V_{1a}$ receptors in liver stimulate glycogenesis; (iv) $V_{1b}$ *receptors* present on corticotropes in anterior pituitary cause increased ACTH secretion.

**$V_2$ receptors** mediate the antidiuretic effect. Insertion of protein water channels (**aquaporin-2**) in the luminal membrane of the collecting duct cells result in increased permeability to water. Aquaporins are stored in endosomes inside the cells and vasopressin causes their rapid translocation to the luminal membrane.

### What is diabetes insipidus and what are its causes? How is it treated?

Diabetes insipidus is associated with large volumes of urine and low specific gravity of urine. Diabetes insipidus may be neurogenic, nephrogenic or gestational. The commonest cause of **neurogenic** diabetes insipidus is surgical hypophysectomy. It occurs 4 to 6 weeks after surgery due to retrograde degeneration of the AVP-secreting neurons. Neurogenic diabetes insipidus can also occur as an autosomal dominant disease. It is treated by administering AVP. **Nephrogenic** diabetes insipidus is usually genetic and may be (i) due to unresponsiveness of V2 receptors to AVP, or (ii) impaired formation of aquaporin-2. **Gestational** diabetes insipidus occurs in pregnancy due to an abnormal increase in plasma *vasopressinase* levels. It is treated by giving *desmopressin*, an analogue of vasopressin that is resistant to inactivation by vasopressinase.

### How is renin secretion activated?

Renin is a protease enzyme. Its primary source is the JG cells (specialized smooth muscle cells) of the kidneys. Renin production also occurs in unspecialized smooth muscle cells in the afferent arteriole up to the interlobular arteries in fetal kidneys and in adults, when there is increased demand for renin secretion (Fig. 69.2).

### What are the factors regulating renin secretion?

The various factors regulating renin secretion are: (i) **Intrarenal vascular baroreceptors**. The JG cells themselves are sensors of intravascular pressure. (ii) **Sodium signal**. Increase in $Na^+$ (or more probably, $Cl^-$) in DCT decreases renin-secretion. The amount of NaCl in the tubular fluid is *sensed by the macula densa*. The information is signaled to the JG cells. Adenosine is a probable mediator of the signal. (iii) **Sympathetic discharge and catecholamines**. These cause *degranulation of renin* from the JG cells. JG cells are innervated by sympathetic fibers. (iv) **Calcium ions**. A decrease in intracellular $Ca^{2+}$ stimulates renin release. (v) **Potassium ions**. A rise in plasma $K^+$ inhibits renin release.

### How does renin activate angiotensin production?

Angiotensin-II (A-II) is formed from angiotensinogen, an $\alpha_2$ globulin plasma protein.

$$\text{Angiotensinogen} \xrightarrow{\quad Renin \quad} \text{Angiotensin-I}$$

$$\text{Angiotensin-I} \xrightarrow{\quad ACE \quad} \text{Angiotensin-II}$$

**Angiotensin converting enzyme (ACE)** is found on the surface of capillary endothelium in the lungs and kidneys.

### What are the actions of angiotensin-II?

The actions of angiotensin-II (A-II) can be classified as *central* effects, *renal* effects and effects on *aldosterone*. The **central effect** is *stimulation of thirst*. A-II acts through angiotensin receptors present in the subfornical organ (SFO) and the organ vasculosum of lamina terminals (OVLT) to increase thirst. The **renal effects** are: (i) *Constriction of both afferent and efferent arterioles*, thereby reducing both GFR and RBF. A-II receptors are present in both afferent as well as efferent arterioles. The efferent arterioles, however, are more sensitive to A-II than are the afferent arterioles. Hence, A-II causes greater constriction of the efferent arterioles, thereby increasing the filtration fraction. (ii) *Mesangial cell hypertrophy* and *stimulation of extracellular matrix production by the mesangial cells*. A-II receptors are present on the mesangial cells. Since both mesangial cell hypertrophy and extracellular matrix expansion are observed in diabetes mellitus, A-II has been implicated in the pathophysiology of diabetes mellitus. ACE inhibitors tend to retard those changes in diabetic nephropathy. (iii) *decreases the pore-size* of the glomerular basement membrane. A-II receptors are present in the glomerular capillaries. ACE-inhibitors have been used in nephrotic syndrome to decrease the proteinuria. Finally, the **effect on adrenal gland** is to *stimulate aldosterone secretion*. AT receptors are present on the zona glomerulosa of the adrenal glands. A-II causes stimulation of aldosterone secretion.

### Where is aldosterone secreted from?

Aldosterone is secreted by the **zona glomerulosa** – the outermost layer of the adrenal cortex. Other zones lack aldosterone synthetase. Adrenal glomerulosa cells do not store aldosterone. Hence, increased synthesis is associated with an immediate increase in secretion. Conversely, chronic increase in aldosterone secretion is associated with hypertrophy of zona glomerulosa.

### What are the factors regulating aldosterone secretion?

The factors regulating aldosterone secretion are: (i) **ACTH**. It increases aldosterone secretion. Hence, stress-producing factors like surgery, trauma, anxiety etc. will also stimulate aldosterone secretion. (ii) **Angiotensin-II**. It increases aldosterone secretion. (iii) **K$^+$**. Even a small increase in plasma K$^+$ (~ 1 mEq/L) can increase aldosterone secretion substantially. (iv) **Na$^+$**. Aldosterone secretion is weakly stimulated by a fall of plasma [Na$^+$].

### What are the actions of aldosterone?

The actions of aldosterone are localized to the distal tubular and collecting duct cells. (i) Aldosterone increases reabsorption of Na$^+$ and with it, of water too. (ii) Increased Na$^+$ reabsorption makes the tubular lumen highly negative. (iii) The highly negative lumen together with the increased apical permeability to K$^+$ promotes K$^+$ secretion.

Aldosterone is the *sole regulator of the external potassium balance*. An increase in plasma K$^+$ stimulates aldosterone secretion, which in turn restores plasma K$^+$ levels by promoting kaliuresis. An absence of this aldosterone-feedback mechanism would result in fatal hyperkalemia (Fig. 77.1).

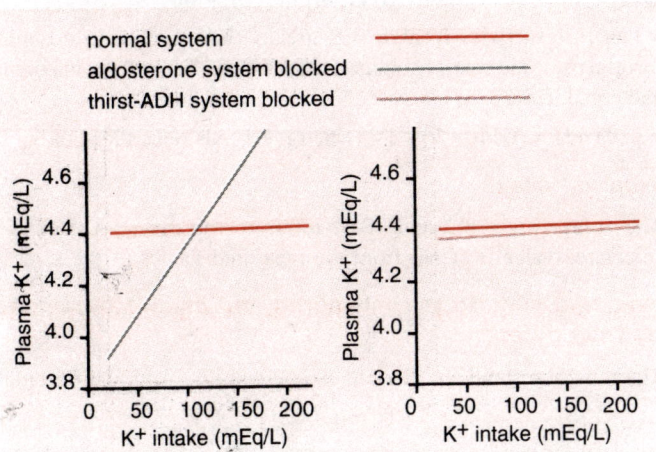

**Fig. 77.1**

Aldosterone is *one of the several regulators* of *body Na$^+$ and water balance*, another important regulator being the thirst-ADH mechanism. In the absence of the aldosterone-feedback mechanism, the thirst-ADH mechanism maintains a near-perfect Na$^+$ balance in the body (Fig. 77.2). In the absence of the ADH-thirst mechanism, however, aldosterone is unable to maintain proper Na$^+$ balance because of the **escape phenomenon**.

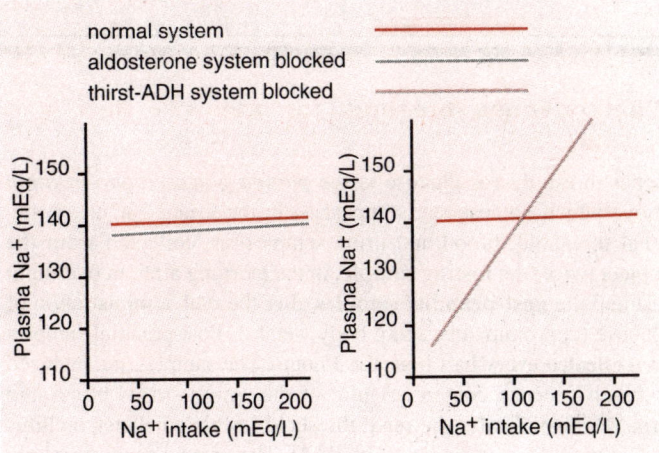

**Fig. 77.2**

### What is the escape phenomenon?

A decrease in plasma Na$^+$ would stimulate aldosterone secretion (provided that the ECF volume is normal). Aldosterone increases the tubular reabsorption of not only Na$^+$ but of H$_2$O too. Water retention expands the ECF volume. Expansion of ECF volume produces natriuresis *through Starling mechanisms* and *sympatho-adrenergic mechanisms*. Hence, aldosterone by itself is unable to produce significant amounts of Na$^+$ and water retention.

### What is the action of PTH on the kidney?

In the kidney, PTH has the following effects: (i) It increases **Ca$^{2+}$** reabsorption in the **distal** nephron and *tends* to decrease the urinary calcium excretion. However PTH also increases the calcium levels through bone reabsorption, which *tends* to produce hypercalcuria. The net effect is hypercalcuria. (ii) It decreases **proximal** tubular reabsorption of **phosphate**. (iii) It stimulates l α-hydroxylase activity (in the mitochondria of the proximal tubular cells) to increase formation of 1, dihydroxycholecalciferol through which the gastrointestinal absorption of calcium and phosphate are controlled.

# 78

# Quantification of Renal Functions

## What is renal threshold for glucose? How is it measured?

Renal threshold for glucose is the *plasma glucose concentration* above which glucose starts appearing in the urine. For measuring renal threshold, blood and urine samples are collected from the subject twice: the **fasting sample**, in the morning after an overnight fast and the **post-prandial samples** after the oral administration of glucose (approximately 2g/kg body weight). Post-prandial samples are collected every half hour for 3 hours. The samples are analyzed for their glucose content. A plot of the simultaneous blood and urine levels indicates the renal threshold (as also diabetes mellitus and alimentary glycosuria) (Fig. 78.1). The normal renal threshold for glucose is 180 mg/dL.

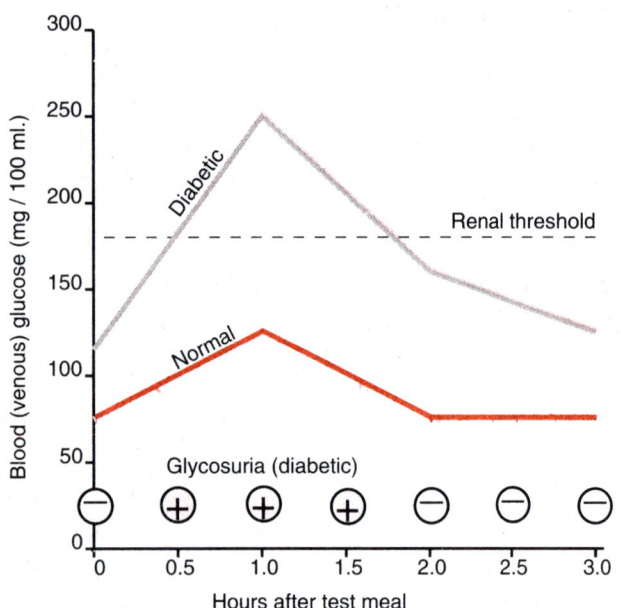

**Fig. 78.1**

## What is TmG? How is it calculated?

Like any active process, the rate of active tubular reabsorption of glucose cannot exceed a certain maximum called the **transport maximum for glucose** or **TmG**. It is about 375 mg/min in males and 300 mg/min in females.

Normally (at plasma levels of 60 – 100 mg/dl), the glucose filtered into the urine is totally reabsorbed. As the plasma level (P) of glucose increases, more glucose is filtered into the tubule and the urinary concentration (U) of glucose rises. But the tubular reabsorption (Tr) of glucose also increases concomitantly so that no glucose appears in urine. However, after the plasma level

exceeds the **renal threshold for glucose**, the amount of glucose filtered into the tubule exceeds the maximal rate at which glucose can be reabsorbed from the tubules (called the **transport maximum for glucose** or **TmG** (Fig. 78.2). Hence, glucose starts appearing in urine. The tubular reabsorption can be calculated from the formula:

$$Tr\,(GFR \times P) = UV$$

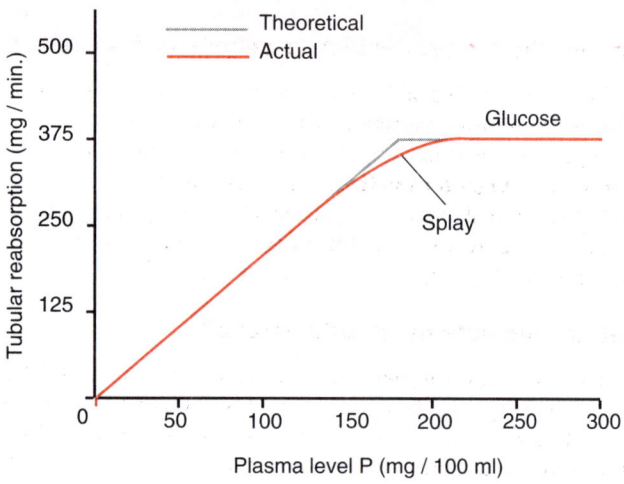

**Fig. 78.2**

*where*

U  = urinary concentration of the solute (glucose)

V  = urinary output per min.

P  = plasma level of the solute (glucose)

Tr = amount of tubular reabsorption of solute (glucose)

When P is sufficiently high (i.e. greater than the renal threshold for glucose), the rate of tubular reabsorption (Tr) will be maximal and equal TmG.

$$\therefore TmG = (GFR \times P) - UV \text{ (when P exceeds renal threshold)}$$

## What is splay?

The splay (Fig. 78.2 and 78.3) refers to the divergence of the calculated value of TmG from the measured values of the same.

## How and why do the measured and calculated values of TmG differ?

The renal threshold for glucose can be deduced from the formula:

$$Tr = (GFR \times P) - UV$$

When the plasma concentration (P) equals renal threshold, the tubular reabsorption (Tr) touches its maximum (i.e., the TmG) and

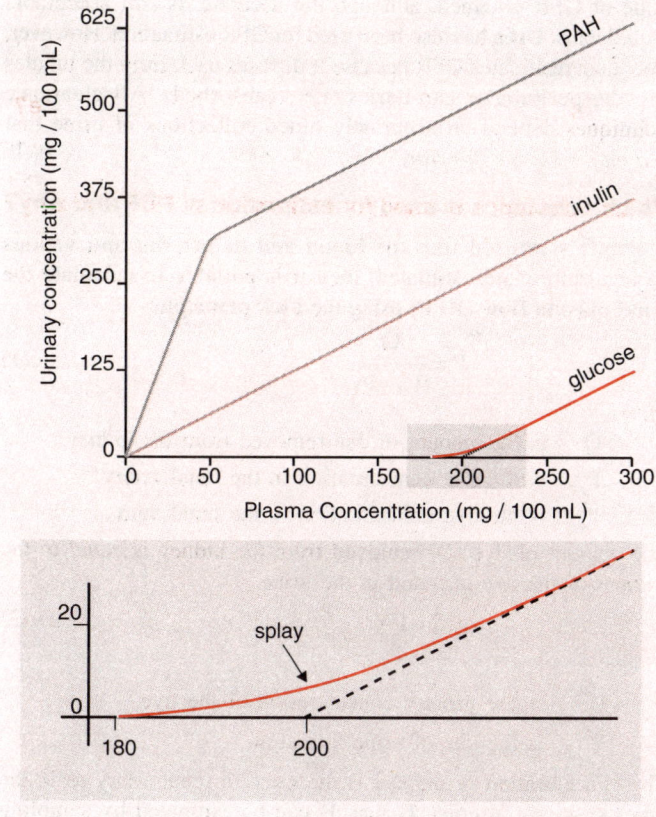

**Fig. 78.3**

exactly balances the filtered load of glucose.

$$\therefore \text{TmG} = (\text{GFR} \times \text{renal threshold})$$

*or* **renal threshold = TmG / GFR**

There is however a discrepancy between the calculated and the observed values of the renal threshold. The renal threshold calculated from TmG would be:

$$375 \text{ mg/min} \div 125 \text{ mL/min} = 3 \text{ mg/mL}$$
$$= 300 \text{ mg/dL}$$

Thus glucose would be expected to appear in urine when the *arterial* concentrations of glucose exceeds 300 mg/dL, which corresponds to a *venous* glucose concentration of about 200 mg/dl. However, the measured value is lesser at about 180 mg/dL.

This is because, the calculated value represents only the *average value of 2 million nephrons*. Several nephrons have TmG that are either higher or lower than the average of 375 mg/min. *Nephrons with lower TmG* will leak glucose into urine at plasma glucose levels lower than the calculated threshold. This discrepancy shows up graphically as the **splay**.

## Define clearance of a substance.

The clearance of a substance is defined as the *volume of plasma that is cleared of that substance completely in 1 minute*. It is a 'virtual volume'. The unit of clearance is ml/min and is calculated by the formula:

$$\frac{UV}{P}$$

*where:* U = urinary concentration of the substance
V = rate of flow of urine
P = plasma concentration of the substance

## What is osmolar clearance?

Osmolar clearance (Cosm) is the volume of plasma that is cleared of *all its electrolytes* in 1 minute. If the urine excreted is isoosmotic to the plasma, then the osmolar clearance is equal to the urinary output in 1 minute.

$$\text{Cosm} = \frac{UV}{P}$$

If U = P
then Cosm = V

Thus, defined in another way, osmolar clearance is the volume of *isotonic urine* that must be excreted per minute for eliminating the same solute load present in the actual urine excreted in 1 minute.

## What is free-water clearance?

Free-water clearance ($C_{H_2O}$) is defined as the amount of water that must be taken away from the urine volume excreted to render it isotonic with plasma. It is given by:

$$\text{Cosm} = V - C_{H_2O}$$
*or*
$$V = \text{Cosm} + C_{H_2O}$$

In other words, the urine volume can be viewed as the sum of the volume of urine passed free of electrolytes ($C_{H_2O}$) and that containing solutes at isoosmolar concentration (Cosm). A **positive free-water clearance** occurs when urine is hypoosmolar and a **negative free-water clearance** when urine is hyperosmolar.

## How does clearance of a substance change with its plasma concentration?

The general formula for urinary excretion of solutes is:

$$UV = (GFR \times P) - Tr + Ts$$

Tr is the amount reabsorbed from the tubule;

Ts is the amount secreted into the tubule;

$GFR \times P$ gives the amount filtered into the tubule per min

$U \times V$ gives the amount of the substance excreted in urine per minute

*Dividing through out by P,*

$$UV/P = GFR - Tr/P + Ts/P$$

Since the values of Tr or Ts cannot increase indefinitely (they are limited by the Tm), at very high values of P, Tr/P and Ts/P approach zero. Hence, the clearance of all substances approaches the value of GFR (inulin clearance) at higher values of P. The clearance of glucose is normally zero since the normal urinary concentration of glucose (U) is zero. However as the plasma level of glucose exceeds the threshold, its clearance exceeds zero and its Tr approaches Tm. At higher plasma levels, the clearance of glucose too (like that of other substances) approaches the value of inulin clearance (Fig. 78.4).

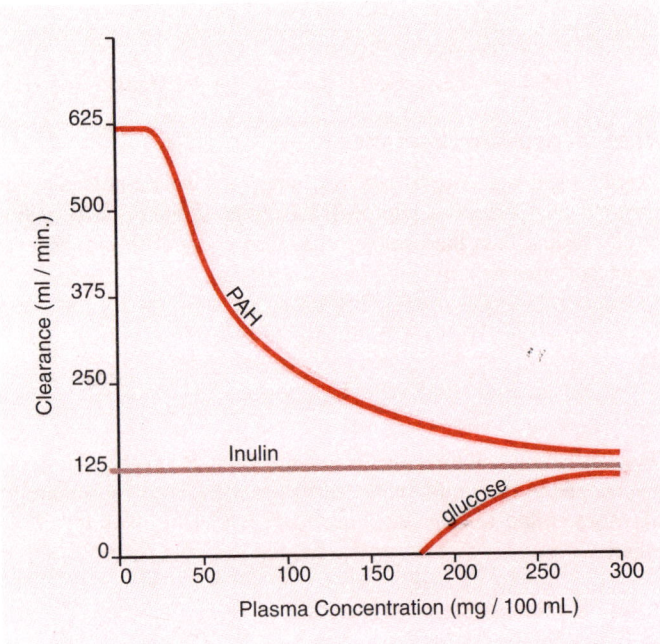

**Fig. 78.4**

### Which substances is used for estimation of GFR and why?

We know that:

$$UV/P = GFR - Tr/P + Ts/P$$

If a substance is neither secreted into nor reabsorbed from the tubule, the formula reduces to:

$$UV/P = GFR$$

**Inulin**, and to a lesser extent **creatinine** meet the above criteria. Hence, GFR can be estimated by measuring inulin clearance or creatinine clearance.

Inulin is a dye (chemically, a polysaccharide). Inulin clearance gives an estimate of the GFR because (i) it is freely filtered into the glomerular filtrate, and (ii) it is neither secreted nor reabsorbed in the kidneys. Also, it satisfies the other elementary requirements of a good indicator dye, i.e., (iii) it is neither metabolized not stored in the kidneys; (iv) neither toxic nor has any effect on the filtration rate itself; and (v) easily estimated in the laboratory. Inulin clearance, or the GFR is given by:

$$\text{Inulin clearance} = GFR = \frac{U\,V}{P_a}$$

*where:*

    U is the urinary concentration of inulin

    V is the rate of urine flow

    $P_a$ is the arterial concentration of inulin.

During estimation, it is important to achieve a fairly constant level of the plasma concentration of inulin. This is achieved by giving a single bolus dose of inulin solution followed by a continuous i/v infusion of the same. GFR is *more easily* but *less accurately* estimated by using **creatinine** as an indicator. Creatinine is an endogenous substance having a fairly constant plasma value (P) of about 0.6-1.5 mg/dl. This eliminates the need for a continuous i/v infusion. Unlike inulin however, creatinine is slightly secreted into the tubules, increasing its urinary concentration (U). The

value of GFR obtained, although not accurate, is still acceptable to clinicians. **Urea** has also been used for GFR estimation. However, urea underestimates GFR because it diffuses back from the tubules into the peritubular capillaries (i.e. reabsorbed). All clearance techniques depend on accurately timed collections of urine that is *a major source of error.*

### Which substance is used for estimation of RBF and why?

If a dye is infused into the blood and its arterial and venous concentrations are estimated, then it is possible to calculate the **renal plasma flow** (**RPF**) using the **Fick principle**:

$$F = \frac{Q}{(Pa - Pv)} \qquad \text{.......(1)}$$

*where*

    Q    is the amount of dye removed from the kidney.

    $P_a$    is the dye concentration in the renal artery

    $P_v$    is the dye concentration in the renal vein

The amount of dye (Q) removed from the kidney is equal to the amount of the dye excreted in the urine.

$$\therefore \qquad Q = UV \qquad \text{......(2)}$$

*where*

    U    is the urinary concentration of the dye;

    V    is the rate of urine formation

The concentration of the dye is the same in renal artery as in the other systemic arteries. Hence, $P_a$ can be estimated by sampling blood from any systemic artery that can be conveniently accessed. However, it is difficult to obtain blood from the renal vein. Hence, it is convenient to use a dye that is completely excreted into the urine in a single passage through the kidney so that the concentration of the dye in renal blood is zero. If $P_v = 0$, then equation (1) reduces to:

$$RPF = \frac{UV}{P_a} \qquad \text{.......(3)}$$

Hence, *RPF equals the renal clearance of PAH.* In practice, the dye that is used for RPF estimation is **para-amino hippuric acid** (**PAH**), which is only 90%, excreted in the urine in a single passage. (In other words, the **extraction ratio** is 90%). Hence, its concentration in renal venous blood is about 10% of its concentration in the renal arterial blood, i.e.,

    $P_v = P_a \times (1 - \text{extraction ratio})$

*or*     $P_a - P_v = P_a \times \text{extraction ratio)} \qquad \text{.........(4)}$

Substituting (4) in (1), we have:

$$RPF = \frac{UV}{(P_a \times \text{extraction ratio})} \qquad \text{..........(5)}$$

The **RBF** (renal blood flow) can then be calculated from the formula:

$$RBF = \frac{RPF}{(1 - \text{hematocrit})} \qquad \text{.......(6)}$$

### What is urea clearance and what is its significance?

In modern medicine, urea clearance has little relevance since the clearance of inulin and creatinine provide far better measures of the GFR. Urea clearance however continues to be taught for its historical significance. The concept of clearance itself developed around efforts to use urea excretion as an index for renal function. Part of the problem in such efforts was that urea excretion even by a normal kidney varies greatly depending on the rate of urinary outflow. Two *empirical indices* were developed, one for urinary flow < 2 ml / min (called the standard clearance), and other, for urinary flow > 2 ml / min (called the maximal clearance). These indices are fairly constant as long as there is no impairment of renal functions.

$$\text{Standard urea clearance} \ \frac{U\sqrt{V}}{B}$$

$$\text{Maximal urea clearance} = \frac{UV}{B}$$

It was realized only later that UV/B actually signified the 'volume of blood' that was cleared of urea per minute. The blood concentration (B) was later replaced by plasma concentration (P) and the term clearance extended to other solutes some of which more accurately indicated the GFR or RBF. Standard urea clearance does *not* denote a 'volume of blood' and therefore, cannot be called 'clearance' according to its present definition.

## What is filtration fraction?

Filtration fraction (FF) is given by the ratio of GFR and RPF. It serves as an approximate index of glomerular filtration coefficient (Kf):

$$FF = \frac{GFR}{RPF}$$

## Compare and contrast renal threshold and transport maximum for glucose.

**SIMILARITIES**

Both are indicative of proximal tubular function.

**DIFFERENCES**

| Renal threshold | TmG |
|---|---|
| It is the plasma level of glucose and is expressed in mg/100 ml | It is the rate of glucose transport and is expressed = mg/min. |
| It is comparatively a less stable index of proximal tubular function. Even a few disordered nephrons can lower the renal threshold (splay) | It is a more stable function of proximal tabular function. A few disordered nephrons do not significantly affect the overall value of TmG |

# 79

# Urine Analysis & Renal Function Tests

## What are the normal physical characteristics of urine?

**Quantity**. The normal volume of urine passed per day ranges from 500 to 2500 ml. It increases after meals, after drinks / alcohol and on exposure to cold and decreases if water intake is low and after excessive sweating.

| | |
|---|---|
| Polyuria | diabetes mellitus<br>diabetes insipidus<br>diuretic phase of ARF |
| Oliguria | ECF volume contraction<br>hypotension<br>acute GN |
| Anuria | lower urinary tract obstruction |

**Color / turbidity.** (i) Urates precipitate in acidic urine on standing, making the urine cloudy. Urinary urate excretion increases when purine metabolism in the body increases, as in gout. (ii) Strongly alkaline urine appears cloudy due to the precipitation of $Ca_3(PO_4)_2$. The cloudy appearance increases on warming the urine that makes it more alkaline as the $CO_2$ bubbles off from it. (iii) Infection increases the pus cells and bacteria in urine, giving it a cloudy appearance. Filtering clears up the urine if it is due to precipitation of phosphates and urates but not if it is due to infection.

| | |
|---|---|
| normal tint | urochrome, uro-erythrine<br>urobilin (formed on standing) |
| cloudy | strongly alkaline urine<br>excessive urates, infection |
| smoky | hematuria (> 0.5 ml/L) |
| frothy | proteinuria |
| milky | chyluria |
| orange | excess urobilin |
| brown | bilirubinuria |
| red-dark brown | porphyrins (on standing)<br>frank hematuria |
| red-dark brown-black | Hemoglobinuria<br>melanin (on standing) |

**Hematuria** means the presence of RBCs in the urine. Hematuria does not necessarily indicate a renal abnormality: the blood can come form the urinary tract. Red cells that enter urine through the damaged glomerulus are usually distorted, which helps in differentiating *glomerular* from *non-glomerular* bleeding. **Hemoglobinuria** refers to the presence of free hemoglobin in the urine.

The **specific gravity** is normally 1.003 – 1.030 and the *normal osmolarity* is 100 – 1000 mOsm/kg. If the early morning urine sample after an overnight fast has an osmolarity of > 600 mOsm/

kg (specific gravity >1.018), then the patient has a normal urine concentrating ability. If the osmolarity is constantly 300 mOsm/kg (SG=1.009) it is called **isosthenuria**. It occurs in CRF.

The **pH** of urine is normally slightly acidic except shortly after a meal due to the post-prandial alkaline tide. Abnormal causes include alkali consumption, impairment of tubular acidification and UTI (urinary tract infection) with urea-splitting organisms.

## What are the different types of proteinuria? Explain their significance.

Up to 150 mg of proteins are excreted daily in urine. Of this, 15 mg is albumin. The rest are **low molecular weight proteins** (LMPW). About 25 mg of LMPW are the **Tamm-Horsfall proteins** derived from cells of the TAL. The rest are derived from plasma proteins e.g. $\beta_2$ microproteins, lysozymes and light chains of immunoglobulin. *Excretion of > 150 mg/day of proteins is called proteinuria.* (i) **Transient proteinuria** can occur in fever and after exercise. A particular form of transient proteinuria is **orthostatic proteinuria**, which occurs only on standing and is not associated with any renal damage. (ii) **Glomerular proteinuria** occurs when the glomerular permeability increases and the filtered loads of albumin and other high molecular weight proteins (HMWP) increase considerably. This is also called **high molecular weight proteinuria**. The filtration of low molecular proteins (LMWP) increases only slightly, since they are quite permeable even normally, and there is little scope for further increase. Massive glomerular proteinuria is called **nephrotic syndrome**. (iii) In tubular proteinuria, low molecular weight proteins (LMWP) that normally enter the glomerular filtrates in fairly large amounts are not reabsorbed. The tubular reabsorption of LMWP is impaired in tubulointerstitial disorders and Fanconi's syndrome, as a result of which large amounts of LMWP is excreted in urine. (iv) In **overflow proteinuria**, the urinary excretion of LMWP increases due to rise in the plasma LMWP e.g., in multiple myeloma, rhabdomyolysis and intravascular hemolysis. The protein reabsorptive capacity of the tubules is exceeded and LMPW appears in urine. (v) In **nephrogenic proteinuria**, damage to the proximal tubular cells releases the tubular enzymes into the urine, e.g. *N-acetyl β-glucosaminidase* (NAG), and *γ-glutamyl transferase* (γGT).

## Which chemical constituents of urine have diagnostic significance?

(i) The significance of high molecular and low molecular **proteinuria** has been discussed. (ii) **Sugars** like glucose, galactose and fructose are normally absent in urine. Lactose and pentose sugars may occur normally in urine. Lactosuria occurs in late pregnancy and lactation. Pentosuria is caused by consuming large quantities of plum, cherries and grapes. Glycosuria may be due to diabetes mellitus, renal glycosuria and alimentary glycosuria. Galactosuria and frutosuria occur due to inborn errors of metabolism. (iii) **Ketones** are normally absent in urine. Ketonuria occurs in diabetic ketoacidosis, starvation and prolonged diarrhea and vomiting. (iv) **Bilirubin** is normally absent in urine. The daily urobilinogen excretion is normally 1 – 3.5 mg. Bilirubinemia occurs in jaundice. (v) **Heme pigments** are normally absent in urine. They appear in urine following intravascular hemolysis and hemolysis in renal tubules. They also appear following crush injury to muscles and in myopathies, which release heme from myoglobin. (vi) Urinary **nitrites** suggest presence of UTI. Urine normally contains nitrates ($NO_3^-$) but not nitrite ($NO_2^-$). Most UTI-causing organisms produce nitrites from urinary nitrates.

### What are casts? Name the different types of casts and mention their significance.

Casts are proteinaceous plugs (made of **Tamm-Horsfall protein**) formed within the nephron and washed out by the flow of tubular fluid. Casts may be cellular or non-cellular. **Cellular casts** may be (i) **Leukocyte casts** that are typically found in acute bacterial pyelonephritis; (ii) **Fatty casts** that are found in nephrotic syndrome. They contain epithelial cells laden with fat droplets; (iii) **Red cell casts** that are pathognomonic of glomerular bleeding and are almost diagnostic of acute GN; or (iv) **Tubular epithelial cell casts** that are most commonly present in ATN.

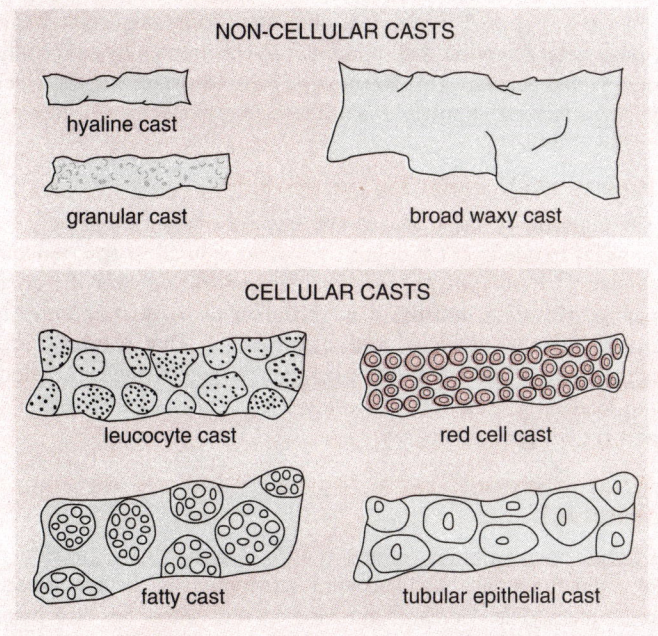

**Fig. 79.1**

**Non-cellular casts** may be (i) **Hyaline casts** that are structureless, transparent proteinaceous plugs, made largely of Tamm-Horsfall proteins. Up to 1 hyaline cast per low power field (×10) is normal. They increase in proteinuria. (ii) **Granular casts** that are similar to hyaline casts except that granular aggregates of proteins are embedded in them. Less than 1 granular cast per LPF should be considered normal. (iii) **Broad waxy casts** (**renal failure casts**) that are formed in chronic renal failure in the dilated nephrons (Fig. 79.1).

### Name the tests that assess glomerular function.

Glomerular function tests include (i) urine analysis for **high molecular weight proteinuria**; (ii) **plasma urea** and **plasma creatinine** concentrations; and (iii) direct GFR estimation by measuring **inulin clearance** or **creatinine clearance**. Neither the blood urea, nor the plasma creatinine rise much until the GFR falls below 30 ml/min. Once GFR falls below 30 ml/min., the plasma creatinine is an accurate and sensitive guide to further changes in renal function.

Although plasma urea is widely used clinically for assessing glomerular function, it may be false high in conditions of low urine flow rates (e.g. dehydration, heart failure, nephrotic syndrome) when urea diffuses out of the tubular lumen to re-enter blood; high protein diet, gastrointestinal bleeding (blood proteins are digested) and catabolic states like infection and steroid therapy. Plasma creatinine levels are less affected by extra-renal causes, although the urinary excretion of creatinine is proportional to the whole body muscle mass.

### Name the tests that assess proximal tubular function.

Proximal tubular function tests include (i) Urine examination for **low molecular weight proteinuria**; (ii) Urinary secretion of **enzymes** present in the cells of the proximal tubule, e.g., N-acetyl β-glucosaminidase (NAG), and γ-glutamyl transferase (γGT), and (iii) **tubular reabsorption of glucose**. It is a *fairly good index* of proximal tubular function. Renal threshold is an easily measurable index of glucose reabsorption in tubules. *TmG is a more stable index* than the renal threshold. (Threshold is affected by the 'splay' but TmG is not.)

### Name the tests that assess distal tubular function.

The distal tubular function tests include (i) tests for *urine concentrating and diluting ability*, like specific gravity of urine, water loading test and water deprivation test. (ii) tests for *urine acidification ability*, like the oral ammonium chloride test.

### Describe the oral water-loading test.

The water-loading test gives accurate information regarding the *urine-diluting ability* of the kidneys. After voiding, the subject drinks 20 ml/kg of body weight of water over 15 minutes. Half-hourly samples are collected over the next 5 hours. Normally, >75% of the administered water load should be excreted by 4 hours. Urine osmolarity should fall to <100 Osm/kg. The ability to produce a dilute urine is lost in: (i) cardiac failure (impaired renal perfusion causes excessive proximal reabsorption of $Na^+$); (ii) progressive liver disease; and (iii) chronic renal failure. The inability to alter the osmolarity of the urine is called **isosthenuria**, in which the urine excreted is always isoosmolar to the plasma.

### Describe the water deprivation test.

The water-deprivation test gives accurate information regarding the *urine-concentrating ability* of the kidneys. Oral fluids are withheld for a period of 12 hours (one normal meal is allowed in between). Urine sample is collected and analyzed for its volume and osmolarity. To prevent serious and life-threatening dehydration, the test should be abandoned if body weight falls by 3% at any time during the test. Normally, osmolarity is > 900 mOsm/L. In diabetes insipidus, it is < 300 mOsm/L. If nephrogenic, subsequent ADH will not improve it. In compulsive water drinking (CWD), the osmolarity would be normal.

# 80

# Renal Syndromes

## Define nephritic syndrome. What are its common causes? What are its clinical features?

Nephritic syndrome is characterized by: (i) hematuria, (ii) red-cell casts in urine, (iii) moderate proteinuria, (iv) edema, (v) hypertension and oliguria (occasionally). Nephritic syndrome occurs due to immunological damage to the glomerular basement membrane. The initiating cause of this immunological damage is mostly unknown except in a particular type that occurs *following an infection with group-A β-hemolytic Streptococci*. It is called **acute post-streptococcal glomerulonephritis**, and occurs due to cross-reaction of anti-streptococcal antibodies with the glomerular basement membrane.

## Define nephrotic syndrome. What are its common causes? What are its clinical features?

Nephrotic syndrome is defined as *proteinuria that exceeds 4g/ day*. Most cases of nephrotic syndrome are of immunologic origin due to unknown causes. The commonest glomerulopathy associated with nephrotic syndrome is **minimal change glomerulonephritis** (lipoid nephrosis). Some cases of nephrotic syndrome are secondary to known causes, like diabetes mellitus, amyloidosis, exposure to allergens (e.g., bee stings) and toxins (e.g. mercury), infections and drugs. The clinical features of nephrotic syndrome include (i) **hypoalbuminemia** (due to heavy proteinuria); (ii) **edema** (plasma oncotic pressure decreases due to hypoalbuminemia); (iii) **hyperlipidemia**; (iv) **microcytic hypochromic anemia** (due to losses of transferrin); (v) **increased tendency to thrombosis**, esp. of renal veins (due to losses of antithrombin III); (vi) **vitamin D deficiency** (due to loss of cholecalciferol-binding protein); (vii) **thyroid abnormalities** (due to loss of thyroid-binding globulin); (viii) **susceptibility to infections** (due to loss of IgG).

|  | Nephrotic Syndrome | Nephritic Syndrome |
|---|---|---|
| **Proteinuria** | Gross | Moderate |
| **Plasma albumin** | Markedly reduced | Slightly reduced |
| **Hematuria** | Absent or traces | Marked |
| **Blood pressure** | Normal or low | Raised |
| **Edema** | Marked | Moderate |
| **GFR** | Normal / increased | Reduced |
| **Urine volume** | Normal / reduced | Reduced |
| **Plasma lipid** | Grossly elevated | Minimal increase |

## Define acute renal failure. What are its common causes?

Acute renal failure is defined as an *abrupt impairment of renal function* that is *always associated* with increase in blood urea and serum creatinine, and is usually *associated with* oliguria and is reversible. In a broad sense, **acute renal failure** (ARF) includes: (i) **pre-renal azotemia**, i.e., inadequate renal perfusion resulting in rise in nitrogenous waste products in the blood, but without causing ischemic necrosis of renal tubules; (ii) **acute (intrinsic) renal failure**, the commonest cause of which is **acute tubular necrosis (ATN)**. (iii) **post-renal azotemia**, i.e., obstruction to the flow of urine causes renal dysfunction and azotemia. In a more restricted sense, *ARF is used synonymously with acute tubular necrosis* (ATN), which is by far the commonest cause of ARF.

## What are the clinical features of acute tubular necrosis?

Acute tubular necrosis goes through the following phases: (i) **Initiating phase** (**stage of onset**) which lasts for ~ 36 hours. The signs of the underlying cause e.g. shock or the toxin, are prominent in this phase. (ii) **Maintenance phase** (**oliguric stage**) lasts for a few days to up to 3 weeks. It is characterized by oliguria < 400ml / day, water retention with dilutional hyponatremia, hyperkalemia, uremia and acidosis. (iii) **Recovery phase** (**diuretic stage**), which is characterized by polyuria, natriuresis, hypokalemia and decrease in blood urea.

## How is acute renal failure treated?

The mainstay of the management, besides treating the underlying cause, is to tide over the oliguric phase so as to allow **spontaneous recovery**. *Hemodialysis* may be required to tide over the crisis period. However, mostly, it is sufficient to (i) *restrict water* to match urinary output and eliminating electrolytes from administered fluids; and (ii) *restricting dietary proteins* to reduce the load on the kidneys while allowing plenty of carbohydrates and fats to provide energy.

## What is chronic renal failure? What are its clinical features?

Chronic renal failure is defined as a slowly progressive impairment of renal function associated with a reduction in the functioning renal mass. The decreased functioning renal mass has two broad effects: decreased excretion and decreased biosynthesis. The metabolites that are most affected by the **decreased excretory capacity** of the kidney are creatinine and urea. **Decreased biosynthetic capacity** of the surviving renal mass results in: (i) decreased activation of vitamin $D_3$; (ii) Decreased erythropoietin secretion, which results in a normocytic, normochromic anemia.

Clinical features of CRF include: (i) azotemia; (ii) fluid imbalance and / or hypertension; (iii) anemia; (iv) hyperkalemia; (v) metabolic acidosis; (vi) renal osteodystrophy. Management of CRF includes *hemodialysis* and *kidney transplantation*.

## What is dialysis?

Dialysis is a term of physical chemistry. It is the process of *separation of colloids from crystalloids* in a complex solution. In medical diction, it refers to the process by which some of the excess crystalloids and other toxic waste products that accumulate in blood in renal failure are eliminated from the plasma while retaining the colloids like plasma proteins and the cellular elements.

**Hemodialysis** is done by interposing a semipermeable membrane between the patient's blood and the *dialysate* (an electrolyte solution with a composition similar to that of the normal plasma). As the blood equilibrates with the dialysate, its crystalloid composition becomes similar to that of the dialysate. By varying the dialysate composition, the plasma composition can be modified as desired by the clinician.

In **peritoneal dialysis**, the dialysate is infused into peritoneal cavity and allowed to equilibrate with blood across the peritoneal membrane, which thereby acts as the dialyzing membrane. Dialysis involves transport of both solute and water. Hence, by appropriately altering the composition of the dialysate, it is possible to use dialysis for removal of extra water from the body.

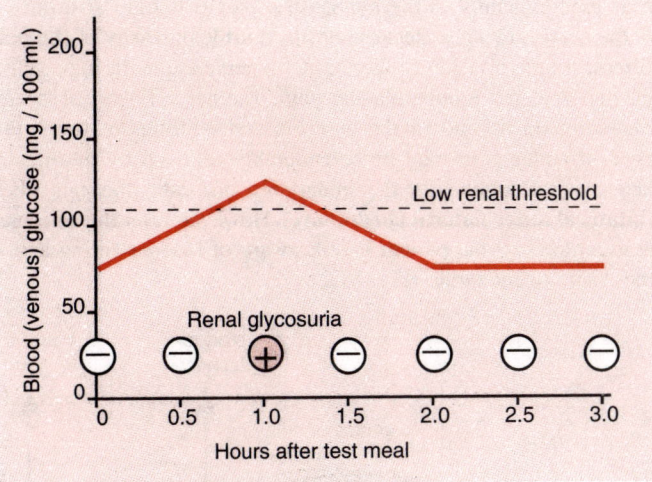

**Fig. 80.1**

## What is renal glycosuria? How is it diagnosed?

Renal glycosuria is an autosomal-recessive disorder in which there is impaired reabsorption of glucose from the tubules. As a result, glycosuria occurs in the presence of normal blood glucose and the measured renal threshold for glucose is low (Fig. 80.1).

Renal glycosuria is of 2 types: (i) *Type A*, which is characterized by a *low TmG*, and (ii) *Type B*, which is characterized by an *increased splay* (Fig. 80.2).

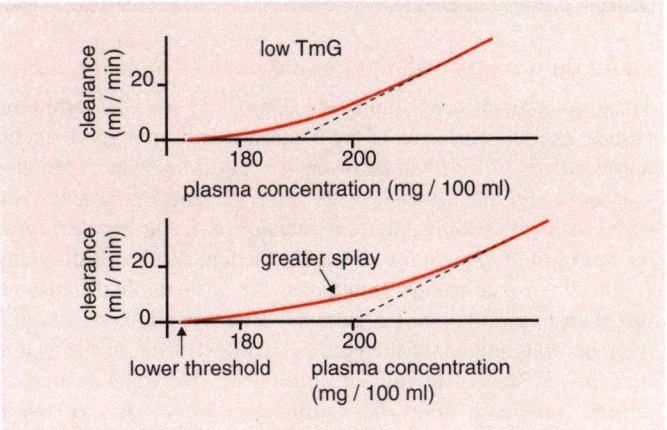

**Fig. 80.2**

## What is renal tubular acidosis?

Renal tubular acidosis (RTA) is a condition in which systemic **acidosis** occurs due to a tubular defect in $H^+$ secretion. The decrease in $H^+$ secretion can be due to (i) inadequate $H^+$ secretion, and (ii) excessive back-diffusion of the secreted $H^+$ from lumen to blood. Due to the decreased $H^+$ secretion, bicarbonate reclamation decreases. As a result, there is a compensatory increase in $Cl^-$ reabsorption that accompanies $Na^+$ reabsorption. Hence, the acidosis is associated with **hyperchloremia**.

## What is Fanconi Syndrome?

Fanconi syndrome refers to a defect in proximal tubular transport of several ions and organic substances like $Na^+$, $K^+$, $HCO_3^-$, $Ca^{2+}$, $PO_4^{3-}$, glucose, uric acid, proteins and aminoacids. It usually occurs as an autosomal recessive disorder.

# 81

# Urinary Bladder & Cystometry

### Name the urinary sphincters and explain their functions.

There are four urinary sphincters (Fig. 81.1): (i) The **sphincter vesicae** encircles the neck of the bladder. It is composed of smooth muscles derived from the detrusor. It is not prominent in females. It is *not essential for continence* as evidenced by patients who undergo prostatectomy. Its real function is in the *prevention of the retrograde ejaculation*. Neurally mediated contraction of the sphincter vesicae occurs simultaneously with seminal emission, just prior to ejaculation. (ii) **Intrinsic leiomyosphincter**, which is the inner longitudinal of the urethra, is an extension of the trigone muscles. It has little role in continence. During voiding, its contraction *pulls open the sphincter vesicae*. (iii) **Intrinsic rhabdomyosphincter (sphincter urethrae)**, which is located inside the urogenital diaphragm and surrounds the membranous urethra. It is the tightest of all the sphincters. It is the main sphincter that *maintains continence at rest (tonic continence)*. (iv) The **extrinsic rhabdomyosphincter** are formed by the *periurethral muscles of the levator ani*. It has mainly fast-twitch, easily fatigued fibers. It is *not essential for tonic continence*. However, it helps maintain urethral closure quickly in response to sharp increases in intravesical pressure such as those that accompany coughing or straining (*phasic continence*). Contraction of this sphincter causes inhibition of detrusor activity through a spinal reflex. Hence, it is especially suitable for *stopping micturition in mid-stream*. After radical prostatectomy, patients have tonic incompe-tence due to lack of the intrinsic rhabdomyosphincter but are still able to voluntarily interrupt urination in mid-stream by contracting the external rhabdomyosphincter.

### Briefly outline the sensory innervation of the bladder and mention its clinical implications.

The sensation of **bladder distension** travel from the detrusor stretch receptors travel to the spinal cord via the pelvic splanchnic nerve (nervi erigentes). They then ascend *in the posterior columns* of the spinal cord (fasciculus gracilis) to the spinal, pontine and suprapontine micturition centers. The sensation of **bladder pain** runs predominantly in the hypogastric plexus but are also present in the nervi erigentes. Because of this **double pathway of the pain fibers**, simple division of the presacral nerve (superior hypogastric plexus) does not relieve bladder pain. The nerve fibers subserving bladder pain ascend in the anterolateral columns of the spinal cord. Bladder pain may be considerably relieved by cutting the anterolateral columns of the spinal cord that carry the pain fibers (**bilateral anterolateral cordotomy**). However, after the anterolateral cordotomy, the patient is still aware of bladder filling and of the desire to micturate (Fig. 81.2).

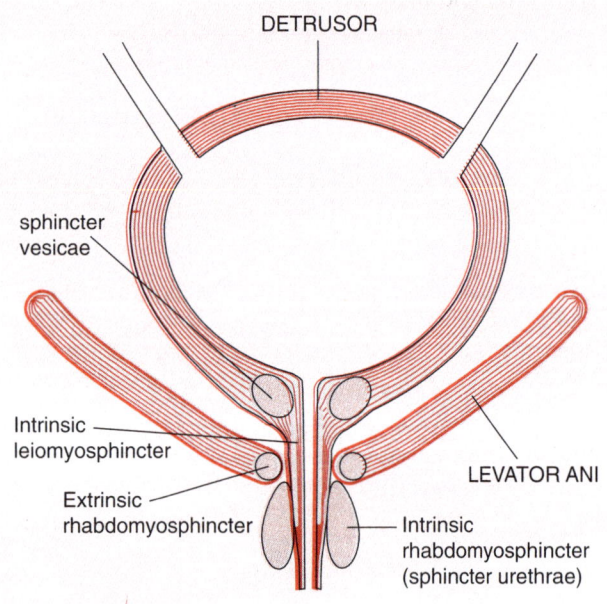

**Fig. 81.1**

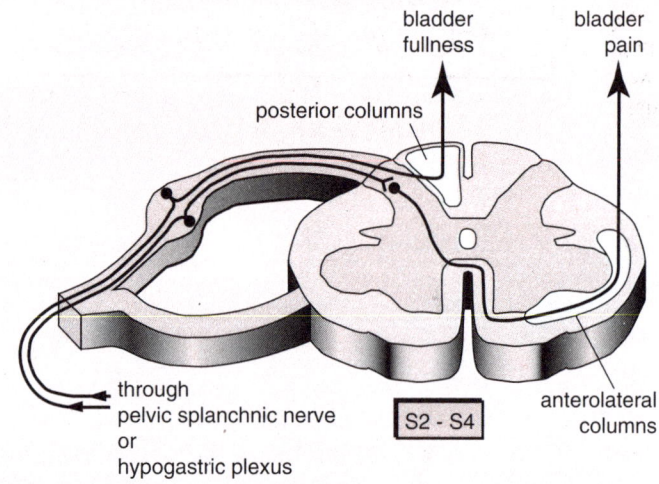

**Fig. 81.2**

### Briefly outline the motor innervation of the bladder.

Sympathetic fibers originate from the intermediolateral gray horn of the spinal at the level of T10 - L2 segments of the cord. They travel via the *hypogastric nerves* to the bladder, bladder neck, and urethra. Sympathetic fibers are inhibitory to the detrusor and excitatory to the sphincter vesicae. If the sympathetic nerves are damaged, *bladder neck closure does not occur with ejaculation.*

Parasympathetic fibers originate from the **sacral detrusor nucleus** – cluster of cell bodies of the preganglionic parasympathetic neurons located in the intermediolateral gray matter of S 2, 3 and 4 (Fig. 81.3). Fibers from the sacral detrusor nucleus leave the cord ventrally and mix with sympathetic efferent fibers to form the *pelvic splanchnic nerve* or the *nervi erigentes.* The parasympathetic efferents relay in the ganglia near or within the bladder and urethra. The postganglionic fibers supply the muscles of the bladder and urethra. The parasympathetic fibers are excitatory to the detrusor muscle and inhibitory to the sphincter vesicae.

The somatic motor nerves to the bladder originate from the **sacral pudendal nucleus**, which is also known as the *nucleus of Onuf.* It is a collection of neurons in the ventral horn of S2 and S3. They reach the *extrinsic rhabdomyosphincter* through the perineal branch of the pudendal nerve (S2, S3 and S4). However, the sphincter itself receives fibers from the S2 and to a lesser degree, from the S3 nerve fibers. They also reach the *intrinsic rhabdomyosphincter* through the inferior hypogastric plexus (pelvic plexus) and the pelvic nerve (nervi erigentes). Hence, pudendal neurectomy does not abolish urethral sphincter spasticity. Damage to the S2 nerve will weaken the external urethral sphincter but leave the detrusor innervation intact. Damage to the S3 nerve will preserve sphincter tone but result in a flaccid detrusor.

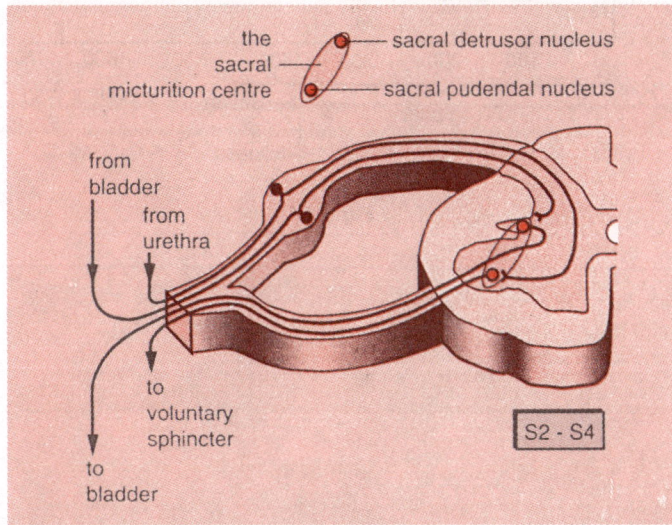

the sacral micturition centre — sacral detrusor nucleus — sacral pudendal nucleus

from bladder

from urethra

to voluntary sphincter

to bladder

S2 - S4

**Fig. 81.3**

### Enumerate the centers for bladder control.

The center for the micturition reflex is the **sacral micturition center**, which consists of the **sacral detrusor nucleus**, and the **sacral pudendal nucleus**. Afferent impulses from the detrusor and urethra travel via the *pelvic splanchnic nerve* and enter the sacral cord through its dorsal root to reach the sacral micturition center where they: (i) excite the sacral detrusor nucleus, thereby causing detrusor contraction; (ii) inhibit the sacral pudendal nucleus, thereby exciting the *intrinsic and extrinsic rhabdomyophincters.*

The sacral micturition center is under the control of the pontine micturition center (PMC). The **PMC** (also called **Barrington's center**) corresponds to the *locus ceruleus* of the rostral pons.

Neurons from the PMC exert control over the sacral micturition center and thoracolumbar sympathetics. The functions of the PMC are to coordinate the activity of bladder and urinary sphincter, and to relay inputs from suprapontine centers. Any lesion between the PMC and the sacral micturition center, will cause: (i) **detrusor-sphincter dyssynergia** (due to disruption of the PMC influence), and (ii) **decreased storage and incomplete voiding** (due to disruption of suprapontine influences). The micturition reflex is also influenced by the *cerebral cortex, basal ganglia and the limbic system.*

### What is detrusor-sphincter dyssynergia?

For proper micturition, it is important that the detrusor contraction and the sphincter relaxation are properly coordinated. In the absence of supraspinal controls, there is loss of coordination between the bladder and distal sphincteric mechanism, which is called **detrusor-sphincter dyssynergia**.

### What are the consequences of deafferenting the bladder?

A deafferented bladder results in a **flaccid (or atonic) neuropathic bladder**. In the absence of the micturition reflex, the bladder gets overfilled till urine starts leaking out (**overflow incontinence**). Due to overfilling, the bladder wall is thin and distended (**flaccid**). The bladder is always full and the *residual urine* is high. However, the intravesical pressure is low.

### What are the consequences of deefferenting the bladder?

A deefferented bladder is also called a *decentralized* or *autonomous* bladder. It results initially in **flaccid neuropathic bladder** with overflow incontinence, similar to the deafferented bladder. However, sooner or later, the detrusor develops denervation hypersensitivity and results in the small, **hypertrophic areflexic bladder**. Due to decreased bladder distensibility, there is a steep pressure rise in the bladder with filling with consequent *overflow incontinence*. The bladder never voids reflexly and always remains full. Residual urine is low.

### What are the consequences of a spinal cord injury that isolates the bladder from the spinal micturition center?

Immediately following the injury, there is abolition of the micturition reflex resulting in a **flaccid neuropathic bladder** with all its attendant features, e.g. overflow incontinence etc. In the initial stages of recovery, the reflex excitability of the striated muscles of the sphincters is restored. The incontinence disappears but there is urinary retention since bladder excitability is still not restored. In the later stages of recovery, the reflex excitability of the detrusor returns and the bladder capacity is reduced. In the absence of supraspinal inhibition, the micturition reflex is exaggerated, resulting in the **spastic neuropathic bladder**. The micturition reflex is triggered whenever the bladder gets distended, resulting in incontinence. Sphincter spasticity and detrusor-sphincter dyssynergia leads to detrusor hypertrophy and high voiding pressures (i.e. intravesical pressure at which voiding is initiated). A few patients develop the ability to empty the bladder reflexly by using trigger techniques, i.e., by tapping or scratching the skin above the pubis or external genitalia.

## Compare and contrast the common types of neuropathic bladders.

| Bladder disorder | Causes | Reflexes | Overflow | Bladder size |
|---|---|---|---|---|
| Flaccid neuropathic | Deafferentation or immediately after deefferentation or spinal cord injury | Absent | Present | Large |
| Hypertrophic areflexic | A few days after deefferentation | Absent | Present | Small |
| Spastic neuropathic | A few days after spinal cord injury | Exaggerated | Absent | Small |

## Enumerate the objectives of cystometry.

Cystometric evaluations are performed to ascertain: (1) **Accommodation:** the ability of the bladder of accommodating large volumes of urine without significant rise in the intravesical pressure; (2) **Total bladder capacity:** the bladder volume at which voiding cannot be prevented; (3) **Bladder contractions**, i.e., (i) the ability of the bladder to *contract when full*; (ii) the ability of the bladder to *sustain a contraction* till the bladder is empty; it is indicated by the **residual urine** left in the bladder at the end of voiding; and (iii) the ability of the bladder to respond to parasympathomimetic drugs. (4) **Voluntary bladder control**, i.e., the ability to initiate voiding even before filling is complete and the ability to inhibit voiding in midstream. (5) **Unstable bladder activity**, i.e. the presence of premature bladder during filling; and (6) **Bladder sensations**, i.e., the ability to perceive fullness of the bladder.

## What is cystometry? What are the two types of cystometry?

Cystometry is one of a battery of tests called the urodynamic studies. **Urodynamic studies** are done to obtain graphic recordings of activity in the bladder functions, urethral sphincteric functions, and urinary flow rate. The urodynamic studies relating to the bladder function are: (a) cystometry and (b) radiographic (cine fluoroscopy) techniques. The radiographic technique is now done only infrequently.

Cystometry is of two types. **Voiding cystometry** allows physiologic filling of the bladder with urine. Recording of the intravesical pressure is started when the patient's bladder is empty and continued until the bladder is full. The patient is then asked to urinate. The disadvantage with this method is that the bladder volume is inferred from the amount of urine voided, with the assumption that there is not residual urine. In **static cystometry**, the bladder is progressively filled with water and the intravesical pressure is recorded. This method permits accurate determination of the bladder volume and pressure at each level of filling. The disadvantage with this method is that the fluid is introduced at a more rapid rate than occurs naturally through urine. That might affect the bladder function.

## Describe a normal cystometrogram.

A normal cystometrogram shows 3 phases of filling: **Phase Ia** is the initial phase of filling up to 50 ml is associated with a slight increase in pressure to about 10 cm of $H_2O$. **Phase Ib** lasts till the bladder volume is about 400 ml. There is almost no change in pressure in this phase. This is because the increase in the bladder volume keeps the pressure unchanged, which is in accordance with the Laplace law. **Phase II** denotes voiding contractions. Normally, the voiding contractions raise the intravesical pressure by about 20 – 40 cm of water. The dotted lines beyond phase II denotes the intravesical pressure changes with further filling if voiding is not initiated.

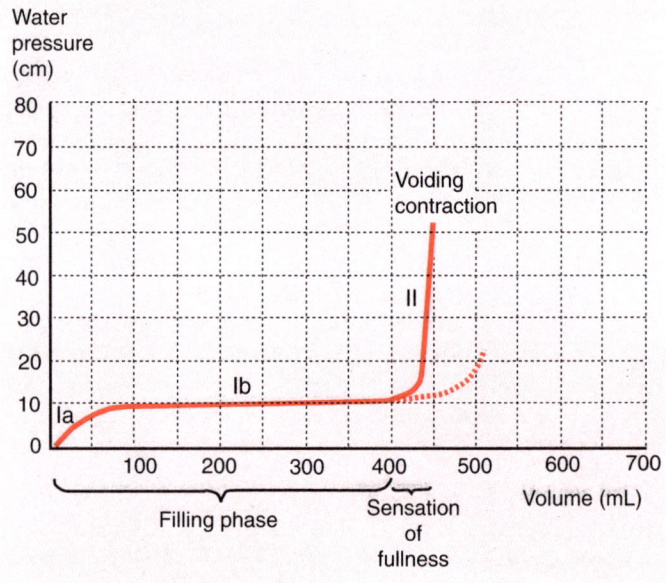

**Fig. 81.4**

# 82

# Events in the Mouth & Esophagus

## What are the muscles of mastication?

The muscles of mastication are masseter, temporalis and the pterygoids.

## Which are the neural centers associated with the swallowing reflex?

The reflex center of the swallowing (**deglutition**) is located in the **nucleus of the tractus solitarius** (**NTS**) and the **nucleus ambiguus**. The afferent arc comprises the trigeminal, glosso-pharyngeal, and vagus nerves. The efferent arc reaches the pharyngeal musculature and the tongue through the trigeminal, facial, and hypoglossal nerves.

## What are the stages of swallowing?

Swallowing has three phases: oral, pharyngeal and esophageal. The *oral phase* is *voluntary* in which the bolus is squeezed out of the oral cavity into the pharynx. This squeezing is made possible through the following steps: (i) The jaws are shut and the lips are closed. (ii) The tongue brings the bolus into the midline between the anterior portion of the tongue and the hard palate. The tip of the tongue then presses firmly against the roof of the hard palate, and limits the bolus anteriorly. (iii) The voluntary contraction of mylohyoid muscle pushes the bolus towards the posterior pharyngeal wall. (iv) The bolus stimulates the sensory nerve endings of the glossopharyngeal nerve in the soft palate and epiglottis and starts off the *swallowing reflex*, which has its center (the deglutition center) in the medulla.

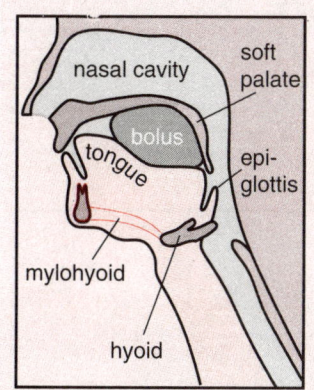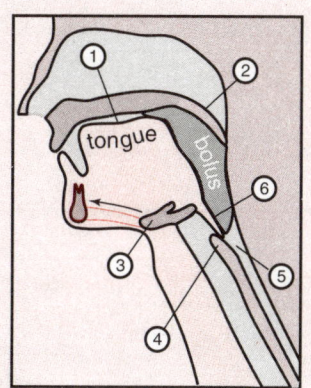

**Fig. 82.1**

In the **pharyngeal phase**, the contact of the bolus with the posterior pharyngeal wall initiates reflex pharyngeal contractions. The pharyngeal reflex is centered in the medulla. It occurs through the following steps: (i) The oral cavity is shut off from the pharynx by the *approximation of the posterior pillars* of the fauces. (ii) The

nasopharynx is shut off from the pharynx by the *elevation of the soft palate*. The soft palate is elevated through the action of the palatopharyngeus muscle. (iii) The glottis is shut off from the pharynx by the approximation of the vocal cords. (iv) The *hyoid is raised* by the contraction of the digastric and the geniohyoid. The *larynx rises with the hyoid* and *brings the epiglottis in the path of the bolus*. (v) The *bolus tilts the epiglottis backwards over the closed glottis*. The lumen of the *esophagus is dragged open* by the forward movement of the larynx and trachea, the posterior walls of which are attached to the anterior walls of the pharynx and the esophagus respectively. (vi) Respiration is arrested. (vii) The hypopharyngeal sphincter (formed by the cricopharyngeus) briefly relaxes and the bolus enters the upper esophagus. (viii) Cricopharyngeus contracts, vocal cords reopen and breathing resumes (Fig. 82.1).

The **esophageal phase** begins once the bolus enters the esophagus. Here, it is propelled by **peristalsis** and aided by **gravity**. The lower sphincter relaxes concomitantly with the relaxation of the hypopharyngeal sphincter. Because of gravity, food travels through esophagus faster in standing than in supine position. However, peristaltic waves are strong enough to propel food against gravity. There are two types of peristaltic waves in the esophagus, primary and secondary.

## What is the difference between primary and secondary peristalsis?

**Primary peristaltic waves** are those that *originate in the pharynx* during the pharyngeal phase of swallowing and travel down the esophagus. The contraction of the cricopharyngeus, which begins when the bolus enters the esophagus, travels at a velocity of 2 - 3 cm/s and involves the lower esophageal sphincter too. **Secondary peristaltic waves** *originate in the esophagus itself* when the esophageal wall is stretched by the bolus. Secondary waves continue to be produced till the bolus is dislodged from the esophagus into the stomach.

## What are the functions of the saliva?

The saliva has the following functions. (i) It keeps the mouth moist and clean. (ii) It acts as a lubricant and thereby aids in speech, chewing and swallowing. (iii) It helps in bolus formation by acting as a glue. (iv) It dissolves food particles, and is therefore necessary for taste. Taste receptors respond only to dissolved substances. (v) It is alkaline and therefore helps to neutralize the gastric juices that might regurgitate into the esophagus. (vi) It contains amylase, which initiates digestion of carbohydrates. (vii) It contains *lysozyme,* an antibacterial enzyme that disinfects the food.

## What is the composition of the saliva? How is it affected as it flows through the salivary ducts?

Saliva is composed of water, electrolytes, enzymes, glycoproteins, and growth factors. The composition of saliva depends on the particular salivary gland, the stimulus, and the rate of flow. The composition of saliva at basal flow rates is as follows:

| Tonicity | Hypotonic |
| --- | --- |
| pH | 7.0 |
| $Na^+$ and $Cl^-$ | Slightly lower than plasma |
| $K^+$ and $HCO_3^-$ | Slightly higher than in plasma |
| Other ions | $Ca^{2+}$, $Mg^{2+}$, $PO_4^{3-}$ |
| Organic substances | Amylase, mucin |

Saliva is formed by *transudation* (pressure filtration) of plasma and therefore is *isotonic when freshly formed*. During its transit through salivary ducts, $Na^+$ and $Cl^-$ are reabsorbed from it while $K^+$ and $HCO_3^-$ are secreted into it. Hence, slower the salivary flow, greater is the change in ionic composition. The absorption of NaCl is more rapid than the secretion of $KHCO_3$. Because the duct epithelium is relatively impermeable to water, the resulting intraluminal fluid is hypotonic. Aldosterone promotes $Na^+$ reabsorption and $K^+$ secretion in the salivary ducts.

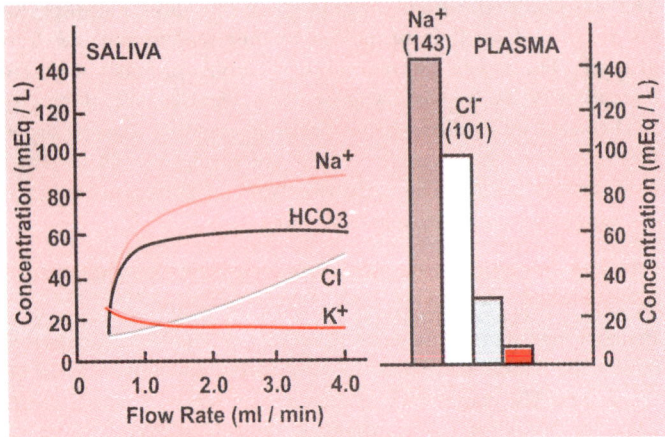

Fig. 82.2

## How are the volume and composition of saliva from the three salivary glands different?

Of the 1 to 2 L of saliva is secreted each day by the three salivary glands, 25% is secreted by the parotid, 70% by the submandibular, and 5% by the sublingual glands. Depending on the type of secretion, salivary acini are categorized into 2 types: (i) *serous acini* secrete the watery saliva containing more than 90% water, and (ii) *mucous acini* secrete a more viscous fluid containing the glycoprotein substance *mucin*, which gives the saliva its characteristic sticky and viscous texture. The parotid gland is purely serous. The sublingual gland is largely mucous and the submandibular is a mixed gland.

## How is salivary secretion regulated?

Salivary secretion is *exclusively under neural control.* The salivary glands are innervated by both parasympathetic cholinergic nerves and sympathetic adrenergic nerves. Some nerve fibers to the salivary glands also contain VIP and substance P. *Parasympathetic discharge* causes *profuse secretion of watery saliva* with a relatively low content of organic material. Parasympathetic nerves are stimulated: (i) through *unconditioned reflex*, e.g., by the presence of food (esp. dry or sour food) in the mouth; (ii) through *conditioned reflex*, e.g., the smell or even the thought of good food. *Sympathetic discharge* causes vasoconstriction and inhibits the secretion of serous saliva. These nerves are stimulated during fear and excitement, when the *mouth becomes dry.*

## What are the salivary enzymes and what are their functions?

Digestive events in the mouth include the actions of two enzymes. (i) **Ptyalin**, an α-*amylase* (optimum pH = 6.7) breaks down the starches by hydrolyzing the 1:4 α linkages. Also called salivary amylase, its action is very short lasting because it gets inactivated by the acidic gastric pH shortly after entering the stomach. (ii) **Lingual lipase** is secreted by Ebner's glands on the dorsal surface of the tongue. The lipase remains active in the stomach and digests as much as 30% of dietary triglycerides.

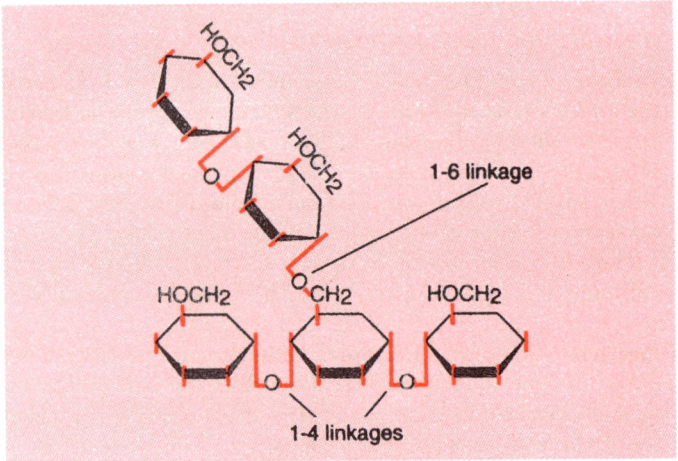

Fig. 82.3

# Events in the Stomach

## What are the functions of the stomach?

The stomach has both motor and secretory functions which are as follows. (i) **Reservoir functions**. The stomach relaxes to accommodate large volumes of food. (ii) **Grinding**. It grinds food to optimal sized particles. (iii) **Mixing**. It mixes the bolus with the gastric juice and converts the bolus into a soup-like *chyme*. (iv) **Partitioning**. It retains the solid portion of the meal until most of the liquid has emptied. (v) **Sieving**. It retains larger particles, permitting more time for their further breakdown. (vi) **Regulating delivery**. It regulates the amount of chyme delivered to the intestine. (vii) **Secretion** of HCl which disinfects the food. (viii) Initiation of protein **digestion**.

## What are MMCs? How are they related to BER?

Migrating motor complexes (MMC) are contraction waves *present in the empty gastrointestinal tract*. They are produced by the electrical activity of the single-unit smooth muscle of the gastrointestinal tract that is called the **basal electrical rhythm (BER)**. This electrical activity originates in pacemaker cells located in the outer circular muscle layer near the myenteric plexus. There is a close correlation of the BER with the MMC. When there are no MMC, the BER consists of rhythmic oscillation of the RMP between about -65 and -45 mV. The oscillations occur due to rhythmic changes in $Ca^{2+}$ and $K^+$ permeabilities. During the MMC, the electrical oscillations are superimposed with spikes. MMCs occur in a cyclical pattern, each cycle lasting 90 min. It shows three phases. **Phase-I** is the phase of quiescence in which there are no contractions, and no spike potentials on the underlying BER. It is the longest phase, lasting about 80 minutes. **Phase-II** is associated with irregular spikes on the BER and irregular

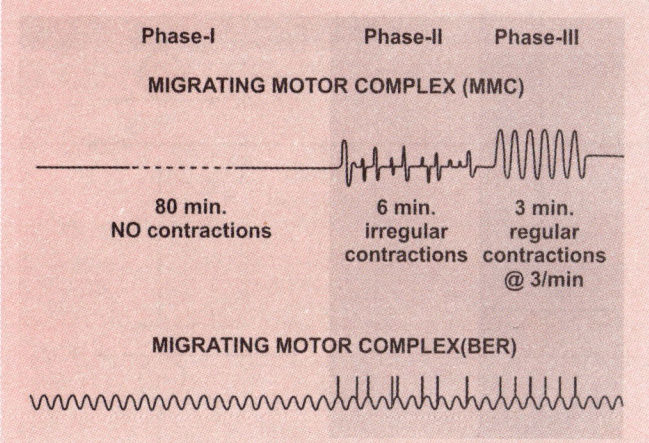

| Phase-I | Phase-II | Phase-III |
|---------|----------|-----------|

**MIGRATING MOTOR COMPLEX (MMC)**

| 80 min. NO contractions | 6 min. irregular contractions | 3 min. regular contractions @ 3/min |

**MIGRATING MOTOR COMPLEX(BER)**

**Fig. 83.1**

contractions. It lasts about 6 minutes. **Phase-III** is associated with regular contractions and regular spike potentials on the BER. It lasts about 3 minutes. The phase-III MMC is associated with a rise in plasma motilin level (Fig. 83.1).

MMCs are of two types. Some originate in the stomach. The phase III of these MMCs have a frequency of 3/min. Others originate in the duodenum. The phase III of these MMCs have a frequency of 11/min. Most MMCs pass along the entire bowel to the terminal ileum with a velocity of 5 cm/min. As soon as one complex reaches the terminal ileum, another starts in the stomach or duodenum.

During MMC, there is an increase in gastric secretion, bile flow and pancreatic secretion. They clear the stomach and small intestine of luminal contents in preparation for the next meal. Hence, they have been called the *interdigestive housekeepers*. MMCs are probably responsible for the hunger contractions.

## Describe the motility of the fed stomach.

When food enters the stomach, the fundus and upper part of its body relax to accommodate the food with little increase in pressure. This is called **receptive relaxation**. Receptive relaxation is vagally mediated and is synchronized with the primary peristaltic waves in the esophagus.

Entry of food in the stomach is associated with *immediate cessation of MMC* although the BER continues as before. In its place appear **peristaltic contractions** that resemble the Phase-II of the interdigestive MMC. Unlike the Phase-II of the interdigestive MMC, these peristaltic waves occur as long as food is present in the stomach and also, these peristaltic waves retain the large particles in the stomach. In contrast, the Phase-III of the interdigestive MMC sweeps out even the large food particles into the duodenum are comparatively weaker.

The peristaltic waves begin near the middle of the body of the stomach and sweep downwards towards the pyloric sphincter. As the wave approaches the pylorus, the sphincter closes. Hence, only a small amount of liquefied chyme squirts through the sphincter into the duodenum, while most of the chyme bounces back off the closed sphincter.

## Describe the factors affecting gastric emptying.

Gastric emptying is regulated mainly from the duodenum through the **enterogastric reflex**. A number of factors initiate this reflex by stimulating duodenal receptors. The reflex is mediated either by local neural circuits or by gastrointestinal hormones. The enterogastric reflex ensures that the gastric chyme does not enter the duodenum too fast. The reflex is initiated by the following factors: (i) **Acid in the duodenum**. It stimulates the release of secretin which reduces gastric motility and increases pyloric sphincteric tone. (ii) **Products of fat digestion**. These stimulate the releases of a number of gastrointestinal hormones like CCK, GIP, VIP and peptide YY, all of which reduce gastric motility. Even before these hormones were identified, the presence of a hormonal mediator was suspected and was provisionally named **enterogastrone**, a term which is obsolete today. (iii) **Products of protein digestion**. These stimulate the release of gastrin, CCK and GIP, all of which slow gastric emptying. (iv) **Osmolarity of the duodenal chyme**. Entry of hyperosmolar chyme into the duodenum reflexly slows gastric emptying. The hormonal mediator of the reflex has not been identified yet. (v) **Mechanical distention of duodenum**. It retards gastric emptying through neural mechanism. (vi) Fats are very effective in inhibiting gastric emptying. Some people consume fats before a cocktail party. The fat keeps the alcohol in the stomach longer, slowing its absorption and reducing the chances of getting intoxicated.

Other factors also affect gastric emptying. (vii) Liquids leave the stomach much faster, flowing around the solid food in the stomach. (viii) Solids with smaller particles leave the stomach faster than solids with larger particles. (ix) Vagotomy slows gastric emptying and cause gastric atony and distention. (x) Excitement speeds up gastric emptying, and fear retards it.

### What are the different types of cells in a gastric gland and what do they secrete?

The gastric mucosa contains several gastric glands. Several of the glands open on a common chamber (gastric pit) that opens in turn on the surface of the mucosa. Mucus and $HCO_3^-$ are secreted by **mucus cells** on the surface of the epithelium between glands. In the body of the stomach, including the fundus, the glands contain **parietal (oxyntic) cells**, which secrete hydrochloric acid and intrinsic factor, and **chief (peptic) cells**, which secrete pepsinogens (Fig. 83.2).

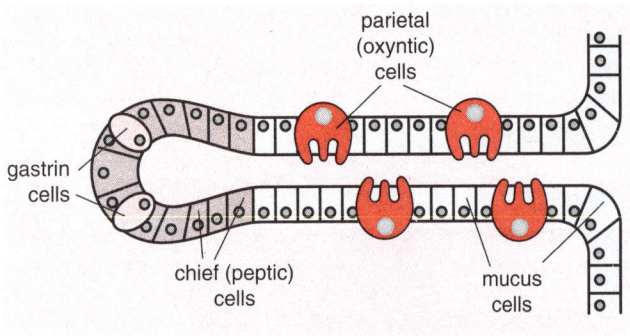

**Fig. 83.2**

About 2.5 L of gastric juice is secreted into the lumen daily. It contains **pepsin** (from chief cells), **acid** (from parietal cells), **mucus** (from mucus cells) and **intrinsic factor** (from parietal cells). Gastric gland also secretes a hormone **gastrin** which is secreted by the **G-cells**.

### What are the functions of gastric acid?

Gastric juice serves the following functions: (i) The acidic gastric juice acts as a good solvent that dissolve iron compounds and other foodstuffs that are not soluble in water. (ii) An acidic pH is required for activation of gastric enzyme pepsin. (iii) Acid is a strong disinfectant, killing bacteria and other microorganisms in the ingested food. (iv) Acid stimulates the duodenum to secrete hormones to release bile and pancreatic juices.

### What are the functions of the gastric enzymes?

The *stomach secretes two enzymes*: pepsin, which digests proteins and gastric lipase, which digests fats. **Gastric lipase** is of little importance in fat digestion except in pancreatic insufficiency. **Pepsin** cleaves food *proteins,* forming small *peptides.* When secreted by the chief *(zymogen)* cells, pepsin is in its inactive form, a larger protein called *pepsinogen.* Acid in the lumen promotes conversion of pepsinogen to pepsin. Pepsin, once formed, also attacks pepsinogen, producing more pepsin molecules *(autocatalysis).*

### Describe the mechanism of HCl secretion by the parietal cells.

Gastric glands secrete a concentrated solution of *hydrochloric acid*, which has a pH of approximately 1.0. Its secretion involves the secretion of $H^+$ ions and the secretion of $Cl^-$ ions. **Secretion of $H^+$ ions** occurs in the following steps (Fig. 83.3). (1) $H^+$ ions are produced inside the cell from metabolic $CO_2$ through the following reaction which is catalyzed by the enzyme *carbonic anhydrase* that is present in the parietal cells in large amounts, i.e., $CO_2 + H_2O = H_2CO_3 = H^+ + HCO_3^-$. (2) The hydrogen ions are secreted by the parietal cell through its apical membrane by a *primary active transport* with coupled antiport of $K^+$ ions. The $H^+$-$K^+$ exchange is obviously electroneutral. (3) The *bicarbonate ($HCO_3^-$)* ions produced is transported out of the parietal cell at the serosal border through *primary active transport* with coupled antiport of *chloride ions* into the cell. The $HCO_3^-$-$Cl^-$ exchange is again electroneutral. The $HCO_3^-$ transported out of the parietal cells enters the blood stream and increases the blood pH (the *postprandial alkaline tide*). The **secretion of $Cl^-$ ions** occurs in the following steps. (4) The $Na^+$-$K^+$ pump located on the basolateral membrane of the parietal cell pumps out three $Na^+$ for every two $K^+$ pumped in. The inside of the parietal cell therefore becomes

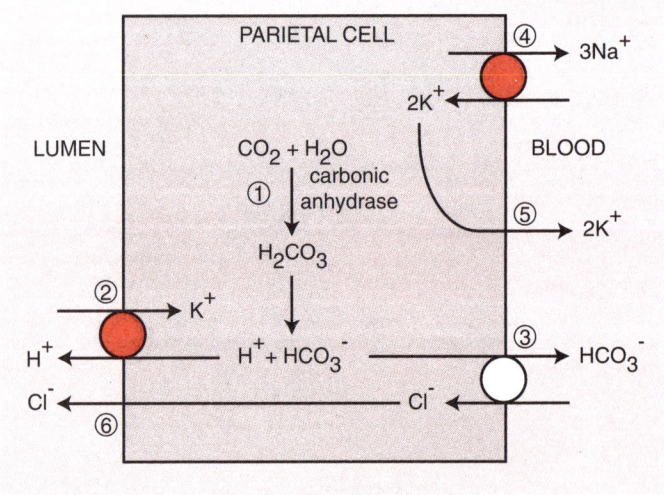

**Fig. 83.3**

negative. (5) The $K^+$ ions that are pumped in diffuse out through the $K^+$ channels present on the basolateral as well as apical membranes. This diffusion further increases the intracellular negativity of the parietal cell. (6) *The high intracellular negativity forces out $Cl^-$ ions* through the $Cl^-$ channels located on the apical membrane.

### What are the receptors involved in the control of gastric acid secretion

The *second messengers* that activate gastric acid secretion are activated by various receptors present on the membrane of the parietal cell. There are 5 types of receptors of which 3 are stimulatory and 2 are inhibitory. (i) **Acetylcholine (Muscarinic) receptors**. When acetylcholine binds to these receptors, the $Gs \rightarrow$ phospholipase-C pathway generates high levels of $IP_3$ and diacylglycerol from membrane phospholipids. $IP_3$ mobilizes $Ca^{2+}$ from intracellular stores while diacylglycerol activates protein kinases. (ii) **Gastrin receptors**. The second messengers associated with gastrin have not been identified with certainty but is unlikely to be $Ca^{2+}$ or cAMP. (iii) **Histamine receptors**. $H_2$ receptor stimulation leads to the formation of cAMP through the $Gs \rightarrow$ adenyl cyclase pathway. The cAMP then activates protein kinase A. (iv) **Prostaglandin ($PGE_2$)** and (v) **Somatostatin receptors**. Somatostatin and prostaglandin $E_2$ bind to specific receptors that act via an inhibitory GTP regulatory protein ($G_i$) in preventing the activation of adenylate cyclase (Fig. 83.4).

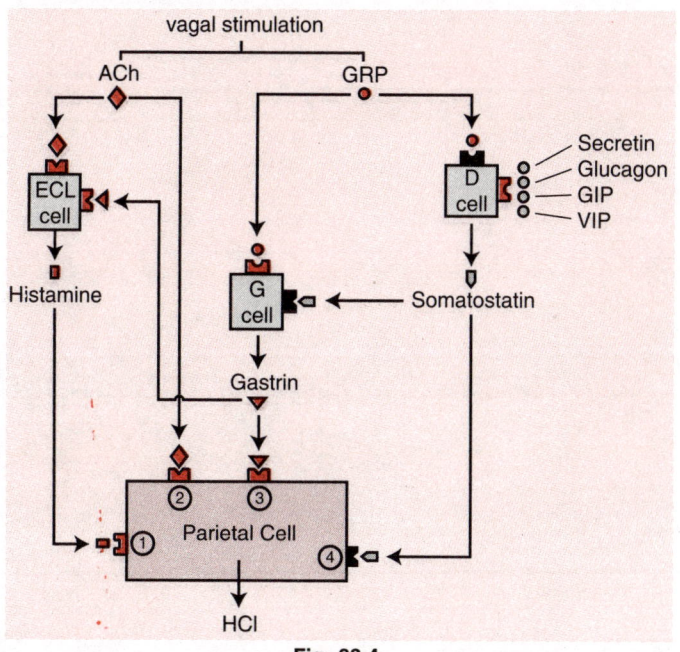

vagal stimulation
ACh    GRP
Secretin
Glucagon
GIP
VIP
ECL cell
D cell
Histamine
G cell
Somatostatin
Gastrin
② ③
Parietal Cell
① ④
HCl

**Fig. 83.4**

### Describe the paracrine cells involved in gastric acid secretion.

The paracrine control of gastric secretion involves the G-cells, D-cells and ECL cells. (i) **G-cells** are located at the base of the gastric glands and are especially abundant in the pyloric gastric glands. It secretes gastrin, which stimulates HCl secretion. Gastrin secretion is *stimulated by GRP* (**Gastrin-releasing peptide**) and *inhibited by somatostatin*. (ii) **D-cells** secrete **somatostatin**, which *inhibits HCl secretion* in two ways: through a direct action on

parietal cells and an indirect action by inhibiting gastrin secretion by G-cells. D-cells are located adjacent to the G-cells or the parietal cells. Secretin, enteroglucagon, GIP and VIP – all inhibit gastric secretion by stimulating somatostatin release. (iii) **Entero-chromaffin-like (ECL)** cells are found in the oxyntic region of the stomach, in the base of the gastric gland. They secrete histamine. The histamine released stimulates HCl secretion from parietal cells. ECL cells bear both gastrin receptors and ACh receptors. They release histamine in response to both circulating gastrin as well as the ACh released by vagal fibers. Stimulation of ECL cells is an important mechanism through which gastrin stimulates acid secretion.

### What is the effect of vagus on gastric secretion?

Vagal fibers to the stomach have two types of neurotransmitters. (i) Some vagal fibers release **gastrin releasing peptide** (GRP). The GRP increases gastrin secretion from G-cells with consequent increase in acid secretion. The GRP also inhibits somatostatin secretion from D cells and thereby disinhibits HCl secretion from parietal cells. (ii) Other vagal fibers release **acetylcholine**, which acts directly on the cells in the glands in the body and the fundus to increase the secretion of acid, pepsin and mucus. Part of the acid secretion is mediated by ECL cells that secrete histamine. Vagotomy does not abolish the secretory response to local stimuli.

### Describe the phases of gastric acid secretion.

There are four phases of gastric secretion: interdigestive, cephalic, gastric and intestinal. In the **interdigestive phase** (basal acid secretion), acid is continuously secreted by the stomach even between meals and during sleep. A circadian rhythm is seen, with basal secretion reaching its peak around midnight and its lowest around 7 in the morning. Interdigestive phase of gastric acid secretion is vagally mediated. Emotional outbursts, tension and anxiety alter basal acid secretion.

Gastric secretion stimulated by **cephalic factors** accounts for up to 50% of the acid secreted in response to a normal meal. It is vagally mediated and is easily conditioned. The unconditioned stimulus is the presence of food in the mouth. Conditioned stimuli include the sight, smell, and thought of food increase gastric secretion. The conditioned reflex involves activation of the anterior hypothalamus and parts of the adjacent orbital frontal cortex. The cephalic phase of gastric secretion is influenced by psychic states: it is *increased with anger and hostility*, and is *reduced in fear and depression*.

The **gastric phase** of acid secretion comes into play when food makes contact with the gastric mucosa. It accounts for up to 50% of the acid secretion in response to meal. Acid secretion in this phase is brought about by: (i) *gastrin secretion*, brought about by the stimulatory effect of the products of protein digestion, mainly amino acids, and (ii) *stretch of the stomach wall* which activates a local reflex arc that terminates on vagal postganglionic neurons.

The **intestinal phase** begins when food enters the intestine. *Gastric secretion is inhibited* by the same intestinal factors that reduce gastric motility through the enterogastric reflex. Briefly, they are: (i) acid in the duodenum; (ii) product of fat digestion; (iii) osmolarity of the duodenal chyme; and (iv) mechanical distension of the duodenum. Products of protein digestion, however, have a slight *stimulatory effect on gastric acid secretion*, and accounts for about 5% of the total gastric acid secretion that occurs following a meal. The hormone *enterogastrone* was thought to mediate the inhibition of gastric secretion in the intestinal phase. The candidates for this non-existent hormone, which might mediate the intestinal inhibition of acid secretion, are *secretin*, *CCK*, *prostaglandins*, *somatostatin*, and *peptide YY*.

Several **other factors** are known to affect gastric secretion. Hypoglycemia stimulates central vagal discharge to stimulate acid and pepsin secretion. Other stimulants include alcohol and caffeine, both of which act directly on the mucosa.

### Define basal acid output. How is it measured?

**Basal acid secretion** (**BAO**) is the rate of acid secretion in the absence of all avoidable stimulations. About 400ml of gastric juice is collected overnight (from 9.00 pm to 9.00 am) through an indwelling nasogastric catheter. The room is made devoid of the physical presence and even the odor of food. Normally, BAO is < 10 mmoles/L in males and < 5 mmoles/L in females.

### How is the gastric epithelium protected from the corrosive effect of acid?

The stomach mucus forms a thick protective coat covering the inner linings of the stomach in order to protect it from mechanical damage and the corrosive actions of the acid in the gastric juice. The breakdown of this coat is one of the causes of ulcers. Gastric wall cells' impermeability to acid, as well as the protective action of the alkaline stomach mucus, prevents ulcers from occurring in healthy individuals. The surface membranes of the mucosal cells and the tight junctions between the cells are also part of the **mucosal barrier** that protects the gastric epithelium from damage. Substances that tend to disrupt the barrier and cause gastric irritation include *ethanol, vinegar, bile salts, aspirin* and other *nonsteroidal anti-inflammatory drugs* (**NSAIDs**). Prostaglandins stimulate mucus secretion, and aspirin and related drugs inhibit prostaglandin synthesis. Some of the resistance of the gastric mucosa to autodigestion is also provided by the presence of acid-resistant peptides called **trefoil peptides** in the mucosa.

# 84

# Events in the Duodenum

## What are the major sources of duodenal secretions?

Duodenal secretions are derived from two main sources: **bile juice** and *pancreatic juice*. In addition, the **Brunner's glands** in the duodenum secrete thick *alkaline mucus* that probably helps *protect the duodenal mucosa from the gastric acid*.

## What are the major constituents of the bile juice?

The major constituents of the bile juice are: (i) **Bile salts** – *taurocholates* and *glycocholates*. (ii) **Bile pigments** – *bilirubin* and *biliverdin*. (iii) **Electrolytes**. The cations $Na^+$, $K^+$ and $Ca^{2+}$ are all present in concentrations about 20% greater than in the plasma. The two major anions are $Cl^-$ and $HCO_3^-$. $Cl^-$ is present in concentrations lesser than in plasma while $HCO_3^-$ is far greater than in plasma, which makes the bile juice considerably alkaline. (iv) **Lipids**. *Cholesterol* is present in a concentration of 60 – 170 mg/L. Other lipids present in bile are *lecithin*, *fatty acids* and *triglycerides*. Of these, only the bile salts are of importance to the digestive system.

## How is bile secretion regulated?

The entry of bile into the duodenum can be increased in two ways. (i) *Increased bile secretion by the liver cells*. Substances that increase bile secretion by liver are called **choleretics**. Examples of choleretics are *secretin* and *bile salts*. *Vagal stimulation* also increases bile secretion. Although bile salts increase the hepatic secretion of bile, it *inhibits the synthesis of new bile salts*. Despite the inhibition of fresh bile salt synthesis, the amount of bile salts in the bile does not decrease. This is because the bile salts secreted into duodenum are reabsorbed from the intestine and resecreted into the bile juice (**enterohepatic circulation**). Drugs that stimulate the liver to increase the output of bile of low specific gravity are called **hydrocholeretic**. (ii) *Release of bile stored in the gall bladder into the duodenum*. Stored bile is released by the contraction of the gall bladder with simultaneous relaxation of the sphincter of Oddi. Substances that cause contraction of gall bladder are called **cholagogues**. A well-known cholagogue is the hormone **cholecystokinin (CCK)**. *Fatty acids and amino acids in the duodenum release CCK*, which causes gallbladder contraction.

## What is the composition of the pancreatic juice? How is it affected during its flow through the pancreatic ducts?

The volume of pancreatic juice secreted per day is about 500 – 1500 mL. It is *highly alkaline* (pH = 8.4) due to its high $HCO_3^-$ content (2 – 5 times higher than the plasma concentration). *As the flow rate of pancreatic juice increases, its $HCO_3^-$ concentration*

*increases and chloride concentration decreases*. The $Na^+$ and $K^+$ concentrations are similar to those of plasma and do not change with flow rate. The reciprocal relationship with flow rate occurs because $HCO_3^-$ *is secreted in the small ducts, but is reabsorbed in the large ducts in exchange for $Cl^-$*. The magnitude of the exchange is inversely proportionate to the rate of flow.

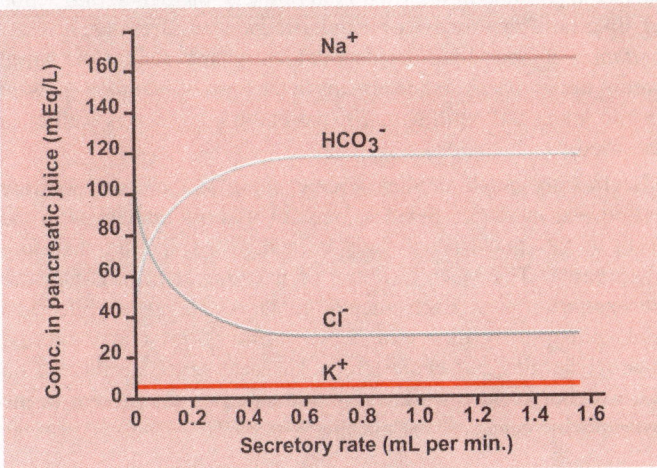

**Fig. 84.1**

## What are the functions of the pancreatic juice?

The pancreatic juice is *the major source of digestive enzymes* that digest all components of the food – proteins, carbohydrates, fats and nucleic acid. Its highly alkaline pH *helps to neutralize the gastric HCl* in the chyme that enters the duodenum.

## Describe the hormonal control of pancreatic secretion

Pancreatic secretion is controlled by secretion and CCK. **Secretin** *acts on the pancreatic ducts* to cause secretion of large amounts of a very alkaline pancreatic juice that is *rich in $HCO_3^-$ and poor in enzymes*. The effect on duct cells is due to an increase in intracellular cAMP. **CCK** *acts on the acinar cells* to cause the release of zymogen granules and production of pancreatic juice *rich in enzymes*. Its effect is mediated by phospholipase C.

Cells secreting these hormones are found at several places but mainly, in the *mucosa of the upper intestine*. The secretion of both is stimulated by the contact of the intestinal mucosa with the *acidic pH* of the chyme and by the *peptides and aminoacids* present in the chyme. Secretin is additionally secreted by the presence of *long chain fatty acids* in the duodenum. Thus, *both CCK and secretin mediate a physiological reflex* wherein the food stimulates the secretion of the digestive juice required to digest it. **Insulin** also has long-term effects on the *regulation of the synthesis of pancreatic enzymes*.

### Describe the neural control of pancreatic secretion.

Stimulation of the vagi causes secretion of a small amount of pancreatic juice rich in enzymes. Vagal stimulation occurs as part of a conditioned reflex in response to the sight or smell of food. The vagal effect is mediated through acetylcholine released by the vagal endings.

### What is the action of the bile juice?

The role of bile salts in fat digestion is three fold: (i) emulsification of fats; (ii) formation of micelles, and (iii) activation of an enzyme called **bile salt activated lipase** which is present in milk.

### What is the difference between emulsification and micelle formation?

**Emulsification** is the division of large lipid droplets into smaller droplets about *1 mm in diameter*. Emulsification increases the surface to volume ratio of the lipid droplets, facilitating the action of lipases. The process of emulsification requires *mechanical agitation* of large lipid droplets (which is provided by the antral part of the stomach) and detergents in the form of *bile salts* (present in bile juice) and *phospholipids* (present in bile juice as well as in the food).

**Micelles** are much smaller – about *5 nm in diameter*, and are cylindrical in shape. Besides, most of its lipid content is in the form of fats that have already been digested and are therefore absorbable. The *main function of micelles is to assist in the absorption of fats*. Each micelle contains *detergents* (bile salts and phospholipids) and *absorbable fats* (fatty acids, monoglycerides and cholesterol). The detergents are located on the micellar surface while the absorbable fats are present in the hydrophobic center of the micelle (Fig. 84.2).

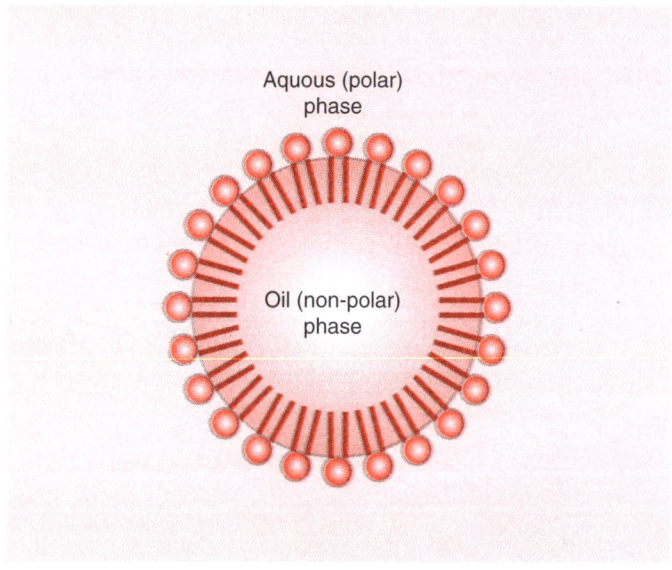

Aquous (polar) phase

Oil (non-polar) phase

**Fig. 84.2**

### Enumerate the pancreatic enzymes that digest proteins.

The pancreatic juice contains three endopeptidases (trypsin, chymotrypsin and elastase) and two exopeptidases (carboxypeptidase A and B). *Endopeptidases* break the peptides somewhere in the middle. *Exopeptidases* break the peptide chain near its end, releasing single aminoacids. **Trypsin** cleaves peptide bonds of basic aminoacids. **Chymotrypsin** cleaves the peptide bonds containing uncharged aminoacid residues, such as aromatic aminoacids. **Elastase** attacks peptide bonds next to small amino acid residues such as glycine, alanine and serine. **Carboxypeptidase A** cleaves the carboxy-terminal aminoacid that have aromatic or branched aliphatic side chains. **Carboxypeptidase B** cleaves the carboxy-terminal aminoacids that have basic side chains.

All the above enzymes are secreted from the pancreas as inactive precursors (**zymogens**). Chymotrypsinogen, proelastase, and procarboxypeptidases are *converted into their active forms by the action of trypsin*. Trypsin itself is activated from trypsinogen by the action of **enteropeptidase** (**enterokinase**) secreted by the intestinal mucosa.

Pancreatic juice also contains **ribonuclease (RNase) and deoxyribonuclease (DNase)** that are responsible for the digestion of dietary nucleic acids.

### Enumerate the pancreatic enzymes that digest carbohydrates.

The pancreatic juice contains *only a single enzyme* that digests carbohydrates – it is the pancreatic α-amylase. **Pancreatic amylase** is similar in action to salivary amylase, *hydrolyzing 1:4α linkages* but spare 1:6α linkages, terminal 1:4α linkages, and the 1:4α linkages next to branching points. Consequently, the end products of α-amylase digestion are mostly: (i) the disaccharide **maltose** (two α-glucose residues linked by 1:4 α bonds); (ii) the trisaccharide **maltotriose** (three α-glucose residues linked by 1:4 α bonds); (iii) oligosaccharides with more glucose residues linked by 1:4 α bonds; and (iv) α-**limit dextrins,** polymers of glucose containing an average of about eight glucose molecules with 1:6 α linkages.

### Enumerate the pancreatic enzymes that digest fats.

The pancreatic enzymes involved in the digestion of fats are: (i) pancreatic lipase; (ii) colipase; (iii) phospholipase $A_2$; (iv) bile salt activated lipase. Phospholipase $A_2$ and colipase are secreted as inactive precursors that are *activated by trypsin*. **Phospholipase $A_2$** hydrolyzes the ester bond in the 2-position of glycerophospholipids of both biliary and dietary origins to form lysophospholipids, which, being detergents, aid emulsification and digestion of lipids. **Pancreatic lipase** specifically hydrolyzes primary ester linkages at positions 1 and 3 of triacylglycerols, yielding mostly *free fatty acids* and *2-monoglycertides*. Pancreatic lipase is inhibited by bile salts. **Colipase** helps overcome this inhibition. **Bile salt-activated lipase** breaks down triacylglycerol completely into glycerol and fatty acids. It also catalyzes the hydrolysis of cholesterol esters, esters of fat-soluble vitamins and phospholipids. **Cholesteryl ester hydrolase** breaks down cholesteryl esters. Most of the dietary cholesterol is in the form of cholesteryl esters, and cholesteryl ester hydrolase hydrolyzes these esters, releasing cholesterol in nonesterified free form.

### What are the major absorptive events in the duodenum?

Significant amounts of absorption occur in the duodenum. In general, *the absorptive pattern in duodenum resembles that in the jejunum*. The duodenum and upper jejunum have the highest capacity to absorb *sugars, dipeptides and tripeptides, and fats*.

$Ca^{2+}$ *and phosphate* absorptions are especially high in the duodenum and ileum. The duodenum is also the principle site of absorption of *non-heme iron*.

### Enumerate some of the pancreatic function tests.

The pancreatic function tests are broadly of two types: (i) *Analysis of stimulated pancreatic secretions*. The pancreas is stimulated either by giving secretin (**secretin test**) or by a standardized meal (**Lundh meal test**). (ii) *Analysis of digestion products*, by microscopic **examination of stool** for undigested meat fibers and fat, **fecal fat quantification** (normally < 7% of the dietary intake), **fecal nitrogen estimation** (normally less than 7g/day).

# 85

# Events in the Small Intestines

## What are the major types of intestinal motility?

In the unfed state, the small intestinal motility is characterized by the MMCs (migrating motor complexes) that pass down from the stomach along the intestine at regular intervals. Following a meal, as in the stomach, the MMCs are replaced by different motility patterns like the segmentation and peristaltic patterns. The *MMCs are much stronger* than the peristaltic waves that occur in their place.

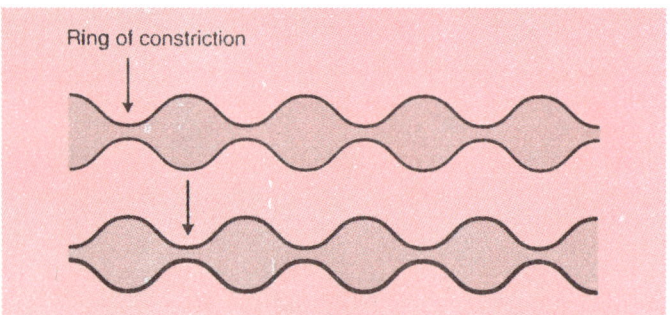

Ring of constriction

**Fig. 85.1**

**Segmentation contractions** are ring-like contractions of the circular smooth muscle of the gut that appear at regular intervals. The intestine gets transiently compartmented into several short segments. The contractions disappear after sometime, only to reappear as another set of ring contractions in the segments between the previous contractions. They move the chyme to and fro and increase its exposure to the mucosal surface. *Segmentation slows down the transit in the small intestine.* This permits longer contact of the chyme with the enterocytes and promotes absorption. **Peristaltic waves** propel the intestinal chyme toward the large intestines. They are contraction rings of the intestine that travel short distances along the intestine at velocities of 2 – 3 cm/s. Very intense peristaltic waves called **peristaltic rushes** are *not seen in normal individuals*, but they occur when the intestine is obstructed.

## Name the intestinal reflexes.

**Peristaltic reflex** is a reflex in which a localized distension of the intestine induces peristaltic contraction proximal to the point of stretch and inhibition distal to it. The peristaltic reflex is *coordinated by the enteric nervous system* of the intestine. In the **gastroileal reflex**, elevated secretory and motor activity of the stomach reflexly increases the motility of the terminal part of the ileum and accelerates the movement of material through the ileocecal sphincter. The reflex is vagally mediated. In the **intestinointestinal reflex**, overdistention of one segment of the intestine relaxes the smooth muscle in the rest of the intestine.

## What is the composition of the succus entericus? How is its secretion regulated?

The intestinal glands secrete an isotonic fluid. Most of the enzymes usually found in this secretion come from the desquamated mucosal cells. *Cell-free intestinal juice contains hardly any enzymes.* Gastrointestinal hormones such as VIP stimulate the secretion of intestinal juice. Vagal stimulation increases the secretion of Brunner's glands (mucus secreting cells abundant in the first part of the duodenum) but has no effect on that of the intestinal glands.

## What are the enzymes for carbohydrate digestion in the small intestine?

There are five enzymes responsible for carbohydrate digestion at the intestinal brush border: (i) **sucrase,** which breaks down sucrose into glucose and fructose; (ii) **maltase** (α glucosidase), which breaks the 1:4 α linkages and releases glucose; (iii) **isomaltase** (α dextrinase), which breaks down the 1:6 α linkages and releases glucose; (iv) **lactase** (β glucosidase), which breaks down lactose into glucose and galactose; and (v) **trehalase,** which hydrolyzes trehalose, a 1:1 α-linked dimer of glucose, into two glucose molecules.

## What are the enzymes for protein digestion in the small intestine?

There are five enzymes responsible for protein digestion at the intestinal brush border. One of them – **enteropeptidase** – is meant only for activating trypsinogen to trypsin. The other four are: (i) **aminopeptidase,** which is an exopeptidase that breaks the peptide bonds next to N-terminal amino acids of peptides; (ii) **carboxypeptidase,** which is an exopeptidase that breaks the last peptide bond towards the C-terminal; (iii) **endopeptidase,** which breaks peptide bonds somewhere in the middle of the polypeptide; and (iv) **dipeptidase,** which splits dipeptides into aminoacids.

## What are the enzymes for fat digestion in the small intestine?

The fat digestion that occurs in the intestine is brought about mostly by the pancreatic juice. However, the intestinal mucosal cells have on them a **phospholipase**, which attacks phospholipids to produce glycerol, fatty acids, phosphoric acid and bases such as choline.

## Describe the mechanisms of proteins absorption in the intestine.

Absorption of amino acids is *more in the jejunum but less in the ileum.* Some amount of aminoacid is reabsorbed through simple diffusion. However, most aminoacids employ transporters. At least seven **specific transport systems** transport different types of amino acids into enterocytes across the brush border. In humans, a *congenital defect in the transport of neutral amino acids* in the intestine and renal tubules causes **Hartnup disease**. A *congenital defect in the transport of basic amino acids* causes **cystinuria**.

Dipeptides and tripeptides are transported across the brush border through secondary active transport. Most of the peptides that enter the enterocyte are split into aminoacids inside the cell. The aminoacids diffuse out of the basolateral membrane into portal blood. However, some peptides diffuse out into blood stream unchanged, possibly using a transporter. Some amounts of proteins can also pass unaltered from the intestine into the blood. *In infants, the IgA present in maternal colostrum are thus able to enter the circulation* to provide passive immunity. In adults, some *food proteins may produce allergy after getting absorbed without digestion.*

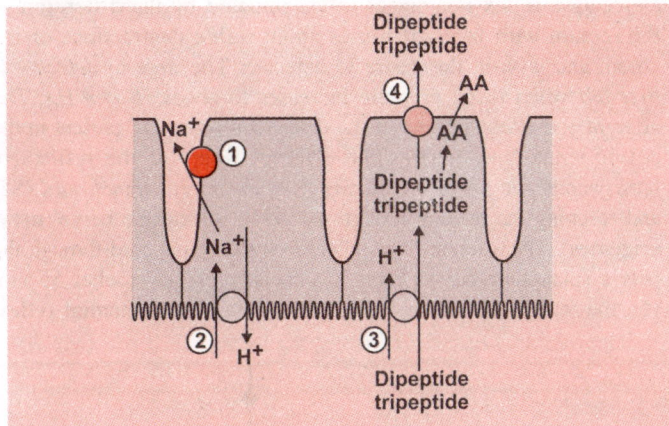

**Fig. 85.2**

## Describe the mechanisms of carbohydrate absorption in the intestine.

Monosacharides are rapidly absorbed from the intestine before the meal reaches the terminal part of the ileum. **Pentoses** are absorbed by simple diffusion. **Glucose** and **galactose** are absorbed by facilitated diffusion employing SGLT-1 and GLUT-2. **Fructose** employs GLUT 5 and GLUT 2 for diffusion across the luminal and basolateral membranes respectively.

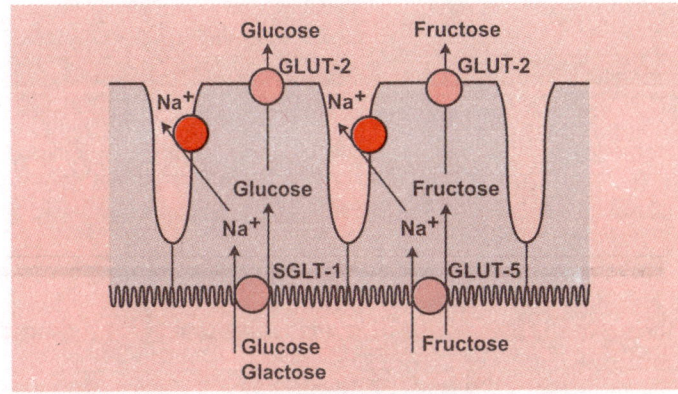

**Fig. 85.3**

## Describe the mechanisms of fat absorption in the intestine.

All fatty acids enter the enterocytes by **facilitated diffusion**. Once inside the mucosal cell, short and long chain fatty acids are dealt with differently. **Short chain fatty acids** containing less than 10-12 carbon atoms pass from the mucosal cells directly into the portal blood. **Long-chain fatty acids** (> 10-12 carbon atoms) enter the mucosal cell and are rapidly reesterified to triglycerides in the mucosal cells, maintaining a favorable diffusion gradient of lipids. The triglycerides are then coated with a layer of protein, cholesterol and phospholipid to form **chylomicrons**. These leave the cell and enter the lymphatics. **Cholesterol** is treated like long-chain fatty acids. They are esterified in the mucosal cells, incorporated into chylomicrons and released into the lymphatics.

# 86

# *Events in the Colon*

### Describe the electrical activity associated with colonic motility.

The movements of the colon are coordinated by the *BER of the colon*. The frequency of this wave, unlike the wave in the small intestine, *increases along the colon*, from about 9/min at the ileocecal valve to 16/min at the sigmoid.

### Describe the pressure changes associated with colonic motility

Pressures changes in the colon are measured by open-tip catheters (which records only pressure) or catheters with balloons (which record both pressure and contraction, but does not distinguish between them). Three types of pressure waves can be discerned in recordings made with water-filled balloons: **Type-I** consists of small pressure variations (about 5 cm saline) that lasts about 5 seconds each, and occur with a frequency of 10/min. In an anxious subject, the frequency increases to 30/min. **Type-II** consists of larger pressure variations that lasts longer – about 30 seconds each, and occur once every few minutes. Sometimes, the rise in pressure is as much as 100 cm saline. These pressure changes are associated with **mass contraction**. **Type-III** consists of a minor pressure elevation that lasts for several minutes. In anxious patients, the pressure may remains elevated above baseline for nearly 50% of the time.

### Describe the cineradiographic patterns of colonic motility.

**Cineradiographic patterns** indicate both the pattern of colonic contractions as well as the movement of the colonic contents. **Haustral shuttling** is the commonest form of movement detected in a subject and at rest. These are similar to the segmentation contractions of the ileum that mix the contents of the colon and, by exposing more of the contents to the mucosa, facilitate absorption. *Haustra* are the sacs of colonic mucosal fold, produced by annular contractions in the colon. **Segmental propulsion** causes the contents of a haustrum to be expelled into the 'next' or the 'next-to-next' haustrum. The direction of propulsion may be aboral or adoral, but retropulsion is only about 2/3 as common as the forward propulsion. **Systolic multihaustral propulsion** (also called **mass contraction**) causes a number of adjacent haustra to contract more or less simultaneously. These contractions move material from one portion of the colon to another. They also move material into the rectum, and rectal distention initiates the defecation reflex.

### How much is the colonic transit time?

A test meal consumed reaches the cecum in about 4 hours, hepatic flexure in 6 hours, splenic flexure in 9 hours and sigmoid colon in 12 hours. From the pelvic colon to the anus, transport is much slower, and as much as a quarter of the residue of a test meal is retained in the rectum for up to 3 days. Complete expulsion of the meal in stool takes more than a week. High residue diet pass more rapidly through the entire gut.

### Describe the defecation reflex.

Defecation reflex is a spinal reflex initiated by the distension of the rectum with feces. It brings about reflex contractions of the colon, and with it, the desire to defecate. The *urge to defecate is first felt* when rectal pressure increases to about *18 mm Hg*. The afferent and efferent fibers of the defecation reflex are present in the pelvic splanchnic nerve. The efferent fibers of the reflex are *parasympathetic fibers originating from the sacral spinal cord* (S2) and reaching the rectum through the pelvic splanchnic nerve (**nervi erigentes**). The afferent fibers also reach the spinal cord through the pelvic splanchnic nerve. When the rectal pressure reaches 55 mm Hg, the *internal sphincter relaxes*. It is called the **rectoanal reflex**.

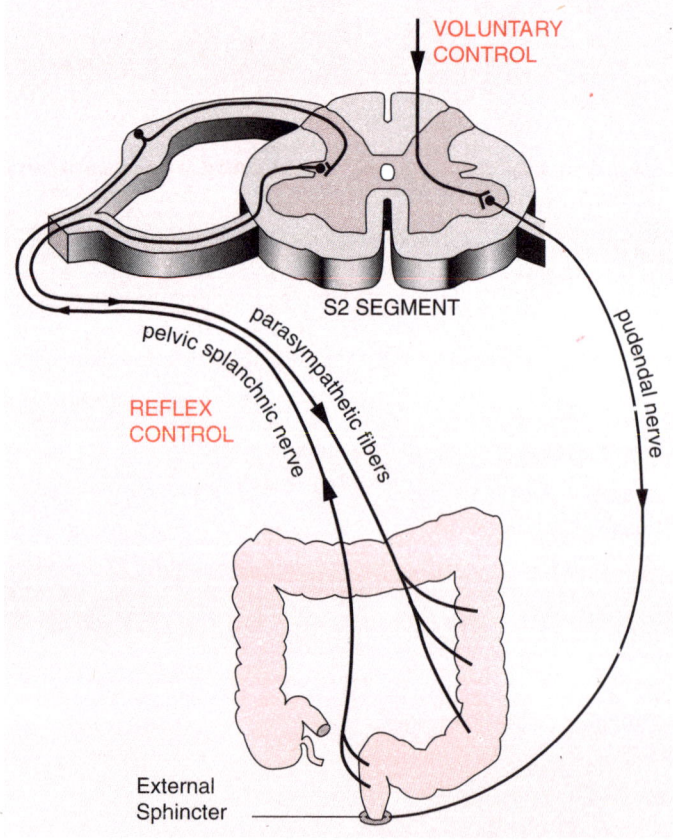

**Fig. 86.1**

The relaxation is mediated by *noncholinergic, non-adrenergic fibers* but the reflex pathway is not known.

*Defecation can be voluntarily inhibited* by keeping the external anal sphincter contracted. Alternatively, the external sphincter can be relaxed voluntarily, allowing the contents of the rectum to be expelled. Chronic spinal patients have no voluntary control on defecation. Evacuation is entirely reflex in them. *Defecation can be voluntarily initiated* anytime when the rectal pressure is between 18 and 55 mm Hg. This is done by voluntarily relaxing the external sphincter and contracting the abdominal muscles (**straining**), thereby aiding the reflex emptying of the distended rectum.

### Name some other colonic reflexes.

**Gastrocolic reflex** is the reflex contraction of the colon brought about by the distension of the stomach. The reflex results in an urge to defecate immediately after a meal. It is *probably not a neural reflex*; rather, it may be mediated by gastrointestinal hormones like *gastrin and cholecystokinin* that are secreted into the blood stream in significant amounts shortly after a meal. Because of this reflex, defecation after meals is the rule in children. In adults, bowel training suppresses this reflex.

### Describe the composition of the feces.

About 75% of stool is water and only 25% of it is solid. The solid part in turn has the following composition.

| | |
|---|---|
| Dead bacteria | 30% |
| Undigested roughage, sloughed epithelial cells and the solid constituents of gastrointestinal secretions, e.g., bile pigments | 30% |
| Fats | 10 – 20 % |
| Inorganic matter | 10 – 20 % |
| Proteins | 2 – 3 % |

The *protein in the stools is not of dietary origi*n but comes from bacteria and cellular debris. Similarly, the *fats in the stools also are mostly not from dietary origin* but are derived from sloughed epithelial cells or from bacterial synthesis. Since a large fraction of the fecal mass is of nondietary origin, fecal composition is relatively unaffected by dietary variations. That is why *appreciable amounts of feces continue to be passed even during prolonged starvation.*

The *pH of stool* is slightly acidic (5.0-7.0) due to the organic acids formed from carbohydrates by colonic bacteria. The *brown color of the stool* is due to the presence of **urobilin**, which is formed by the oxidation of urobilinogen (colorless). Urobilinogens are formed from bilirubin by the action of colonic bacteria. Darkening of feces upon standing in air is due to the oxidation of residual urobilinogens to urobilins. When bile fails to enter the intestine, the stools become white (**acholic stools**). The *odor of stool* is due to substances like *indole, skatole, mercaptans and hydrogen sulfide*, which are formed in colon through bacterial action on food.

### What are dietary fibers? What is their importance?

Dietary fiber or roughage is defined as the parts of plant materials in our diet that are resistant to digestion in the gut. Crude fiber is made up of two broad categories depending on their solubility in hot water: *Insoluble fibers*, e.g., **celluloses** and **lignin**. Wheat bran and other whole grain are rich in insoluble fiber. (ii) *Soluble fibers*, e.g., **hemicelluloses, gums, mucilages, and pectin**. Oat bran, peas, and beans are rich in soluble fiber. Except lignin, which is made up of phenyl propane units, almost all other dietary fibers are carbohydrates.

Fibers absorb and retain water, and thereby swell up and increase the bulk and consistency of fecal matter. Increased bulk of stool decreases intestinal transit time. *Anaerobic bacterial fermentation of fiber* in the colon results in the formation of water, carbon dioxide, hydrogen, and short-chain fatty acids, such as acetic, propionic, and butyric acids. Such short-chain fatty acids are absorbed *avidly* by the colon, provide an important nutrient source for colonic mucosa, and in addition promote the absorption of water, sodium, and chloride. Anaerobic fermentation of fiber also speeds up colonic transit.

If the amount of dietary fiber is small, the diet is said to lack bulk. When the bulk of fecal matter in the colon is small, the colon is inactive and bowel movements are infrequent. In addition, starvation and parenteral nutrition lead to atrophy of the mucosa of the colon, and this is reversed when substances like pectin are placed in the colon.

### What are the different types of bacteria normally present in the colon?

Colonic bacteria include both harmless ones such as *Escherchia coli* and *Enterobacter aerogenes* but also the potentially dangerous ones like *Bacleroides fragilis* and gas gangrene bacilli, which can cause serious disease in tissues outside the colon. In immunosuppressed individuals, these colonic bacteria are able to enter the blood stream in large numbers and produce fatal septicemia. Even in normal subjects, the spread of *E.coli* to the urinary tract causes severe infection.

Some colonic bacteria can be beneficial as they *synthesize vitamin K, vitamins B's*, and *folic acid*. Some of these are absorbed in significant amounts and supplement dietary intake. Unabsorbed carbohydrates are converted to short-chain fatty acids by colonic bacteria. Some of the short-chain fatty acids produced have a trophic effect on the colonic mucosa. Colonic bacteria can be harmful as some of them consume nutrients like *vitamin C, vitamin $B_{12}$ and choline*, and lead to deficiency symptoms unless these are supplemented in adequate amounts in the diet.

Colonic bacteria also *produce ammonia*, which is absorbed by blood but is quickly detoxified in the liver. Hence, in liver dysfunction, hyperammonemia results, causing neurological symptoms (**hepatic encephalopathy**). Colonic bacterial activity is associated with higher plasma LDL and cholesterol levels. Poorly absorbed antibiotics (luminal antibiotics) like neomycin that modifies the intestinal flora lowers LDL and the plasma cholesterol level.

Colonic bacteria synthesize substances like *indole, skatole, mercaptans and hydrogen sulfide* that contribute to the fecal odor. Even *methane* is formed in some individuals. Colonic bacteria also *form hydrogen from unabsorbed carbohydrates*. The hydrogen is absorbed and expired in breath. In lactose intolerance, breath hydrogen increases following a dictary load of lactose, and is used as a diagnostic test (the **hydrogen breath test**).

# 87

# Gastrointestinal Hormones

### Enumerate the GIT hormones.

The three main GIT hormones are gastrin, cholecystokinin (CCK) and secretin. Other gastrointestinal hormones include (i) gastric inhibitory peptide (GIP) (ii) vasoactive intestinal peptide (VIP) (iii) peptide YY (iv) motilin (v) neurotensin (vi) substance P (vii) gastrin-releasing polypeptide (GRP) (viii) somatostatin, (ix) glucagon.

### What are the principal actions of gastrin?

Gastrin (i) stimulates gastric acid and pepsin secretion; (ii) inhibits gastric emptying, and (iii) stimulates the growth of the mucosa of the stomach and small intestines (**trophic action**).

### What are the principal actions of cholecystokinin?

Cholecystokinin causes (i) contraction of the gall bladder; (ii) secretion of an enzyme-rich pancreatic juice, and (iii) potentiates the action of secretin on pancreatic juice secretion.

### What are the principal actions of secretin?

Secretin (i) stimulates the secretion of watery, alkaline pancreatic juice, rich in bicarbonates; (ii) decreases gastric acid secretion, and (iii) potentiates the action of CCK on pancreatic juice secretion.

### What is enterogastrone?

It has long been known that the presence of fats in the duodenum brought about a reflex inhibition of gastric motility and secretion. This lead to the search for a hormone that could mediate the feedback mechanism. The hormone, when identified, was to be named **enterogastrone**. It turned out however that several hormones could, at least theoretically, bring about the feedback inhibition and that no single hormone could lay claim to the name enterogastrone. The candidates for the name enterogastrone are CCK, GIP, VIP and peptide YY, all of which reduce gastric motility. **Peptide YY** seems to be the strongest candidate.

### Describe some of the feedback control of gastrointestinal exocrine secretion mediated by GI hormones.

(i) Acid in the duodenum inhibits gastrin secretion. This effect is the basis of a negative feedback loop regulating gastrin secretion. Increased secretion of the hormone increases acid secretion, but the acid then feeds back to inhibit further gastrin secretion.

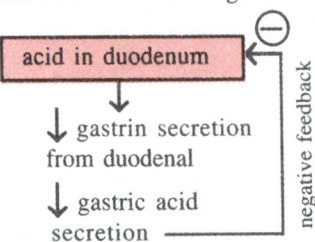

(ii) The release of secretin by acid is another example of feedback control. Secretin causes alkaline pancreatic juice to flood into the duodenum, neutralizing the acid from the stomach and thus stopping further secretion of the hormone.

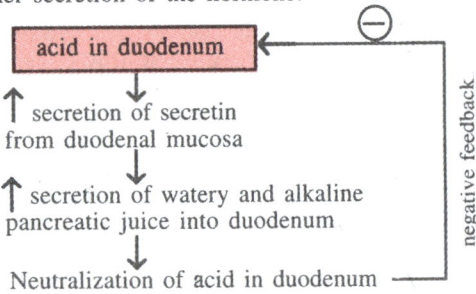

(iii) Similarly, bile and pancreatic juice enters the duodenum in response to CCK. These juices promote the digestion of protein and fat. The products of this digestion stimulate further CCK secretion, thus resulting in a positive feedback that stops only when the products of digestion move on to the lower portions of the gastrointestinal tract.

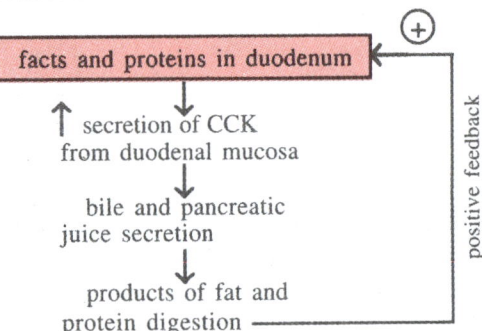

(iv) GIP, glucagon and the three major hormones – gastrin, CCK and secretin – are all known to stimulate insulin secretion. Thus, they mediate a mechanism through which not only glucose, but even proteins and fats in diets can stimulate insulin secretion.

## Summary of Gastrin, Secretin & Cholecystokinin.

| | GASTRIN | CHOLECYSTOKININ | SECRETIN |
|---|---|---|---|
| Discovery | Gregort and Tracy (1960) | Mutt and Jorpes (1960) | Bayliss and Starling (1902) |
| Secreted by | 1. G-cells in antral and duodenal mucosa;<br>2. TG-cells throughout stomach and small intestine;<br>3. Pancreatic islets;<br>4. Hypothalamus and pituitary;<br>5. Medulla and vagus. | 1. Mucosa of upper intestine;<br>2. Nerves in distal ileum and colon;<br>3. Cerebral cortex. | 1. S-cells in ileal mucosal glands |
| Stimulated by | 1. Peptides and aminoacids in stomach and duodenum;<br>2. Distension of stomach;<br>3. Vagus (GRP);<br>4. $Ca^{2+}$ in blood;<br>5. Epinephrine. | 1. Peptides and aminoacids in small intestine;<br>2. Acids;<br>3. Fatty acids (>10 C) in duodenum;<br>4. $Ca^{2+}$ in blood. | 1. Peptides and aminoacids in small intestine;<br>2. Acid in small intestine. |
| Inhibited by | 1. Acid in duodenum;<br>2. Secretin, GIP, VIP, CCK peptide YY;<br>3. Glucagon;<br>4. Calcitonin. | | |
| Effects on exocrine secretions | 1. ↑es gastric acid secretion;<br>2. ↑es pepsin;<br>3. ↑es pancreatic enzyme secretion (+)<br>4. ↑es pancreatic bicarbonate secretion (+) | 1. ↓es gastric acid secretion (effect on pepsin not known);<br>2. ↑es pancreatic enzyme secretion;<br>3. ↑es enterokinase (from duodenum);<br>4. ↑es succus entericus secretion. | 1. ↑es pepsin and ↓es acid secretion in gastric juice;<br>2. ↑es pancreatic $HCO_3^-$ secretion;<br>3. ↑es $HCO_3^-$ secretion from duct cells of gall bladder (choleretic);<br>4. ↑es succus entericus secretion. |
| Effects on endocrine secretions | 1. ↑es insulin secretion;<br>2. ↑es glucagon secretion. | 1. ↑es insulin secretion;<br>2. ↑es glucagon secretion;<br>3. Potentiates secretin action. | 1. ↑es insulin secretion;<br>2. ↓es glucagon secretion;<br>3. Potentiates CCK action. |
| Effect on gastrointestinal motility | 1. LES tone (+)<br>2. Proximal stomach motility (-)<br>3. Distal stomach motility (+)<br>4. Pyloric sphincter tone (+)<br>5. Gastric emptying (-)<br>6. Small intestine motility (-)<br>7. Ileocecal sphincter tone (-) | 1. LES tone (-)<br>2. Proximal stomach motility (-)<br>3. Distal stomach motility (+)<br>4. Gastric emptying (-)<br>5. Gall bladder (+)<br>6. Small intestine, colon motility (+) | 1. LES tone (-)<br>2. Pyloric sphincter tone (+)<br>3. Gastric emptying (-)<br>4. Small intestine motility (-)<br>5. Ileocecal sphincter tone (+) |
| Other effects | Trophic effect on gastrin mucosa | Trophic effect on pancreas | |

## Summary of GIP, VIP & Motilin.

| | GIP | VIP | MOTILIN |
|---|---|---|---|
| Secreted by | 1. K-cells in duodenal and jejunal mucosa | 1. Gland cell and nerves throughout GIT;<br>2. Blood;<br>3. Brain;<br>4. Cholinergic nerves. | 1. Duodenal and jejunal mucosa. |
| Stimulated by | 1. Glucose in duodenum;<br>2. Fat in duodenum;<br>3. Acid in duodenum. | 1. Vagal stimulation; | |
| Inhibited by | | | |
| Effect of exocrines | 1. ↓ acid;<br>2. ↓ pepsin;<br>3. ↑ succus entericus. | 1. ↑ intestinal secretion of electrolytes and water (++++);<br>2. ↑es salivary secretion by potentiating ACh.;<br>3. ↓es gastric acid and pepsin secretion;<br>4. ↓es pancreatic enzymes;<br>5. ↑es pancreatic $HCO_3^-$. | 1. ↑es gastric acid and pepsin secretion;<br>2. ↑es pancreatic enzymes;<br>3. ↑es pancreatic $HCO_3^-$;<br>4. ↑es bile flow. |
| Effect on endocrines | 1. ↑ insulin secretion;<br>2. ↓ gastrin secretion. | | |
| Effect on GIT motility | 1. ↓ gastric motility. | 1. ↓es gastric motility;<br>2. ↓es gall bladder motility;<br>3. ↓es small intestine motility. | 1. ↑es gastric motility;<br>2. ↑es gall bladder motility;<br>3. ↑es small intestine motility |

# 88

# Gastrointestinal Disorders

## What is xerostomia? What are its causes?

Xerostomia is *dryness of mouth due to impaired salivary secretion*, which results in difficulty with speech and swallowing, extensive dental caries, and disturbances of taste. It occurs when the salivary gland secretion are inhibited temporarily with infections or drugs such as anticholinergic agents. Permanent inhibition of secretion occurs following therapeutic irradiation, and in **Sjogren's syndrome**, an autoimmune disorder affecting the salivary glands.

## What is achalasia? How is it treated ?

Achalasia is a condition in which the esophagus becomes massively dilated due to accumulation of food in it. It results from the increased tension of the **lower esophageal sphincter** (LES), and incomplete relaxation of this sphincter on swallowing due to a *deficient myenteric plexus* at the LES. There is defective release of NO and VIP at the LES. The condition is treated by dilation of the sphincter or incision of the esophageal muscle (myotomy). Injection of botulinum toxin into the LES also produces relief that lasts for several months.

## Describe the vomiting reflex.

Vomiting is the rapid ejection of gastric contents effected by *reverse peristalsis in the intestine* aided by simultaneous contraction of abdominal muscles and diaphragm. The sequence of events during vomiting is as follows: (i) The breath is held in mid-inspiration followed by the closure of glottis, both of which guard against the aspiration of vomitus. The hyoid moves upward and forward, resulting in the pulling open of the upper esophageal sphincter. (ii) Next, a reverse peristaltic wave originating in the middle of the intestine propels the chyme into the duodenum. The stomach and its pyloric sphincter relax to receive the duodenal contents. (iii) Finally, an increase in the abdominal pressure forces the chyme into the esophagus and out of the mouth. The coordinated response is controlled by a **vomiting center** in the reticular formation of the medulla. The center lies close to the nucleus of tractus solitarius (NTS) in the medulla. It actually consists of a scattered group of neurons that control the peripheral components of the vomiting act through the 5th, 7th, 9th, 10th and 12th cranial nerves.

## What are the factors causing vomiting?

There are different ways in which the vomiting center is stimulated. (i) **Irritation of upper GIT mucosa** is a common cause of vomiting. Vomiting can also be initiated through the gag reflex, by physical stimulation of the back of the throat. These afferent impulses reach the vomiting center by way of the 9th and 10th cranial nerves.

(ii) **Drugs acting on the CNS** (like apomorphine, ipecac) can trigger vomiting. These initiate responses from a **chemoreceptor trigger zone** located in or near the **area postrema** in the medulla oblongata. It is located outside the blood-brain permeability barrier and therefore accessible to activation by blood-borne substances. Impulses from the chemoreceptor trigger zone are relayed to the vomiting center. The vomiting that occurs in uremia and in radiation sickness is also mediated through the chemoreceptor trigger zone and occur due to the endogenous production of emetic substances. (iii) **Motion sickness** is associated with vomiting. The stimuli causing such vomiting originate in the vestibular apparatus. The afferent impulses relay in the vestibular nuclei and then in the chemoreceptor trigger zone before finally reaching the vomiting center. (iv) **Raised intracranial tension** stimulates the vomiting center directly, causing **projectile vomiting** – *a rapid, forceful vomiting not accompanied by nausea*. (v) **Psychic stimuli**, like sickening sights and noisome odors cause vomiting. Such vomiting does not involve the chemoreceptor trigger zone. The neural pathways involved in such vomiting reaches the vomiting center from the limbic system. (vi) **Severe visceral pain** of any kind is known to cause vomiting, even when the pain does not involve the GIT. Thus, the severe pain associated with testicular torsion can produce vomiting.

## What are the factors predisposing to peptic ulcer?

Peptic ulcers are produce by an imbalance between the gastroduodenal mucosal defense mechanisms and/or the damaging forces that tend to breach the mucosal barrier. Factors that are damaging to the mucosal barrier are: (i) Excessive acid-pepsin secretion. (ii) *H.pylori* infection. (iii) Cigarettes, alcohol. (iv) NSAID, aspirin, and (v) Stress. Psychological stress predispose to ulcers. Also, patients with an anxiety personality disorder are also prone to get these ulcers.

## What is dumping syndrome?

In gastrectomized patients, there is *rapid and unregulated dumping of the chyme into the intestine*. This has two consequences: one immediately after a meal (the early dumping syndrome) and the other about 2 hours after meals (the late dumping syndrome). In both types, the attacks last for about half an hour. **Early dumping syndrome** occurs due to *hypovolemia and hypotension*. This happens as the hypertonic chyme entering the duodenum rapidly extracts large amounts of fluid from circulation into the intestinal lumen. **Late dumping syndrome** occurs due to *hypoglycemia*. It occurs because the rapid entry of the chyme into the intestine also results in rapid absorption of glucose from the intestine. The resultant hyperglycemia induces an abrupt rise in insulin secretion, which overcorrects the hyperglycemia, causing hypoglycemia. The symptoms include weakness, dizziness, and sweating after meals. (Apart from the dumping syndrome, gastrectomy is also associated with intrinsic factor deficiency that must be corrected by parenteral injection of cyanocobalamin).

### What is adynamic ileus? How does it compare with intestinal obstruction?

In both adynamic ileus and intestinal obstruction, the *intestinal contents do not move* and the intestine becomes irregularly distended by alternate pockets of fluids and gases that appear as "**multiple fluid levels**" in radiographs. **Adynamic ileus** is caused by reduced intestinal motility, as occurs following injury or peritonitis. It is *painless*. It is commonly seen after abdominal operations. Intestinal peristalsis normally returns 6-8 hours after an operation. *Passing of flatus* by a post-operative patient signifies the resumption of his colonic activity. **Intestinal obstruction** on the other hand *causes severe cramping pain*. Proximal to the obstruction, the luminal pressure rises, and the blood vessels in the intestinal wall are compressed, causing *ischemia*. There is reflex sweating, hypertension and severe vomiting. If the obstruction is not relieved, the condition is fatal.

### What is steatorrhea?

Steatorrhea is the presence of *excess undigested fats in stool* as a result of which the *stools become bulky, pale, foul smelling, and greasy*. A common cause of steatorrhea is **exocrine pancreatic insufficiency**. Pancreatic lipase is the principal enzyme that digests fats. In its absence, not only are fats not digested but the digestion of other foods also suffers. This is because undigested fat forms a coating over the chyme and prevents the penetration of the chyme by proteolytic and glycolytic enzymes. The absorption of fat-soluble vitamins (A, D, E & K) also suffers.

### What is blind loop syndrome?

It is a condition that is prominent in patients with surgically created blind loops of small intestine. The resulting stasis of the intestinal contents encourages *massive overgrowth of intestinal bacteria*. The overgrowth of bacteria within the intestinal lumen causes steatorrhea due to excessive hydrolysis of conjugated bile salts by the bacteria. There is also vitamin $B_{12}$ deficiency due to binding of vitamin $B_{12}$ by anaerobic bacteria.

### What is sprue?

Sprue is a disorder of mucosal absorption from the intestine. It is of two types: the non-tropical and tropical. **Tropical sprue** occurs in residents of, and visitors to tropical countries. Its cause is unknown. **Non-tropical sprue** is also called *celiac sprue* or *gluten-induced enteropathy*. Gluten is a high-molecular protein found especially in wheat that is incompletely digested in individuals lacking in their intestinal mucosa the specific aminopeptidases for hydrolyzing gluten. The incompletely digested *gluten damages the intestinal mucosa*, either by releasing some toxic substances or by initiating an immunological reaction to the mucosa.

### What are the major causes of malabsorption syndrome?

The term malabsorption syndrome encompasses the following broad categories of disorders, all of which impair absorption. (i) Inadequate digestion, as in exocrine pancreatic insufficiency, or in deficiency of oligosaccharidases present on the intestinal brush border. (ii) Reduced intestinal bile salt concentration as occurs in liver diseases. It affects the absorption of fats by impairing the formation of micelles. Impaired absorption of fats result in steatorrhea. (iii) Blind loop syndrome (iv) Inadequate absorptive surface as when more than half the small intestine is resected or affected by diseases (**short bowel syndrome**); (iv) Mucosal absorptive defects like **gluten-induced enteropathy,** and (v) lymphatic obstruction.

### What is Hirschsprung disease?

Also called **aganglionic megacolon**, this disease occurs in children due to *congenital absence of the ganglion cells* in both myenteric and submucous plexuses of a segment of the *distal colon*. The absence of peristalsis causes feces to pass the aganglionic region with difficulty and children with the disease may defecate as infrequently as once every 3 weeks. The clinical features include abdominal distention and anorexia. The condition is relieved if the *aganglionic portion of the colon is resected* and the portion of the colon above it anastomosed to the rectum.

### Define diarrhea and enumerate its possible causes.

Diarrhea is both a symptom (what the patient complains) and a sign (what the physician observes). *As a symptom* the term diarrhea means an increase in stool frequency or volume or decreased stool consistency. *As a sign*, diarrhea is defined as an increase in stool weight of more than 250 g/24 h.

About 9 liters of fluid, (2 liters from the diet and 7 liters representing secretions from the gut and pancreas) enters the gastrointestinal tract each day. All but 100 to 200 ml of this fluid is absorbed. Diarrhea results when there is an *imbalance between absorption and secretion* in the intestine. Diarrhea can occur due to decreased digestion, decreased absorption, increased secretion or increased intestinal motility. (i) **Impaired digestion** (and therefore absorption) of dietary carbohydrates results in diarrhea (**osmotic diarrhea**) due to increased luminal osmolality. Such diarrhea stops on fasting. **Lactose intolerance** is an example of a diarrheal disorder caused by increased luminal osmolality. (ii) Diarrhea due to decreased absorption is very unusual and mostly represents congenital absence of a specific transport process. (iii) **Secretory diarrhea** is caused by bacterial enterotoxins (as in cholera), neurohumoral agents (as in carcinoid syndrome and hyperthyroidism) and detergents (diarrhea caused by laxatives). (iv) Increased intestinal motility is the most unlikely cause of diarrhea.

### What causes gallstones? What are its different types?

Gallstone afflicts up to 20% of the population, and are mainly prevalent in *f*at, *f*ertile (multiparous), *f*latulent *f*emales in their *f*orties. Gallstones are mostly made of cholesterol (**cholesterol gall stones**) while others are made of bilirubin calcium salts (called **pigment gallstones**). The most prominent symptom of gallstone is an excruciating *biliary pain*. Other effects of gallstones include obstructive jaundice, steatorrhea, and bleeding tendencies due to defective absorption of vitamin K.

Gallstone are mostly of two types: cholesterol gallstones or pigment gallstones. **Cholesterol gallstones** are formed when bile is supersaturated with cholesterol. Cholesterol is normally rendered soluble in bile by aggregation with water-soluble bile salts and water-insoluble lecithins, both of which act as detergents. When cholesterol concentrations exceed the solubilizing capacity of bile (*supersaturation*), it starts forming solid **cholesterol monohydrate crystals** (*nucleation*). Supersaturation is promoted by gall bladder stasis. Nucleation is promoted by the presence of microprecipitates of inorganic or organic calcium salts, which may serve as nucleation sites for cholesterol stones. **Pigment gallstones** are formed by the precipitation of calcium salts of *unconjugated bilirubin*. In hemolytic anemias, there is a rise in deconjugated bilirubin in bile, predisposing to pigment stones. Moreover, infection of the biliary tract, as with *Escherichia coli*, roundworm or liver fluke causes deconjugation of conjugated bilirubin.

## What is constipation? What are its causes?

Idiopathic constipation is as defined by infrequent defecation (<2 bowel movements weekly). The mechanisms suggested for it include decreased dietary fiber intake, decreased water intake, decreased physical activity, increased serum progesterone levels in women, failure to respond to the urge to defecate, or damage to colonic nerves induced by chronic ingestion of stimulant laxatives. None of these theories are supported by available scientific information. Contrary to popular belief, *fiber supplementation does not normalize stool output and frequency* in patients with idiopathic constipation.

# Liver

## What are the functions of the liver?

The function of the liver are: (1) **storage**, of glycogen, fat and vitamins; (2) **synthesis**, of plasma proteins (including coagulation proteins) and heparin; (3) **excretion**, of bile; (4) **detoxification**, of exogenous drugs and endogenous waste; (5) **hemopoiesis** and destruction of erythrocytes (6) **metabolism**, of protein, carbohydrate and fat.

## What are the effects of extirpation of the liver?

Complete extirpation of the liver results in (1) hypoglycemia, (2) fall in blood urea and rise in aminoacid levels in blood, (3) hyperbilirubinemia and jaundice and (4) bleeding tendencies due to low plasma levels of coagulation factors, specially prothrombin and fibrinogen.

## Enumerate the various tests for hepatic function.

The hepatic function tests are broadly of four categories: (A) *Tests for hepatic conjugation and excretion.* It includes estimation of (i) serum bilirubin – total, conjugated and unconjugated; (ii) urine bilirubin; (iii) urine urobilinogen; (B) *Test for hepatic synthesis* which includes estimation of (i) serum albumin and globulin, (ii) coagulation factors, especially prothrombin; (iii) serum cholesterol and triglycerides; (C) *Tests for hepatic metabolic reactions* which includes (i) Galactose tolerance test (normally, much of ingested galactose gets converted into glucose, so that little of it appears unchanged in blood in the galactose form); serum ammonia (normally, all the ammonia is effectively cleared from the blood by the liver which consumes it in the urea biosynthesis); and (D) *Tests for integrity of hepatic cells,* which includes the estimation of (i) serum aspartate aminotransferase (AST); serum alanine aminotransferase (ALT) and serum alkaline phosphatase.

## How much is the normal serum bilirubin? How is it estimated? •

The normal **total serum bilirubin** is 0.3 - 1.0mg%. Of this, **conjugated bilirubin** constitutes 0.1 - 0.3mg% and **unconjugated** 0.2 - 0.7mg%. Jaundice is usually apparent *when the serum bilirubin exceeds 2.0 mg%* (hyperbilirubinemia). If the more than 50 % of the bilirubin is conjugated, it is called **predominantly conjugated hyperbilirubinemia**. If less than 15 % is conjugated, it is called **predominantly unconjugated hyperbilirubinemia**.

Serum bilirubin is estimated by using the **Van den Berg's method**. A mixture of sulphanic acid, hydrochloric acid and sodium nitrite (diazo reagent) is added to the serum containing excess bilirubin glucuronide, a reddish violet color results, the maximum color being reached within 30 seconds. This is the "direct reaction". If the bilirubin in the serum is unconjugated, no color develops until alcohol is added whereupon the reddish color appears. This is the "indirect reaction". (The alcohol dissolves the water-insoluble bilirubin allowing the reaction to occur.)

## What is the normal urine urobilinogen? How is it estimated?

The normal urine urobilinogen is 1.0 - 3.5mg in 24 hours. An excess of urobilinogen in the urine can be detected by **Ehrlich's aldehyde test** or by the **Urobilistix** modification of this reaction. Since urobilinogen is readily oxidized to urobilin on exposure to air at room temperature, only fresh urine samples should be used.

## How much is the normal serum cholesterol and triglycerides?

The normal level of total serum cholesterol is 130 - 230 mg%. Cholesterol esters comprise 50 - 70% of the total cholesterol. Serum triglycerides level is 40 - 145 mg%. In hepatic *parenchymal diseases*, the total serum cholesterol as well as the percentage of esters decrease. In *cholestasis*, the total serum cholesterol and the triglyceride levels decrease while there is a decrease in the percentage of esters.

## What are the normal levels of serum ALT, AST and alkaline phosphatase? What is their clinical significance?

**Serum aspartate aminotransferase (AST)** was earlier called serum glutamic oxaloacetic transaminase (SGOT). Its normal level is 10 – 40 Karmen Units. It is found in all body tissues, specially the heart, liver and skeletal muscle. It catalyzes the reaction:

Aspartic acid + $\alpha$-ketoglutaric acid = oxaloacetic acid + glutamic acid

**Serum alanine aminotransferase (ALT)** was earlier called serum glutamic pyruvic transaminase (SGPT). Its normal level is 10 - 40 Karmen units. It is found mainly in the liver and to a lesser extent, in the kidney and skeletal muscle. It catalyzes the reaction:

Alanine + $\alpha$-ketoglutaric acid = pyruvic acid + glutamic acid

Whenever **liver** cells are damaged or killed, these enzymes are liberated into the blood. Both are very sensitive but *ALT is more specific for hepatocellular damage.*

**Serum alkaline phosphatase** is derived mainly from the bone and the liver and to a lesser extent from the intestine and the placenta. In the liver, it is situated principally in the canalicular and the sinusoidal membrane. Its normal level is 4 - 13 King-Armstrong units. It *increases greatly in cholestasis*. It may also be increased in adolescents, hyperparathyroidism, rickets and in the third trimester of pregnancy.

### Define Respiratory Quotient.

The respiratory quotient (RQ) is the ratio of the volume of $CO_2$ evolved from the lungs over the volume of $O_2$ absorbed from the lungs in one minute. RQ gives an approximate information about metabolic processes in the body.

### How is RQ affected by the metabolism of different types of foodstuff?

*With pure carbohydrate,* the RQ is 1. This is easily deduced from the chemical equation for carbohydrate oxidation, which shows that the volume of $CO_2$ evolved is equal to the volume of $O_2$ used.

$$C_6H_{12}O_6 + 6O_2 = 6CO_2 + 6H_2O$$

*With fatty acids,* the RQ is about 0.7. The equation of fatty acid oxidation shows that 18 moles of $CO_2$ are released for every 26 moles of $O_2$ consumed.

$$C_{17}H_{35}COOH + 26O_2 = 18CO_2 + 18H_2O.$$
$$\therefore RQ = 18/26 = 0.693.$$

*With proteins,* the RQ is about 0.8.

If the RQ is determined over a period of time, the value obtained will indicate the mixture of foodstuffs undergoing oxidation. For example, if the predominant foodstuff being oxidized is carbohydrate, the RQ will approximate to 1. If more fat is oxidized, the RQ will be about 0.7. Thus, *the diabetic patient shows a low RQ* due to the increased dissimilation of fats and the decreased dissimilation of carbohydrate.

### How is RQ affected by pulmonary ventilation?

The RQ is affected by pulmonary ventilation independently of the nature of foodstuffs oxidized. Voluntary hyperpnoea raises RQ as it washes out excessive quantities of $CO_2$ without increase in $O_2$ consumption. Metabolic acidosis raises the RQ as it stimulates hyperpnoea with increase in $CO_2$ output but again without corresponding rise in $O_2$ consumption. The same is true for the hyperpnoea associated with raised body temperature. Conversely, the RQ falls in metabolic alkalosis.

### How is RQ affected by exercise?

The RQ of *moderate exercise* is about the same as pre-exercise RQ, i.e., ~ 0.85. It suggests that the body uses various foodstuffs in exercise in roughly the same proportions as at rest. During *severe exercise*, lactic acid released by muscles into bloodstream. In blood, the lactate gets buffered by plasma $HCO_3^-$ and liberates large volumes of $CO_2$ that are eliminated from the lungs. The $CO_2$ liberated by lactate buffering represents an additional amount over the $CO_2$ that is released through respiration. With the $CO_2$ liberated greatly exceeding the $O_2$ consumed, the *RQ may then exceed 2.0.* During recovery from exercise, the plasma bicarbonate

(that had got depleted due to lactate buffering) is regenerated by the hydration of $CO_2$. Due to excess consumption (and consequent reduction in exhalation) of $CO_2$, the RQ falls to a very low value.

### Define BMR.

**Basal metabolic rate (BMR)** is the energy output of an individual under standardized resting conditions, i.e. at complete bodily and psychical rest, 12-18 hours after a meal (post-absorptive period) and in an equable environmental temperature. Under such conditions a proportion of the energy liberated is used to maintain the activities of vital organs like the heart, brain, or glands, but the greater part is converted into heat so as to maintain body temperature and prevent it from falling below the normal level.

Clinically, BMR is expressed as a percentage above or below the accepted normal standard for the individual taking into account his age, height, weight, etc. Thus a BMR of +30 means one that is 30% above the normal average for that person.

### How is BMR estimated?

The amount of energy released by oxygen depends on the type of foodstuff metabolized. 1 liter of oxygen releases ~5 kcal of energy when the fuel is pure carbohydrate (RQ = 1), and ~4.8 kcal when the fuel is pure fat (RQ = 0.7). It has been estimated, considering the foodstuff mixture that is metabolized *at the usual RQ of 0.8,* that *1 L of $O_2$ releases ~ 4.875 kcal of energy.*

The amount of heat released by the body can therefore be calculated once the $O_2$ consumed by the body is measured. In such calculations, the RQ is often assumed to be 0.8. For more precise estimates, the RQ is measured, and the calorific value of 1 liter of oxygen is obtained from a table. Thus, if the RQ = 0.8 (calorific value per 1 liter $O_2$ = 4.875), and the $O_2$ consumption per minute is 0.25 liter, then the heat production per minute is 0.25 × 4.875 = 1.22 kcal.

Clinically the BMR is calculated from the $O_2$ consumption alone. It is measured under conditions of complete rest and fasting. $O_2$ consumption is determined most readily by means of the **Benedict-Roth apparatus** (Fig. 90.1), which consists essentially of tank filled with oxygen and suspended in water. It is connected by means of tubing through a soda-lime column to the patient's mouth (the nose is clipped). The patient rebreathes from the tank. The $CO_2$ formed is removed by means of the soda lime, and the decrease in the volume of oxygen in the tank is a direct measure of the oxygen consumption. The $CO_2$ output (and therefore, the RQ) cannot be measured by this method.

### What are the factors affecting BMR?

**Surface area**. The basal metabolism is most closely related to the

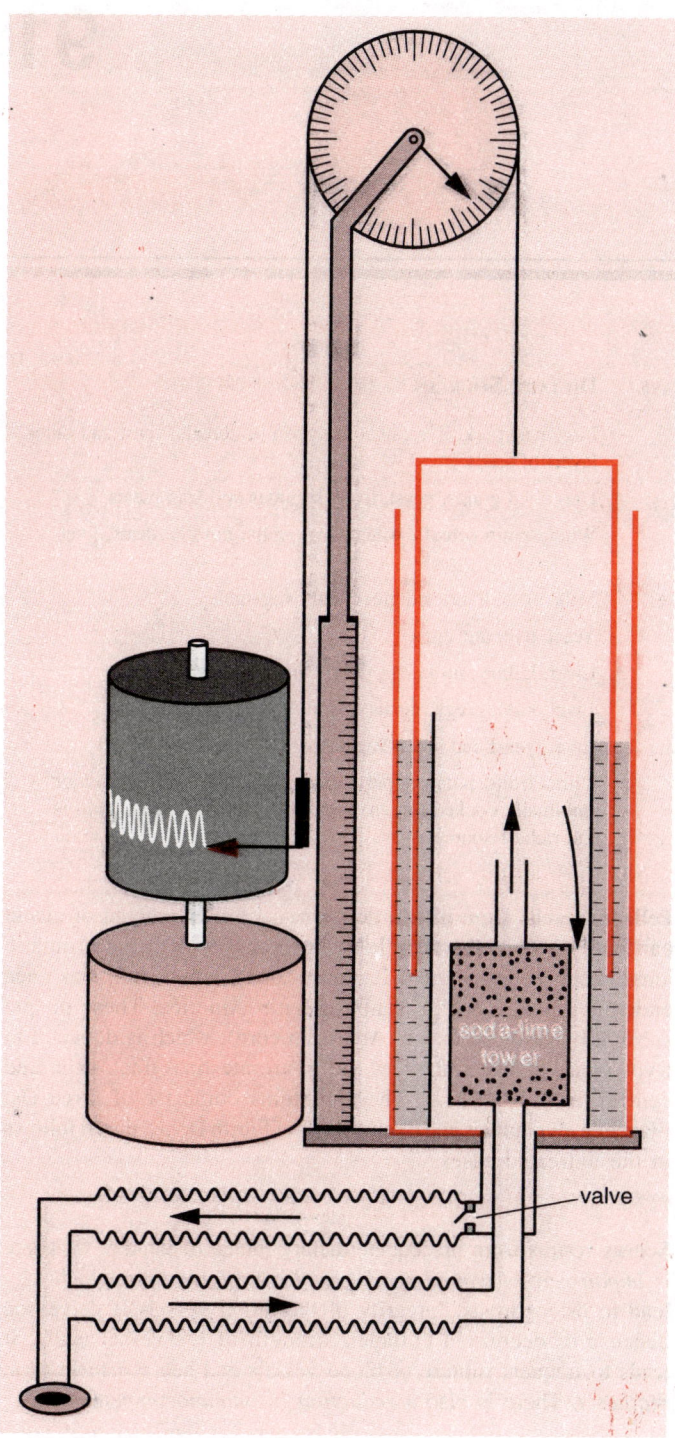

surface area and is less directly related to height or weight. In the male 40 kcal (165 kJ), and in the female about 37 kcal (155 kJ), are given off every hour per square meter of body surface. The surface area of an average adult is about 1.8 m$^2$ **Age.** The basal metabolism is considerably greater per sq meter of surface in children than in adults. There is a further gradual fall in the metabolism during adult life as age advances. **Starvation** or prolonged undernutrition decreases the metabolic rate. This decreases in the metabolic rate explains why, when an individual tries to shed weight, the weight loss is initially rapid but slows down thereafter. **Body temperature.** For every rise of 0.5 °C in the internal temperature of the body, the basal metabolism increases by 7%. This is because the chemical reactions of the body, like any other chemical reactions, are speeded up by a rise of temperature.. **Ambient temperature.** Exposure to cold increases the metabolism. Prolonged exposure to heat decreases the metabolic rate. **Hormones.** *Thyroid hormones* act as a general catalyst, speeding up the metabolic activities of the tissues. The BMR increases in thyrotoxicosis, and decrease in myxedema. *Adrenalin* increases the metabolic rate. The *anterior pituitary* influences the metabolic rate indirectly through its thyrotrophic hormone. **Emotions.** Anxiety and tension elevates BMR because they cause epinephrine secretion and tensing of the muscles. On the other hand, apathetic, depressed patients may have low BMRs. **Specific dynamic action.** Metabolism is stimulated by the consumption of food. This effect is greatest with protein (a 10 – 35 % increase) and is termed its *specific dynamic action*. The increase in metabolism is due to the stimulation of cellular metabolism of the fatty acid residues that are left after the NH$_2$ groups have been removed from the aminoacids. **Exercise.** Muscular work increases the metabolism. During very violent exercise, the BMR may increase over 16 times.

**Fig. 90.1**

# *Vitamins*

**Summarize the dietary sources and daily requirements of water-soluble vitamins and their deficiency diseases.**

| Water Soluble Vitamin | Daily Requirement | Deficiency Disease | Dietary Sources |
|---|---|---|---|
| Thiamine, vitamin $B_1$ | 1.0- 1.5mg | Beriberi | Legumes, pork, liver, nuts the germ of cereals, yeast and outer layers of seeds. |
| Niacin, vitamin $B_3$ | 12-20 mg | Pellagra | Unrefined grains, yeast, liver, legumes and lean meats. |
| Pyridoxine, vitamin $B_6$ | 2 mg | Rare | Whole-grain cereals, wheat, corn, nuts, muscle meats, liver and fish. |
| Riboflavin. vitamin $B_2$ | 1.1-1.5 mg | Ariboflavinosis (rare) | Milk, eggs, liver, and green leafy vegetables. |
| Pantothenic acid. Vitamin $B_5$ | 5-10 mg | Rare | Yeast, liver and eggs. |
| Biotin, vitamin H | 50ug/1000kcal | Widespread injury | Liver, kidney, milk, egg yolk, corn, and soya milk. |
| Cobalamin, Vitamin $B_{12}$ | 3 µg | Pernicious anemia | Liver, kidney, egg. meats and milk. |
| Folic acid: pteroylglutamic acid | 400 µg | Megaloblastic anemia | Liver, yeast and green vegetable. |
| Ascorbic add. Vitamin C | 45 mg | Scurvy | Citrus fruits, potatoes particularly skin, strawberries, raw or minimally cooked (green) vegetables and tomatoes; *amla* is the richest source. |

## Outline the clinical features of beriberi.

Beriberi results from severe thiamine deficiency and are of three types. (1) In **dry beriberi**, neuromuscular symptoms predominate. In long standing cases, there is degeneration and demyelination of sensory and motor nerves and severe wasting of muscles. (2) In **wet beriberi**, cardiovascular manifestations and edema are notable features. These signs and symptoms are largely accounted by inadequate metabolism and therefore accumulation of pyruvic acid and its reduced form, lactic acid. (3) In **infantile beriberi** develops in breast-fed infants mostly between the second and the fifth months in the areas where beriberi is endemic. Thiamine deficiency in alcoholics does not result in beriberi but rather in **Wernicke-Korsakoff syndrome**. The acute stage of this disease, known as **Wernicke's encephalopathy**, is characterized by mental derangements, delirium and ataxia. In the chronic stage, known as **Korsakoff psychosis**, the patient has anterograde amnesia.

## Outline the clinical features of pellagra.

Pellagra results from **niacin** deficiency. Limited amount of niacin can be synthesized in the body from tryptophan, an aromatic amino acid. Pellagra (from Italian meaning rough skin) was once endemic among poor peasants of Latin America. These people subsisted chiefly on maize (American corn), which is deficient in tryptophan. Pellagra involves the gastrointestinal tract, skin, and central nervous system. The symptoms comprise of three Ds: **diarrhea**, **dermatitis** and **dementia**. The fourth D, i.e., **death** follows in the untreated cases.

## Outline the clinical features of scurvy.

Scurvy results from inadequate dietary intake of vitamin C. There is *impairment of wound healing and bone formation*, which may lead to osteoporosis. Integrity of the blood vessels is decreased because of decreased collagen strength of the vessel walls. It leads to frequent rupture of blood vessels and hence *hemorrhagic diathesis*. There is also a *reduction in immunocompetence*.

**Summarize the dietary sources and daily requirements of fat-soluble vitamins and their deficiency diseases.**

| Water Soluble Vitamin | Daily Requirement | Deficiency Disease | Dietary Sources |
|---|---|---|---|
| Vitamin A | 4.5 g carotene or 1.1 mg retinol equivalents | Night blindness; skin lesions. | Liver, kidney, butter fat, oils, egg yolk, green leafy vegetables, fruits. |
| Vitamin D | 400 IU (10 µg Vitamin $D_3$) | Rickets in children, osteomalacia in adults. | Saltwater, liver, egg yolk and butter. |
| Vitamin E (tocopherol) | 10 – 30 mg | Liver atrophy; red blood cell hemolysis; neurologic disorders | Vegetable seed oils, liver and eggs. |
| Vitamin K | 1 µg | Coagulation disorder | Spinach, cabbage, egg yolk and liver. |

### Define a reference man and woman.

Nutritional requirements vary depending on the age, sex, height and work of the individual. These variables have been defined in the **reference man** and **reference woman** so that his/her nutritional requirement can be stated. The criteria for reference man and woman in India are given below.

### Criteria for reference man and woman in India

| Criteria | Reference man | Reference woman |
|---|---|---|
| Health status | Normal health | Normal health |
| Weight (kg) | 60 | 50 |
| Age (yrs) | 20-39 | 20-39 |
| Occupational work | Sedentary | Sedentary |
| Surface area (m$^2$) | 1.62 | 1.40 |
| BMR (kcal/hr/m$^2$) | 35.5 | 31.6 |

### How much is the caloric requirements for sedentary, moderate and heavy work?

| | Caloric requirement in a reference man | Caloric requirement in a reference woman |
|---|---|---|
| Sedentary work | 2425 | 1875 |
| Moderate work | 2875 | 2225 |
| Heavy work | 3800 | 2925 |

### Define a balanced diet.

A balanced diet is one that consists of a variety of foods and provides all the macronutrients and micronutrients, recommended for individual's age/sex/occupation category. Special allowances should be made in the formulation of balanced diet for stressful physiological conditions (pregnancy, lactation etc.) or diseases.

### What are the special nutritional requirements in pregnancy?

Fetal life is a phase of fast growth, tissue differentiation and rapid cellular turnover. All this requires energy which is met by mother's nutritional resources. All through the period of pregnancy, there is a marked increase in the requirements of *energy, protein, calcium, iron* and *folate. Iodine* requirement also increases. However, the pregnancy does not create an additional demand for vitamins A and C, which are additionally required during lactation.

### What are the special nutritional requirements in lactation?

As in pregnancy, in lactation too, there is raised demand of energy, protein, calcium and folate. In lactation, however, *iron requirement reverts to normal* and *vitamins A and C are required additionally.*

### What are the special nutritional requirements in infancy?

Infants have highest per Kg energy and protein requirements than any other age group. Breastfeeding is essential for normal development during infancy as well in subsequent years. A yellowish secretion from the breast during initial 3 days after the childbirth is called **colostrums**. It must be given to the neonate. It is very rich in proteins and vitamin A, provides immune protection and helps in developing certain digestive enzymes.

For *first 4 months*, mother's milk is sufficient to furnish all the nutritional requirements of the child. Its caloric yield and fat, protein, calcium and other mineral contents are lower than the bovine milk but it is richer in vitamin C. Though human milk lacks iron, routine supplementation is not needed for breastfed infants. Even water is not needed during this phase. This is the basis behind **exclusive breast feeding**, which recommends that for initial 4 months only mother's milk be given to the child. Anything else, including prelacteal feeds and water, is not only unnecessary but hazardous also.

**Weaning** is a process of gradual shift from mother's milk towards adult diet. After the 4$^{th}$ month, mother's milk needs to be supplemented by other liquid and semi-solid food items. Weaning, therefore, should start in 5$^{th}$ month while continuing the breastfeeding as long as possible. The process should be slow and gradual, from liquids to semi-solids to solids, avoiding sudden changes. Home available convenient weaning foods should be preferred over market preparations. Boiled bovine milk and soft cooked *khichri* (rice, pulse, vegetables mix) are good weaning foods for Indian households. The 'hunger demand' of the infant should be followed rather than adhering to a strict timetable.

### Outline the clinical features of protein-energy malnutrition (PEM).

Insufficient input of protein and/or energy causes loss of both body mass and adipose tissue. Primarily two syndromes of PEM have been distinguished: marasmus and kwashiorkor. **Marasmus** results from catabolism and *depletion of somatic protein compartment* represented by the skeletal muscles. There is reduction in the input of protein as well as energy. Visceral protein compartment is depleted only marginally. It is for this reason that *serum albumin levels remain normal* or only slightly decreased. Subcutaneous fat is also mobilized resulting in *emaciated extremities* and *monkey-like facies*. The skin appears dry and inelastic. In comparison *head appears too large* for the body. The main brunt of disease process falls on weight gain and the *weight for age is below the cut-off point.* In **kwashiorkor**, *protein deprivation is relatively greater* than reduction in total calories. Unlike marasmus, marked protein deprivation is associated with *severe loss of visceral protein compartment* represented by protein stores in the visceral organs, mainly liver. This leads to *hypoalbuminemia* and consequently generalized or dependent *edema*. Compromised weight for age may be masked by fluid retention and *relative sparing of subcutaneous fat and muscle mass*. Fatty liver is often present. Hairs are sparse, brittle and depigmented.

The commonest form of PEM is borderline undernutrition or mild PEM where the classical picture of marasmus/kwashiorkor is not seen. In India, marasmus is the most frequent presentation of severe PEM. Cases of pure kwashiorkor are seldom seen in India. What is seen is mostly **marasmic kwashiorkor**.

## Compare and contrast kwashiorkor and marasmus.

**SIMILARITIES**

Both occur due to insufficient intake of protein and/or energy.

Both show apathy, inactivity and irritability.

Both show growth retardation

**DIFFERENCES**

| Kwashiorkor | Marasmus |
|---|---|
| Usually seen in recently weaned infants | Usually seen in children who have been weaned early or have never been breast-fed. |
| Visceral protein compartment is depleted | Somatic protein compartment is depleted |
| Hypoalbuminemia present | Serum albumin normal or slightly decreased. |
| Edema is characteristically present. | Edema not present. |
| Body weight remains normal | Severe cachexia is present. |
| Face puffy and moon-shaped | Face shriveled and monkey-like |
| Impaired appetite | Voracious appetite |

# 93

# The Pituitary Gland & Growth Hormone

### Explain briefly the mechanism of the hypothalamic-hypophysial-target gland axis.

The anterior lobe of the pituitary releases a set of hormones called the **tropic hormones**, which increase the secretory activity of the target glands. For example, ACTH (adrenocorticotropic hormone) increases the secretory activity of the adrenal cortex while TSH (thyroid stimulating hormone) increases the secretory activity of the thyroid gland. The secretion of tropic hormones by the anterior lobe is controlled by **hypothalamic hormones** (releasing or inhibiting hormones), which reach the pituitary (hypophysis) through the **hypothalamic-hypophysial portal system**.

Unbound circulating hormones produced by target endocrine organs (thyroid gland, adrenal cortex, gonads) inhibit the hypothalamic-pituitary system, causing a decrease in the secretion of pituitary tropic hormones, which, in turn, control the secretion by the endocrine target glands. This is called **negative feedback control** and it occurs at three levels(Fig. 93.1). (i) **Long-loop feedback.** Peripheral gland hormones and substrates arising from tissue metabolism can exert long-loop feedback control on both the hypothalamus and the anterior lobe of the pituitary gland. Long-loop feedback, which usually is negative but occasionally can be positive, is particularly important in the control of thyroid, adrenocortical, and gonadal secretions. (ii) **Short-loop feedback.** Negative feedback also can be exerted by the anterior pituitary tropic hormones on the synthesis or release of the hypothalamic releasing or inhibiting hormones. (iii) **Ultrashort-loop feedback.** Hypothalamic hormones may inhibit their own synthesis and secretion via a control system referred to as ultra-short-loop feedback.

### What is the hypothalamo-hypophysial portal system?

The hypothalamo-hypophysial portal system is formed by the **superior hypophysial artery**, which divides into *two sets of capillary plexuses*, one in the **medial eminence of the hypothalamus** and the other in the **anterior lobe of the pituitary**. The two capillary plexuses are connected by the **long portal vessels**, and constitute a portal system that is important for transport of hypothalamic releasing hormones to the pituitary (Fig. 93.2).

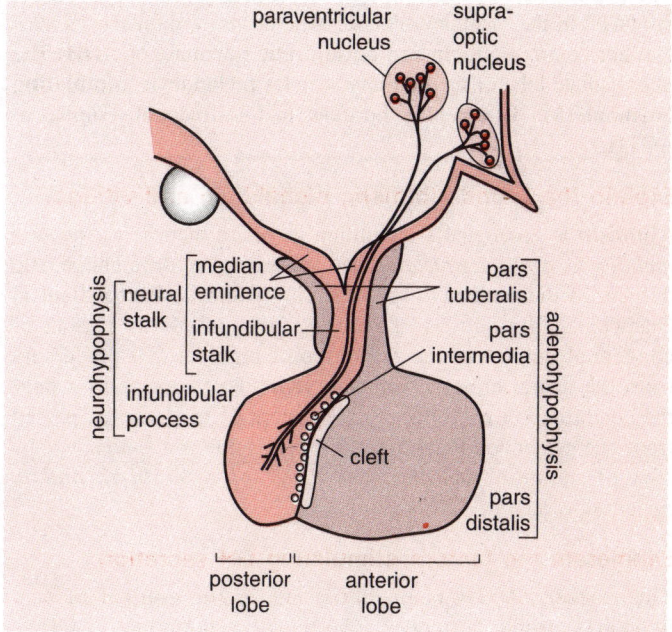

**Fig. 93.2**

### Enumerate the pituitary hormones and name the cells that secrete them.

Two major types of cells are found in equal numbers in the anterior lobe: the chromophobes and the chromophils. The *chromophobes* do not have any physiological significance. The *chromophils* (granular secretory cells) exist in two forms. acidophils (80%) and basophiles (20%). *Acidophils* (eosinophils) are the source of **prolactin** and **growth hormone** (GH). *Basophils* are the source of **thyroid-stimulating hormone (TSH)**, **adrenocorticotropic hormone (ACTH)**, **luteinizing hormone (LH)**, **follicle-stimulating hormone (FSH)**, and β-**lipotropic hormone (β-LPH).**

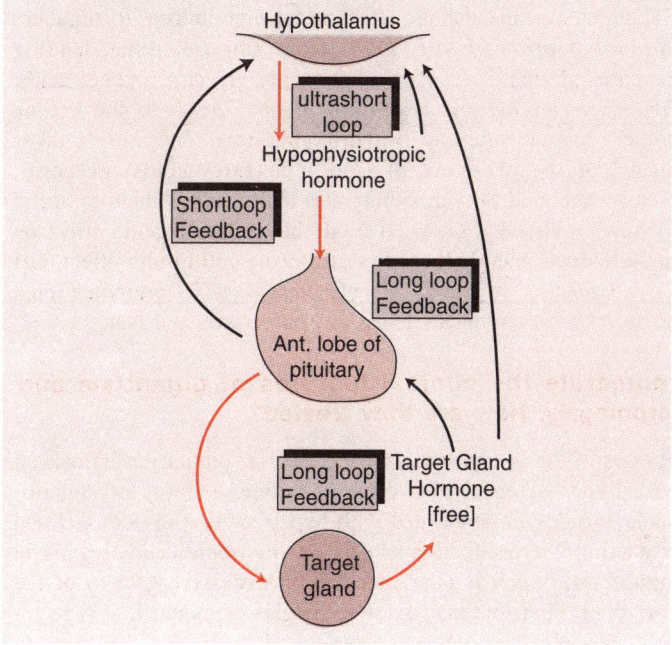

**Fig. 93.1**

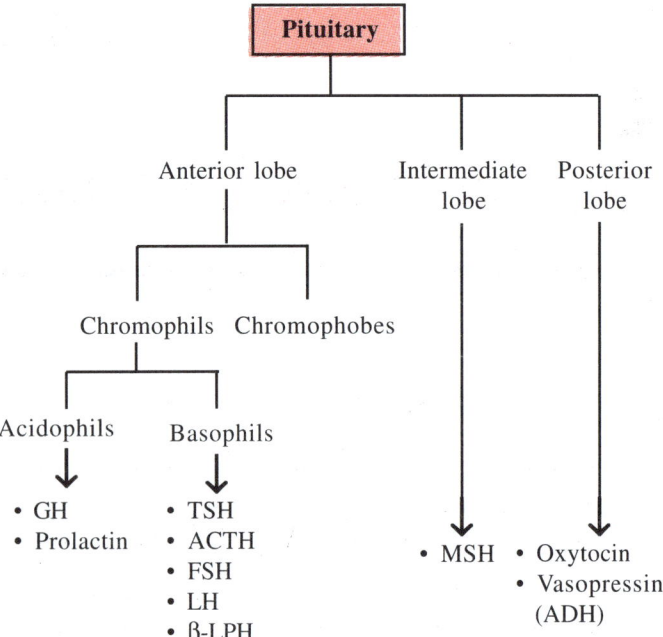

The posterior lobe is made of *neurosecretory neurons* originating in **supraoptic** and **paraventricular nuclei** of the hypothalamus. The posterior lobe is the storage and secretory site for hormones produced in the median eminence. The posterior pituitary secretes two hormones: **oxytocin** and **antidiuretic hormone** or **ADH**. The intermediate lobe of the pituitary secretes **melanocyte stimulating hormone (MSH),** a peptide hormone that is structurally similar to ACTH.

## Explain the terms albinism, piebaldism and vitiligo.

**Albinism** is a congenital condition in which there is a *complete inability to synthesize melanin* due to a variety of different genetic defects in the pathways for melanin synthesis. **Piebaldism** is characterized by *patches of skin that lack melanin* as a result of congenital defects in the migration of pigment cell precursors from the neural crest during embryonic development. Not only the condition but even the precise pattern of the losses is passed from one generation to the next. **Vitiligo** is due to a *similar patchy loss* of melanin, but the loss *develops after birth and is progressive.*

## Enumerate the factors stimulating GH secretion.

The release of GH is primarily under the control of two hypophysiotropic hormones. The releasing hormone for GH is **somatotropin releasing hormone (SRH)**. Other factors stimulating GH release include (i) *bromocriptine* (a dopamine agonist), enkephalins, endorphins (β-endorphin), and opiates. (ii) *hypo-glycemia*, increased plasma concentrations of *amino acids* (arginine, leucine, lysine, tryptophan, and 5-hydroxy-tryptophan), and *decreased free fatty acid* concentrations. (iii) *estrogens.* (iv) *Stress stimulates GH secretion.* Stressful situations include moderate-to-vigorous exercise, emotional stress and stress resulting from fever, surgery, anesthesia, trauma, pyrogen administration, and repeated venipuncture. Fasting or starvation leads to elevated GH secretion after 2 or 3 days. A regular nocturnal peak in GH secretion occurs during deep sleep.

## Enumerate the factors inhibiting GH secretion.

GH inhibits its own secretion via a short-feedback loop mechanism that operates between the anterior lobe and the median eminence. GH secretion is also inhibited by (i) **somatostatin.** (ii) It is also inhibited by **somatomedin,** which inhibits GnRH secretion through negative feedback. Somatomedin also stimulates somatostatin secretion, which in turn, inhibits GH secretion. (iii) Obesity decreases GH secretion. (iv) Glucocorticoids decrease GH secretion. (v) A decline in GH secretion is observed in late pregnancy.

## What is somatostatin?

Somatostatin is also called **somatotropin-inhibiting hormone (SIH)** It is secreted by neurosecretory neurons of the *median eminence*. It also is found in other parts of the brain, in the *gastrointestinal tract*, and in the *delta cells of the pancreatic islets*. It inhibits the synthesis and release of GH and TSH. It also inhibits the secretion of insulin, glucagon, and gastrin and reduces the intestinal absorption of glucose. These effects produce a state of hypoglycemia.

## Enumerate the physiological effects of GH.

(i) The effects of GH on **bone, cartilage and connective tissue** are mediated by **somatomedins** that are also called **insulin-like growth factors (IGFs)**. These are synthesized mainly in the liver. Somatomedin has *insulin-like effects* on tissues, including lipogenesis in adipose tissue and increased glucose and amino acid transport by muscle. Through somatomedin, GH *stimulates proliferation of chondrocytes* and the *appearance of osteoblasts*. The increase in the thickness of the epiphysial (cartilaginous) end plate accounts for the *increase in linear skeletal growth.*

(ii) GH has predominantly anabolic effects on **protein metabolism**. In skeletal and cardiac muscle, it stimulates protein synthesis. GH reduces circulating levels of amino acids and urea, i.e., it promotes nitrogen retention and results in positive nitrogen balance. (iii) GH has an overall catabolic effect on **fat metabolism**. It stimulates the *mobilization of fatty acids* from adipose tissue, leading increased plasma levels of free fatty acids, glycerol, and ketoacids. GH *increases hepatic oxidation of fatty acids* to the ketone bodies, acetoacetate and β-hydroxybutyrate. The muscle takes up all of the products of lipolysis (fatty acids, glycerol, acetoacetate, and β-hydroxybutyrate) and converts them to acetyl coenzyme A (acetyl-CoA). (iv) GH has a diabetogenic effect on **carbohydrate metabolism**. Because of its anti-insulin effect, GH has a tendency to cause *hyperglycemia.* (v) GH promotes renal reabsorption of **minerals** like $Ca^{2+}$, phosphate, and $Na^+$.

## Enumerate the clinical features of gigantism and acromegaly. How are they treated?

Tumors of the *somatotropes* of the anterior pituitary is associated with hypersecretion of growth hormone. Tumors of somato-mammotropes are associated with hypersecretion of both GH and prolactin. Overproduction of GH *during adolescence* results in **gigantism,** which is characterized by excessive growth of the long bones. Patients may grow to heights of as much as 8 feet.

Acromegaly occurs due to excessive GH secretion *during*

*adulthood*, after the epiphysial (growth) plates of long bones have fused, causing growth in those areas where cartilage persists. The principal features in acromegaly are those related to the *local effects of the tumor* i.e., enlargement of the sella turcica. headache, visual disturbances. Others are those due to growth hormone secretion, i.e., *enlargement of the hands and feet* (*acral* parts: hence the term acromegaly) and a *protrusion of the lower jaw* (**prognathism**) and prominent brows. Body hair is increased in amount. There is soft tissue hypertrophy e.g., cardiomegaly, hepatosplenomegaly, and renomegaly. About a quarter of the patients have *abnormal glucose tolerance* and a few develop lactation in the absence of pregnancy.

Acromegaly is treated by selective *surgical extirpation* of the pituitary adenoma without damage to other pituitary functions. *Bromocriptine*, a stimulator of GH secretion in normal individuals, is effective in suppressing GH levels in most acromegalic patients. *Somatostatin* is also effective in the treatment of long-term acromegaly.

### Compare and contrast acromegaly and gigantism

| SIMILARITIES |
| --- |
| Both occur due to hypersecretion of GH. |
| Both are associated with the consequences of GH hypersecretion like soft-tissue hypertrophy and hyperglycemia. |
| Both are associated with the local effects of the GH-secreting tumor, like enlargement of the sella turcica, headache and visual disturbances. |

| DIFFERENCES | |
| --- | --- |
| **Acromegaly** | **Gigantism** |
| Occurs during adulthood, after the epiphyseal plates of long bones have fused. | Occurs during adolescence, before the epiphyseal plates of long bones have fused. |
| There is no abnormal increase in height. However, there is enlargement of hand and feet and a protrusion of the lower jaw (prognothism). | Patients become abnormally tall. Proportions of body parts remain normal. |

### Enumerate the causes and clinical features of pituitary dwarfism.

Hyposecretion of GH causes dwarfism. GH deficiency is usually a part of an overall lack of anterior pituitary hormones (**panhypopituitarism**). Selective GH deficiency is rare in adults. Decreased GH secretion in immature persons leads to stunted growth, or **dwarfism,** which is accompanied by sexual immaturity, hypothyroidism, and adrenal insufficiency. Impaired hair growth and a tendency toward fasting hypoglycemia are also present. Also, in contrast to the *mandibular* prognathism, which characterizes acromegaly, there is *maxillary* prognathism in hyposecretion of GH.

# 94

# *Thyroid Hormones*

### Name the hormones secreted by the thyroid gland.

The thyroid gland secretes two hormones, which are *iodothyronines*. The major secretory product of the thyroid gland is **3,5,3,`5'-tetraiodothyronine** (**thyroxine** or $T_4$). The other thyroid hormone is **3,5,3'-triiodothyronine** ($T_3$) which is secreted in smaller amounts. Most of the $T_3$ in the plasma is derived from mono-deiodination of $T_4$ by the action of *5'-deiodinase* found in peripheral tissue. Only $T_4$ and $T_3$ have biologic activity. A third iodothyronine called the **reverse 3,3',5'-triiodothyronine** ($rT_3$) is a biologically inactive thyronine formed by peripheral conversion catalyzed by 5-deiodinase. The term **thyroid hormone** denotes both thyroxine ($T_4$) and triiodothyronine ($T_3$).

### What are the differences between $T_3$ and $T_4$?

(i) $T_4$ is secreted in larger amounts. (ii) $T_4$ is more stable, being bound to plasma protein in greater proportion and more avidly. (iii) $T_4$ is an extracellular hormone while $T_3$ penetrates cells readily. (iv) $T_4$ is largely converted to $T_3$ in the body. $T_4$ therefore acts as a prohormone. (v) $T_3$ is much more potent than $T_4$ in all the hormonal actions including the feedback inhibition of TSH.

### Briefly outline the steps of thyroid synthesis and release.

The thyroid gland accumulates or 'traps' iodide by secondary active transport involving a **Na⁺-I⁻ symporter** that is linked to the $Na^+$-$K^+$-ATPase pump. Inside the thyrocyte, iodide is *oxidized* by **thyroid peroxidase** into iodine. Iodine is then **organified**

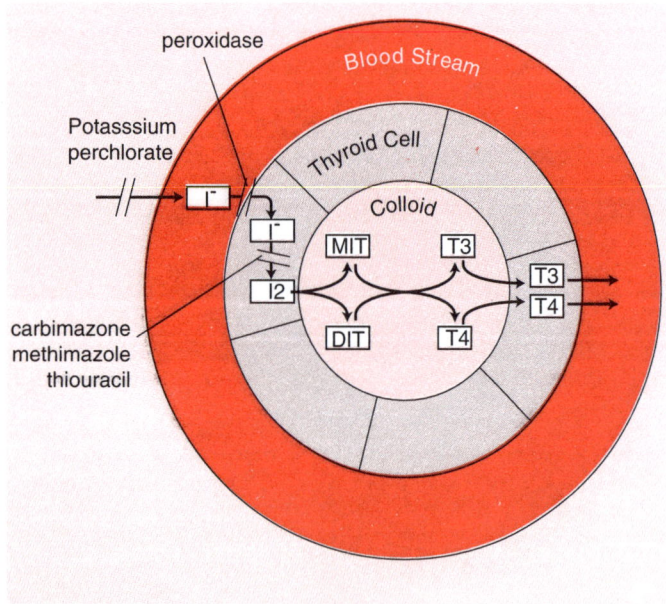

**Fig. 94.1**

(covalently bound) to the tyrosyl residues of **thyroglobulin**. Iodination also requires thyroid peroxidase. Organification results in the formation of monoiodotyrosine (MIT) and diiodotyrosine (DIT). Biologically active thyronines ($T_3$ and $T_4$) are formed by **coupling** (condensation) of iodotyrosines mediated by thyroid peroxidase. $T_4$ synthesis requires the coupling of two DIT molecules, and $T_3$ synthesis requires the coupling of an MIT molecule with a DIT molecule (Fig. 94.1).

### Name the thyroid binding proteins in blood.

Thyroxine is mainly associated with two of the three binding proteins: (i) **Thyroxine-binding globulin** (**TBG**) binds about 75% of the plasma $T_4$ and nearly all the plasma $T_3$. (ii) **Thyroxine-binding prealbumin** (**TBPA**) binds about 20% of the circulating $T_4$. (iii) **Thyroxine-binding albumin** (**TBA**) binds the remaining $T_4$.

### How is TH secretion regulated?

TSH secretion is regulated mainly by the **thyroid releasing hormone (TRH)**, which is synthesized in the *arcuate nucleus* of the hypothalamus. It is transported to the median eminence, where it is stored. From there, it is released into the hypophysial portal system and is carried to the anterior lobe of the pituitary gland. TRH stimulates the **thyrotropes** (basophils) in the anterior pituitary to secrete **thyroid stimulating hormone** (TSH). TRH secretion by the hypothalamus is decreased by $T_3$. **TSH** stimulates the thyroid follicle to secrete thyroid hormone by stimulating. (i) iodide transport into the thyroid cells; (ii) iodination of tyrosine; (iii) condensation of iodotyrosines; and (iv) release of iodotyrosines and iodothyronines. Both TRH and TSH secretions are inhibited by $T_3$.

Thyroid function is also regulated by an intrinsic control system. High concentrations of intrathyroidal **inorganic iodide** lead to the inhibition of organification of iodide and therefore, reduced TH synthesis (**Wolff - Chaikoff effect**). High concentrations of **organic iodide** (thyroid hormone) lead to a decrease in iodide uptake. Both of these effects reduce the fluctuation in thyroid hormone secretion when an acute change occurs in the availability of iodide.

### What are the other factors affecting thyroid hormone secretion?

(i) **Iodine deficiency** reduces TH synthesis. However, the TH secretion gets restored by the operation of the axis. (ii) **Iodine** decreases the proteolytic release of TH from a hyperactive thyroid by inhibiting glutathione reductase. In Graves's disease, it reduces thyroid hyperplasia and hyper-vascularity. Iodine is commonly administered before thyroid surgery for reducing its vascularity. (iii) **Plasma protein levels,** when elevated, reduce the free level of TH due to increased protein binding. This triggers the 'axis', which restores the free TH level to normal by augmenting TH secretion. This characteristically occurs *in pregnancy*. (iv) **Goitrogens** are present in certain vegetables e.g. plants of the *Brassica* family. When ingested, they produce goiter by impairing hormonal synthesis. (v) *Estrogens* enhance TSH secretion. (vi) *Somatostatin* inhibits TSH secretion. (iv) Dopamine and bromocriptine decrease the secretion of TSH. (vi) **Genetic enzyme deficiency** impairs TH secretion.

## Enumerate the physiologic effects of thyroid hormone.

The physiologic actions of thyroid hormone are growth, differentiation, calorigenesis, and TSH (and TRH) suppression. (i) **Basal metabolic rate**. Thyroid hormone increases the BMR of most cells in the body. The increase in BMR accounts for the thermogenic calorigenic effect of thyroid hormone. (ii) **Growth**. Thyroid hormone is essential for ossification of cartilage and *bone growth*. It is also important for the normal *myelination* and synaptic development in the CNS. In hypothyroidism, there is a marked decrease in the myelination of neurons in the brain. If hypothyroidism is untreated, mental retardation occurs (cretinism). TH also promotes erythropoiesis. TH is also essential for normal onset of puberty, fertility and lactation. (iii) **Carbo-hydrate metabolism**. In physiologic amounts, the actions of thyroid hormone include both hypoglycemic and hyperglycemic effects. High levels of thyroid hormone lead to hyperglycemia. **Protein metabolism**. Thyroid hormone is required in association with other anabolic hormones, notably growth hormone, for normal protein synthesis. Thyroid hormone has a potent protein anabolic effect. In large doses, thyroid hormone has a protein catabolic effect. (iv) **Fat metabolism**. Thyroid stimulates both hormone-sensitive and lipoprotein lipases. Hormone-sensitive lipase mobilizes fat from adipose tissues, increasing the plasma concentrations of FFA and glycerol. The elevated levels of FFA and glycerol promote *hepatic triglyceride synthesis*. The FFA released is also oxidized to generate energy for **thermogenesis**. However when the triglycerides synthesized in the liver are released into circulation, they are again broken down into FFA and glycerol by lipoprotein-lipase. Thyroid hormone also enhances *de novo* cholesterol synthesis as well as bile acid synthesis. On a net basis, the *lipolytic effect is greater than the lipogenic effect*. Hence, elevated thyroid hormone levels are associated with *decreases in blood triglycerides, phospholipids and cholesterol,* and *increases in plasma free fatty acids and glycerol*. (v) **Vitamin metabolism**. Thyroid hormone is required for the hepatic synthesis of vitamin A from carotene and the conversion of vitamin A to retinene. In hypothyroid states, the serum carotene is elevated, and the skin becomes yellow. This skin condition differs from that observed in jaundice in that the sclera of the eye is *not* yellow.

## Explain why thyroid hormone has both hyperglycemic as well as hypoglycemic effects.

The *hypoglycemic* effects are (i) enhancement of peripheral utilization of glucose and (ii) potentiation of the action of insulin with consequent promotion of glycogenesis and glucose utilization. The *hyperglycemic* effects are (i) potentiation of the glycogenolytic effect of epinephrine, causing glycogen depletion;

(ii) stimulation of gluconeogenic, thereby increasing the availability of lactates and glycerol for glucose production; and (iii) acceleration of intestinal glucose absorption, which is partly due to an increase in bowel motility. (iv) It also increases food intake, possibly in response to the increased glucose utilization.

## What is goiter?

Any enlargement of the thyroid gland is called a **goiter**. A goiter does not specify the functional state of the thyroid gland. Hence, a goiter may be associated with a hypothyroidism or hyperthyroidism.

## What are goitrogens?

Goitrogens are antithyroid substances that produces goiter by blocking the synthesis of thyroid hormone. When a goitrogen reduces TH secretion, TSH secretion is enhanced which leads to thyroid gland enlargement (goiter) and the restoration of plasma thyroid hormone levels. Cabbage and some other vegetables of the *Brassicaceae* family contain **progoitrin** that is activated to **goitrin** (a goitrogen) in the intestine by intestinal bacteria. Thus excess consumption of cabbage can lead to goiter (**cabbage goiter**).

## What is the recommended iodine intake?

The daily dietary iodine intake is ~500µg. The recommended minimum intake is 150 µg per day (about 1 mg per week) to maintain euthyroidism because iodine is added to salt and iodate is sometimes added to bread. During pregnancy the recommended intake is 200 µg per day. The minimum intake required to prevent goiter is 75 µg per day. The neonatal iodide requirement is 40 µg per day.

## Enumerate the causes and clinical features of hypothyroidism.

Hypothyroidism can occur in the following situations. (i) Iodine deficiency ranks as the most common cause of thyroid biosynthetic failure worldwide. It is associated with a hypothyroid goiter. With lesser degrees of iodine deficiency a euthyroid goiter is more likely other causes are (ii) diseased or maldeveloped thyroid; (iii) genetic enzyme deficiency; and (iv) antithyroid therapy; (v) goitrogens in diet.

The signs and symptoms of hypothyroidism include fatigue, lethargy and sleepiness, muscular weakness, bradycardia, decreased cardiac output, decreased blood volume, weight gain, constipation, mental sluggishness, reduced hair growth and scaliness of the skin, huskiness of voice and in severe cases, an edematous appearance through out the body, called **myxedema**. Myxedema is not due to fluid retention. It is due to the *deposition in the interstitial fluid of large quantities of gel-like substances* (proteins mixed with hyaluronic acid and chondroitin sulfate). Hence instead of the usual pitting-edema that occurs due to increase in interstitial volume, in myxedema, there is **non-pitting edema**. Hyperthyroidism is associated with a rise in blood cholesterol with a consequent increased predisposition to atherosclerosis, with all its complications: peripheral vascular disease, deafness and coronary artery disease.

When thyroid deficiency occurs during fetal life, infancy or childhood, the result is **cretinism**. Skeletal growth in the cretin is more inhibited than is soft tissue growth. Therefore *soft tissues enlarge excessively*, producing the characteristic appearance of cretins.

### Enumerate the causes and clinical features of hyperthyroidism.

The most common cause of hyperthyroidism is **Grave's disease,** an autoimmune disease in which autoantibodies are formed against TSH receptors. The TSH receptors get activated by the auto-antibodies and bring about hypersecretion of thyroid hormone. Hyperthyroidism can also occurs due to a TSH-secreting tumor of the anterior pituitary.

Clinical features of hyperthyroidism include rise in BMR, intolerance to heat, excessive sweating, weight loss, muscle weakness, diarrhea, nervousness and psychic disorders, inability to sleep and tremors of the hands. Patients of Grave's disease develop **exophthalmos**, i.e., protrusion of the eyeballs. In this condition, the eyelids do not close completely when the person blinks or is asleep. It occurs due to the swelling of the extraocular muscles, and to lesser degree, the connective tissue within the rigid bony walls of the orbit. Treatment of hyperthyroidism includes surgical removal of the thyroid and use of antithyroid drugs.

### Enumerate the thyroid function tests.

**Radioactive iodide ($I^{131}$) uptake** by the thyroid gland is a useful therapeutic index of the functional status of the thyroid gland. A 24-hour uptake normally ranges between 5% and 35% of the administered dose. The uptake is increased in hyperthyroidism and reduced in hypothyroidism. **Scintiscanning** is done using the radioisotope pertechnetate-99m. Scintiscanning localizes sites of accumulation of the radionucleotides and thereby detects localized areas of thyroid hyperactivity or hypoactivity. **Radioimmunoassay** of the plasma concentrations of thyroid hormones indicates thyroid function status. **TRH stimulation test**.

The basal concentration of serum TSH increases in response to TRH administration and decreases on the administration of thyroid hormone. **Thyroid suppression test**. Exogenous TH suppresses pituitary TSH resulting in a decrease of radioactive iodine uptake to 50% of normal. Lack of suppression indicates autonomous production. *Non-specific indices* include **basal metabolic rate** (-15 to +5%), **serum cholesterol** (120-220 mg%) and **systolic ejection time** (shortened in hyperthyroidism and lengthened in hypothyroidism). Tests for detecting damage to the thyroid gland include **serum thyroid globulin concentration** (in carcinoma of thyroid, thyroglobulin is released into blood stream). The presence of **autoantibodies** to the thyroid gland indicates thyroid disorders, e.g., antimicrosomal antibodies (suggests Hashimoto's disease) and antithyroglobulin antibodies (suggests Graves disease).

### Name the antithyroid drugs and explain their mechanism of action.

Antithyroid drugs are grouped into two classes: agents that *block iodide transport* and agents that *inhibit the coupling of iodotyrosyl residues* in thyroglobulin. **Pertechnetate** ($TcO_4^-$), **perchlorate** ($ClO_4^-$), **thiocyanate** ($SCN^-$), and **nitrate** ($NO_3^-$) are drugs that *block the uptake of iodide* into the thyroid. These anions are competitive inhibitors of iodide transport. $SCN^-$ and $ClO_4^-$ are no longer used because of their toxicity. **Thionamides** (propylthiouracil, methimazole, and carbimazole) compete with tyrosyl residues for iodide, thereby reducing iodination of tyrosine residues. Thionamides also *inhibit the coupling reactions* mediated by thyroxine peroxidase. Propylthiouracil also *inhibits 5'-deiodinase*, leading to a reduction in the extrathyroidal synthesis of $T_3$. Other drugs that affect thyroid function include **radioiodine $I^{131}$** (the most common treatment of Graves' disease), **lithium carbonate**, which inhibits organification of iodide and may cause goiter and hypothyroidism, and **excess iodide** which leads to hypothyroidism.

# 95

# Calcitropic Hormones

## Enumerate the role of Ca²⁺ in physiologic processes.

(i) $Ca^{2+}$ is necessary for the activation of clotting enzymes in plasma. (ii) $Ca^{2+}$ controls *membrane excitation*, and $Ca^{2+}$ influx occurs during the excitatory process of nerve and muscle. (iii) $Ca^{2+}$ is bound to cell surfaces and has a role in the *stabilization of the membrane* and *intercellular adhesion*. (iv) $Ca^{2+}$ is necessary for *muscle contraction*. (v) $Ca^{2+}$ is essential in all *excitation-secretion processes*, both endocrine and exocrine. It also is essential for *neurotransmitter release*. (vi) $Ca^{2+}$ is necessary for the *production of milk* and the *formation of bone and teeth*. (vii) $Ca^{2+}$ acts as *a second messenger in the cytosol*. (viii) $Ca^{2+}$ has an essential role in the **mineralization of bone**.

## What are the different forms in which Ca²⁺ exists in the body?

$Ca^{2+}$ is present in the plasma as (i) ionized or free (45%); (ii) complexed with $HPO_4^{2-}$, $HCO_3^-$, or citrate ion (10%), and (iii) bound to protein (primarily to albumin) (45%). The plasma concentration of total (ionized and nonionized) $Ca^{2+}$ is about 10 mg/dl. Ionic $Ca^{2+}$ has a plasma concentration of about 5mg/dl.

## What are the various Ca²⁺ pools in the body?

Total body $Ca^{2+}$ is present as two major pools. The larger $Ca^{2+}$ pool, which contains 99% of the total $Ca^{2+}$ (about 1 kg) consists of stable (mature) bone. This represents the **skeletal pool** that is not readily exchangeable, but can be mobilized only through the action of the parathyroid hormone.

The smaller $Ca^{2+}$ pool (~4g), which contains about 1% of the total body $Ca^{2+}$, consists of labile (young) bone. This $Ca^{2+}$ pool is readily exchangeable with the ECF and is called the **ECF pool**. The pool consists of calcium phosphate salts, and provides an immediate reserve for sudden decreases in blood $Ca^{2+}$.

## What is the composition of bones?

Dry, fat-free bone is *two thirds mineral (inorganic) matrix* and *one-third organic matrix*, mostly collagen. The Ca: P ratio in the mineral matrix is about 1.7:1. Bone $Ca^{2+}$ is found in the form of **hydroxyapatite crystals**. Fluoride ion can replace the OH⁻ group in hydroxyapatite and form **fluorapatite**.

## Name the hormones involved in Ca²⁺ metabolism. How is their secretion regulated?

$Ca^{2+}$ regulation involves *3 tissues*: bone, intestine, and kidney; *3 hormones*: PTH, calcitonin, and calcitriol; and *3 cell types*: osteoblasts, osteocytes, and osteoclasts. PTH is secreted by the chief cells of the parathyroid gland. Calcitonin is secreted by the parafollicular (c) cells of the thyroid gland. The pituitary gland does not play a major role in $Ca^+$ metabolism.

*PTH and calcitonin secretions* are controlled mainly by serum $Ca^{2+}$ levels. Hypocalcemia stimulates PTH secretion while hypercalcemia stimulates calcitonin secretion. Stimuli for calcitonin secretion also include gastrointestinal hormones such as gastrin, pentagastrin, and enteroglucagon. Somatostatin inhibits calcitonin secretion. *Calcitriol synthesis* is controlled by PTH and hypophosphatemia, both of which directly activate renal $1\alpha$-hydroxylase, which catalyzes the conversion of calcidiol to calcitriol.

## What is the effect of parathyroid hormone on Ca²⁺ metabolism?

PTH regulates only the plasma $Ca^{2+}$ and not the phosphates. However, it is controlled by both $Ca^{2+}$ and phosphates. PTH is the **hypercalcemic hormone** of the body and exerts its effects on the bone, intestine, and kidney.

An inverse linear relationship exists between plasma $Ca^{2+}$ and PTH secretion: when plasma $Ca^{2+}$ falls, PTH secretion increases. Conversely, as plasma $Ca^{2+}$ increases, PTH secretion decreases. High $Ca^{2+}$ causes inhibition of PTH secretion, inhibition of renal synthesis of calcitriol, decreased intestinal active transport of $Ca^{2+}$, increased renal excretion of $Ca^{2+}$, decreased excretion of phosphate, and a decrease in bone resorption.

Phosphates increase PTH secretion, suppress renal synthesis of $1,25(OH)_2D_3$, and inhibit bone resorption. An increase in plasma phosphate concentration also can indirectly reduce plasma $Ca^{2+}$ concentration, which also enhances PTH secretion.

## What is the effect of calcitonin on Ca²⁺ metabolism?

Calcitonin is the **hypocalcemic hormone** of the body. It exerts a biologic effect on the bone, intestine, and kidney. A positive linear relationship exists between plasma $Ca^{2+}$ and calcitonin secretion: as plasma $Ca^{2+}$ increases, calcitonin secretion increases. Conversely, when plasma $Ca^{2+}$ decreases, calcitonin secretion decreases.

## Can vitamin D be called a hormone?

The term vitamin D denotes both vitamins $D_2$ and $D_3$. The only difference between vitamin $D_2$ (ergocalciferol) and vitamin $D_3$ (cholecalciferol) is structural. Structurally, vitamin $D_3$ is a steroid hormone. *Vitamin $D_3$ is both a vitamin and a hormone*: it is a vitamin when ingested from nutritional sources and a hypercalcemic hormone when it is produced in the skin and activated sequentially in the liver and kidney. Therefore, vitamin $D_3$ is not a true vitamin, unless there is a deficiency of it. Exposure of the skin to sunlight for 15-20 minutes daily has an antirachitic effect. Vitamin $D_3$ exerts biologic activity only after in has been converted to its active metabolites, i.e., calcidiol and calcitriol.

## How is active vitamin D₃ synthesized in the body?

In the epidermis (stratum corneum), the **provitamin $D_3$**, (7-dehydrocholesterol) is converted into vitamin $D_3$ (cholecalciferol) by nonenzymatic photoactivation by solar radiation in the ultraviolet-B frequency range (290 and 315 nm). Vitamin $D_3$ enters the circulation and is bound to the vitamin $D_3$-binding protein (globulin) and transported to the liver where it is converted to 25-hydroxycholecalciferol (**calcidiol**) by hepatic *25-hydroxylase*. Calcidiol is the major blood form of vitamin $D_3$. It is two to five times more effective than vitamin $D_3$ in preventing rickets.

Calcidiol is transported to the kidney, where it is metabolized to 1, 25 dihydroxycholecalciferol (**calcitriol**) by *1α-hydroxylase*. PTH and hypophosphatemia are the major inducers of this enzyme. Calcitriol is 100 times more potent than calcidiol. All target tissues for vitamin $D_3$ contain a nuclear receptor for calcitriole.

### Describe the actions of vitamin $D_3$.

*In the bones*, vitamin $D_3$ apparently has two physiologically opposite effects: an **antirachitic effect** leading to enhanced mineralization, and an **increase in bone resorption**. Vitamin $D_3$ promotes mineralization of osteoid laid down by osteoblasts by maintaining the extracellular $Ca^{2+}$ and phosphorus concentrations within the normal range. This results in the deposition of calcium hydroxyapatite into the bone matrix. Paradoxically, vitamin $D_3$ also acts directly on bone to promote resorption that mimics the effects of PTH. This is because vitamin $D_3$ induces the transformation of osteoblasts into osteoclasts. *In the intestine*, vitamin $D_3$ stimulates $Ca^{2+}$ absorption, which occurs mainly in the duodenum. *In the kidney*, vitamin $D_3$ stimulates phosphate reabsorption in the proximal tubule and $Ca^{2+}$ reabsorption in the distal tubule. It also inhibits 1α-hydroxylase activity in the kidney, resulting in a negative feedback inhibition of its own production.

### Describe the actions of PTH.

*In the bone*, PTH increases osteoclastic cell number and activity. The bone reabsorption is associated with increased mobilization of $Ca^{2+}$ and inorganic phosphate, and increased urinary secretion of hydroxyproline. Paradoxically, PTH also exerts an anabolic action by increasing the formation of trabecular bone. PTH stimulates release of insulin-like growth factors (IGF I) from osteoblasts. IGFs enhance bone collagen and matrix synthesis. IGFs also decrease collagenase activity and inhibit bone-collagen degradation. *In the intestine*, there is increased $Ca^{2+}$ and phosphate absorption. The effect is mediated through calcitriol, whose production is increased by PTH.

*In the kidney*, (i) PTH increases $Ca^{2+}$ reabsorption in the distal nephron and *tends* to decrease the urinary calcium excretion. However PTH also increases the calcium levels through bone resorption, which *tends* to produce hypercalcuria. The net effect is hypercalcuria. (ii) It decreases proximal tubular reabsorption of phosphate. (iii) It stimulates 1 α-**hydroxylase activity** (in the mitochondria of the PCT and PST cells) to increase formation of calcitriol through which the gastrointestinal absorption of calcium and phosphate are controlled. In addition, calcitriol can decrease the renal excretion of $Ca^{2+}$ and phosphate.

### Describe the actions of calcitonin.

*In the bone*, calcitonin inhibits osteoclastic bone resorption, and thereby tends to produce hypocalcemia and hypophosphatemia. It does not promote bone formation or mineralization. *In the intestine*, calcitonin has no effect on $Ca^{2+}$ absorption from the intestines but may decrease absorption of phosphorus. *In the kidney*, calcitonin decreases the renal threshold for urinary reabsorption of calcium and phosphorus. This, added to the presence of high phosphate levels in plasma, promotes increased urinary phosphorus excretion.

### Enumerate the clinical features of hypoparathyroidism.

**Primary hypoparathyroidism** is caused by a deficient secretion of PTH by the parathyroid glands or removal of parathyroid tissue during thyroid surgery. PTH deficiency results in low plasma $Ca^{2+}$ and high phosphate concentrations. The low plasma $Ca^{2+}$ results in increased and spontaneous excitability of nerves and muscles – a condition called **hypoparathyroid tetany**. Tetany is characterized by: (i) **Chvostek's sign**: Percussion of the facial nerve just anterior to the ear lobe results in ipsilateral contractions of the facial muscle. (ii) **Trousseau's sign**: Occlusive pressure applied with a blood pressure cuff results in a *carpal spasm*, appearing as thumb adduction, metacarpophalangeal joint flexion, and interphalangeal joint extension.

**Secondary hypoparathyroidism** is caused by the feedback suppression of PTH secretion by increased plasma $Ca^{2+}$ concentration, e.g., by excessive intake of vitamin D.

### What is pseudohypoparathyroidism?

**Pseudohypoparathyroidism** is a disorder characterized by target tissue unresponsiveness to the biological actions of PTH. The biochemical findings in these patients are identical to those observed in patients with surgical hypoparathyroidism (i.e., hypocalcemia and hyperphosphatemia), except that in most patients the plasma PTH is increased.

### Enumerate the clinical features of hyperparathyroidism.

In **primary hyperparathyroidism**, there is excess secretion of PTH by a tumor of the parathyroid gland or by ectopic parathyroid tissue. Excess PTH leads to: (i) increased plasma $Ca^{2+}$ and decreased plasma inorganic phosphate concentrations; (ii) increased urinary excretion of phosphate (phosphaturia), cyclic AMP, and hydroxyproline; and (iii) muscle weakness and fatigability.

In **secondary hyperparathyroidism**, the increased secretion of PTH occurs in response to hypocalcemia caused by: (i) vitamin D-deficient diet; (ii) poor absorption of fat, leading to the concomitant decreased absorption of fat-soluble vitamins (A, D, E, and K); (iii) impaired synthesis of calcitriol due to renal disease; (iv) increased demand for $Ca^{2+}$ as during pregnancy and lactation.

### Define the terms osteoporosis, osteomalacia and rickets.

**Osteoporosis** is the most common metabolic bone disease. It is characterized by a reduction in bone mass with a normal ratio of mineral to organic matrix. The term **osteopenia** is sometimes used to describe reduced bone mass in the absence of symptoms or signs of osteoporosis. It occurs in estrogen deficiency following menopause (**postmenopausal osteoporosis**) and following prolonged immobilization (**immobilization osteoporosis**).

**Osteomalacia** is characterized by an excess of unmineralized bone, which results from the failure of the organic matrix (osteoid) to mineralize normally.

**Rickets** is a failure of normal mineralization of the epiphyseal plate in children. It is caused by inadequate mineralization of both osteoid and cartilage.

# 96

# Corticosteroid Synthesis & Secretion

## Name the zones in the adrenal cortex and their secretions.

The adrenal cortex consists of three distinct zones of cells. **Zona glomerulosa** is the outermost layer, and is the site of *aldosterone* and *corticosterone* synthesis. These two hormones regulate the effects on the $Na^+$, $K^+$ and $H_2O$ homeostasis of the body and are called the *mineralocorticoids*. **Zona fasciculata** is the wider, middle zone. **Zona reticularis** is the innermost layer. The two inner zones of the adrenal cortex constitute a single functional unit, where *glucocorticoids*, (the most important of which is *cortisol*) and *androgens* (*androstenedione*, *DHEA* and *testosterone*) are synthesized. The hormones secreted by the adrenal cortex as a whole are called *corticosteroids*.

The adrenal cortex thus secretes *two glucocorticoids* (cortisol and corticosterone), *one mineralocorticoid* (aldosterone), *three biosynthetic precursors* of the end products (progesterone, 11-deoxycorticosterone, and 11-deoxycortisol), and *one androgen* dehydroepiandrosterone or DHEA. The adrenal cortex *does not secrete physiologically effective amounts of testosterone or estradiol.*

## Explain the biosynthesis of corticosteroids diagrammatically.

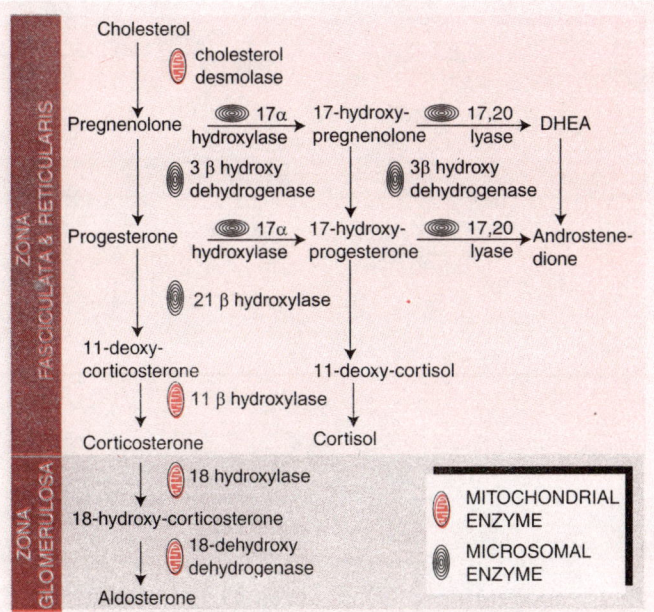

**Fig. 96.1**

## What are the cortisol-binding proteins?

About 90% of the plasma cortisol is bound to **cortisol-binding globulin** (CBG transcortin), which is an α-globulin. About 6% of the plasma cortisol is bound to plasma **albumin,** and about 4% is **unbound** and represents the physiologically active steroid. The bound cortisol represents the metabolically inactive pool, which serves as a reservoir for free hormone.

## How are corticosteroids metabolized?

The liver is the major extra-adrenal site of corticosteroid metabolism. Corticosteroid is mostly inactivated to **tetrahydrocortisol**. Conjugation with glucuronic acid forms a water-soluble metabolite that is readily excreted by the kidney. Some of the cortico-steroids is converted into **17-ketosteroids** that are conjugated with sulfates.

## Describe the regulation of adrenocortical secretion.

The hypothalamus releases **corticotropin-releasing hormone** (CRH), which stimulates the secretion of ACTH from the anterior lobe of the pituitary gland via the hypophysial portal system. Normally, blood ACTH levels are higher in the morning than in the evening. This accounts for the **diurnal rhythms** in cortisol secretion (**hypophysial-adrenocortical rhythm**). ACTH is also increased by **stress**. Among the stresses shown to induce increased activity are severe trauma, pyrogens, hypoglycemia, histamine injection, electroconvulsive shock, acute anxiety, burns, hemorrhage, exercise, infections, chemical intoxication, pain, surgery, psychological stress, and cold exposure.

**ACTH** stimulates the output of aldosterone as well as that of glucocorticoids and sex hormones. As a negative feedback, corticosteroids inhibit secretion of both CRH and ACTH. Of the endogenous corticosteroids, *only cortisol has ACTH-suppressing activity*. The negative feedback of cortisol is exerted at the level of both the pituitary gland and the hypothalamus. In the presence of excess free cortisol, ACTH secretion is suppressed and the adrenal cortex undergoes disuse atrophy. Conversely, if plasma free cortisol levels are subnormal, the pituitary is released from inhibition by cortisol, ACTH secretion rises, and the adrenal cortex secretes more cortisol and becomes hypertrophic. The synthetic glucocorticoid, **dexamethasone,** is a potent inhibitor of ACTH secretion and, therefore, of endogenous glucocorticoid secretion.

## How is aldosterone secretion regulated?

The *three principal stimuli* that increase aldosterone secretion are *ACTH, angiotensin II,* and *hyperkalemia*. (i) **ACTH** stimulates the output of both aldosterone and deoxycortisone. However, *the effect on aldosterone is transient* – lasting a day or two – because a rise in aldosterone produces hypervolemia (which inhibits angiotensin-II production) and hypokalemia. Both these factors tend to lower aldosterone secretion. In other words, *in the* *presence of stronger controllers* of aldosterone secretion (angiotensin-II, hyperkalemia), *ATCH does not act as an important controller of aldosterone.* Thus, after hypophysectomy, the basal rate of aldosterone secretion is not immediately affected. However, *chronic ACTH deficiency results in atrophy of the zona glomerulosa* and leads to hypoaldosteronism. (ii) **Angiotensin-II** stimulates secretion of aldosterone. Angiotensin-II has an *early action on the conversion of cholesterol to pregnenolone*, and a *late action on the conversion of corticosterone to aldosterone.* (iii) **Hyper-kalemia** is the most potent stimulator of aldosterone secretion. Like angiotensin II, $K^+$ also stimulates the *conversion of cholesterol to pregnenolone* and the conversion of *corticosterone to aldosterone.*

Other factors affecting aldosterone secretion are as follows: (iv) **Plasma Na⁺ concentration**. A sharp fall in plasma $Na^+$ of about 20 mEq/L stimulates aldosterone secretion, but such changes are rare. (v) **Posture**. Plasma aldosterone concentration increases on prolonged standing. This increase is due to a decrease in the rate of removal of aldosterone from the circulation by the liver and an increase in aldosterone secretion due to a postural increase in renin secretion. (vi) **Diurnal variations**. There is a circadian rhythm of aldosterone and renin secretion, with the highest values in the early morning before awakening. (vii) **Atrial natriuretic peptide (ANP)**. It inhibits renin secretion and decreases the responsiveness of the zona glomerulosa to angiotensin II.

### What are the different subtypes of congenital adrenal hyperplasia?

**Congenital adrenal hyperplasia** (CAH) (also known as **adrenogenital syndrome**) results from enzyme deficiencies that produce *low levels of cortisol, elevated ACTH* (due to feedback), and *adrenocortical hyperplasia* (due to excess ACTH). Hypersecretion of ACTH results in *excessive production of those substrates that are proximal to the deficient enzymes.* The possible enzyme deficiencies and their consequences are tabulated below.

|  | Gluco-corticoid effect | Mineralo corticoid effect | Androgenic effect |
|---|---|---|---|
| 3β dehydrogenase | Low | Low: salt-losing | Low:feminizing in males; virilizing in females |
| 21β-hydroxylase | Low | Low: salt-losing | High: virilizing |
| 11β-hydroxylase | Low | Moderate: hypertensive | High: virilizing |
| 17α-hydroxylase | Low | Excess: hypertensive | Low:feminizing |

# 97

# Actions of Corticosteroids

## Enumerate the physiologic actions of glucocorticoids.

**Effect on blood cells** Glucocorticoids stimulate hematopoiesis and increases the total blood count and the total white blood cell count (TLC) because they *increase* the numbers of *erythrocytes*, *neutrophils* and *platelets*. Glucocorticoids increase the number of circulating neutrophils due to the *accelerated release from bone marrow and a reduced migration* from the circulation. Steroids also inhibit the ability of neutrophils to marginate to the vessel wall. Glucocorticoids *reduce* the number of circulating *lymphocytes, monocytes, eosinophils,* and *basophils,* primarily due to their *relocation from the vascular compartment into the lymphoid tissue* (e.g., spleen, lymph nodes, bone marrow).

**Anti-inflammatory effects.** Glucocorticoids inhibit inflammatory and allergic reactions in several ways. (i) They *stabilize lysosomal membranes* and thereby inhibit the release of proteolytic enzymes. (ii) They *decrease capillary permeability*, thereby inhibiting diapedesis of leukocytes. Decreased capillary permeability also *lessens edema formation* and thereby, *reduces inflammatory swellings*. (iii) Glucocorticoids also decrease the release of secretory products of granulocytes, mast cells, and macrophages, which release inflammatory mediators like serotonin, histamine and hydrolases.

**Anti-immunity effects.** Glucocorticoids cause *involution of the lymph nodes, thymus, and spleen*. In high doses, they *decrease antibody production* by reducing the proliferation of B-cells and also *suppress cell-mediated immunity* by reducing the number of T-lymphocytes and inhibiting cytokine release. Glucocorticoids are therefore *administered to organ transplant recipients* for reducing the immune response. However, treatment with large doses of glucocorticoids predispose to infections, making *antibiotics a necessary adjunct to the steroid therapy.*

**Anti-allergenic effects.** The decrease in circulating basophils accounts for the *fall in blood histamine levels* and a reduction in the allergic response.

**Renal effects.** Glucocorticoids facilitate rapid excretion of a water load (increases free-water clearance) and also enhance uric acid excretion.

**Gastric effects.** Cortisol increases gastric acid secretion, and decreases gastric mucosal cell proliferation. Hence, chronic cortisol treatment predisposes to peptic ulceration. Stress, which is always associated with excessive glucocorticoid secretion, often results in gastric ulcers (*stress ulcers*).

**Psychoneural effects.** High cortisol levels can cause insomnia, mood changes, reduced memory function and lower seizure threshold.

**Antigrowth effects.** Large doses of cortisol reduce absorption of $Ca^{2+}$ from the gut (by antagonizing DHCC), inhibit mitosis of fibroblasts, and cause degradation of collagen. These effects lead to *osteoporosis*, i.e., a reduction in bone mass per unit volume with a normal ratio of mineral-to-organic matrix. The breakdown of collagen leads to an *increase in urinary hydroxyproline excretion*. Glucocorticoids *inhibit the anabolic actions of growth hormone* (GH) and insulin-like growth factor-1 (IGF-1), particularly in bone. Excess glucocorticoids suppress GH secretion and *inhibit somatic growth*. Glucocorticoids *delay wound healing* because of the reduction of fibroblast proliferation. Connective tissue is reduced in quantity and strength. Glucocorticoids increase the ability of muscle to perform work. However in large doses, glucocorticoids cause *muscle atrophy* and muscular weakness.

**Vascular effects.** Cortisol *enhances catecholamine synthesis* by activating phenolethanolamine-N-methyl-transferase (PNMT). In pharmacological doses, cortisol enhances the vascular responsiveness to vasoactive substances like norepinephrine, and thereby *helps maintain the normal arterial systemic blood pressure and blood volume*. Absence of cortisol results in vasodilatation and hypotension.

**Stress adaptation.** Various stresses like trauma, cold, illness and starvation are *associated with increased ACTH secretion* and consequent increase in glucocorticoid secretion. The physiological significance of this is however poorly understood because *resistance to stress is not increased by the administration of glucocorticoids*.

**Effects on carbohydrate metabolism.** Cortisol is *a carbohydrate-sparing, hyperglycemic hormone*. Cortisol also *promotes hepatic glycogenesis*, thereby increasing the glycogen content of the liver. Although increased glycogenesis should reduce blood glucose levels, a hyperglycemia occurs because cortisol *promotes gluconeogenesis*.

Cortisol is a *diabetogenic hormone*: it exerts *an anti-insulin effect* by blocking glucose transport in muscle and adipose tissue and inhibiting the glycolytic enzymes – glucokinase, phosphofructokinase, and pyruvate kinase. These effects result in glucose intolerance or eventual *steroid diabetes*. The hyperglycemia associated with glucocorticoids causes compensatory hyperinsulinemia.

**Effects on protein metabolism.** Cortisol enhances the *release of amino acids from proteins in skeletal muscle* and other extrahepatic tissues, including the protein matrix of bone. The amino acids released are transported to the liver and converted to glucose through gluconeogenesis. The deamination reactions associated with gluconeogenesis results in increased urea production and *increased urinary nitrogen excretion.*

The amino acids taken up by the liver are used not only for gluconeogenesis and glycogenesis, but also for *synthesis of new protein.* This *protein anabolic effect* at the level of the liver is in contrast to the *overall protein catabolic effect* of cortisol. Moreover, glucocorticoids also inhibit the *de novo* synthesis of protein, probably at the translational level, which is called the *antianabolic effect.*

**Effects on fat metabolism.** Glucocorticoids are *lipolytic hormones.* The cause lipolysis by stimulating hormone-sensitive lipase which mobilizes fatty acids from adipose tissue. They also potentiate the lipolytic actions of other hormones such as GH, catecholamines, glucagon, and thyroid hormone. Increased oxidation of the fatty acid that is mobilized may lead to *ketosis.*

### Name the hormones with mineralocorticoid activity.

**Aldosterone** is the principal mineralocorticoid secreted by the adrenal, although **corticosterone** is secreted in sufficient amounts to exert a minor mineralocorticoid effect. **Deoxycorticosterone,** which is secreted in appreciable amounts only in abnormal situations, has about 3% of the activity of aldosterone. Large amounts of **progesterone** and some other steroids also have some mineralocorticoid-like activity but they do not have any physiological role in the control of Na+ excretion.

### Enumerate the physiologic actions of mineralocorticoids.

The principal role of mineralocorticoids is the *regulation of Na+ and K+ excretion.* Mineralocorticoids increase the reabsorption of Na+ from the urine, sweat, saliva, and gastric juice. Sodium ions move out of urine (and other transcellular fluids) into the interstitial fluid where they are retained so that the *ECF concentration of Na+ increases.*

The actions of aldosterone are localized to the distal tubular and collecting duct cells of the kidney. (i) Aldosterone increases reabsorption of Na+ and with it, of water too. (ii) Increased Na+ reabsorption makes the tubular lumen highly negative. (iii) The highly negative lumen together with the increased apical permeability to K+ promotes K+ secretion.

Aldosterone is the *sole regulator* of the **external potassium balance**. An increase in plasma K+ stimulates aldosterone secretion, which in turn restores plasma K+ levels by promoting kaliuresis. An absence of this aldosterone-feedback mechanism would result in fatal hyperkalemia. Aldosterone is *one of the several regulators* of *body Na+ and water balance*, another important regulator being the thirst-ADH mechanism. In the absence of the aldosterone-feedback mechanism, the thirst-ADH mechanism maintains a near-perfect Na+ balance in the body. In the absence of the ADH-thirst mechanism, however, aldosterone is unable to maintain proper Na+ balance because of the **escape phenomenon**.

### Which part of the adrenal gland, the cortex or the medulla, is essential for life, and why?

The adrenal cortex is essential for life; the adrenal medulla is not. Following adrenalectomy, the mineralocorticoid deficiency results in hypotension, circulatory insufficiency, and, eventually, fatal shock.

### Outline the clinical features of Addison's disease. How does it differ from secondary adrenal insufficiency?

In Addison's disease (also called **primary adrenal insufficiency**), there is *deficiency of three adrenal hormones*—cortisol, aldosterone, and DHEA. (i) *Deficiency of cortisol* results in *hypoglycemia* due to increased peripheral glucose utilization associated with increased sensitivity to insulin, with impaired gluconeogenesis, hepatic glucose production, and glycogen synthesis. Cortisol deficiency also causes a *feedback increase in ACTH secretion.* The high levels of ACTH cause *hyperpigmentation of skin.* (ii) *Deficiency of aldosterone* causes anorexia, weakness, weight loss, vomiting, hyperpigmentation, *hyponatremia (natriuresis), hyperkalemia, hypotension, metabolic acidosis,* increased plasma ADH, hypoosmotic dehydration, and elevated plasma ACTH. (iii) *Deficiency of androgens* leads to the loss of pubic hair, reduced muscle mass, and loss of libido in men and women. Amenorrhea may also occur.

**Secondary adrenal insufficiency** occurs when there is inadequate stimulation of the adrenals by ACTH. It results in the *deficiency of two adrenal hormones* – cortisol and DHEA. The secretion of aldosterone remains nearly unaffected. The clinical features are *similar to those of primary insufficiency.* However, there is *absence of hyperpigmentation* (since there is no hypersecretion of ACTH). Also, since there is no aldosterone deficiency, *fluid and electrolyte disturbances do not occur,* and the *hypotension* that occurs occasionally is attributable to cortisol deficiency.

### Explain why Addison's disease is associated with hyperpigmentation of skin.

In Addison's disease, the cortisol deficiency causes a feedback increase in ACTH. The hyperpigmentation is caused by ACTH which is structurally similar to melanocyte stimulating hormone (MSH) and also has MSH activity.

### Compare and contrast primary and secondary adrenal in sufficiency.

| SIMILARITIES |
| --- |
| Both are associated with deficiencies of cortisol and DHEA. |

| DIFFERENCES | |
| --- | --- |
| **Primary adrenal deficiency** | **Secondary adrenal deficiency** |
| Occurs due to destruction of adrenals by tuberculosis, cancer or autoimmune diseases | Occurs due to decreased ACTH secretion |
| Associated with aldosterone deficiency | Not associated with aldosterone deficiency |
| Associated with skin pigmentation due to high circulating levels of ACTH | Not associated with skin Pigmentation |

### Outline the clinical features of Cushing's syndrome.

Cushing's syndrome can be caused by partially autonomous pituitary tumors secreting ACTH (**ACTH-dependent Cushing's syndrome**) or by autonomous adrenal or ectopic tumors secreting cortisol (**ACTH-independent Cushing's syndrome**). ACTH-independent Cushing's syndrome is associated with feedback suppression of ACTH secretion.

Major clinical manifestations of Cushing's syndrome (**hypercorti-solism**) include *hypertension* due to Na$^+$ retention, *hyperglycemia* (due to gluconeogenesis insulin resistance, and hyper-insulinemia), *increased plasma levels of DHEA* and *increased urinary excretion of 17-ketosteroids*. Other features include *osteoporosis*, weight gain with *centripetal obesity, muscle wasting* and weakness. *Sex-related problems* include amenorrhea and hirsutism (in women) impotency (in men) and decreased libido (in both). *Psychological problems* include depression, irritability, insomnia, psychosis, manic depression.

Overall, glucocorticoids bring about a redistribution of fat together with an increase in total body fat. There is characteristic centripetal distribution of fat i.e., an accumulation of fat in the central axis of the body (**truncal obesity**) with wasting of the extremities. As the thin skin of the abdomen is stretched by the increased subcutaneous depot, the subdermal tissues rupture to form prominent **reddish-purple stria**. The deposition of fat in the facies is called "**moon face**." The deposition of fat in the suprascapular region is referred to as "**buffalo hump**" or "**dowager's hump**" (dowager = elderly woman). Excessive fat distribution leads to a *pendulous abdomen*. Chronic excess of glucocorticoids lead to *hyperlipidemia and hypercholesterolemia*.

### Outline the clinical features of Conn's syndrome.

Conn's syndrome (**primary aldosteronism**) results from the excessive aldosterone secretion in patients with *aldosterone-producing adenoma* (APA). Patients of Conn's syndrome have *hypokalemia*, which impairs insulin secretion and results in *glucose intolerance* or overt diabetes. Although aldosterone causes salt and water retention, patients of Conn's syndrome *rarely exhibit edema* owing to Na$^+$ "escape," – the **escape phenomenon** – in which the Na$^+$-retaining effects of chronic aldosteronism are lost, possibly mediated by a compensatory increase in atrial natriuretic peptide (ANP) secretion.

### What is secondary hyperaldosteronism?

Secondary hyperaldosteronism occurs in conditions like *congestive heart failure, nephrosis* and *cirrhosis of liver*. These conditions are associated with the activation of renin–angiotensin system. The high levels of circulating angiotensin-II stimulate aldosterone secretion.

### What are the indications and precautions of cortico-steroid therapy?

Adrenocorticosteroids are used for **substitution therapy** in primary or secondary *adrenal insufficiency*. They are also used in numerous non-endocrine conditions. Corticosteroids have both anti-inflammatory and immunosuppressive effects and therefore are used in the treatment of *chronic inflammatory disorders with immunologic etiology* like rheumatoid arthritis, collagen disorders etc. Due to their anti-allergic effects, they are used in *bronchial asthma* and *skin diseases*. Due to their antilymphocytic effect, they are used in malignancies like *lymphocytic leukemias and lymphomas*. They are also used in *breast cancers*, which are aggravated by estrogens. This is because corticosteroids suppress adrenocortical activity by feedback inhibition of ACTH secretion. The adrenal cortex therefore produces less androgens that are precursors to estrogens.

Since corticosteroids reduce edema, they are used in *cerebral edema*. Patients of *cerebral stroke* are administered corticosteroids almost immediately on their arrival to the emergency wards. The stress associated with the cerebral stroke tends to cause stress ulcers, and the administration of corticosteroids aggravates them. Hence, antacids are administered *simultaneously with steroid therapy*. Since glucocorticoids enhance the vascular responsiveness to vasoactive substances like norepinephrine, they are frequently administered in *circulatory shock* along with other drugs.

An important precaution that has to be observed during long-term therapy with corticosteroids is that the therapy should not be stopped suddenly. *Abrupt cessation of steroid therapy is associated with life-threatening adrenal insufficiency*. Hence, the dose of the steroid must be slowly decreased i.e., *tapered*. Full recovery from hypothalamic-hypophysial-adrenocortical suppression may require as long as 1 year following cessation of all steroid therapy.

# 98

# Adrenomedullary Hormones

### What are the secretions of the adrenal medulla?

The adrenal medulla synthesizes and secretes bioactive amines called **catecholamines**. The catecholamines secreted by the adrenal medulla are epinephrine and norepinephrine. **Epinephrine** is produced almost exclusively in the adrenal medulla, with smaller amounts synthesized in the brain. **Norepinephrine** is widely distributed in neural tissues, including the adrenal medulla, sympathetic postganglionic fibers, and central nervous system (CNS).

### Outline the synthesis of catecholamines.

The precursor of all catecholamines is **L-tyrosine**, which is *derived from the diet* or from the hepatic *hydroxylation of L-phenylalanine* by **phenylalanine hydroxylase**. Tyrosine is hydroxylated to L-dopa in the cytoplasm by **tyrosine hydroxylase**. *Tyrosine hydroxylase is the rate-limiting enzyme* in the overall biosynthesis of epinephrine. Dopa is converted in the cytosol to **dopamine** by **dopa decarboxylase**. *Dopamine enters the chromaffin granule, where it is converted to **L-norepinephrine** by **dopamine-β-hydroxylase**, which exists exclusively in the chromaffin granules of the adrenomedullary chromaffin cells and sympathetic nerve endings.

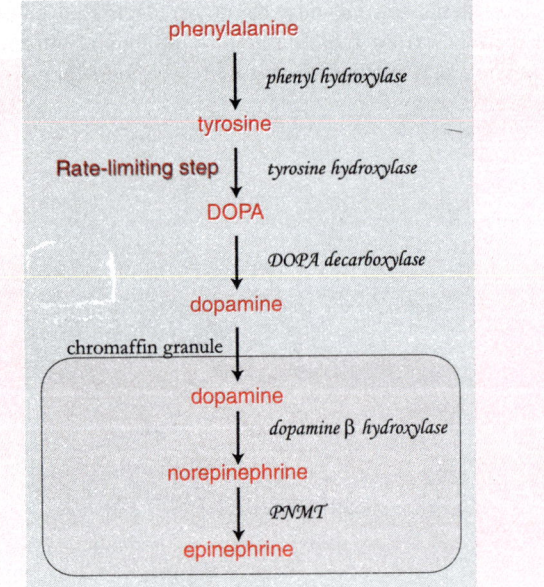

**Fig. 98.1**

In about 80% of chromaffin cells, norepinephrine is further methylated by **phenylethanolamine-N-methyltansferase** (PNMT) to **epinephrine**. Epinephrine is not secreted in significant amounts by neurons. This is because *PNMT is present in significant concentrations only in the adrenal medulla* (Fig. 98.1).

### What are the facts stimulating catecholamine secretion regulated?

The adrenal medulla and the sympathetic nervous system are in emergency (**fight-or-flight**) situations. Stimuli activating the sympathetic nervous system are fear, anxiety, pain, trauma, hemorrhage and fluid loss, asphyxia and hypoxia, changes in blood pH, extreme cold or heat, severe exercise, hypoglycemia, and hypotension. Anger is associated with increased norepinephrine secretion. Anxiety is associated with increased epinephrine secretion. In asphyxia and hypoxia, more norepinephrine is secreted. In hemorrhage, more epinephrine is secreted. In emotional stresses to familiar situations, norepinephrine secretion increases. In emotional stresses to uncertain situations, epinephrine secretion increases.

### What are the metabolites of catecholamines?

Catecholamines are sequentially metabolized by two enzymes: **catechol-O-methyltransferase (COMT)** and **monoamine oxidase (MAO)**. After both enzyme-system have acted, the final products are **VMA** (vinillyl-mandelic acid) and **MHPG** (3-methoxy-4 hydroxy phenylglycol). However, depending upon which of them acts first, the intermediate metabolites are either **DOMA** (dihydroxymandelic acid) and **DHPG** (dihydroxyphenyl glycol) or **metanephrines** and **normetanephrine** (Fig. 98.2). Circulating catecholamines are mostly excreted as metanephrine and normetanephrine. Norepinephrine in nerve ending is mostly excreted as VMA and MHPG.

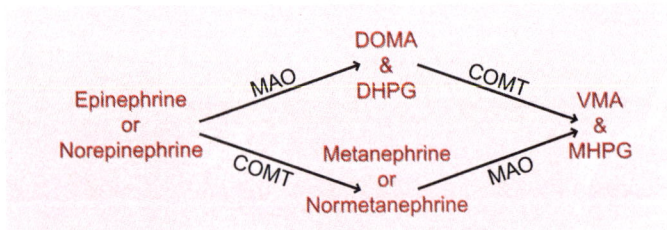

**Fig. 98.2**

### What is the importance of adrenergic receptors?

The effects of adrenomedullary stimulation and sympathetic nerve stimulation generally are similar. However, in some tissues, epinephrine and norepinephrine produce different effects owing to the existence of two types of adrenergic receptors, **alpha** (α) and **beta** (β) receptors, which have different sensitivities for the various catecholamines and, therefore, produce different responses. Epinephrine acts equally on both α and β receptors.

Norepinephrine acts practically on α-receptors alone. The α-**adrenergic receptors** are mostly excitatory but they inhibit gastrointestinal motility. The β-**adrenergic receptors** are associated with most of the inhibitory functions of the body (through $\beta_2$ receptors) but are excitatory to the myocardium (through $\beta_1$ receptors).

### What are the physiological actions of catecholamines?

Catecholamines help to prepare the individual to cope with emergencies but are *not* essential for life. In general, epinephrine and norepinephrine mimic the effects of sympathetic nervous discharge. The effects broadly comprise the *cardiovascular and metabolic* ones. They also have *central nervous* effects. Both *increase alertness*. Epinephrine evokes anxiety and fear.

**Cardiovascular effects.** *Epinephrine* stimulates both α and β receptors. The α-induced vasoconstriction is more than nullified by the β-induced vasodilatation. Hence, the *peripheral resistance and diastolic BP remain unchanged or fall slightly*. The β-induced increase in stroke volume and heart rate results in higher cardiac output, a rise in systolic BP and a widening of pulse pressure. *Norepinephrine* has much greater effect on α than on β receptors. Hence, it produces vasoconstriction with a *rise in peripheral resistance and diastolic BP*. Due to weak β-activation, direct cardiac stimulation are insignificant. Rather, there is *reflex decrease in heart rate* due to the rise in diastolic BP.

**Metabolic effects.** (i) Catecholamines stimulate **glycogenolysis**. α-*adrenergic* receptor stimulates glycogenolysis *in the liver* while β-*adrenergic* receptor stimulates glycogenolysis *in muscle*. Liver *contains* glucose-6-phosphatase, and hence hepatic glycogenolysis is associated with *release of free glucose into blood stream*. Muscle *lacks* glucose-6-phosphatase, and epinephrine-induced glycogenolysis in muscle *does not release free glucose into blood stream*. Instead, glycogenolysis ends with the formation of glucose-6-phosphate. However, the glucose-6-phosphate is metabolized to lactate or pyruvate, which is *converted to glucose by the liver* and released into blood.

(ii) Epinephrine *suppresses insulin secretion* (α-adrenergic effect) and *stimulates glucagon secretion* (β-adrenergic effect). It also *inhibits insulin-mediated facilitated diffusion of glucose* by muscle and adipose tissue. (iii) Epinephrine stimulates **lipolysis** by stimulating *hormone-sensitive lipase* via β-adrenergic receptor. Free fatty acids mobilized from stores in adipose tissue are converted in the liver to acetoacetate and β-hydroxybutyrate. These are released in the blood stream and reach the peripheral tissues, where they are quantitatively important as energy sources. (iv) Catecholamines cause a biphasic (a large, immediate and a small, delayed) rise in the **metabolic rate** and **body temperature**. The immediate rise is possibly due to increased muscular activity, and/or due to cutaneous vasoconstriction, which decreases heat loss leading to a rise in body temperature. The delayed rise that is probably due to oxidation of lactate (released during muscle activity) in the liver.

### Compare and contrast the cardiovascular effects of epinephrine and norepinephrine.

| Epinephrine | Norepinephrine |
|---|---|
| Stimulates the heart through β-receptors. | Due to weak β-activation, cardiac stimulation is insignificant. |
| Due to stimulation of both α and β receptors, peripheral resistance and diastolic BP remains unchanged or falls slightly. | Due to predominant α activation, peripheral resistance and diastolic BP increases. |
| Due to direct stimulation of heart, there is increased stroke volume and heart rate. | The reflex inhibition of sympathetic discharge (due to high diastolic BP) results in reduced heart rate and stroke volume. |

### What is pheochromocytoma? Outline its clinical features.

Pheochromocytoma is a **chromaffin-cell tumor** that secretes large amounts of catecholamines. Most pheochromocytomas secrete predominantly norepinephrine. 90% of pheochromocytomas are benign. They are treated by surgical removal of the tumor. Pheochromocytoma patients have **hypertension** and are prone to **orthostatic hypotension**. The hypersecretion of catecholamines is also associated with severe headache, sweating (**cold sweating** or **adrenergic sweating**), palpitations, chest pain, extreme anxiety, pallor of the skin caused by vasoconstriction, and blurred vision. If epinephrine is secreted primarily, the *heart rate is increased*. If norepinephrine is the predominant hormone, the *heart rate decreases reflexly* in response to marked hypertension. The *urinary excretion of catecholamines, metanephrines, and VMA are increased* in pheochromocytomas.

# 99

# Pancreatic Hormones

### Name the cells of endocrine pancreas and the hormones they secrete.

The endocrine pancreas consists of approximately one million islets of Langerhans, each islet consists of approximately 3000 cells. Four types of cells have been identified in the islets: **A cells** make up about 25% of the islet cells and are the source of glucagon. **B cells** constitute about 60% of the islet cells and are associated with insulin synthesis. **D cells** form about 10% of the islet cells and are the source of somatostatin. **Pancreatic polypeptide** (PP or F) **cells** form approximately 5% of the islet cells and synthesize a polypeptide that inhibits digestion of food in several ways.

### How is insulin secretion controlled?

**Carbohydrates**. The *principal stimulus for insulin release is glucose*. As the blood glucose level rises above 80 mg/dl, it stimulates the release and synthesis of insulin.

**Aminoacids**. B cells are also stimulated by certain essential amino acids like arginine, lysine, and phenylalanine.

**Hormones**. Gastrointestinal hormones, like gastrin, secretion, cholecystokinin and gastric inhibitory peptide (GIP) stimulate insulin secretion. Glucagon and growth hormone (GH) stimulate insulin secretion and somatostatin inhibits insulin secretion. Several hormones, like corticosteroids, estrogens, progesterone and parathyroid hormone have an anti-insulin effect and thereby induce a compensatory increase in insulin secretion.

**Other factors**. Both $K^+$ and $Ca^{2+}$ are necessary for normal insulin response to glucose. Hypokalemia leads to glucose intolerance. *Obesity is associated with insulin resistance* and compensatory hyperinsulinemia. cAMP is a releaser of insulin.

### Explain why oral glucose or aminoacid stimulates greater insulin release than when administered intravenously.

Oral glucose stimulates the secretion of gastrointestinal hormones like gastric inhibitory peptide (GIP), gastrin, secretin and cholecystokinin (CCK). These hormones potentiate insulin release. GIP is the main gastrointestinal potentiator of insulin release. Gastrin, secretion and CCK also potentiate the insulin secretion stimulated by orally administered aminoacids.

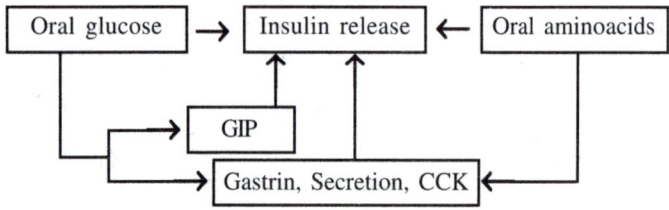

### Enumerate the effects of insulin on carbohydrate metabolism.

(1) In the **liver**, insulin *diminishes hepatic glucose output* by activating glycogen synthetase and by inhibiting gluconeogenesis. (2) In **muscle**, insulin (i) promotes glucose uptake by stimulating GLUT-4 and thereby increasing the facilitated diffusion of glucose; (ii) increases glycogen synthesis by stimulating glycogen synthetase; (iii) increases glucose utilization by stimulating phosphofructokinase. (3) In **adipose tissue**, insulin increases glucose uptake by stimulating GLUT-4. Increased glucose uptake leads to increased glucose metabolism in fat cells and formation of $\alpha$-glycerophosphate, which is a precursor for triglyceride synthesis.

### Enumerate the effects of insulin on fat metabolism.

Insulin is a *lipogenic* and an *antilipolytic* hormone. (1) In the liver, insulin (i) promotes fat synthesis; (ii) exerts a potent antiketogenic effect. (iii) promotes the synthesis and release of **lipoprotein lipase,** which is an extracellular enzyme that hydrolyzes both chylomicron and very-low-density lipoprotein (VLDL) triglyceride into fatty acids and glycerol. (2) In adipose tissue, insulin-stimulated glucose uptake in human fat cells provides $\alpha$-glycerophosphate for esterification of free fatty acids.

### Enumerate the effects of insulin on amino acid and protein metabolism.

Insulin is an important *protein-anabolic hormone* and is necessary for the assimilation of a protein meal. Insulin increases uptake of most amino acids into muscle and increases the incorporation of amino acids into protein. Insulin increases body protein stores through four mechanisms: (i) increased tissue uptake of amino acids; (ii) increased protein synthesis; (iii) decreased protein catabolism; and (iv) decreased oxidation of amino acids.

### What is the effect of insulin on electrolyte metabolism?

Insulin lowers serum $K^+$ concentration and also has an antinatriuretic effect. The hypokalemic action of insulin is caused by stimulation of $K^+$ uptake by muscle and hepatic tissue. Diabetic patients tend to develop hyperkalemia as $K^+$ move out of the cells into the ECF.

### How is glucagon secretion controlled?

The two main controllers of glucagon secretion are metabolic substrates and gastrointestinal hormones. (1) Glucagon secretion is stimulated by hypoglycemia. Amino acids like arginine and alanine also stimulate glucagon release. Fatty acids inhibit glucagon release. (2) CCK, gastrin, secretin, and gastric inhibitory peptide stimulate glucagon secretion. The potentiation of glucagon secretion by the ingestion of a protein meal is mediated by CCK secretion.

## What are the metabolic actions of glucagon?

The major site of action of glucagon is the liver. In almost all aspects the actions of glucagon are the exact opposite to those of insulin. (1) Glucagon has a hyperglycemic action, resulting from stimulation of hepatic glycogenolysis and gluconeogenesis. (2) Glucagon is a lipolytic hormone because of its activation of hormone-sensitive lipase (triglyceride lipase) in adipose tissue. Glucagon causes an elevation in the plasma level of fatty acids and glycerol. The glycerol is utilized as a gluconeogenic substrate in the liver. The fatty acids are oxidized to provide energy, thereby accounting for the glucose-sparing effect of glucagon. Glucagon is also essential for the ketogenesis brought about by the oxidation of fatty acids. (3) Glucagon causes increased amino acid oxidation and urea formation (proteolytic effect) and inhibits protein synthesis (antianabolic effect), leading to a net negative nitrogen balance.

## What is somatostatin and what are its functions?

Somatostatin is a decapeptide secreted by the D cells of the pancreatic islets and similar D cells in the gastrointestinal mucosa. It is also secreted by the neurosecretory neurons of hypothalamus and other areas of the nervous system. Most of the factors that stimulate insulin secretion (e.g., glucose, arginine, leucine, CCK) also stimulate the secretion of somatostatin. In the nervous system, somatostatin functions as a peptidergic neurotransmitter. Somatostatin inhibits the secretion of several hormone including GH, TSH, insulin, glucagon and gastrin. It also reduces intestinal absorption of glucose. It produces a decrease in blood glucose concentration.

Somatostatin is secreted not only into the blood stream but also into the gastric lumen. Its secretion is stimulated by acid in the lumen. The somatostatin secreted into the gastric lumen mixes with the gastric juice. Thereafter, it acts on the gastric mucosa to inhibit gastrin secretion. It is probable that the inhibitory effect of gastric acid on gastrin secretion is mediated by somatostatin.

The above action of somatostatin is an example of **paracrine control**, wherein a secretion diffuses though the ECF to affect neighboring cells some distance away. Somatostatin also inhibits pancreatic exocrine secretion, gastric acid secretion and motility, gallbladder contraction and the absorption of glucose, amino acids, and triglycerides.

Acid in the gastric lumen

↓

Stimulation of D cells in gastric mucosa

↓

Somatostatin secretion into gastric lumen

↓

Stimulation of gastric mucosa by somatostatin

↓

Inhibition of gastrin secretion

## Outline the pathophysiology and clinical features of diabetes mellitus.

In diabetes mellitus, **hyperglycemia** occurs due to reduced entry of glucose into the cells (*decreased peripheral utilization*) and more importantly, due to the *deranged glucostatic functions of the liver*. (2) The hyperglycemia causes **glycosuria** and osmotic diuresis leading to **polyuria** and **polydipsia**. (3) Intracellular glucose deficiency, which occurs in all cells of the body, also occurs in the cells of hypothalamic satiety center, resulting in **polyphagia**. (4) The rate at which aminoacids are catabolized to $CO_2$ and $H_2O$ is increased and protein synthesis is reduced, leading to a **negative nitrogen balance**, protein depletion and wasting. Protein depletion is also associated with **poor resistance to infection**. (5) The plasma cholesterol level is elevated which plays a role in the accelerated development of **atherosclerosis** and vascular diseases. (6) Due to accelerated lipid breakdown, there is excess formation of acetyl CoA that is converted in the liver to acetoacetate, resulting in **ketosis** and **acetone breath**. (7) The large amounts of acetoacetic acid and β-hydroxy butyric acid (ketone bodies) result in **acidosis**. The acidosis stimulates hyperventilation, known clinically as **Kussmaul breathing**. (8) **Coma** results from acidosis, dehydration and hyperosmolarity of plasma.

## Compare and contrast type 1 and type 2 diabetes mellitus.

| Characteristic | Type 1 | Type 2 |
|---|---|---|
| Earlier names | Insulin-dependent diabetes mellitus (IDDM), auto-immune diabetes | Non-insulin-dependent diabetes mellitus (NIDDM). |
| Circulating islet cell antibodies | Present | Absent |
| Body weight | Nonobese | Obese |
| Onset | Abrupt | Slow |
| Age at onset | Usually < 30 years | Usually > 40 years |
| Ketoacidosis | Common | Rare |
| Circulating insulin levels | Low | Sometimes elevated |
| Inflammatory cells in islets | Present | Absent |
| Islet cell mass | Markedly decreased | Normal or slightly decreased |
| Insulin response | Sensitive | Resistant |
| Cardinal signs | Polyuria, polydipsia, polyphagia | Obesity, hyperphagia, and physical inactivity. |

# 100

# Testicular & Ovarian Hormones

### Name the major hormones secreted by the testis.

The hormone secreting cells in the testis are the *Leydig cells* and *Sertoli cells*. The major hormones produced by the testes are **testosterone, dihydrotestosterone** (DHT) and **androstenedione**. Most of the DHT is however produced peripherally by the action of *5α reductase* on testosterone. The testis also produces **estradiol** in small amounts. It is produced by the action of *aromatase* on testosterone.

### How are androgens synthesized?

Testicular steroidogenesis occurs in the Leydig cell and is similar to the biosynthetic pathway for adrenocortical steroids (Fig. 100.1).

produced by the Sertoli cells inhibit testosterone production by Leydig cells. (ii) High intratubular testosterone levels are essential for normal spermatogenesis. **Endocrine**. (i) FSH is necessary for normal spermatogenesis. FSH promotes the synthesis of androgen-binding protein (ABP) by Sertoli cells. ABP binds testosterone, increasing its local concentration, which supports spermatogenesis. (ii) FSH indirectly affects testosterone synthesis by increasing the number of LH receptors on the Leydig cell. (iii) GnRH controls testosterone secretion by stimulating the release of *both* LH and FSH from the anterior pituitary. GnRH secretion is pulsatile occurring at a frequency of 8 to 14 pulses per day. (iii) LH stimulates the Leydig cells and increases

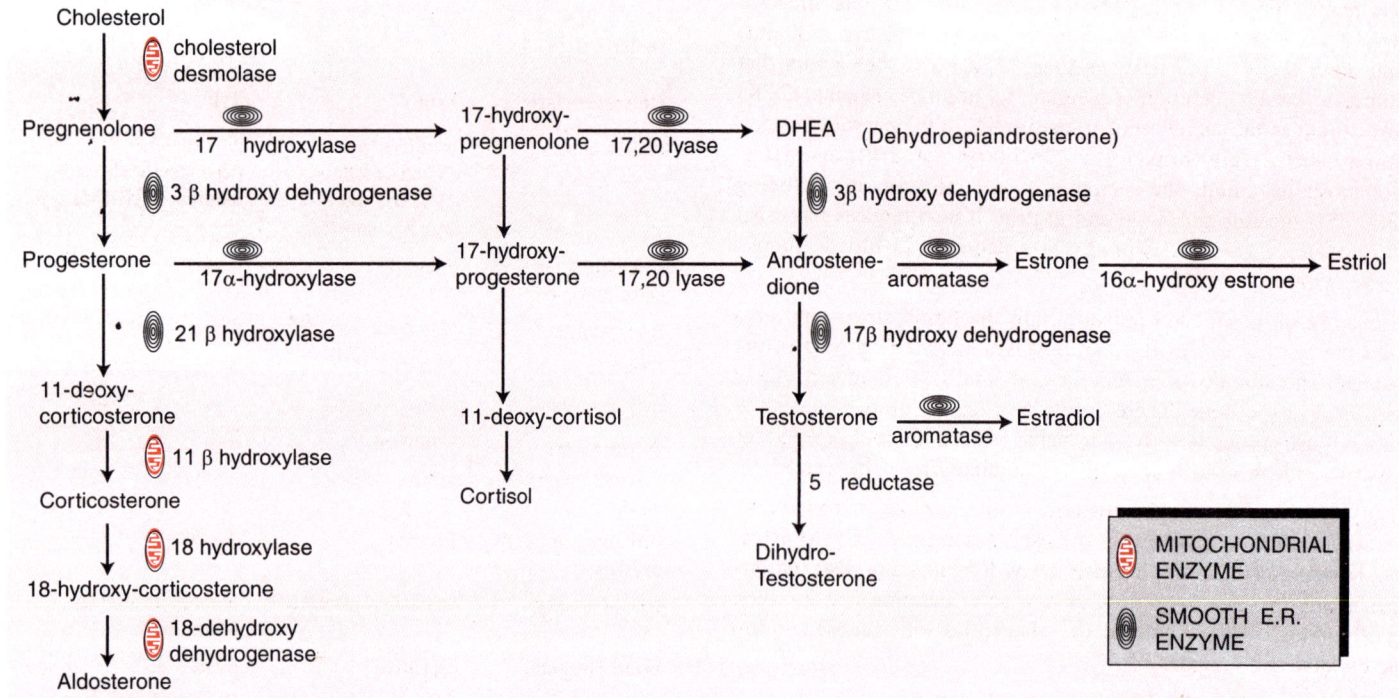

**Fig. 100.1**

### Name the metabolites of testosterone.

Testosterone is metabolized into *active metabolites* like DHT and estradiol as well as *inactive metabolites* like 17-ketosteroids. DHT too ultimately metabolized to 17-ketosteroids.

### Enumerate the factors affecting testosterone secretion

The factors affecting testosterone can be categorized as autocrine, paracrine, endocrine and neuroendocrine. **Autocrine**. Androgens produced by the Leydig cells exert autocrine control on its own testosterone biosynthesis. **Paracrine**. (i) Inhibin and estrogens

testosterone synthesis. (iv) Insulin, prolactin and thyroxin have direct stimulatory effects on Leydig cells. **Neuroendocrine**. Opiates, neuropeptides and neurotransmitters affect GnRH secretion and thereby, the secretion of testosterone.

### Why does normal spermatogenesis require both FSH and LH?

Neither LH nor FSH acts on the spermatogonia themselves. Yet, *normal spermatogenesis requires both LH and FSH*. This is because normal spermatogenesis requires a high local concentration of testosterone. The testosterone is secreted by the Leydig cells, which are *stimulated by LH*. The maintenance of a high local concentration of testosterone requires the secretion of (ABP) by the Sertoli cells, which are *stimulated by FSH* (Fig. 100.2).

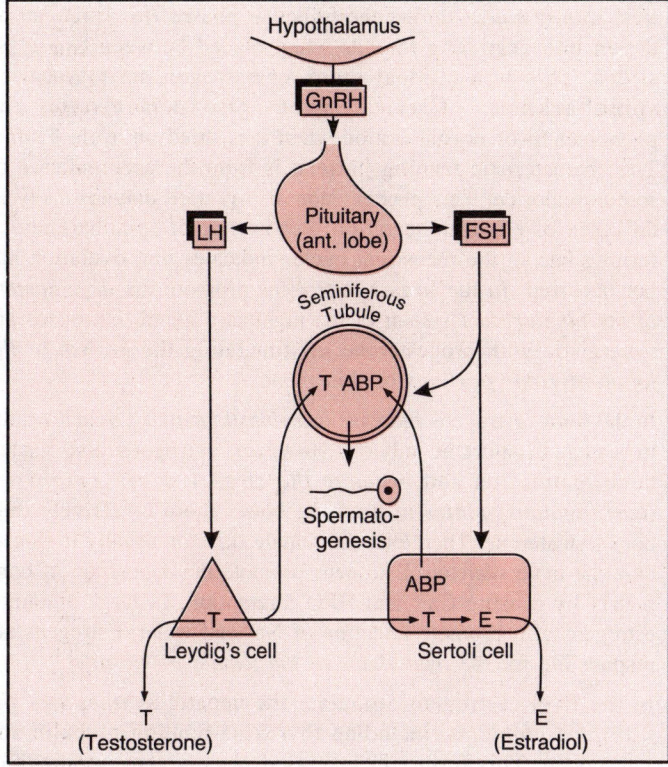

**Fig. 100.2**

# What are the feedback mechanisms involved in the hormonal control of testicular functions?

(i) There is *feedback inhibition of LH secretion* by testosterone and estradiol. The negative feedback effects of estradiol are at both the hypothalamic (GnRH) and pituitary (LH) levels, while that of testosterone is mainly at the hypothalamic (GnRH) level. (ii) FSH promotes the synthesis of **inhibin** by Sertoli cells. At the same time, there is *feedback inhibition of FSH secretion by inhibin*, which acts at the level of pituitary. Inhibin does not suppress GnRH secretion. The rise in plasma FSH levels following damage to seminiferous tubules occurs due to reduced inhibin secretion. Physiologic levels of *testosterone do not produce significant feedback inhibition* of FSH secretion (Fig. 100.3).

## Does exogenous testosterone promote spermatogenesis?

*Exogenous* testosterone *does not promote* spermatogenesis. Spermatogenesis requires that a high concentration of testosterone be produced locally by LH action on Leydig cells. Rather, by inhibiting LH secretion, exogenous testosterone tends to depress spermatogenesis.

## Describe the physiologic effects of testosterone.

(1) Testosterone stimulates the **differentiation** of the male *internal* genitalia. It stimulates differentiation of the Wolffian duct system into the epididymis, vas deferens, and seminal vesicles. (2) During

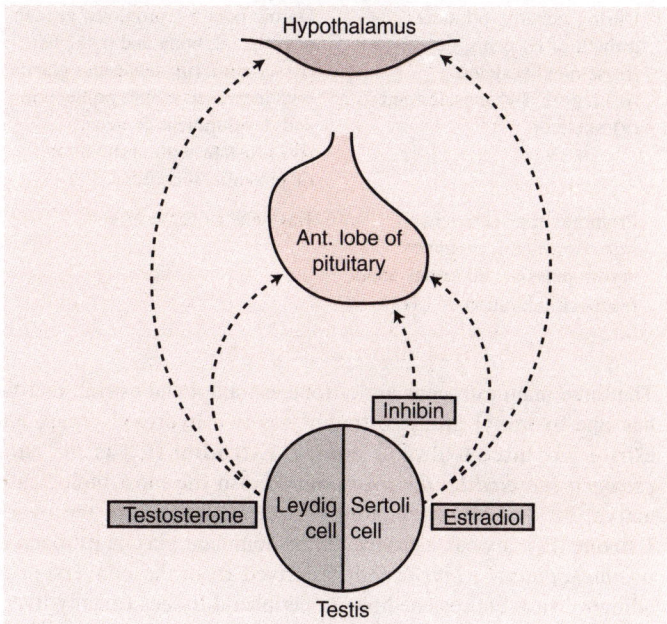

**Fig. 100.3**

puberty, it stimulates the development of the **secondary sexual characteristics**, libido and potency (erectile functions). (3) Testosterone is essential for normal **spermatogenesis**. In the absence of an adequate local concentration of testosterone in the testis, the sperm count decreases. (4) Testosterone is a **protein anabolic hormone**. It stimulates cell division as well as tissue growth and maturation. The anabolic effect in muscle is referred to as the *myotrophic effect*. In the adolescent, it produces linear growth, muscular development, and retention of nitrogen, potassium, and phosphorus. Testosterone also accelerates epiphysial fusion of the long bones. Testosterone is responsible for the broad shoulders in males. Treatment with testosterone prevents bone loss and osteoporosis. (5) Testo-sterone stimulates **erythropoiesis** directly and by stimulating erythropoietin secretion. (6) Testosterone inhibits LH secretion.

## What is DHT and how is DHT formed?

DHT (dihydrotestosterone) is the active metabolite of testosterone. It is formed in some target cells by the action of 5α reductase on testosterone. The enzyme 5α reductase exists in two forms: type-1 and type-2. Type-1 is present in the skin, especially the scalp. Type-2 is present in genital tissues. It brings about differentiation of the external genitalia in the fetus. During puberty, it brings about the skin changes.

## Compare and contrast the effects of testosterone and DHT.

**SIMILARITIES**

Both are androgens that are important in sexual differentiation of the male fetus and later, in male pubertal changes.

**DIFFERENCES**

| Testosterone | Dihydrotestosterone |
|---|---|
| Necessary for the differentiation of the internal genitalia | Necessary for the differentiation of the external genitalia. |

| | |
|---|---|
| During puberty, promotes growth of (i) penis, (ii) seminal vesicles, (iii) larynx, (iv) muscles and (v) skeleton. | During puberty, promotes growth of (i) facial, body and pubic hair, (ii) scrotum, (iii) sebaceous glands with increased sebum production and development of acne, (iv) prostate with stimulation of prostatic secretions. |
| Promotes spermatogenesis, increases libido, promotes erythropoiesis, and brings about feedback inhibition of LH. | Has none of these effects. |

### What are the three main estrogens?

The three main estrogens are estrone, estradiol and estriol. Estrone has one hydroxyl group, estradiol has two hydroxyl group, and estriol has three hydroxyl groups. **Estradiol** ($E_2$) is *the main estrogen secreted by the ovary* and is also the most biologically active. 90% of the circulating estradiol comes from the ovary. **Estrone** ($E_1$), a weak estrogen, is the dominant plasma estrogen *in postmenopausal women*, and is derived from the conversion of adrenocortical androstenedione in peripheral tissues (mainly liver). In premenopausal women, it is much lesser, and is derived mostly from estradiol. **Estriol** ($E_3$), which is the dominant plasma estrogen *during pregnancy*, is secreted by the placenta. *Estriol is not secreted by the ovary.* In non-pregnant women, estriol is formed in small amounts in the liver from estradiol and estrone.

### Which are the ovarian cells that secrete hormones?

Three types of ovarian cells are involved in hormone secretion: the granulosa cells, luteal cells and thecal cells (cells of theca interna). The **thecal cells** produce androstenedione and testosterone. These are converted in the **granulosa cells** to estrone and estradiol respectively by the enzyme *aromatase*. **Luteal cells** produce progesterone and some estradiol.

### Briefly outline the hormonal control of ovarian function.

The development of the ovarian follicle is largely under the control of FSH. *Ovulation is caused by LH.* Under the influence of LH, the ruptured *Graafian follicle luteinizes* and the corpus luteum that is formed *secretes progesterone.* Depending on the dose and timing estrogen can either inhibit or stimulate the secretion of LH through both negative and positive feedback controls. Progesterone can also either stimulate or inhibit GnRH secretion.

### Enumerate the physiologic effects of estrogens.

Estrogens have important **protein anabolic effects**. Estrogens mediate the *growth and development of the maternal reproductive organs*, especially, that of the gravid uterus. They also promote cellular proliferation in the mucosal linings of these structures. The estrogenic effects of pregnancy are primarily caused by estradiol, the most potent of the estrogens.

In the **endometrium**, estrogens stimulate the *regeneration of the stratum functionalis* during the proliferative phase of the endometrial cycle by increasing mitosis. The water content and blood flow to the endometrium are increased markedly. The *spiral arterioles of the stratum functionalis grow rapidly.* In the myometrium, estrogens increase the amount of contractile proteins (i.e., actin and myosin) and thereby, *increase spontaneous muscular contractions.* Estrogens also *sensitize the myometrium to the action of oxytocin*, which promotes uterine contractility. In the **cervix**, estrogens stimulate the secretion of large amounts of *thin, watery mucus* during the follicular phase. This fluid can be drawn into very long threads when placed between two glass slides. This is a clinical index of estrogen activity called **spinnbarkheit**. Cervical mucus also demonstrates the phenomenon of crystallization when it is dried on a glass slide. The characteristic **ferning pattern** is from the accumulation of sodium chloride. This phenomenon also is used diagnostically as an index of estrogen secretion. Persistence of spinnbarkheit or ferning late in the menstrual cycles indicates that ovulation has not occurred. In the **breast**, estrogens promote the *development of the tubular duct system* of the mammary gland. Estrogens are synergistic with progesterone in stimulating the *growth of the lobuloalveolar portions* of this gland.

In the **bone**, estrogens *increase osteoblastic activity*, which results in a growth spurt at puberty. However, estrogens also hasten bone maturation and *promote the closure of the epiphysial (cartilaginous) plates* in the long bones more effectively than does testosterone. Therefore, the female skeleton usually is shorter than the male skeleton. Estrogens promote the deposition of bone matrix by causing $Ca^{2+}$ and $HPO_4^{2-}$ retention. In large amounts, estrogens also promote retention of $Na^+$ and water. Estrogens are responsible for the *oval shape of the female pelvic inlet.*

In the **liver**, estrogens stimulate the hepatic *synthesis of the transport globulins*, including thyroxine-binding globulin and transcortin. This results in increased plasma concentrations of thyroxine and cortisol but unchanged amounts of free thyroxine. Pregnant women often are in a state of mild hyperadrenocorticism because the elevated placental progesterone competes with cortisol for binding sites on transcortin, thus *increasing plasma free cortisol.*

### Enumerate the physiologic effects of progesterone.

(i) The **endometrium**, which proliferates under the influence of estrogens, becomes a secretory structure under the influence of progesterone. The *endometrial glands become elongated and coiled* and secrete a glycogen-rich fluid. It also converts the secretory endometrium of the luteal phase of the menstrual cycle to the decidua during pregnancy. Progesterone is essential for *implantation and maintenance of the decidua*. (ii) In the **cervix**, the *mucus secreted becomes thick and viscid* under the influence of progesterone. This consistency of cervical mucus indicates that ovulation and luteinization have occurred. (iii) In the **myometrium**, progesterone *inhibits uterine motility* by hyperpolarization of the uterine myometrium. (iv) In the **breast**, progesterone promotes *lobuloalveolar growth* in the mammary gland. (v) In the **fetus**, progesterone contributes to the growth and development by acting as a *precursor for corticosteroid synthesis* by the fetal adrenal cortex.

**Compare and contrast the effects of estrogen and progesterone.**

| ESTRADIOL | PROGESTERONE |
|---|---|
| **General**<br>Promotes development of female secondary sexual characteristics | **General**<br>Serves as a precursor for steroid hormones<br>Increases basal body temperature |
| **Pituitary-hypothalamus**<br>Inhibits FSH secretion by negative feedback<br>Sensitizes pituitary to secrete prolactin<br>Inhibits (at high levels) LH secretion by negative feedback<br>Stimulates midcycle surge of LH (and FSH) by positive feedback on pituitary | **Pituitary-hypothalamus**<br>Inhibits LH secretion by negative feedback<br>Stimulates midcycle FSH peak |
| **Vagina**<br>Causes thickening of vaginal mucosa | |
| **Mammary Glands**<br>Promotes development of lactiferous ductal system | **Mammary Glands**<br>Promotes alveolar growth and development of ductal system |
| **Ovary**<br>FSH increases FSH receptors on granulosa cells;<br>FSH (in presence of estradiol) increases LH receptors on granulosa cells; LH stimulates theca cells<br>Proliferation and development of granulosa cells | **Ovary**<br>Stimulates theca cells to secrete androgens<br>Inhibits further follicular development |
| **Uterus**<br>Promotes uterine growth: hypertrophy of myometrium and hyperplasia of endometrium<br>Causes thinning of cervical fluid (spinnbarkheit)<br>Up-regulates estradiol and progesterone receptors<br>Promotes uterine motility | **Uterus**<br>Arrests endometrial mitosis<br>Inhibits myometrial contraction<br>Induces secretory activity of endometrium<br>Increases viscosity of cervical fluid<br>Promotes maturation and differentiation of endometrium<br>Down-regulates estradiol and progesterone receptors |
| **Kidney**<br>Promotes renal $Na^+$ retention ("ferning" of cervical fluid) | **Uterus in Pregnancy**<br>Causes implantation (nidation) of the fertilized ovum (blastocyst)<br>Causes formation of decidua (decidualization) of maternal endometrium |
| **Bone**<br>Enhances bone growth, density, and maturation leading to epiphyseal closure | **Kidney**<br>Antagonizes the action of aldosterone on the kidney |

# Puberty & Gametogenesis

### Define the terms puberty, thelarche, pubarche, adrenarche and menarche.

**Puberty** or **adolescence** is that stage of development when the endocrine and gametogenic functions of the gonads develop, for the first time, to the point where reproduction is possible. It coincides with *a surge of sex hormone secretion* resulting in the development of the **secondary sexual characteristics**. In girls, the most striking events associated with the onset of puberty are **thelarche** (the development of breasts) followed by **pubarche** (development of axillary and pubic hair) and **menarche** (the first menstrual period). **Adrenarche** is *an increase in the secretion of adrenal androgens* occurring during puberty.

### What is meant by the term secular changes in pubertal onset?

Puberty generally occurs between the ages of *8 and 13 in girls* and *9 and 14 in boys*. It however seems that over the past couple of centuries, the age of onset has been declining at the rate of 1 – 3 months per decade. Such changes are called **secular changes**.

### Outline the salient male and female secondary sexual characters.

The male secondary sexual characteristics are as follows. **Genitalia**. Penis and scrotum increase in size and become pigmented; rugal folds appear in scrotal skin. **Hair**. Mustache and beard develop; scalp hair line undergoes temporal recession; pubic hair develops as a triangle with apex up; axillary and body hair appear. **Growth**. Pubertal growth spurt occurs; androgens interact with growth hormone to increase somatomedin levels. Shoulders broaden. **Accessory sex organs**. Prostate and seminal vesicles enlarge, and secretion begins. **Skin**. Sebaceous gland secretion thickens and increases, predisposing to acne. **Voice**. The pitch is lowered because of enlargement of larynx and thickening of vocal cords. **Psyche**. More aggressive attitudes are manifest; interest in opposite sex develops. **Muscle mass**. Muscle bulk and strength increase; there is positive nitrogen balance.

The female secondary sexual characteristics are as follows. **Genitalia**. Development of external genitalia; onset of menstruation. **Hair**. Pubic hair develops as a triangle with apex below; axillary hair appears. **Growth**. Pubertal growth spurt occurs; there is a female pattern of fat deposition. **Breast**. Development of breast occurs. **Psyche**. Interest in opposite sex develops.

### What is the mechanism of pubertal onset?

Till puberty, the GnRH secretion from the hypothalamus is highly sensitive to feedback inhibition by testosterone/estrogens. As a result, the level of testosterone/estrogen is never able to rise sufficiently high to induce puberty. From birth to puberty, the sensitivity of the hypothalamus to feedback inhibition by testosterone or estrogens decreases. By puberty, the hypothalamus does not remain highly sensitive to feedback inhibition by testosterone/estrogen and therefore is secreted in substantial amounts, and shows the normal pulsatile release of GnRH.

### What is the role of leptin in pubertal onset?

It is observed that young women often stop menstruating when they lose weight and resume menstruation once they regain weight. It therefore seems that a *critical body weight* is required for puberty to occur, and that **leptin**, a satiety-producing hormone secreted by fat cells, may be inhibitory to pubertal changes.

### What is precocious puberty and what causes it?

Early development of *secondary sexual characteristics without gametogenesis* is caused by abnormal exposure of immature males to androgen or females to estrogen. This syndrome is called **precocious pseudopuberty** to distinguish it from **true precocious puberty** due to an early but otherwise normal pubertal pattern of gonadotropin secretion from the pituitary. Hypothalamic diseases are frequently associated with precocious puberty. Some cases of precocious puberty occur without adequate gonadotropin secretion. These are called **gonadotropin-independent precocity** and are due to increased LH secretion from the anterior pituitary in response to stimulation by GnRH.

### What is the difference between primary and secondary amenorrhea?

Puberty is considered to be pathologically delayed if *menarche fails to occur by the age of 17* or *testicular development fails to occur by the age of 20*. Failure of maturation can occur in panhypopituitarism, and Turner's syndrome as well as in some individuals with no discernable problems.

### What is that condition in male that is equivalent to primary amenorrhea in females?

In males, the clinical picture that is equivalent to primary amenorrhea in females is called **eunuchoidism.**

### Where are the Leydig cells located? What do they secrete?

The **interstitial cells of Leydig** are located between the coils of seminiferous tubules. They are the endocrine cells *secreting testosterone*.

## What forms the blood-testis barrier? What is its significance?

The blood-testes barrier is formed by tight intracellular junctions between adjacent Sertoli cells in the seminiferous tubule (Fig. 101.1). The barrier separates the basal and adluminal compartments of the seminiferous tubule. All substances passing from the basal to the adluminal compartment therefore must pass through the cytoplasm of the Sertoli cell. Thus, the *germ cells also cross the barrier* as they pass from the basal compartment to the adluminal compartment. The tight junctions between Sertoli cells loosen up to enable passage of the maturing germ cells through the junction, only to tighten up after they have passed.

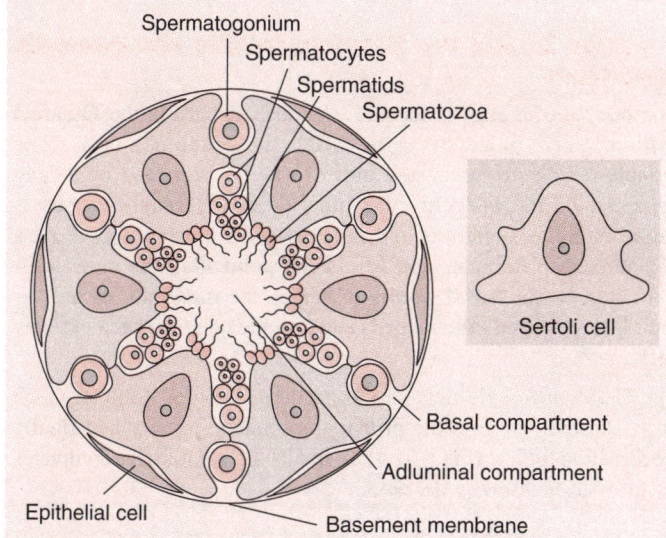

**Fig. 101.1**

The blood-testis barrier *protects the spermatocytes, spermatids and spermatozoa* from blood-borne toxic substance and circulating antibodies. It also *prevents byproducts of gametogenesis from entering circulation* lest they should stimulate an autoimmune reaction. Not unexpectedly, the breakdown of the barrier sometimes leads to autoimmune response against the germ cells. *Steroids penetrate the barrier with ease.*

The blood-testis barrier enables the seminiferous tubule to maintain a somewhat different composition of fluid inside its lumen. The fluid in the lumen of the seminiferous tubules contains very little protein and glucose but is rich in androgens, estrogens and $K^+$ ions.

## Enumerate the functions of the Sertoli cells.

(1) They stimulate the early mitosis and meiosis of the developing spermatozoa and provide them nourishment. Sertoli cells serve numerous functions. (2) The intercellular junctions between adjacent Sertoli cells *constitute the blood-testis barrier.* (3) They produce **inhibin**; (4) they secrete **androgen-binding globulin** (**ABP**) which has high affinity for testosterone and is responsible for the maintenance of high intra-tubular testosterone levels by concentrating testosterone in tubular lumen. (5) They produce **mullerian duct inhibiting factor** (**MIF**); (6) They also secrete **transferrin** for transporting iron to tubular cells; **ceruloplasmin** for transporting copper to the tubular cells; and **plasminogen activator** which may mediate proteolytic reactions important for

migration of maturing germ cells from the basal compartment to the adluminal compartment. (7) Sertoli cells *secrete small amounts of* **estrogens**. They *produce aromatase*, the enzyme which converts androgens produced by the Leydig cells to estrogens which although contribute little to the circulating pool, may play intra-testicular roles, e.g., it binds to specific receptors in the Leydig cells and inhibit androgen production. (8) They *absorb the unnecessary cellular organelles that are cast off from the spermatozoa.* (9) They have receptors for (and hence, are stimulated by) both FSH and LH.

## What are the 3 phases of spermatogenesis? Name the cells that are precursors to the mature spermatozoa.

The male gametes or the sperms are formed inside the **seminiferous tubules.** Male gametogenesis or **spermatogenesis** is the formation of mature sperms from the primitive germ cells or spermatogonia. Spermatogenesis has 3 phases: (i) mitotic multiplication of spermatogonia (stem cells) to form primary spermatocytes; (ii) meiosis leading to the formation of primary spermatids; and (iii) spermiogenesis, resulting in the formation of primary spermatozoa. Mature spermatozoa differentiate from spermatids (spermiogenesis), and cast off residual cytoplasm (Fig. 101.2).

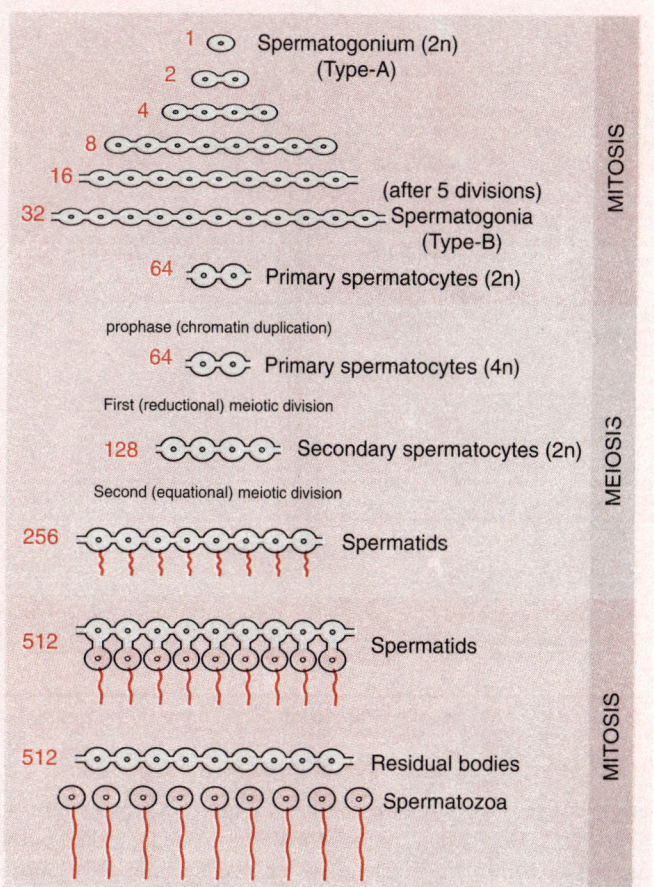

**Fig. 101.2**

## Define spermiogenesis. Enumerate the changes associated with spermiogenesis.

The term **spermiogenesis** refers to the *transformation of the spermatids into mature spermatocytes or sperms.* It is androgen-dependent. The spermatids mature into spermatozoa *inside the recesses in the membrane of the Sertoli cells.* Mature spermatozoa are released from the Sertoli cells and become free in the lumens of the tubules. Spermiogenesis involves the following transformation. (i) The Golgi apparatus is transformed to the acrosomes. (ii) The centrioles and mitochondria are transformed to the flagellae (sperm tails). (iii) Nuclear condensation protects the genome from the deleterious effects of mutagens in the foreign environment. (iv) Unnecessary cellular organelles are cast off from the spermatozoa as residual bodies. (v) The spermatozoa do not grow or divide any further.

### Describe the structure of a mature sperm.

Each sperm is a motile cell, rich in DNA, with a head that is made up mostly of chromosomal material. Covering the head like a cap is the **acrosome,** a lysosome-like organelle rich in enzymes involved in sperm penetration of the ovum and other events involved in fertilization. The motile tail of the sperm is wrapped in its proximal portion by a sheath holding numerous mitochondria. Mitochondria generate energy and are therefore important for movement of the spermatozoa. The flagella of the sperm tail originate from the basal body, which is a modified centriole (Fig. 101.3).

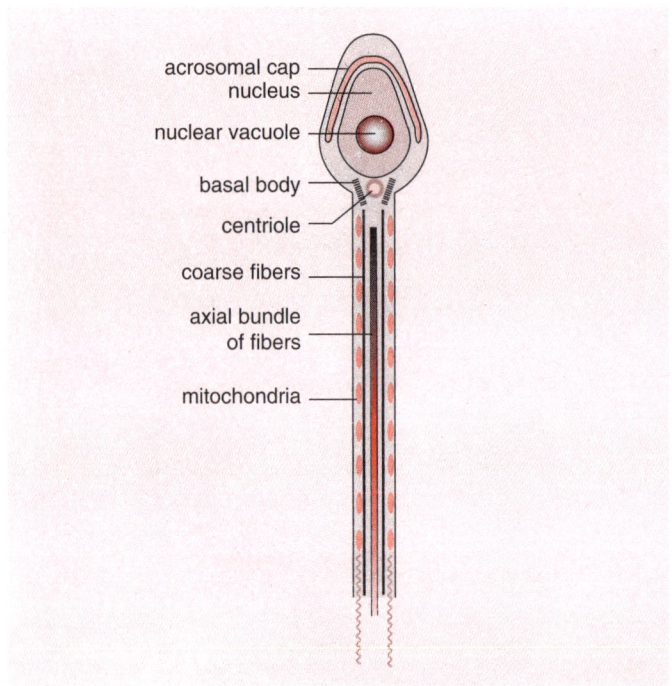

**Fig. 101.3**

### Enumerate the factors affecting spermatogenesis.

**Temperature**. Proper spermatogenesis requires a temperature of about 32°C. Hot baths and tight underwears reduce the sperm count. The following mechanisms ensure that the developing sperms are maintained at a body temperature lower than the body temperature. (i) The testes are located in the scrotum, which is outside the body cavity. Failure of testicular descent (**cryptorchidism**) results in sterility because of thermal damage to the spermatogonia. (ii) The temperature inside the scrotum is kept low by *evaporative cooling*. (iii) Warm arterial blood at 37°C

flowing into the testes tends to increase the testicular temperature. However, this tendency is minimized by the *countercurrent heat-exchanger mechanism* operating between the spermatic arteries and veins. **Seasonal variations**. There is a seasonal effect in men, with sperm counts being greater in the winter regardless of the temperature to which the scrotum is exposed. **Local testosterone concentration** must be adequate for normal spermatogenesis. It is maintained at high levels through the *counter current androgen exchange* between the spermatic arteries and veins. Androgen binding protein (ABP) also helps to maintain a high local concentration of testosterone **Age**. Sperm production continues till age 80 or 90, although the production rate slows down after age 40.

### Describe briefly the Graafian follicle and name its precursors.

The **oocyte** (the egg) is located eccentrically inside the Graafian follicle, surrounded by cells called the granulosa cells. The granulosa cells are organized into two layers separated by a fluid space called the **antrum**. The inner layer of granulosa cells is called cumulus oophorus and is separated from the oocyte by a structureless membrane called the **zona pellucida**. The outer layer is limited by the **basal lamina**. Outside the basal lamina are the multilayered **theca interna cells** and a single layer of **theca externa cells**.

The Graafian follicle develops from the primordial follicle which grow successively into the primary, secondary, tertiary and finally the Graafian follicle (Fig. 101.4). A small batch of follicles completes its growth *once every 28 days*.

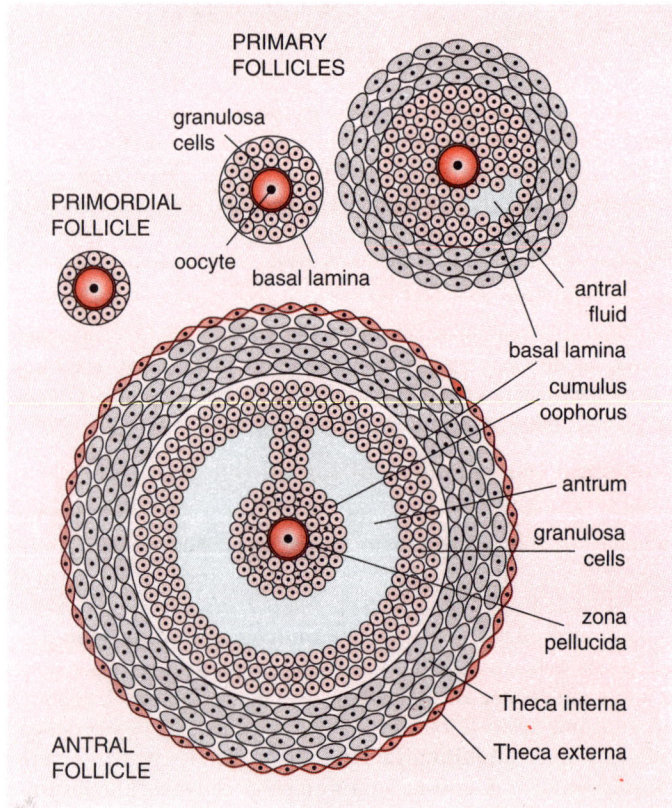

**Fig. 101.4**

## Describe briefly the ovarian cycle.

On about the sixth day, one of the follicles in one ovary starts growing rapidly and outgrows all the others, which then gradually start regressing through apoptosis. At about the *14th day of the cycle, the distended follicle ruptures*, and the ovum is extruded into the abdominal cavity. This is the process of **ovulation**. The ovum is *picked up by the fimbriated ends of the uterine tubes* and is transported to the uterus. If fertilization does not occur, the ovum is passed out through the vagina. The follicle that ruptures at the time of ovulation promptly fills with blood, forming a **corpus hemorrhagicum**. The granulosa and theca cells of the follicle lining promptly begin to proliferate, and the clotted blood is rapidly replaced with yellowish, lipid-rich **luteal cells**, forming the **corpus luteum**. The luteal cells secrete estrogens and progesterone. The fate of the corpus luteum depends on whether or not pregnancy occurs: *If pregnancy occurs*, the corpus luteum persists and serves as the major source of estrogen and progesterone till the 3rd month of pregnancy when the placenta takes over its endocrine function. *If there is no pregnancy*, the corpus luteum begins to degenerate about 4 days before the next menses (24th day of the cycle) and is eventually replaced by scar tissue, forming a **corpus albicans**.

# 102

# Menstrual Cycle

## What is the normal duration of the menstrual cycle? What is the usual timing of ovulation?

The menstrual cycle is conventionally *counted from the first day of menstrual bleeding* (menstruation). A typical cycle has a length of 28 days (25-30 days). The length of the postovulatory period is remarkably constant at approximately 14 days. Therefore, the time of ovulation can be estimated by subtracting 14 days from the duration of the menstrual cycle (Fig. 102.1).

## What are the ovarian changes during the menstrual cycle?

The preovulatory phase of the ovarian cycle is called the follicular phase. The follicular phase is marked by *follicular growth and maturation*. It begins with the onset of menstruation and ends with ovulation. *Ovulation is the extrusion of the secondary oocyte from the Graafian follicle into the peritoneal cavity.* The ruptured follicle promptly fills up with blood forming the **corpus**

|  | 1 | 2 | 3 | 4 | 5 | 6 | 7 | 8 | 9 | 10 | 11 | 12 | 13 | 14 | 15 | 16 | 17 | 18 | 19 | 20 | 21 | 22 | 23 | 24 | 25 | 26 | 27 | 28 |
|---|---|---|---|---|---|---|---|---|---|---|---|---|---|---|---|---|---|---|---|---|---|---|---|---|---|---|---|---|
| Ovary | | | | | | | | Follicular phase | | | | | | | O | Luteal phase | | | | | | | | | | | | |
| Uterus | Menstrual bleeding | | | | Proliferative endometrium | | | | | | | | | | Secretory endometrium | | | | | | | | | | | | | |
| Cervix | | | | | Watery mucus secretion | | | | | | | | | | Thick mucus secretion | | | | | | | | | | | | | |
| Vagina | | | | | Cornified epithelium | | | | | | | | | | Proliferative epithelium with leukocytic infiltration | | | | | | | | | | | | | |

**Fig. 102.1**

## What are the indicators of ovulation?

Ovulation is invariably followed by formation of corpus luteum and progesterone secretion. Tests for ovulation are essentially tests for confirming an increased progesterone secretion during the postovulatory phase. While these can be confirmed by direct *hormonal assay* or *endometrial biopsy*, two simple methods are the basal body temperature charting and the cervical mucus test. (i) **Basal body temperature charting**. Progesterone is associated with a 0.2°C-0.5°C rise in basal body temperature, which occurs immediately following ovulation and which persists during most of the luteal phase. The basal body temperature dips during the follicular phase. This temperature increment is used clinically as an index of ovulation. (ii) **Cervical mucus test**. The cervical epithelium secretes a watery mucus in response to estrogen stimulation. During the preovulatory phase, estrogen makes the cervical mucus thinner and more alkaline. The *mucus is thinnest at the time of ovulation*, and its elasticity, or **spinnbarkheit,** increases so much that by mid-cycle, *a drop can be stretched into a 8-12 cm long, thin thread*. In addition, it dries in an arborizing, **fern-like pattern** when a thin layer is spread on a slide. In the postovulatory phase, progesterone makes the cervical mucus *thick, tenacious, and cellular*. It fails to form the fern pattern on drying and the spinnbarkheit is no longer possible. *Anovulatory cycles are indicated by the persistence of spinnbarkheit and fern pattern.*

**hemorrhagicum**. The blood gets clotted and subsequently replaced by yellowish, lipid-rich luteal cells (derived from the granulosa and thecal cells), forming the **corpus luteum**. Hence, the postovulatory phase of the ovarian cycle is called the **luteal phase**. *If fertilization does not occur, the corpus luteum begins to degenerate by day-24*, and is eventually replaced by fibrous tissue forming the **corpus albicans.** *If conception occurs, the functional lifespan of the corpus luteum is extended under the tropic influence of HCG from the placenta*, and it continues to secrete estradiol and progesterone at increasing rates during the first 6-8 weeks gestation.

## What are the uterine changes during the menstrual cycle?

During the **preovulatory period**, the uterus goes through two phases: menstrual phase and proliferative phase. During **menstruation**, the *endometrial lining of the uterus is shed along with blood and uterine secretions*. Menses, beginning on day 1 of the following cycle, starts with *vasoconstriction of the spiral arterioles, which causes ischemia and necrosis*. The average duration of menstrual flow is 4 days. The necrotic tissue releases vasodilator substances, causing vasodilatation. The *necrotic walls of the spiral arterioles rupture, causing hemorrhage* and shedding of cells over a period of 4-6 days. During the **proliferative phase**, estrogens stimulate mitosis of the stratum basale (*endometrial proliferation*), which regenerates the stratum functionale. The *endometrium grows from 0.5 to 5 mm in depth.* Estrogens stimulate angiogenesis (*neovascularization*) in the stratum functionale as well as stimulate the *growth of secretory glands*. The *blood vessels become the spiral arterioles* that perfuse the stratum functionale. The glands contain glycogen but are nonsecretory at this time. In the **postovulatory period**, the uterus enters its **secretory phase** during which the endometrium is prepared for the possible implantation of the fertilized ovum. The endometrium during this secretory phase is *hyperemic* and has a "Swiss cheese" appearance. Progesterone halts endometrial mitosis but causes maturation and differentiation of the endometrium, including *elongation and coiling of the mucous glands* (which secrete a thick viscous fluid containing glycogen) and *spiraling of the blood vessels*.

### What is the cause of menstrual bleeding?

The endometrial shedding occurs *due to the sudden drop in estrogen and progesterone* levels from a previous high. Hence, the bleeding is called **withdrawal bleeding**.

### Which hormonal event is associated with ovulation?

Ovulation is triggered by a sharp rise in the LH level – the **LH surge** – that occurs 24 hours before ovulation. It occurs because when the plasma estradiol concentration reaches its peak, it suddenly exerts a *positive feedback* (instead of the usual negative feedback) on the hypothalamic-hypophysial axis, causing a reflex release of GnRH and a concomitant surge in pituitary LH secretion 24 hours later, on day 14. A lesser increase in plasma FSH secretion also occurs simultaneously. The midcycle LH surge requires a plasma estradiol concentrations of ~150 pg/ml for at least 36 hours. The onset of the *LH surge is a fairly precise indicator of ovulation*. LH initiates the process of luteinization of the theca and the granulosa cells and enhances progesterone secretion. The rising estradiol levels also causes a *FSH surge*. FSH increases the granulosa cell LH receptors (Fig. 102.2).

### What are the hormonal changes before and after ovulation?

The **preovulatory phase** is associated with the *secretion of large amounts of estradiol by the developing follicle* in response to FSH secretion from the pituitary. This phase generally lasts 10 days, by the end of which one follicle reaches the final stage of growth. The **postovulatory period** is characterized by secretion of *both progesterone and estradiol* by the corpus luteum under the effects of FSH and LH that remains elevated for a few days after ovulation. However, progesterone is secreted in greater amounts and therefore, the postovulatory phase is also called the **progestation phase**. LH and FSH levels continue to decline during the luteal phase due to negative feedback of progesterone and estrogens respectively.

### What are the vaginal changes associated with the menstrual cycle?

In the *preovulatory phase*, the *vaginal epithelium becomes*

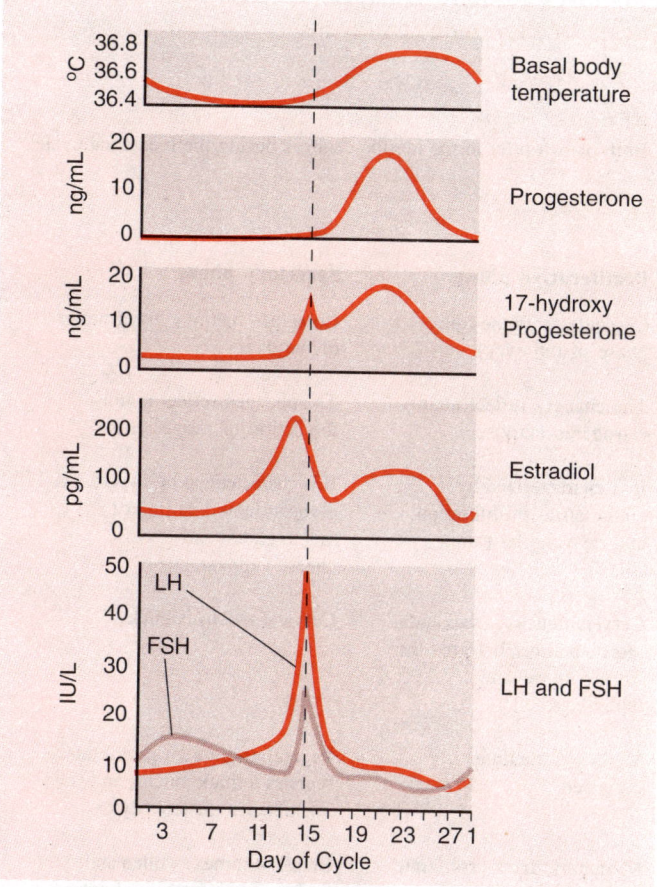

**Fig. 102.2**

*cornified* under the influence of estrogens. The cornified epithelial cells can be identified in the vaginal smear. In the *postovulatory phase*, under the influence of progesterone, a thick mucus is secreted. The *epithelium proliferates and becomes infiltrated with leukocytes*.

### What are the breast changes associated with the menstrual cycle?

In the *preovulatory phase*, there is *proliferation of mammary ducts* under the influence of the high estrogen levels. In the *postovulatory phase*, there is breast swelling, tenderness, and pain during the last 10 days of the menstrual cycle due to *distention of the ducts, hyperemia, and edema of the interstitial tissue* of the breast.

### Define the terms menarche and menopause.

The onset of menstruation at puberty is called **menarche**. It normally occurs between the ages of 12 and 14 years. Prior to menarche, minimal amounts of estrogen are produced by the peripheral conversion of androgens. In early adolescence, the cycle is characterized by *irregular menses and anovulation*. **Menopause** refers to the cessation of menses, which typically occurs at about the age of 50 years. Menopause is a result of cessation of ovarian steroid secretion and is associated with an increased gonadotropin (predominantly FSH) secretion.

## Compare and contrast the proliferative and secretory phases of the menstrual cycle.

### SIMILARITIES

Both phases refer to the uterine changes during the menstrual cycle.

### DIFFERENCES

| Proliferative phase | Secretory phase |
|---|---|
| Coincides with the follicular phase of the ovary | Coincides with the luteal phase of the ovary |
| The changes reflect mainly estrogenic activity | The changes reflect mainly the action of progesterone |
| It is characterized by endometrial proliferation and neovascularization | It is characterized by hyperemia, elongation and coiling of mucus glands and a "swiss cheese" appearance |
| Cervical mucus is thin and more alkaline. It forms the 'fern pattern' and 'spinnbarkheit'. | Cervical mucus is thick |
| Vaginal epithelium cornified | Vaginal epithelium proliferates, secretes a thick mucus, and is infiltrated with leukocytes. |
| Mammary ducts proliferate | Breast becomes swollen and tender due to interstitial edema, hyperemia and distension of ducts. |

# 103

# Sperm Maturation & Fertilization

## What are the four stages of sexual arousal?

The four stages of sexual arousal are **excitement, plateau, orgasm** and **resolution.** All four stages of sexual arousal occur in both males and females.

## What is the difference between emission and expulsion? How are they brought about?

**Ejaculation** is mediated by parasympathetic fibers and is aided by contraction of the bulbocavernous muscles, leading to forcible ejection of sperm from the urethra. At the same time, ascending impulses give rise to the sensation of **orgasm.** *Ejaculation in the male involves two processes*: emission and expulsion of ejaculatory fluid. Both the processes last only a few seconds. **Emission** is the *entry of the ejaculatory fluid into the urethra.* It is stimulated by increased sympathetic nerve activity and is produced by rhythmic muscular contractions of the vas deferens, seminal vesicles, and prostate. Once these contractions have begun, they cannot be stopped until ejaculation is complete. **Expulsion** is the *forcing of ejaculatory fluid out of the tip of the penis.* It is brought about by rhythmic muscular contractions of the urethra. The sphincter vesicae contracts during ejaculation, sealing off the entrance to the bladder and preventing urine from mixing with ejaculatory fluid.

## Enumerate the role of the epididymis in sperm maturation.

Sperms take 2–11 days to pass through the epididymis. During this transit, the epididymis subserves four major functions: *sperm maturation*, *sperm storage*, *decapacitation*, and *sperm protection from immunological damage.* The motility of the sperm, which is acquired in the head and body of the epididymis, is suppressed (**decapacitated**) again in the tail of the epididymis by the lactates in the epididymal fluid that diffuse into the sperm, lowering the pH. Spermatozoa show motility only after they are ejaculated (Fig. 103.1).

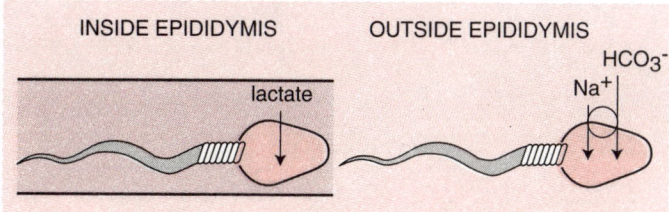

INSIDE EPIDIDYMIS    OUTSIDE EPIDIDYMIS

lactate    HCO₃⁻  Na⁺

**Fig. 103.1**

## What is capacitation and what is its mechanism?

Capacitation is *a reversal in the female tract of a mechanism in the male tract (mainly epididymis) to keep sperm quiescent* before the right moment and place of fertilization. Once a sperm cell is capacitated, its tail shows **hyperactivation** and its head shows the **acrosome reaction** and it acquires the capability to interact with the egg. For capacitation to occur, the **decapacitation factors** acquired in the epididymis and seminal vesicle secretions are first removed during sperm transport through uterus and oviduct. The *follicular fluid that* enters the female tract during ovulation contains sterol-binding proteins that *extract cholesterol from the sperm membranes.* The *decapacitation factors are lost with the cholesterol.*

## Define fertilization. What are steps in fertilization after the sperm comes in contact with the ovum?

**Fertilization** is the fusion of the haploid chromatin content of the male and female gametes, resulting in the formation of a new individual. It occurs normally in the ampulla of the fallopian tube. For fertilization to occur, the sperm has to *pass through two layers of egg-coatings* before it can contact the oocyte directly. (i) The outer coat is the **cumulus oophorus** which *consists of granulosa cells* embedded in a *matrix composed mainly of hyaluronic acid.* (ii) The inner coat is the **zona pellucida** of the oocyte which is acellular and *consists of a meshwork of the glycoproteins.* The penetration of the cumulus oophorus is made possible by the *hyperactivation of the sperm* and the *hyaluronidase present on the sperm surface.* Penetration of the zona pellucida is made possible by the *acrosome reaction, which is stimulated by contact with the zona pellucida.* The acrosome reaction involves release of a protease called **acrosin** from the acrosome that *aids the passage of the sperm through the zona pellucida* (Fig. 103.2).

## What is the mechanism of prevention of polyspermy?

Sperm enters the ovum after fusion of the egg membrane with the sperm membrane at the equatorial region. This action at the membrane stimulates *calcium release from intracellular egg reserves.* The calcium promotes the exocytosis of **cortical granules** that are superficially situated in the unfertilized ovum. The *cortical granules act to inhibit polyploidy* by preventing a second sperm entering the egg by action at two levels, the vitellus and the zona. (i) Firstly, when the cortical granules fuses with the vitelline membrane, large parts of the vitelline membrane get replaced by the membranes of the cortical granules, for which sperm have no affinity. This constitutes the **vitelline block to polyspermy.** (ii) Secondly, the contents of the granules are released into the perivitelline space. Proteases present in these granules degrade the glycoprotein present in the zona pellucida so that it is unable to bind to acrosome-reacted spermatozoa. This constitutes the **zona block to polyspermy.**

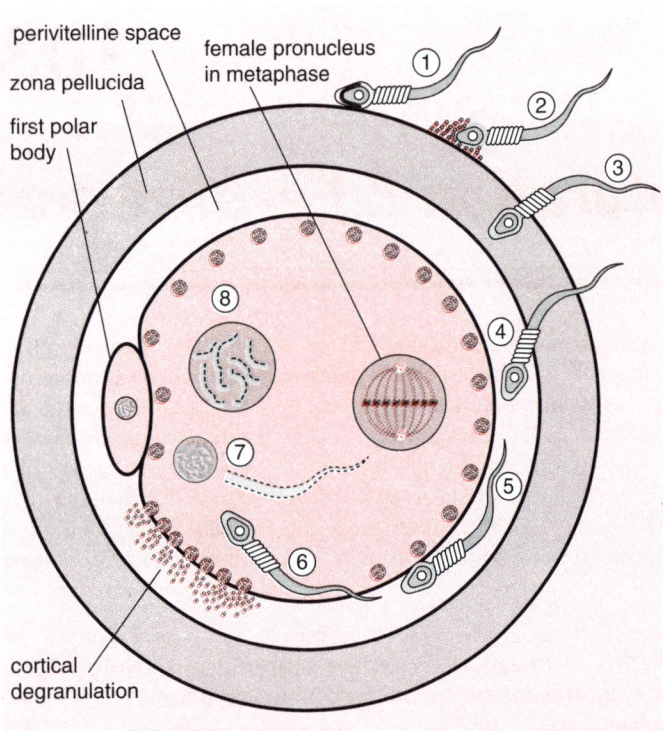

perivitelline space
zona pellucida
first polar body
female pronucleus in metaphase
cortical degranulation

**Fig. 103.2**

**1. Sperm head binding to zona pellucida 2. sperm head undergoes acrosomal reaction 3. sperm penetrates zona pellucida 4. sperm head enters perivitelline space 5. sperm head binds to oolemma 6. sperm in ooplasm 7 sperm tail disappears and the nucleus decondenses 8. nucleus decondenses further to form the male pronucleus.**

### What is implantation?

By the time the fertilized ovum reaches the uterus, it is already a *morula* but is still surrounded by the zona pellucida, which prevents it from sticking to the walls of the uterine tube. The trophoblast tends to invade any tissue it comes in contact with. *Once the zona pellucida disappears, the trophoblast sticks to the uterine endometrium*. This is called **implantation**. The trophoblast invades the endometrium and the blastocyst *burrows deeper into the uterine mucosa* till the whole of it gets buried in the endometrium. This is called **interstitial implantation** to differentiate it from the central implantation occurring in some other mammals where the blastocyst remains in the uterine cavity.

### What is the normal composition of the semen?

Seminal fluid analysis is performed after 24 to 36 hr abstinence on samples obtained by masturbation into a glass container. Analysis is performed within an hour.

The normal ejaculate volume is greater than 2 ml. Immediately after ejaculation, coagulation of the seminal fluid occurs, followed within 15 to 30 min by liquefaction. Normal semen is white or opalescent in color with a specific gravity of 1.028 and a pH of 7.35 - 7.50. The normal sperm count is 40 - 100 million/ml with fewer than 20% having abnormal morphology. For normal fertility, the sperm count should be at least 20 million/ml and at least 60% of the sperm should be motile and of normal morphology. The major secretions of the sex organs that appear in seminal plasma include **fructose** from seminal vesicles; **zinc, acid phosphatase, citric acid, prostate-specific antigen** from the prostate, and **carnitine, glycero-phosphocholine, neutral α-glucosidase** from the epididymis.

The *prostate contributes about 20% to the volume* of the semen. It is slightly acidic (pH 6.5) due to the presence of citric acid. It contains substances important for sperm mobility, notably, **albumin** and the proteolytic enzymes **fibrinolysin** and **fibrinogenase**. It also contains **acid phosphatase** and an **antibacterial substance** of low molecular weight.

The *seminal vesicle contributes 70% to the volume* of the semen. It contains **fructose, citrate, ascorbic acid,** prostaglandins and various enzymes. The fructose is a source of energy for the spermatozoa. It is broken down into lactate through anaerobic glycolysis. The function of **prostaglandins** is not understood. Seminal fluid contains **hyaluronidase**, which acts on hyaluronic acid found in mucus, and so *allows the sperms to pass more readily through the cervix* to the uterus and the tubes.

### What is the cervical mucus contact test?

The cervical mucus secreted during ovulation favors the passage of sperm cells. The same mucus however *prevents the passage of antibody-coated spermatozoa* as well as *morphologically abnormal spermatozoa*. This forms the basis of the *in vitro* **cervical mucus contact test** in which the motility of sperm is observed after bringing them in contact with the cervical mucus.

# 104

# Differentiation of the Sexes

### Outline the time course of sexual differentiation in the fetus.

The normal sex differentiation in the embryo proceeds sequentially. First, the **chromosomal (genotypic) sex** is established at fertilization itself. The chromosomal sex determines the **gonadal sex**, i.e., it causes the indifferent gonad to develop into an ovary or testis. The gonadal sex determines **phenotypic sex**, i.e., the internal genital tracts, the urethras, and the external genitalia.

### How is chromosomal sex determined?

The *chromosomal sex is established at the moment of fertilization*. All ova contain 22 + X chromosomes. However, the spermatozoa are of two types: 50% of the spermatozoa are the X-bearing type having 22 + X chromosomes, while the remaining 50% are the Y-bearing type having 22 + Y chromosomes. An ovum can be fertilized by either type of spermatozoa. If the sperm is X-bearing, the zygote has 44 + 2X chromosomes and its chromosomal sex becomes female. On the other hand, if the sperm is Y-bearing, the zygote has 44 + XY and its chromosomal sex becomes male.

### What is time course of gonadal sex differentiation?

*Till the 6th week* of intrauterine life, the fetal gonads are bipotential: they have the rudiments of both male and female gonads. The bipotential gonad consists of germ cells embedded in a layer of cortical epithelium surrounding a core of medullary mesenchymal tissue. In the genetic male, the *medulla* of the bipotential gonad begins to differentiate into testis at about the *6th week*. The cortical region (from which the female gonad develops) undergoes regression. The testicular differentiation is triggered by the **testis-determining factor (TDF)**, which is encoded by the **SRY gene** (*S*ex-determining *R*egion of the *Y* chromosome) located near the tip of the short arm of the human Y chromosome. TDF causes Sertoli cell differentiation. *In the absence of testis determination, the cortex of bipotential gonad differentiates into the ovaries by the 10th week.*

### What are the factors determining internal genitalia?

*Till the 7th week* of intrauterine life, the internal genitalia of the fetus have the rudiments of both male internal genitalia (the **Wolffian ducts**) and the female internal genitalia (the **Mullerian ducts**). A genetic male fetus with functional testes secretes **testosterone** and **Mullerian inhibiting substance** (**MIS**) that result in differentiation of the genital ducts along male lines. The testosterone (secreted from Leydig cells in the testes) stimulates the development of the Wolffian ducts into vas deferens and related structures. MIS causes regression of the Mullerian ducts by apoptosis on the side on which it is secreted. In the absence of MIS, the Mullerian ducts proliferate and form the oviducts, uterus, and upper two thirds of the vagina. The development of the female external genitalia is independent of ovarian influence. The female internal genitalia are functionally committed to become female as early as 8 weeks. In the absence of androgen, the Wolffian ducts degenerate and the external genitalia maintain the neutral, female form.

### What are the factors determining external genitalia?

*Till the 8th week* of intrauterine life, the external genitalia of the fetus is bipotential, i.e., it can develop along either male or female lines. Unlike the internal genitalia which have distinct male and female components, the *external genitalia in both sexes develop from common rudiments*, viz., the urogenital sinus, the genital sinus, the genital tubercle, the genital swelling, and the genital (urethral) folds. *In the absence of any hormones, the fetal external genitalia develop along female lines.* On the other hand, if the embryo has functional testes secreting testosterone, the testosterone metabolite **dihydrotestosterone** *transforms the fetal external genitalia along male lines.*

### What is Barr body and what is its significance?

Soon after cell division begins during embryonic development, one of the two X chromosomes becomes functionally inactive. In normal cells, the *inactive X chromosome condenses and is seen near the nuclear membrane*, as the **Barr body** or the **sex chromatin**. In females but not in males, the inactive X chromosome is also visible as a small "drumstick" of chromatin projecting from the nuclei in up to 15% of the neutrophils. The Barr body is conveniently employed in **sex determination tests**.

### Explain the origin of chromosomal aberrations.

Abnormalities of chromosomal sex usually arise due to **chromosomal nondisjunction** during gametogenesis, i.e., a pair of chromosomes fails to separate, so that both go to one of the daughter cells during meiosis. Four of the abnormal zygotes that can form as a result of nondisjunction of one of the X chromosomes during oogenesis are shown in Fig. 104.1.

The XXX ("superfemale") pattern is second in frequency only to the XXY pattern and may be even more common in the general population, since it does not seem to be associated with any characteristic abnormalities. The YO combination is lethal.

### What is mosaicism?

Meiosis is a two-stage process, and although nondisjunction usually occurs during the first meiotic division, it can occur during

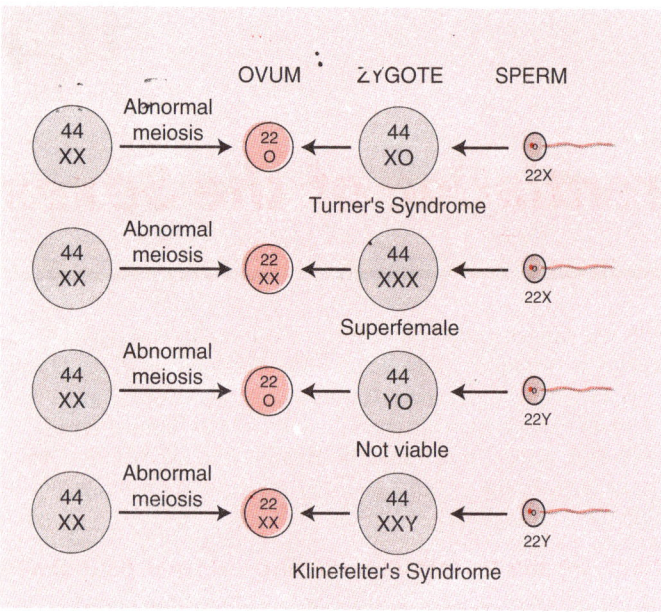

**Fig. 104.1**

the early mitotic divisions after fertilization. The result of *faulty mitosis in the early zygote* is the production of a **mosaic**, an individual with two or more populations of cells with different chromosome complements.

### Describe the clinical features of Klinefelter Syndrome.

Also called **seminiferous tubule dysgenesis**, it has an incidence of 1 in 500 males and is characterized by the genotype of XXY. It occurs in two forms: the classical form and the mosaic form. The **classical form** is due to chromosomal nondisjunction during gametogenesis, i.e., *during meiosis*. Hence it is called **meiotic nondisjunction**. The **mosaic form** occurs due to chromosomal nondisjunction *after zygote formation*. Hence, it is also called **mitotic nondisjunction**. Klinefelter syndrome is characterized by the following features: (i) normal male internal and external genitalia and psychosexual characters; (ii) underdeveloped testes, hyalinization of tubules, azoospermia and infertility; (iii) low levels of testosterone, with high levels of gonadotropins and estradiol; (iv) increased height (due to increase in lower body segment) and obesity; (v) varicose vein, diabetes mellitus, thyroid abnormalities, pulmonary diseases; (vi) mental deficiency.

### Describe the clinical features of Turner Syndrome.

It has an incidence of 1 in 2500 females. Most of them have the karyotype of 45XO due to **meiotic disjunction** in either parent. Others have the karyotype 46XX/45XO mosaicism due to **mitotic disjunction**. Turner syndrome is characterized by the following features: (i) normal female internal and external genitalia and psychosexual characters; (ii) bilateral streak gonads with infertility and primary amenorrhea and amastia; (iii) characteristic facies, with low hairline, ptosis, epicanthus, low set ears, fish-like mouth and micrognathia (small jaw); (iv) short stature; webbed neck, shield-like chest and cubitus valgus; (v) coarctation of aorta.

### What are the features of a true hermaphrodite?

True hermaphrodites *have both male and female gonads*. Some of them have testes on one side and ovary on the other. Others have **ovotestes**, i.e., gonads containing both ovarian and testicular tissues. The internal genitalia correspond to the ipsilateral gonad. The external genitalia are ambiguous. Most true hermaphrodites have the genotype 46XX. The rest have either 46XY or mosaics.

### What are the features of a pseudohermaphrodite?

A pseudohermaphrodite is an individual with the *genetic constitution and gonads of one sex and the external genitalia of the other*. A **female pseudohermaphrodite** is a genetic female with female gonads but male external genitalia. A **male pseudohermaphrodite** is a genetic male with male gonads but female external genitalia.

### What are the causes leading to a female pseudohermaphrodite?

A genetic female exposed to androgens from some other source during the 8th to the 13th weeks of gestation becomes a **female pseudohermaphrodite**. The exposure to androgens may be due to *congenital virilizing adrenal hyperplasia*, or it may be caused by androgens administered to the mother. In the presence of testosterone, the external genitalia develop along male times. The Wolffian duct develops into male internal genitalia only if exposed to testosterone sufficiently early. The Müllerian duct develops into female internal genitalia.

### What are the causes leading to a male pseudohermaphrodite?

If a genetic male fetus has impaired testosterone secretion from its embryonic testes, it turns into a **male pseudohermaphrodite**.

| Hermaphroditism | Female Internal Genitalia | Male Internal Genitalia | External Genitalia |
|---|---|---|---|
| Female pseudo-hermaphroditism | **Present, because MIS** is abscent | **Absent** usually, because exposure to testosterone usually occurs late | **Male**. |
| Male pseudo-hermaphroditism | | | |
| Impaired testosterone secretion | **Present** if MIS secretion is also impaired. **Absent** if MIS secretion is unaffected | **Absent** because testosterone is absent | **Female** because DHT is not formed |
| 5α-reductase deficiency. | **Absent** because MIS is present | **Present** because testosterone secretion in normal | **Female** because DHT is not formed |
| Receptor defect | **Absent** because MIS is present | **Absent** because testosterone is ineffective | **Female** because DHT is ineffective |
| Persistent Mullerian Duct Syndrome | **Present** because MIS is present | **Present** because testosterone is present | **Female** because DHT is present |

Defective testosterone can occur due to defective testis, or due to defective steroidogenesis, as in 17α-hydroxylase deficiency. *In the absence of testosterone, the Wolffian duct fails to develop into the male internal genitalia.* The female internal genitalia is not formed either, because the MIS secretion by testes is usually not affected. When MIS secretion too is impaired, it results in the **persistent Mullerian duct syndrome**. Another cause of male pseudohermaphroditism is **5α-reductase deficiency**, in which the formation of dihydrotestosterone, the active form of testosterone, is decreased. Yet another cause is **androgen resistance** due to mutations in the androgen receptor gene. When the loss of receptor function is complete, it results in the **testicular feminizing syndrome**. In this condition, MIS is present and testosterone is secreted at normal rates. The internal genitalia are therefore male but the external genitalia are female. The vagina ends blindly because there are no female internal genitalia. Individuals with this syndrome develop enlarged breasts at puberty and usually are considered to be normal women until they are diagnosed when they seek medical advice because of lack of menstruation.

# 105

# *Feto-placental Unit & Placental Hormones*

## Enumerate the placental hormones.

The placental hormones are secreted by the **syncytiotrophoblast** of the placenta. They are: (i) human chorionic gonadotropin (HCG); (ii) human chorionic somatomammotropin (HCS); (iii) human chorionic thyrotropin (HCT) and (iv) Placental estrogens.

## What is the source of HCG? What is its clinical significance?

Human chorionic gonadotropin (HCG) is *secreted soon after fertilization by the syncytiotrophoblast*. It is *detectable in maternal blood as early as 6-8 days after conception*. HCG reaches a plasma *peak between 60 and 90 days gestation*. After this the concentration falls to a much lower level that is maintained till just before labor when it falls to zero. If the fetus dies early HCG disappears from serum and urine. The presence of HCG in the urine forms the basis of all pregnancy diagnosis tests. HCG measurement in maternal blood is *a useful index of the functional status of the trophoblast.*

## What are the actions of HCG?

*HCG has actions similar to those of LH.* It is a **luteotropic hormone** that *maintains the function of the corpus luteum up to 7 weeks after conception*, i.e., until the fetoplacental unit is able to synthesize its own estrogens and progesterone. It converts the corpus luteum of menstruation into the corpus luteum of pregnancy, thereby extending the lifespan of the corpus luteum. HCG stimulates the corpus luteum of early pregnancy to secrete 17α-hydroxyprogesterone, which reaches a peak 3-4 weeks postconception. The blood level of *17α-hydroxyprogesterone is an excellent indicator of corpus luteal function* because the *placenta lacks significant 17α-hydroxylase activity.*

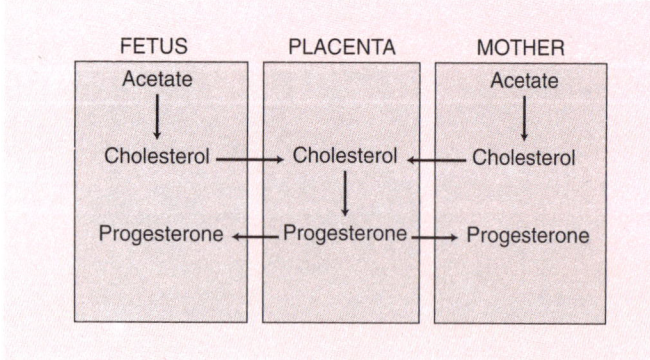

**Fig. 105.1**

## What is fetoplacental unit? What is its physiological significance?

The fetus, placenta, and mother are interdependent and constitute a functional unit called the **feto-placento-maternal unit** or simply, the **fetoplacental unit**. The secretion of hormones by the placenta involves the *shuttling of many of the hormonal substrates back-and-forth between the placenta, fetal circulation and maternal circulation*. Following are the major examples of this shuttling.

(1) The *placenta cannot synthesize cholesterol from acetate*. However, both mother and fetus can do so and the cholesterol so formed diffuses into the placenta, which possesses the enzymes needed to convert cholesterol to progesterone via pregnenolone. The *progesterone formed in the placenta diffuses back into the maternal circulation* and exerts its physiological actions. *Placental progesterone also diffuses into the fetus* where it is converted to corticosteroids (Fig. 105.1).

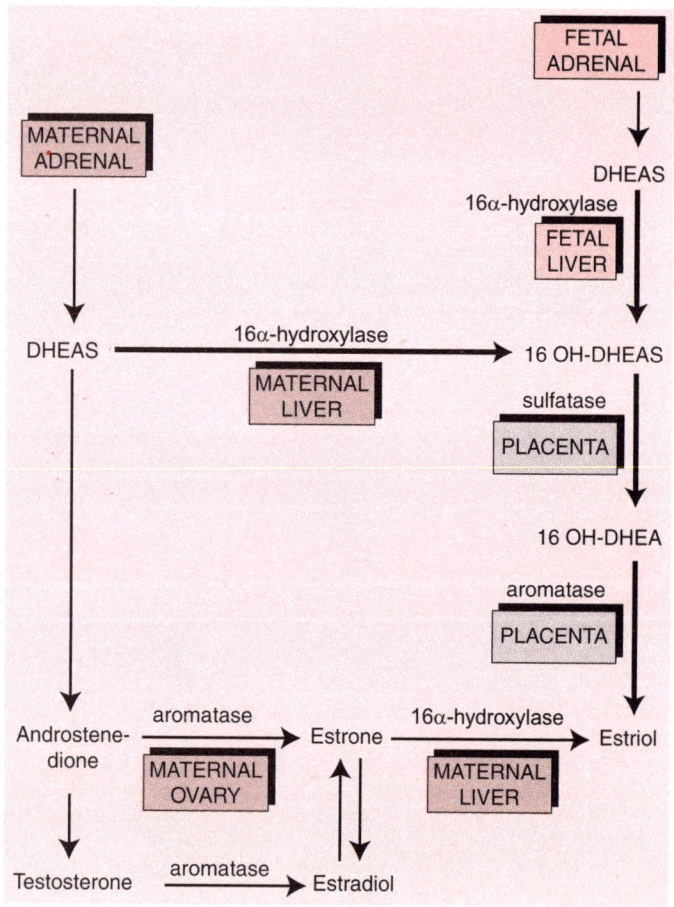

**Fig. 105.2**

(2) The enzyme 17, 20 lyase is essential for the synthesis of DHEA (dehydroepiandrosterone), which is the precursor to all estrogens. *17, 20 lyase is absent in the placenta*. Hence, for estrogen synthesis, the *placenta obtains DHEAS from the maternal and fetal circulation*. DHEAS (dehydroepiandrosterone sulfate) is deconjugated to DHEA in the placenta before it is converted to estriol.

(3) Estriol, the major circulating hormone in pregnancy is synthesized from DHEAS. The conversion requires mainly two enzymes: *16α hydroxylase* and *aromatase*. However, *16α-hydroxylase is absent in the placenta*. The placenta therefore takes up 16 OH-DHEAS from maternal and fetal circulation, deconjugates it into 16 OH-DHEA and converts it into estriol. *Fetal 16 OH-DHEA is the major source of placental estriol* and therefore, the *urinary excretion of estriol in mother is an index of the health of the fetus* (Fig. 105.2).

### Enumerate the pregnancy diagnostic tests. Describe the Gravindex test for pregnancy diagnosis.

All pregnancy diagnostic tests are based on the presence of HCG in urine, which can be detected 14 days after conception. The accuracy of these tests is of the order of 99%. The **biological tests** are tabulated below. Although very sensitive, they have been abandoned as they are quite cumbersome.

| Test | Criterion | Time required |
|---|---|---|
| Aschheim-Zondek (A-Z) Test | Ovulation in immature mice | 5 days |
| Friedman Test | Ovulation in virgin rabbit | 18 hours |
| Hogben Test | Release of ova in female toad *Xenopus laevis* | 24 hours |
| Galli-Mainini Test | Release of sperms in male toads or frogs | 3 hours |
| Immunological | Inhibition of agglutination of sheep red cells or latex particles coated with HCG | 2 hours |

The **immunological tests** (e.g., the **Gravindex test**) are cheap, reliable, and accurate enough to replace biological methods. The kit consists of Gravindex antigen (latex particles coated with HCG), Gravindex antibody (serum containing HCG antibodies), dark slide, sticks and a pipette.

If a serum containing antibodies to HCG is allowed to react with HCG-coated red cells or latex particles, agglutination of the red cells or latex particles occurs. But if the serum is allowed to react with urine containing HCG prior to the reaction with red cells or latex particles, the agglutination of red cells or latex particles is inhibited, since the antibodies are used up by HCG of the urine. Hence *inhibition of agglutination confirms pregnancy*.

# 106

# Pregnancy, Parturition & Lactation

## Enumerate the cardiorespiratory changes in pregnancy.

The elevation of diaphragm by the gravid uterus displaces the heart (and the apex beat) laterally and upward. The ECG shows **left axis deviation**. The marked **peripheral vasodilatation** of pregnancy results in increase in venous return, cardiac output and heart rate. There is marked **fluid and Na⁺ retention**, resulting in increase in blood volume. The diastolic pressure falls while the systolic blood pressure remains unchanged. There is marked increase in pulmonary blood flow and **hyperventilation**, leading to a decrease in the $P_{CO_2}$. The decrease in $P_{CO_2}$ facilitates transfer of $CO_2$ from fetus to the mother. The hyperventilation is due to *stimulation of respiratory center by progesterone*.

The hyperventilation of pregnancy causes **respiratory alkalosis**. The rise in blood pH shifts the maternal oxygen dissociation curve to the left (Bohr effect). However, alkalosis also increases the 2, 3 DPG level, which shifts the same curve to the right.

## Enumerate the renal changes in pregnancy.

The rise in cardiac output results in marked increase in renal blood flow and GFR. **Glycosuria** is normal during pregnancy. There is also increase in *plasma vasopressinase* that reduces the plasma levels of ADH and results in **gestational diabetes insipidus**. Protein excretion also increases during pregnancy and **proteinuria** should be diagnosed only if it exceeds 500 mg in 24 hours.

## Enumerate the hematological changes in pregnancy.

The increase in **blood volume** (30%) is disproportionately higher than the increase in RBC volume. Thus there is hemodilution and **physiological anemia of pregnancy**. Hence, there is reduction in various hematological indices like hemoglobin, volume of packed red cells and RBC count. It also results in moderate **erythroid hyperplasia** and an increase in reticulocyte count. Total white cell count (TLC) also increases during pregnancy predominantly because of **neutrophilia**. Plasma levels of several coagulation factors increase during pregnancy with decrease in fibrinolytic activity. **Fibrinogen** increases by about 50%. This increase causes a marked increase in **ESR** during pregnancy. **Plasma globulin** concentration increases and **plasma albumin** concentration falls reversing the A:G ratio.

## Enumerate the endocrinal changes in pregnancy.

Increase in plasma proteins causes increased protein binding of hormones. The resultant fall in the free hormone concentration increases hormone secretion through negative feedback and restores the free hormonal concentration to normal. The total hormonal concentration in plasma (free + bound) however remains elevated. This is true for thyroid and adrenocortical hormones as well as other hormones that are transported in plasma bound to plasma proteins.

Due to increase in the estrogen and progesterone, there is decrease in maternal serum levels of gonadotropins (FSH and LH). Prolactin levels increase and growth hormone secretion decreases. The sensitivity to insulin increases in the initial half of pregnancy and decreases in the latter half (**gestational diabetes mellitus**). The trophoblast cells produce ACTH and CRF. Renin, angiotensin and aldosterone levels increase.

## Briefly describe the changes in mineral metabolism.

The **iron** requirement increases in pregnancy. Hence, serum iron and ferritin levels fall while serum iron binding capacity (TIBC) increases.

There is increased requirement of calcium during pregnancy. To meet the requirement, there is increase in the absorption of **calcium** from the gut and decreased excretion through the kidneys. This is achieved by increase in parathyroid hormone that increases vitamin $D_3$ (calcitriol).

## What is the mechanism of parturition onset?

The *onset of parturition is triggered by a high estrogen : progesterone ratio*. Towards term, the plasma concentration of estrogen rises steeply while that of progesterone falls sharply. As a result, the estrogen : progesterone ratio rises (Fig. 106.1) and initiates parturition by stimulating the uterine smooth muscles (myometrium).

Once labor starts, uterine contractions dilate the cervix by pushing the fetal head into it. The dilatation sets up signals in afferent nerves that increase oxytocin secretion from posterior pituitary

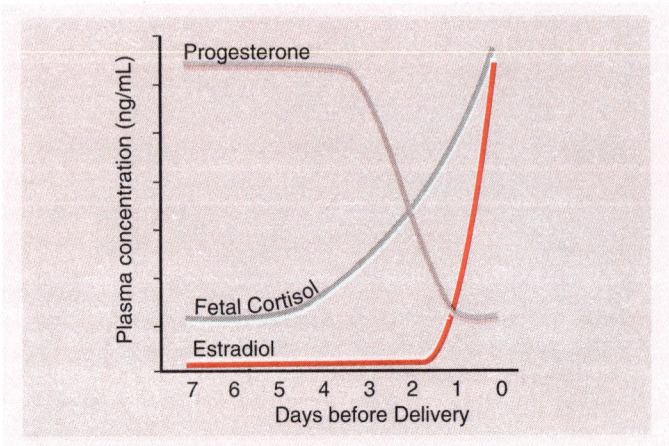

**Fig. 106.1**

(the **Ferguson reflex**). The oxytocin released contracts the myometrium further, increasing the intensity of labor pain.

### Why does the estrogen : progesterone ratio rise towards term?

Towards term, the CRH secretion in the fetus increases, resulting in increase in ACTH secretion and a consequent increase in secretion of androgens from the fetal adrenal cortex. These androgens are converted to estrogens in the placenta. The placental estrogens diffuse out into maternal circulation and raise the estrogen levels in plasma.

The fetus also produces large amounts of dehydroepiandrosterone sulfate (DHEAS) and cortisol. These inhibit the conversion of fetal pregnenolone to progesterone. The maternal progesterone levels falls due to decreased contribution from fetal progesterone.

### Why is parturition favored by high estrogen and low progesterone levels?

*Estrogen* causes (i) increased release of oxytocin from maternal pituitary; (ii) increased synthesis of oxytocin receptors in myometrium and decidua; (iii) increased synthesis of prostaglandins in the decidua, which increase the formation of gap junctions in the myometrium, enabling coordinated muscle activity; (iv) increased synthesis of myometrial contractile protein. On the other hand, *progesterone* relaxes the uterine smooth muscles.

### Where is oxytocin secreted from? What are the factors influencing its secretion?

Oxytocin is secreted from the paraventricular and supraoptic nuclei of the hypothalamus, and is stored in the posterior lobe of the pituitary gland. Its *secretion is stimulated by* (1) stimulation of cervix during parturition or coitus; (2) stimulation of the nipples, and (3) sight and sound of the baby, in case of nursing mothers. Oxytocin *secretion is inhibited by* (1) pain, emotional stress and fright; (2) sympathetic discharge and catecholamines; and (3) alcohol consumption.

### What are the actions of oxytocin?

Oxytocin has two important physiological actions. (1) It *stimulates the myoepithelial cells of the breast*, causing milk ejection. (2) It *stimulates the uterine smooth muscles* towards the term. Oxytocin has been *used for induction of labor*. (3) It aids in the involution of the uterus. It is used therapeutically for controlling uterine bleeding.

### Where is prolactin secreted from? What are the factors influencing its secretion?

Prolactin is synthesized in the pituitary acidophils. Normally, the control of prolactin secretion is under constant inhibition of the **prolactin inhibiting factor (PIF)**. This PIF is now known to be **dopamine**, which is secreted into the hypophysial portal vessels. Prolactin stimulates the secretion of dopamine from the median eminence of the hypothalamus, and thereby *inhibits its own secretion*. Prolactin secretion is *stimulated by TRH*.

Prolactin secretion increases (1) during suckling and stimulation of nipple, (2) during coitus, (3) during sleep, (4) during exercise, (5) during surgical and psychological stresses, and (6) during hypoglycemia.

### What is the suckling reflex?

Suckling is associated with (1) an increase in oxytocin secretion and (2) increase in prolactin secretion. The release of hormones from the hypothalamus is triggered reflexly by the stimulation of the nipples.

### What are the physiological actions of prolactin?

Actions of prolactin include (1) mammogenesis (development of the mammary glands), (2) lactogenesis (milk production) and (3) inhibition GnRH secretion.

### What are the consequences of hyperprolactinemia? How is it treated?

In women, elevated serum prolactin manifests as galactorrhea, infertility and amenorrhea. In men, hyperprolactinemia causes impotence and decreases libido. Treatment of hyperprolactinemia includes administration of **bromocriptine**, a dopamine agonist.

### Describe briefly the composition of human milk and colostrum.

Mature human milk contains 7% carbohydrates (mainly lactose), 4% fat and 1% protein. Its energy content is 60-75 kCal/100mL. Colostrum has twice as much protein as mature milk. Colostrum also contains secretory IgA, the consumption of which confers passive immunity to the infant.

### What are the stages of lactation?

Lactation is divided into four phases: (1) **mammogenesis**, or the preparation of the breasts; (2) **lactogenesis**, or milk production; (3) **galactokinesis**, or milk ejection; and (4) **galactopoiesis**, or maintenance of lactation.

### What are the factors important for mammogenesis?

Mammogenesis involves both duct growth and lobulo-alveolar growth. **Duct growth** is brought about by *estrogen, growth hormone* and *glucocorticoids*. **Lobulo-alveolar growth** requires, in addition to the hormones mentioned, *progesterone* and *prolactin* (Fig. 106.2).

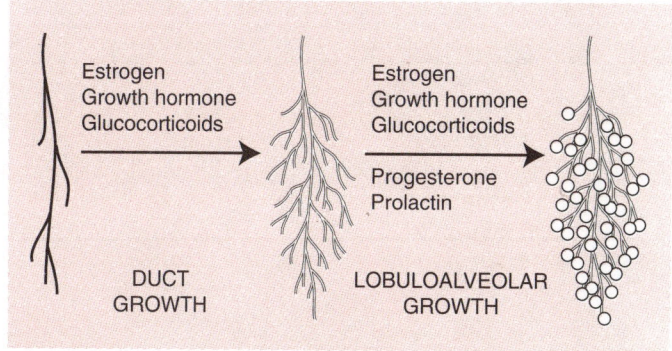

**Fig. 106.2**

### What causes lactogenesis?

*Prolactin* causes lactogenesis. Prolactin stimulates the activity of the enzyme *galactosyl transferase*, leading to the synthesis of lactose. *Growth hormone* and *thyroid hormone* also increase milk production. These hormones have been administered to dairy animals to increase the yield of milk.

### Why does lactogenesis occur after parturition and not before?

Lactogenesis is brought about by the action of prolactin on the breast that has been adequately prepared by estrogen, progesterone and other hormones. During pregnancy, the high levels of estrogen and progesterone cause mammogenesis. They also cause *increased proliferation of lactotrophs* in the pituitary and thereby increase prolactin secretion. Even then, *there is no milk secretion because estrogen and progesterone have a direct inhibitory action on lactogenesis*. After parturition, there is a sharp fall in estrogen and progesterone levels. This removes the inhibitory effect on lactogenesis. Since the prolactin level is still high and mammogenesis is complete, lactogenesis occurs.

### What causes galactokinesis?

*Oxytocin* causes galactokinesis. The oxytocin is released from the supraoptic and paraventricular nuclei of the hypothalamus. It causes milk ejection by stimulating contraction of myoepithelial cells in the mammary alveoli and ducts. Oxytocin is released when the nipple is stimulated during suckling. Spontaneous release of oxytocin also occurs when a lactating woman is allowed to play with her infant or upon hearing the infant cry. Such spontaneous release is called the **milk letdown**. During milk letdown, there is no increase in prolactin secretion; only the oxytocin secretion increases.

### What causes galactopoiesis?

Lactation is maintained by *prolactin*. After parturition, the estrogen and progesterone levels fall, and with it, the prolactin level also declines. However, there are periodic surges of prolactin that are associated with each episode of suckling (Fig. 106.3). These surges maintain lactation. In fact, lactation can continue indefinitely as long as the suckling is continued, as in **wet nurses** who offer themselves on hire for suckling another's child.

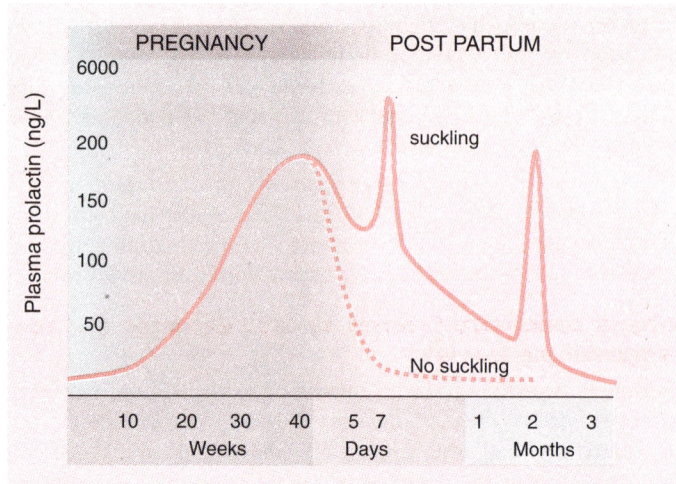

**Fig. 106.3**

### What is the cause of lactation amenorrhea.

Suckling stimulates prolactin secretion. The *high levels of prolactin inhibit GnRH secretion*, resulting in low levels of FSH and LH. Hence, there is anovulation and amenorrhea.

# Contraceptives

## Enumerate the various methods of male contraception.

Male contraceptive methods include: (i) coitus interruptus; (ii) condoms; (iii) thermal methods: hot bath and suspensories; (iv) vas occlusion methods like injection of medical-grade polyurethane or medical-grade silicone rubber; (v) reversible inhibition of sperm under guidance (RISUG); (vi) drugs: androgens, cypropterone, gossypol, *Trypterigium wilfordii*, nifedipine; (vii) vasectomy.

## What is RISUG and how does it work?

RISUG is the newest technology in vas occlusion methods. It uses SMA (**styrene malic anhydride**), a copolymer that can be injected in combination with dimethyl sulphoxide, using a no-scalpel procedure into the vasa deferentia, where it coats the walls and partially blocks the lumen. RISUG is more than a vas-occlusive device. It has three contraceptive effects. First, the basic (high) pH of the compound *interferes with the acidic (low) pH of sperm*. Second, the positive electric charge associated with SMA causes the *membranes of passing sperm to rupture*. Third, the compound *partially blocks the lumen* of the vas deferens. SMA can be removed by flushing the vasa deferentia with an injected solvent. A newer, totally noninvasive reversal technique is to manually squeeze it out into the urethra whence it gets flushed out during micturition. Even multiple occlusions and reversals are possible with RISUG. It is also being tested for use as a spermicide, (which will make it as an effective female contraceptive) and its antimicrobial effects (for possible prevention against AIDS). RISUG is the invention of Sujoy Guha.

## Enumerate the various methods of female contraception.

Female contraceptive methods include: (i) diaphragm and cervical caps; (ii) spermicidal foams and jellies; (iii) intrauterine contraceptive devices (IUCD); (iv) contraceptive pills and (v) tubectomy.

## What is the mechanism of action of IUCD?

IUCDs are inserted into the endometrial cavity to provide long-term contraception (up to several years). These devices generally have been made of plastics with either a serpentine shape (**Lippe's loop**) or a T-configuration of polypropylene with helically shaped arms. Currently available IUCDs have greater efficacy with added progesterone or copper (the **copper-T**). IUCDs act to prevent implantation and growth of the fertilized egg by sterile inflammatory response of the endometrium, with sperm being consumed through phagocytosis. They also alter the tubal transport of sperm and thereby prevent fertilization.

## What is the mechanism of action of contraceptive pills?

The administration of estrogen or progesterone or both inhibits ovulation, and therefore, pregnancy. *Estrogens stop the secretion of FSH* from the pituitary and the presence of *progesterone prevents the release of LH*. Ovulation can therefore be prevented either by stopping the stimulus of ovulation or by preventing follicle growth and either of the steroids will be effectively do this. Hence, either estrogen or progesterone should alone be sufficient to prevent ovulation. In practice, however, both of these are usually combined. The *estrogen inhibits ovulation* and *progesterone ensures that withdrawal bleeding will be short and prompt.*

# Spinal Cord & Brainstem

## What are Rexed laminae?

The spinal gray matter shows an anteroposterior organization into distinct zones called the **Rexed laminae**. There are 10 Rexed laminae (Fig. 108.1). **Laminae I to VI** correspond to the **posterior horn**, which receive cutaneous sensations from the dorsal nerve roots. **Lamina II** corresponds with the **substantia gelatinosa**, which is thought to be the site of gating of pain by touch fibers. **Lamina III to VI** correspond with the **nucleus proprius**, which is the origin of the 2nd order fibers for pain, temperature and crude touch. **Lamina VII** correspond to the lateral horn. It accommodates the autonomic preganglionic neurons and the Renshaw cells. **Lamina VIII to X** correspond to the **anterior horn**. It contains α and γ motor neurons, some β neurons and numerous interneurons.

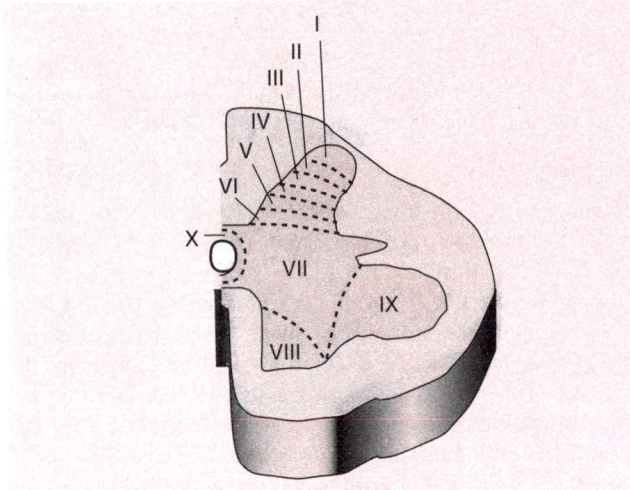

**Fig. 108.1**

## Enumerate the long ascending and descending spinal tracts.

| Ascending | Anterolateral Funiculus | Lateral spinothalamic tract |
| | | Anterior spinothalamic tract |
| | | Spinocervicothalamic tract |
| | | Spinoreticular tract |
| | | Spinotectal tract |
| | | Spinocerebellar tracts |
| | | Dorsolateral tract of Lissauer |
| | Posterior Funiculus | Fasciculus Gracilis |
| | | Fasciculus Cuneatus |
| | | Corticospinal tract (Anterior and Lateral) |
| | | Rubrospinal tract |
| | | Vestibulospinal tract |

| Descending | Anterolateral Funiculus | Reticulospinal tract |
| | | Tectospinal tract |
| | | Olivospinal tract |
| | | Descending autonomic fibers |
| | | Raphe spinal tract |
| | Posterior Funiculus | |

## What is a dermatome?

The area of the skin supplied by the peripheral branches of a spinal nerve is known as **dermatome**.

## Name the cranial nerves and state their origin.

| I | Olfactory | Limbic cortex |
| II | Optic | Thalamus (lateral geniculate body) |
| III | Oculomotor | Midbrain |
| IV | Trochlear | |
| V | Trigeminal | Pons |
| VI | Abducent | |
| VII | Facial | |
| VIII | Vestibulocochlear | |
| IX | Glossopharyngeal | |
| X | Vagus | Medulla oblongata |
| XI | Spinal accessory | |
| XII | Hypoglossal | |

## Describe the pyramidal tract.

The pyramidal tract (also called the **corticospinal tract**) originates mostly from the **pyramidal cells of Betz** in area 4 and area 6 of the motor cortex. They descend in the internal capsule and the crura cerebri to the medulla oblongata where they pass through the medullary pyramids. *Pyramidal fibers are called so because they pass through the medullary pyramids.* In the lower part of the pyramids, the majority of corticospinal fibers decussate and occupy the lateral funiculus as the **lateral corticospinal tract**. The uncrossed corticospinal fibers descend in the anterior funiculus as the **anterior corticospinal tract**.

## What is the effect of a pure pyramidal lesion?

All clinical lesions of pyramidal fibers also affect extrapyramidal fibers too. **Pure pyramidal lesions** that are produced experimentally result in *decrease in muscle tone in the limbs*. Tone in the back, neck and thorax decreases very little. The deep reflexes become slow but are not abolished. The superficial reflexes are abolished initially but return after sometime. There is *marked weakness of the contralateral limbs*, the skilled movement of the hands and fingers being the most affected.

### Describe the four lemnisci.

The lemnisci are ascending tracts from the spinal cord that terminate in the thalamus. There are four lemnisci: from medial to lateral side, they are— medial lemniscus, trigeminal lemniscus, spinal lemniscus and lateral lemniscus. The **medial lemniscus** is the upward continuation of the dorsal column fibers carrying fine touch and proprioception that have decussated in the medulla. It terminates in the ventro-postero-lateral nucleus (VPL) of the thalamus. The **trigeminal lemniscus** is the upward continuation of the decussated $2^{nd}$ order sensory neurons from the contralateral nuclei of the trigeminal nerve. The **spinal lemniscus** is the upward continuation of the lateral spinothalamic tract and conveys pain and thermal senses from the contralateral side of the body. The **lateral lemniscus** is the ascending tract concerned with hearing, which terminates in the medial geniculate body.

### Describe the clinical features of tabes dorsalis.

In tabes dorsalis, there is *bilateral degeneration of dorsal nerve roots* and of *posterior funiculi*, especially fasciculus gracilis. There are loss of position sense, vibratory sense, sense of stereognosis and discriminative touch on the same side at and below the level of cord lesion. There is **sensory ataxia**: the patient walks on a broad base with the legs apart, eyes are fixed to the ground for correcting the steps, associated with raising of the legs excessively high and slapping the feet on the ground. **Romberg's sign** is positive, i.e. the ataxia of tabes dorsalis may be corrected by vision, unlike that of cerebellum.

### Describe the clinical features of syringomyelia.

This rare condition is characterized by **gliosis** (excessive overgrowth of neuroglial tissue) accompanied by *cavitation of the gray matter around the central canal*. Fibers subserving *pain, temperature and crude touch, which decussate in the gray commissure, are destroyed*, resulting in loss of these sensations. However, fibers carrying fine touch ascend which in the dorsal column escape damage. Hence, syringomyelia is characterized by **dissociated anesthesia**, i.e., loss of pain and temperature with retention of touch sensation. The deficiency is bilateral and *usually occurs in the hands and arms* because syringomyelia *mostly affects the cervical enlargement of the cord*.

At later stages, the gliosis and cavitation may spread to involve the anterior horn cells, causing *flaccid paralysis of the upper limb muscles*. As the lesion spreads to the adjacent corticospinal tract, it results in *upper motor neuron paralysis of the legs*.

### Describe the salient features of lower motor neuron paralysis.

Lower motor neuron paralysis is produced by a complete *degeneration of ventral root fibers*. The lesion interrupts fibers of $\alpha$ and $\gamma$ motor neurons. The paralysis is typically observed in **poliomyelitis**, because the *poliovirus selectively affects the lower motor neurons of spinal cord and brain stem*. The manifestations of lower motor neuron paralysis are as follows. (1) **Segmental paralysis** of all voluntary movements. (2) **Segmental areflexia** – loss of all superficial and deep reflexes at the affected level.

(3) **Atonia** due to abolition of the stretch reflex. (4) Within two or three weeks after denervation, the paralyzed muscles show **fibrillation** and **fasciculation** (spontaneous contractions due to hypersensitivity of the denervated muscle to circulating chemical mediators) followed by muscle **atrophy**.

### Describe the salient features of upper motor neuron paralysis.

An upper motor neuron lesion (UMNL) is the *interruption of the corticospinal (pyramidal) tract and associated extrapyramidal fibers*. It is characteristically associated with **spastic paralysis** of muscles. Pure pyramidal lesions causes hypotonia rather than spasticity. Hence, the *spasticity of UMNL is actually due to the interruption of the descending extrapyramidal fibers*.

A lesion above the pyramidal decussation affects the contralateral side while a lesion below the decussation affects the ipsilateral side. The effects of a unilateral UMNL include the following. (1) Loss of voluntary movement in the form of **hemiplegia** (paralysis of upper and lower extremities on one side), (2) **Atonia** (flaccidity) and **areflexia** immediately after the lesion. (3) **Spasticity** (*increased muscle tone* and *exaggerated deep tendon reflexes*) occurs after a few days or weeks, due to augmented $\gamma$-motor discharge. On testing the muscle tone by feeling the resistance to passive movements, the characteristic **clasp-knife** effect is observed. (4) **Superficial reflexes** (abdominal, cremasteric and plantar reflexes) are lost because their reflex pathway are transcortical and the efferent path is formed by the corticospinal tract. In place of the plantar reflex appears the **Babinski sign**.

### Compare and contrast upper and lower motor neuron lesions.

**SIMILARITIES**

Voluntary movements are abolished in both.

Atonia and areflexia occurs in LMNL as well as in the initial stage of UMNL.

Superficial reflexes are lost in both.

**DIFFERENCES**

| UMNL | LMNL |
|---|---|
| Muscles affected in groups, never individually. | Individual muscles may be affected. |
| Muscle atrophy can occur due to disuse but is not marked. | Muscle atrophy is marked. |
| Muscles are spastic and deep tendon reflexes are exaggerated. Clasp-knife effect present. | Muscles are flaccid and deep tendon reflexes are absent. Clasp-knife effect absent. |
| Babinski sign (extensor plantar reflex) present. | Plantar reflex absent if $L_5$-$S_1$ are affected. Otherwise normal. |
| Muscle fasciculations are not present. | Muscle fasciculations may be present. |
| Electromyogram normal. | Electromyogram shows fibrillations and reduced numbers of motor units. |

## What is clonus?

Clonus is a sustained series of rhythmic muscle jerks when a quick stretch is applied to a tendon. **Ankle clonus** is usually observed in upper motor neuron lesion by sudden dorsiflexion of the foot.

## What is Babinski sign?

When the lateral aspect of the sole of foot is scratched with a blunt point, the usual response is the **plantar reflex** in which the toes are plantar flexed. In UMNL, the plantar reflex is abolished and in its place appears the **Babinski sign** (reflex in which the great toe is dorsiflexed and other toes fan out). The Babinski sign is also positive in normal infants prior to the myelination of the corticospinal tract.

## Describe the salient features of Brown Sequard syndrome.

It is a rare clinical condition in which there is segmental damage on one side of the spinal cord (**hemisection**) due to traumatic injury, or compression of extramedullary tumors. (1) *At the level of the lesion* the effects include: (i) radicular pain and parasthesia due to *damage of spinal segment and dorsal nerve root.* (ii) flaccid paralysis of the ipsilateral muscles due to *damage to the ventral root.* (2) *Below the level of the lesion*, the effects include (i) Ipsilateral loss of position and vibratory senses, disturbances of stereognosis and tactile discrimination below the level of lesion due to *damage of posterior funiculus*; (ii) Ipsilateral spastic paralysis with exaggerated tendon reflexes and positive Babinski sign due to *damage to the pyramidal tract*; (iii) Contralateral and segmental loss of pain one of two segments below the level of lesion due to *damage of the lateral spinothalamine tract* (Fig. 108.2).

## Describe the features of spinal cord transection.

Complete transection of the cord results in (1) loss of all sensations below the level of lesion; (2) voluntary movements below the level of lesion; (3) initial loss of muscle tone and reflexes followed by their recovery and exaggeration later. Immediately after injury, there is a period of **spinal shock**, which may last from a *few days to several weeks*. During this period, all somatic and visceral reflex activities are abolished. Thereafter, the reflex activities are returned and the muscles become spastic with exaggerated tendon reflexes.

*In transaction above $S_2$*, voluntary control over the bladder and bowel functions are lost. Immediately following the injury, there is abolition of the micturition reflex resulting in a **flaccid neuropathic bladder** with overflow incontinence. Following recovery, the reflex excitability of the detrusor returns and the bladder capacity is reduced. The micturition reflex is exaggerated, resulting in the **spastic neuropathic bladder**. The micturition reflex is triggered whenever the bladder gets distended and hence the bladder is called an **automatic bladder**. A few patients develop the ability to empty the bladder reflexly by triggering **mass reflex**, i.e., by tapping or scratching the skin above the pubis or external genitalia.

*In transection above $T_1$* i.e. above the thoracolumbar sympathetic outflow, the sympathetic and somatic thermoregulatory mechanisms do not remain under hypothalamic control. Some local vasodilatation and sweating may still be possible through spinal reflexes, but these are too weak for effective control of body temperature. Such patients have to depend largely on conscious behavioral thermoregulatory mechanisms.

*In transection below $C_5$*, the patient becomes **quadriplegic**. When the transection takes place between the cervical and lumbosacral enlargements, the patient becomes **paraplegic**. In paraplegia, when extensor spasms predominate, it is known as **paraplegia-in-extension,** which indicates that the transaction is functionally incomplete. **Paraplegia-in-flexion** takes place when the transection is complete in which flexor spasms predominate.

*In transection above $C_5$*, the patient is unable to survive due to paralysis of respiratory muscles following involvement of phrenic nerve nucleus.

## What is mass reflex?

Mass reflex is seen in the recovery phase of UMNL. In such patients, *afferent stimuli radiate from one reflex center to another*. Even a minor noxious stimulus like pinching of the thigh produces withdrawal response of all the limbs. The stimulus also radiates to autonomic centers and produces evacuation of bladder and rectum, sweating and blood pressure swings. Mass reflex is employed by paraplegic patients to periodically evacuate their bladder and bowel.

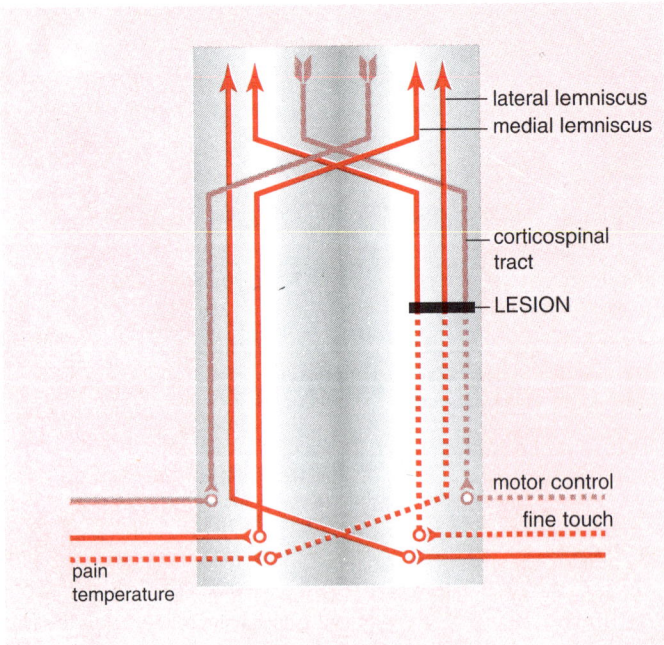

lateral lemniscus
medial lemniscus

corticospinal tract

LESION

motor control
fine touch

pain
temperature

**Fig. 108.2**

### Outline the phylogenetic subdivisions of the cerebellum.

Phylogenetically, the cerebellum is divided into the archicerebellum, paleocerebellum and neocerebellum. (1) The **archicerebellum** (vestibular cerebellum) includes the flocculonodular lobe and the lingula, and is concerned with the *maintenance of equilibrium, tone and posture of trunk muscles*. (2) The **paleocerebellum** (spinal cerebellum) includes the anterior lobe except lingula, and the pyramid and uvula. It is important for the *maintenance of muscle tone and posture of the limbs*. (3) The **neocerebellum** (cerebropontine cerebellum) neocerebellum includes rest of the cerebellum, and is concerned with the *smooth performance of skilled acts* by coordination of movements.

### Briefly outline the longitudinal subdivisions of the cerebellum.

The cerebellum is subdivided longitudinally into three zones—a vermal or median zone, a pair of paravermal or intermediate zones, and a pair of hemispheric or lateral zones. (1) The cortex of **median zone** projects into the nucleus fastigii and is concerned with the *movements of the trunk and extensor muscle tone* through the vestibulospinal and reticulospinal tracts. (2) The **intermediate zone** projects into the nucleus interpositus (nucleus globosus and nucleus emboliformis), and modifies ipsilateral movements and flexor muscle tone through the rubrospinal tracts. Together, the median and intermediate zones are concerned with *postural control of axial and limb muscles for gait*. (3) The **lateral zone** projects into the dentate nucleus and regulates the *coordination of distal limb muscles for skilful prehensile acts*. This is done through the dentato-rubro-thalamocortical pathways, and descending corticospinal and rubrospinal tracts.

### Enumerate the functions of the cerebellum.

The cerebellum receives *sensations at unconscious level*. The inputs are derived from the vestibular system, stretch receptors of muscle spindle and Golgi tendon organs, tactile and pressure receptors of the head and body, and sensations from the visual and auditory system. It uses these inputs for maintaining equilibrium, muscle tone, and posture and adjusts coordination of skilful volitional movements by regulating the relative muscle tension of agonist and antagonist muscles. The cerebellum has been called the **head ganglion of the proprioceptive system**.

(1) The **anterior lobe** of the cerebellum acts like a mode-changing switch, making muscles contract either in the $\alpha$-led mode or $\gamma$-led mode. (2) The **vermal cerebellum** and **flocculonodular lobe** are mainly concerned with *body equilibrium*. (3) The **paravermal regions** regulate *locomotion* and *movements of exploratory nature*. (4) The **hemispheric regions** supervise *skilful learned movements*. (5) The cerebellum *coordinates the* rhythmic *action of agonist and antagonist muscles*, as in diadochokinesia. It is also important in motor learning and conditioning. (6) The cerebellum also influences autonomic functions through the hypothalamus and reticular formation. Stimulation of the anterior lobe produces sympathetic response while stimulation of tonsils produce parasympathetic response.

### Describe the clinical features of neocerebellar disorder.

Neocerebellar (or lateral cerebellar) disorder results in diminished muscle tone, disturbances of muscular coordination, and tremor. In unilateral lesion, the motor disorders are expressed on the same side as the lesion. Neocerebellar manifestations are as follows. (1) **Hypotonia** occurs due to reduction of the facilitatory cerebellar output to the descending inhibitory reticular formation. (2) **Asynergia,** or a loss of muscular coordination, is the characteristic sign of neocerebellar lesion. In cerebellar dysfunction the synergy between the agonists and antagonists becomes defective and these impairments are expressed in various forms. (i) **Ataxia** takes place due to incoordination of muscles of trunk, pectoral and pelvic girdles. There is a tendency to fall on the side of the lesion. To avert the fall, the patient stands or walks on a broad base (drunken gait). (ii) **Dysmetria** means inability to measure the distance for reaching an intended goal, and is expressed by over-shooting to the side of the lesion (**past pointing**). (iii) **Decomposition of movements—**Normally an act such as in bringing a finger to the tip of the nose is produced by series of coordinated movements. In decomposition, the act breaks up into isolated movements at the joints concerned, resembling the movements of puppet. (iv) **Dysdiadochokinesia** or **adiadochokinesia** signifies inability to execute alternate movements in rapid succession, such as pronation and supination of the forearm. (v) **Rebound phenomenon** may be observed in cerebellar lesion when the patient is unable to check the action of agonist muscles by the corresponding antagonists. This happens sometimes when a patient is asked to produce active flexion of the forearm and then the hand is held somewhat away from the face. When released suddenly, unlike a normal individual, he hits his face by the hand due to loss of normal check of the antagonist muscles. (vi) **Dysarthria** or **scanning speech** takes place due to incoordination of muscles concerned with speech. The speech is slurred, prolonged and explosive, with pauses at wrong places. (vii) **Nystagmus** or oscillation of eyeball due to incoordination of extraocular muscles. Nystagmus is not conspicuous in neocerebellar lesion. (viii) **Intention tremor** is evident during purposeful movements, and is diminished or absent with rest. These tremors are coarse, arrhythmic and are observed at the end of the movement. The tremors are significantly observed when the efferent pathways of superior cerebellar peduncles are involved.

### Explain why the cerebellum exerts control over ipsilateral movements.

Cerebellar control over muscles is mostly indirect through the motor cortex. The cerebellum sends corrective signals to the *contralateral* red nucleus and motor cortex through the dentatorubral and rubrothalamocortical fibers respectively, both of which decussate in the lower midbrain. The red nucleus controls contralateral muscles through the rubrospinal tract, which decussates in the upper midbrain. Similarly, the motor cortex controls the contralateral muscles through the corticospinal tract, which decussates in the lower medulla. Hence in effect, the cerebellum controls the ipsilateral musculature (Fig. 109.1).

### Briefly outline the internal structure of the cerebellum.

The cerebellum consists of the cortex and the medulla. The **cerebellar cortex** consists of three layers—outer molecular, intermediate Purkinje and inner granular. The *outer molecular layer* contains two types of neurons—the **stellate** and **basket cells**. It also contains large number of **parallel fibers**, which are the axons of the granule cells. The *intermediate Purkinje layer* is composed of a single layer of **Purkinje cells**. The Purkinje cells are stimulated by the parallel fibers, and their axons stimulate the deep cerebellar nuclei. The *inner granular layer* contains the cell bodies of **granule cells** and **Golgi cells**. Out of five types of neurons in the cerebellar cortex, only the granule cell is *excitatory*: it releases the excitatory neurotransmitter *glutamate*. All the other cells are inhibitory and release the inhibitory neurotransmitter *GABA*.

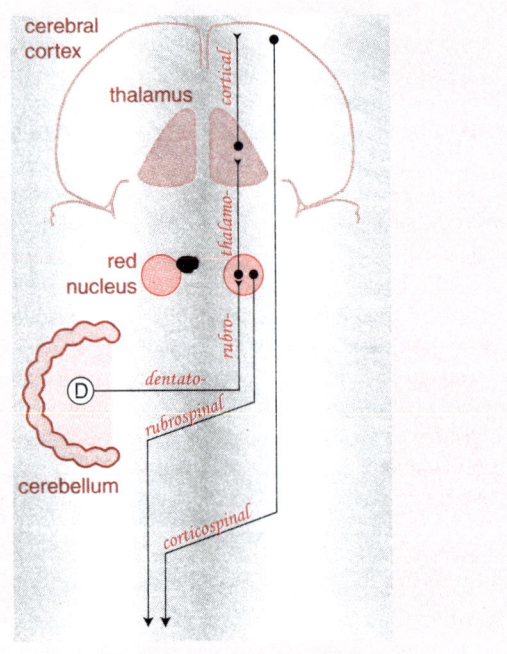

**Fig. 109.1**

The cerebellar input consists of two types of sensory fibers, the climbing fibers and mossy fibers. The climbing fibers are derived from the cells of the *inferior olivary nucleus*. All other afferents reach the cerebellum as the *mossy fibers*. Thus *a climbing fiber directly excites a single Purkinje cell, whereas a mossy fiber*

*through granule cells and parallel fibers fires thousands of Purkinje cells*. Both the climbing and mossy fibers of sensory input exert *excitatory* influence (Fig. 109.2).

The **deep cerebellar nuclei** are the *fastigial, globose, emboliform* and *dentate nuclei*. These nuclei receive axon terminals of Purkinje cells from the cerebellar cortex and collaterals from the climbing and mossy fibers. The axons of the deep cerebellar nuclei are projected as the *final efferent pathways* to the thalamus, red nucleus, brain stem reticular nuclei, inferior olivary and vestibular nuclei. The **fastigial nuclei** receives projections from the *vermal cortex* and their efferents are connected with the vestibular and medullary reticular nuclei. The **globose** and **emboliform nuclei** are collectively called the **nucleus interpositus**. Both of them receive projections from the *paravermal cortex*. Their efferents establish connection with the contralateral red nucleus, brain stem reticular nuclei and inferior olivary nucleus. Each **dentate nucleus** receives projections from the *hemispheric* or *lateral cortex*. The axons of dentate nucleus form *dentatorubrothalamic fibers*.

### Briefly outline the functional significance of the internal cerebellar circuitry.

The deep cerebellar nuclei maintain a continuous excitatory output due to the excitation by climbing and mossy fibers. This tonic excitatory output decreases when there is discharge of the inhibitory Purkinje cells of the cerebellar cortex.

There are *three minor circuits* inside the cerebellum that are meant for ensuring that the discharge of the granule cells and Purkinje cells are extremely precise and short-lasting (**neural sharpening**). This helps in accurate timing of action potentials. These circuits are as follows. (1) When the granule cell discharges, it excites the Purkinje cell. However, the excitation is extremely short lasting. This is because the granule cell inhibits the Purkinje cell (through the basket cell) shortly after stimulating it (feed-forward inhibition). (2) The mossy fiber stimulates the granule cell. However, the stimulation is extremely short-lived. This is because the mossy fiber inhibits the granule cell (through the Golgi cell) shortly after stimulating it. (3) The mossy fiber causes a brief excitation of the granule cell. The duration of excitation of the granule cell is further reduced through feedback inhibition, i.e. the discharge of the granule cells brings about its own inhibition through the Golgi cells.

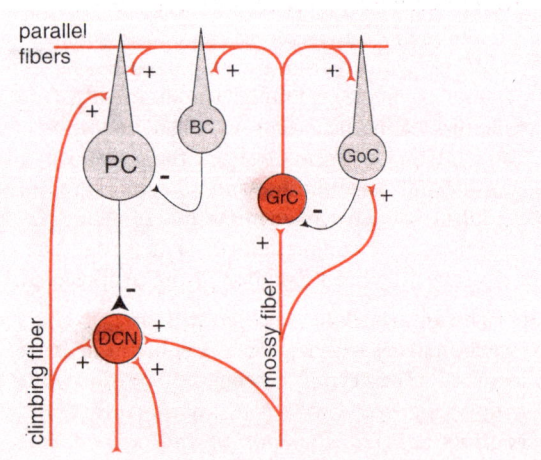

**Fig. 109.2**

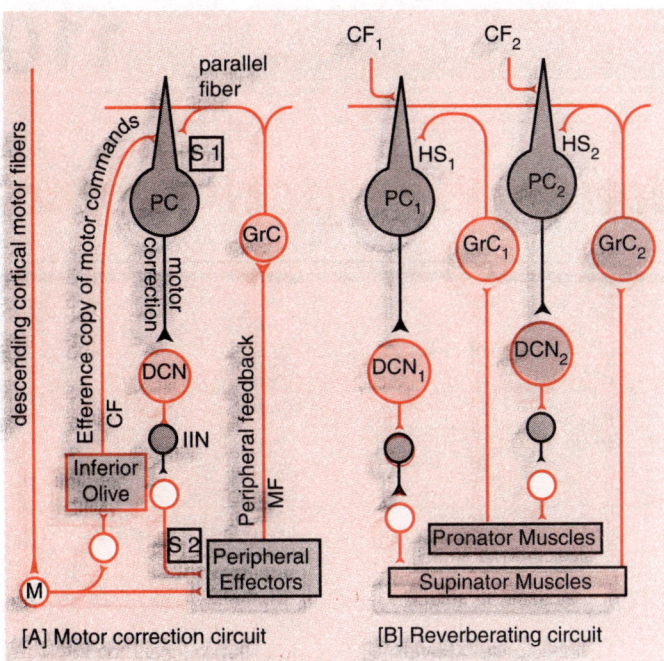

**[A] Motor correction circuit**     **[B] Reverberating circuit**

**Fig. 109.3**

There are *two major circuits* in the cerebellum whose functions are identifiable. These are the motor correction circuit and the reverberation circuit (Fig. 109.3). The **motor correction circuit** helps the cerebral cortex in achieving precision in motor control. When the cortex issues a motor command to the muscles, the cerebellum receives a copy (the *efference copy*) of the command. The cerebellum also receives peripheral feedback from the muscles indicating to what extent the cortical motor commands have been carried out. The cerebellum compares the efference copy and the peripheral feedback to calculate the error in motor effect and accordingly issues a motor correction signal to compensate for the error. The main function of the **reverberating circuit** is to form **Hebbian synapses**. New synapses are formed (rather, non-functional synapses are revived and strengthened) when two neurons repeatedly discharge synchronously. This principle was first enunciated by Hebb and hence, synapses strengthened through repeated use are called Hebbian synapses. The reverberating circuit can explain why the cerebellum is required for alternately supinating and pronating the hand rhythmically (**diadochokinesia**). This capability is impaired in cerebellar disorders and is called **adiadochokinesia**.

# 110

# Thalamus & Hypothalamus

## Name the various parts of the diencephalon.

The diencephalon (interbrain) is a complex mass of gray matter around the cavity of third ventricle. It is continuous caudally with the mid brain. The third ventricle divides the diencephalon into two symmetrical halves. The diencephalon comprises the following parts: (1) **dorsal thalamus** (or simply called thalamus); (2) epithalamus (the **pineal body**); (3) **metathalamus** (medial and lateral geniculate body); (4) hypothalamus; and (5) subthalamus. Functionally, the subthalamus belongs to the basal ganglia (Fig. 110.1).

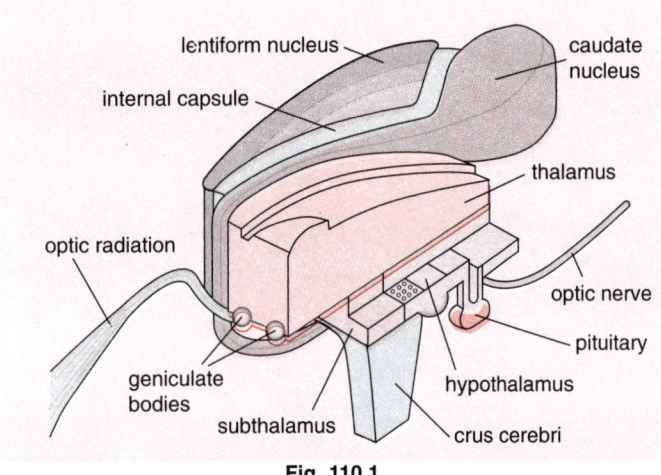

**Fig. 110.1**

## How are thalamic nuclei classified?

Six groups of nuclear masses with many subgroups are present in the thalamus. These are the anterior group, medial group, ventral group, lateral group, intralaminar group and the reticular nuclei (Fig. 110.2). On the basis of fiber connections and functions the thalamic nuclei are grouped into specific relay nuclei, association nuclei, and nonspecific nuclei. The **specific relay nuclei** receive inputs from the ascending sensory pathways and subcortical nuclei. They include most of the nuclear masses of the ventral group—VA (ventroanterior), VL (ventrolateral), VP (ventroposterior), MG (medial geniculate) body and LG (lateral geniculate) body. **Association nuclei.** These have reciprocal connections with the association areas of the cerebral cortex and include the nuclei of the dorsal group, i.e., LD (lateral dorsal), LP (lateral posterior) and pulvinar, and the DM (dorsomedial nucleus) nuclei. **Non-specific nuclei.** These do not have direct connections with the cerebral cortex and include the intralaminar nuclei, midline nuclei and reticular nucleus of thalamus.

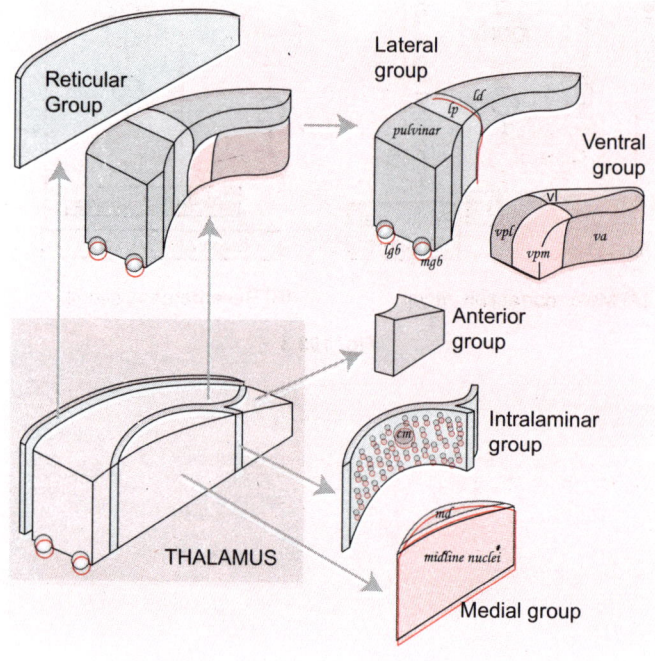

**Fig. 110.2**

## What is the importance of the ventroposterior group of nuclei?

This nuclear mass (also called the **ventrobasal complex**) is subdivided into ventral posterolateral (VPL) and ventral posteromedial (VPM) components. These nuclei are the thalamic relay station for the 2nd order sensory neurons. The **VPL** receives fibers from the medial lemniscus and the spinal lemniscus. The **VPM**, also called **arcuate nucleus**, receives input from the trigeminal lemniscus and solitariothalamic tract. The former conveys general sensory modalities from the face and head. The latter conveys taste sensation from the nucleus of tractus solitarius.

## Enumerate the functions of the thalamus.

(1) The thalamus acts as *a relay station* of *all sensory pathways, except the olfactory senses*, before being transmitted to the cerebral cortex. Here the sensory information is processed and integrated with the activities of the forebrain. (2) The thalamus is concerned with the *conscious interpretation of crude touch, pain and temperature*. The final discrimination of sensations however takes place in the sensory cortex. (3) The thalamus has a significant role in the ascending reticular activating system for *arousal or alertness*. This is mainly mediated by the nonspecific nuclei. (4) The interconnections of the thalamus with the limbic system,

hypothalamus and prefrontal cortex are important for appreciating the *emotional content of sensations.* (5) The thalamic neurons modulate the *synchronization and desynchronization of the brain waves.* (6) The thalamus *regulates the activities of the motor pathways* by linking the cerebellum and globus pallidus with the motor cortex through the VA and VL nuclei of the thalamus.

### Enumerate the clinical features of the thalamic syndrome.

The thalamic syndrome is a disturbance of thalamic function due to a lesion of the thalamus, usually after the thalamogeniculate artery is blocked. It results in a transitory hemiparesis with a severe sensory loss (deep and cutaneous) on the contralateral side of the body (**contralateral hemianesthesia**). Loss of sense of position may results in ataxia. After the lapse of a few weeks, the sensations begin to return and the patient may complain of insufferable pain on the affected side. Minor painful stimuli, such as a pinprick may cause quite severe pain on the affected side. The threshold for pain is actually raised but the reaction to pain is exaggerated (**thalamic pain**). A pleasant music may create annoyance to the affected individual. The reason for the overreaction to pain is unknown. Sometimes the patient with eyes closed is unable to locate the position of a limb or may develop an illusion that the limb is lost. This is known as the **thalamic phantom limb**.

Thalamic lesion may be associated with abnormal involuntary movements in the form of athetosis or intension tremor, when the projection fibers from the basal ganglia or cerebellum to the VA and VL nuclei of the thalamus are involved.

### Describe the subdivisions of the hypothalamus and enumerate the various nuclei in it.

The hypothalamus is subdivided into two zones—lateral and medial. The most medial part of the medial zone is sometimes called the periventricular zone. The nuclear masses of these zones are arranged rostrocaudally into four regions—preoptic, supraoptic, tuberal and mamillary.

(1) The **preoptic region** is important in the *regulation of body temperature.* (2) The **supraoptic region** is further subdivided into (i) the **supraoptic nucleus** which secretes *ADH*; (ii) the **paraventricular nucleus** which secretes the hormone *oxytocin*, *CRF* (corticotrophin releasing hormone) *somatostatin* and lesser amounts of *ADH* (antidiuretic hormone) and *dopamine* (prolactin inhibiting hormone). The axons of both groups of nuclei form the *hypothalamo-hypophysial tract*, which reaches the neurohypophysis where the neurohormones are released from the axonal endings (**neurosecretion**) into the capillary bed; (iii) **suprachiasmatic nucleus** forms a small group of neurons just above the optic chiasma. It receives direct projections from the retina as the **retino-hypothalamic fibers** and is important for regulation of *circadian rhythms.* (3) The **tuberal region** consists of: (i) **ventromedial nucleus**, which is concerned with the regulation of food intake and is called the **satiety center**; (ii) **dorsomedial nucleus**, which together with the ventromedial nucleus, is involved in the regulation of growth, feeding, maturation and reproduction; (iii) **arcuate**

nucleus (infundibular nucleus), which synthesizes and releases *GnRH* (gonadotropin releasing hormone), *GRH* (growth hormone releasing hormone), *TRH* (thyrotropin releasing hormone) and *dopamine* (prolactin inhibiting hormone). **Posterior hypothalamic nucleus** contains groups of large histaminergic neurons that are concerned with *stimulating sympathetic activity, regulation of sleep-wakefulness* and *activation of thermoregulatory mechanisms.* **Lateral hypothalamic nucleus** is important for regulation of food intake and is called the **feeding center.** (4) The **mamillary region** is a relay station in the Papez circuit and is important in the physiology of emotions (Fig. 110.3).

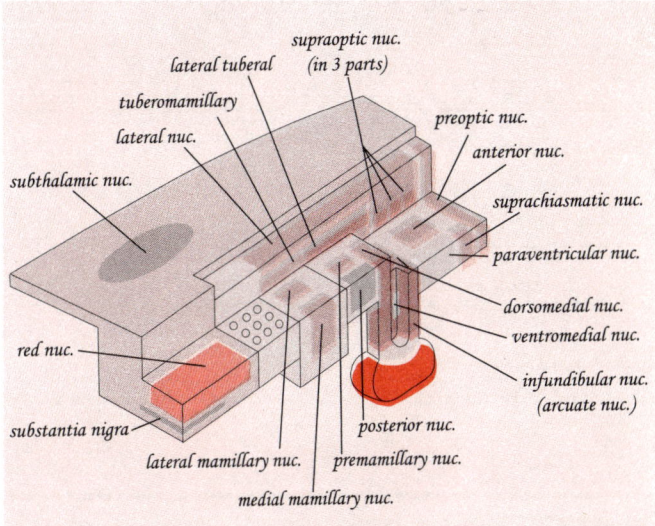

**Fig. 110.3**

### Enumerate the broad functions of the hypothalamus.

The hypothalamus acts as the *'head ganglion' of the autonomic nervous system.* The basic drives of life – hunger, thirst and sex, originate in the hypothalamus. The hypothalamus is central to the maintenance of **homeostasis**. The functions of the hypothalamus include (1) **Autonomic control**. Its anterior and medial parts (*preoptic and supra-optic areas*) *control the parasympathetic activity,* while the *posterior and lateral parts of the hypothalamus regulate the sympathetic activity.* (2) **Control of pituitary**. The hypothalamus regulates the function of posterior lobe through the hypothalamo-hypophysial tract, and modulates the secretion of anterior lobe hormones through the hypothalamo-hypophysial portal system. (3) **Temperature regulation.** The hypothalamus is the principal integrating center for thermoregulation, bringing about a balance between heat production and heat loss. (4) **Regulation of feeding behavior**. The ventromedial nucleus acts as a satiety center, whereas the lateral nucleus serves as the feeding or hunger center. (5) **Regulation of sexual behavior**. The tuberal region of hypothalamus maintains the basal secretion of gonadotropin releasing hormone (GnRH), and its connection with the preoptic area is essential for the cyclical surge of gonadotropin before ovulation. (6) **Emotional behavior**. While emotions are mainly regulated by the limbic cortex, the physical adjuncts of emotions (palpitation, cutaneous flushing, piloerection, sweating etc.) are mediated by the hypothalamus through the autonomic nervous system. Stimulation of the ventromedial nucleus produces aggressive behavior and that of the lateral nucleus induces a flight response. The *lateral hypothalamus* close to the feeding center represents a 'pleasure-center', because electrical stimulation of this area encourages the animal to seek more of such stimulation. The *medial hypothalamus* seems to act as a 'punishment center', since the experimental animal avoids further stimulation. (7) **Circadian rhythm.** The suprachiasmatic nucleus of hypothalamus is central to the maintenance of all circadian rhythms. (8) **Sleep and wakefulness.** The anterior hypothalamus is considered to be a *sleep facilitatory center* while the posterior hypothalamus acts as a *waking center*.

# 111

# Basal Ganglia

## Outline the parts of the basal ganglia.

The **corpus striatum** is divided almost completely by the fibers of internal capsule into a medial part, the **caudate nucleus** and a lateral part, the **lentiform nucleus** (Fig. 110.1). The head of caudate nucleus and lentiform nucleus are connected by a band of gray matter and the whole nuclear mass presents a striated appearance and is called the **corpus striatum**. The lentiform nucleus is further subdivided by an external medullary lamina into an outer part, the **putamen**, and an inner part, the **globus pallidus**. The globus pallidus is further separated into an outer segment (GPo) and inner segment (GPi) by an internal medullary lamina. Structurally as well as functionally, the caudate nucleus and putamen are similar and they are collectively called the **neostriatum** or for short, the **striatum**. The globus pallidus, which provides the chief efferent projection fibers of basal ganglia, is known as the **paleostriatum** or for short, the **pallidum**.

From the physiological viewpoint, the basal ganglia includes in addition to the corpus striatum, the **subthalamic nucleus** and **substantia nigra**. The **raphe nuclei** and **red nucleus** in the midbrain are also functionally connected to the basal ganglia.

## Outline the circuitry of the basal ganglia.

The afferents to the corpus striatum come from the cerebral cortex (**corticostriate** and **corticopallidal**), the thalamus (**thalamostriate** and **thalamopallidal**) and the substantia nigra (**nigrostriate**, **nigropallidal**). Most the afferents reach the neostriatum, which gives a robust projection to the globus pallidus. The efferents arise mostly from the globus pallidus (**pallidofugal**) and go the thalamus, the substantia nigra, the red nucleus and the midbrain reticular formation.

Physiologically, the connections of the corpus striatum are best understood in terms of *functional circuits or loops*. While considering the circuits, it is observed that (i) the corpus striatum does not have any direct connections with the spinal cord – either afferent or efferent. (ii) the globus pallidus internus (GPi) and the substantia nigra pars reticulata (SNpr) behave as the lateral and medial parts of a single functional entity (GPi/SNpr).

(1) The main connection of the corpus striatum is **cortex → striatum → GPi/SNpr → thalamus → SMA**. This circuit has *two inhibitory neurons*: the one running from *striatum to the globus pallidus* internus (GPi) and the other, from *globus pallidus to thalamus*. Thus, the striatum disinhibits the thalamus, and the *effect of the entire circuit is excitatory*. The part of the circuit that passes through the caudate nucleus is called the *caudate loop* while the part which passes through the putamen of the striatum is called the *putamen loop*. (2) There is another *indirect pathway via the subthalamic nucleus*. This circuit contains three inhibitory neurons: one from the

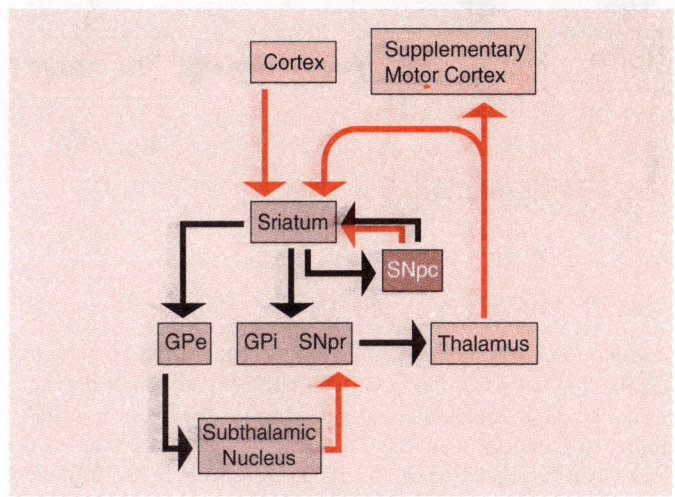

**Fig. 111.1**

striatum to GPe, another from GPe to subthalamic nucleus, and the third from GPi to thalamus. Thus, the striatum disinhibits the subthalamic nucleus (STN). The STN in its turn stimulates GPi, which then increases its inhibitory output to the thalamus. The *overall effect of the circuit is therefore inhibitory*. (3) The third circuit involving the substantia nigra pars compacta (SNpc). The SNpc is inhibited by the striatum through the **striatonigral pathway**. The SNpc in turn exerts both a facilitatory as well as an inhibitory effect on the striatum. The facilitatory effect is exerted on **excitatory striatopallidal pathway** that goes directly to the GPi, while the inhibitory effect is exerted on the **inhibitory striatopallidal pathway** that reaches the GPi through the GPe and STN (Fig. 111.1).

## Enumerate the neurotransmitters present in the basal ganglia and mention their roles.

The neurotransmitter secreted by the nigrostriatal pathway is **dopamine**. Dopamine exerts an excitatory effect when it acts through $D_1$ dopamine receptors, while it exerts an inhibitory effect when it acts through $D_2$ receptors. These receptors are present on excitatory **cholinergic** interneurons. In other areas of the basal ganglia, excitatory neurotransmission is through **glutamate** while inhibitory neurotransmission is mostly through **GABA** (Fig. 111.2). The other inhibitory neurotransmitters involved are enkephalins and substance P.

## Outline the etiology and pathophysiology of Parkinson's disease.

This condition was first described by James Parkinson in 1817. Dopamine and dopamine receptors generally decreases with age. In Parkinson's disease, *aging* is associated with an *accelerated loss of*

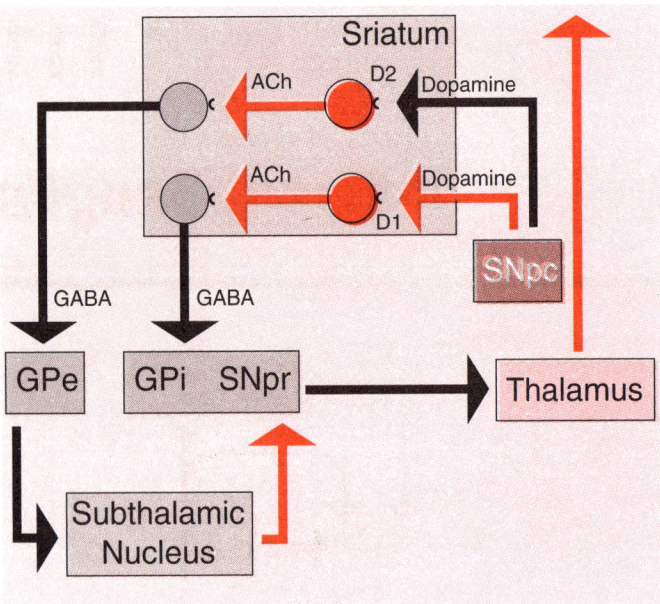

**Fig. 111.2**

*dopamine and dopamine receptors.* Degenerative changes are observed in the *substantia nigra* with marked reduction of dopamine in the striatum and substantia nigra. In the absence of dopamine, there is a decrease in the excitatory output from the direct striatothalamic circuit while there is an increase in the net inhibitory output from the indirect striatothalamic circuit via the subthalamic nucleus. Both results in hypokinetic features (Fig. 111.3).

The term Parkinsonism refers to some other conditions that result in symptoms similar to those in Parkinson's disease. These include certain viral infections and treatment with certain drugs (phenothiazines) which blocks dopamine $D_2$ receptors. Experimental Parkinsonism can be produced by the drug **MPTP** (methyl-phenyl-

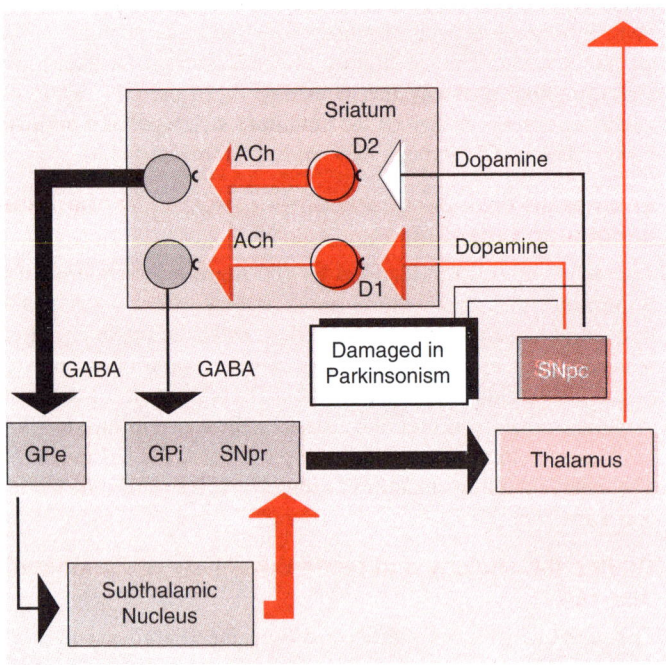

**Fig. 111.3**

tetrahydro-pyridine). MPTP is converted into MPT+ by monoamine oxidase-B (MAO-B). MPT+ is a potent oxidant that is taken up by dopaminergic neurons in the substantia nigra, which then get destroyed. MAO-B inhibitor **diprenyl** protects against MPT+ induced Parkinsonism. The fact that diprenyl slows down the progress of Parkinson's disease even when there is no apparent exposure to MPTP suggests that Parkinson's disease may be caused by some MPT+ like metabolite that is endogenously produced in the body.

## Describe the clinical features of Parkinson's disease.

Clinically, Parkinson's disease is characterized by the triad of *akinesia, rigidity and tremor* (A-R-T). Of these, akinesia is a hypokinetic feature while rigidity and tremors are hyperkinetic features. **Akinesia** includes the following features. (i) Delayed motor initiative, as evident from prolonged reaction time. (ii) Slow performance of voluntary movement (**bradykinesia**), measured by movement times (i.e., the time needed to perform a simple stereotyped movement). (iii) Difficulty reaching a target with a single continuous movement (**hypokinesia**). The movement must stop and resume to touch the intended objective. (iv) Rapid fatigue with repetitive movement. (v) Inability to execute simultaneous actions, e.g., the patient can salute when seated but not when walking. (vi) Inability to execute sequential actions. (vii) Defective kinetic automatism, i.e., the loss of associated movements like reduced facial expression and hand gestures during speech, arm swinging during gait, etc. The patient possesses masked face appearance with no emotional response. (viii) Patient *walks with short, quick steps* and experiences difficulty in taking initial steps and in terminating the movements. The possible cause of akinesia is because of the *dysfunction of the caudate loop, which hampers the smooth transition from one motor program to another difficult.*

The **rigidity** takes place due to increased muscle tone of both agonist and antagonist muscles. During passive flexion or extension of a limb, the muscular resistance increases and decreases alternately as if it is overcoming a series of catches (**cog-wheel rigidity**). Sometimes, there may be a more uniform resistance to passive flexion (**lead-pipe rigidity**). Rigidity probably results from *withdrawal of facilitation of inverse-stretch (Golgi tendon) reflex.* In Parkinson's disease, the increased inhibitory output from the globus pallidus reduces the descending facilitatory influences on the inhibitory interneuron in the Golgi tendon reflex pathway. Since the Golgi tendon reflex is inhibitory to muscle tone, reduction of supraspinal facilitatory inputs to the reflex results in increase in muscle tone. The resulting rigidity is different from spasticity, which results from excessive facilitation of the stretch reflex.

**Tremor at rest** is a prominent sign in Parkinson's disease. The frequency of tremors range from 3 – 6 Hz. The tremor activity is usually suppressed during voluntary movements and sleep, and is exaggerated by stress and anxiety. The tremor occurs with regular frequency, when the subject is at rest. It is characterized by **pill-rolling** movement of the hand. The tremor disappears during movement and is increased in emotion. The tremor seems to occur due to a pacemaker activity in the *nucleus ventralis intermedius of the thalamus.* Thalamic neurons have an intrinsic autorhythmicity and it is possible that this automaticity gets unmasked by the increase in the inhibitory input from the globus pallidus. The *thalamic pacemaker activity induces oscillations in the long-loop reflex pathways*. Long-loop reflex pathways originate from muscle spindle. The reflex path runs through the thalamus up to the cortex and then loops back to extrafusal muscle fibers along the corticospinal tract.

### Outline the treatment of Parkinson's disease.

Parkinsonism is treated by administration of **L-dopa,** which in low doses diminishes rigidity and in high doses reduces tremor. L-dopa crosses the blood brain barrier and gets converted into dopamine. **Bromocriptine** and other dopamine agonists that cross the blood brain barrier to activate dopamine receptors are also useful in treatment. *Dopamine itself is unable to cross the blood brain barrier and therefore is of no therapeutic use.* Surgical destruction of the globus pallidus (**pallidotomy**) or ventrolateral nucleus of thalamus also ameliorates the symptoms of Parkinson's disease. **Anticholinergic drugs** also bring about some improvement. **Diprenyl**, a MAO-B inhibitor, slows down the progress of the disease. **Transplantation** of the adrenal medulla or fetal basal ganglia tissue on the caudate nucleus is associated with significant improvement.

### What is choreoathetosis and what are its causes?

**Chorea** is characterized by brisk, jerky, purposeless and graceful movements of the distal parts of the extremities, and is usually associated with twitchings of the face. A slower version of chorea is **athetosis** that is characterized by slow, worm-like writhing movements of the extremities, affecting chiefly the fingers and the wrists. Choreoathetosis is associated with the *degeneration of the indirect striatopallidal pathway via subthalamic nucleus*. Since the overall effect of this pathway is inhibitory, damage to this pathway results in **hyperkinesia**. Athetosis is frequently seen in *damage of putamen* as a result of birth-injury while chorea is mostly due to damage to the *caudate nucleus* (Fig. 111.4).

Chorea may be genetically inherited or acquired. Examples of chorea that are *genetically inherited* are Huntington's chorea

and Wilson's disease. **Huntington's chorea** is associated with degeneration of caudate nucleus (most affected), putamen (moderately affected) and globus pallidus (least affected). **Wilson's disease** (earlier called hepatolenticular disease) is the widespread manifestation of copper toxicity that occurs due to impaired biliary excretion of dietary copper. The toxic effects are most pronounced in the liver and the brain. In brain, the lesions are widespread. However, the changes are most marked in the putamen and to a lesser degree, in the globus pallidus and caudate nucleus. Wilson's disease is characteristically associated with low plasma levels of **ceruloplasmin**. This is because the increase in copper in liver cells inhibits the binding of copper to apoceruloplasmin: the two must be in an optimum proportion for the hepatic synthesis of ceruloplasmin.

*Acquired chorea is mostly immunological in origin.* One of these is the **Sydenham's chorea**, which occurs following streptococcal infection. Antibodies to β-hemolytic streptococci cross react with neurons of the corpus striatum and damage them.

### What is hemiballismus?

It is a rare disease manifested by wild, flail-like movements of one arm, and is caused by *degeneration of subthalamic nucleus* on the opposite side. Damage to the subthalamus reduces the inhibitory output from the GPi/SNpr, resulting in the disinhibition of the thalamic output (Fig. 111.5).

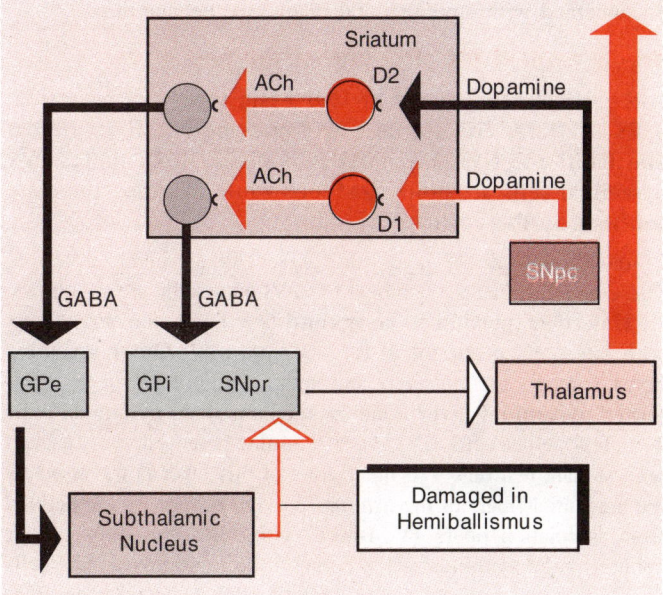

**Fig. 111.5**

### How does Parkinson's tremor differ from cerebellar tremor?

| Parkinson's Tremors | Cerebellum Tremors |
| --- | --- |
| Fine tremors | Coarse tremors |
| 6-8 Hz | 2-4 Hz |
| Rhythmic | Arrhythmic |
| Occurs at rest | Occurs at the end of a movement |

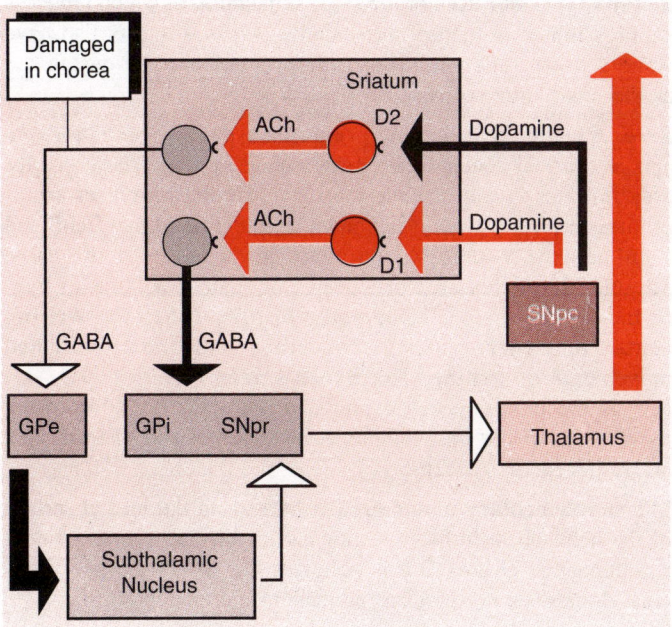

**Fig. 111.4**

# 112

# Cerebral Cortex

### Briefly outline the phylogenetic divisions of the cerebral cortex.

Phylogenetically, the cerebral cortex (**pallium**) is subdivided into two parts—**allocortex** or old cortex, which forms about 10% of the entire cortex, and isocortex or **neocortex**, which comprises remaining 90%. The allocortex is further subdivided into: (i) the **archipallium** (ancient cortex), which includes hippocampus and dentate gyrus; (ii) the **paleopallium** (old cortex) comprises uncus and part of parahippocampal gyrus which belong to the piriform area of olfactory cortex, and (iii) the **mesocortex**, which is the transitional zone between allocortex and isocortex, and comprises the cingulate gyrus, part of parahippocampal gyrus and subiculum. Since most of the allocortex is located around the peripheral margin of the diencephalon, it is also called the **limbic cortex**. In conjunction with the thalamus and hypothalamus, the limbic cortex is concerned with emotions and instinctive behavior.

### Briefly explain the structure of the neocortex.

The cortical neurons are of four basic types: (i) pyramidal cells of Betz, (ii) stellate (granule) cells, (iii) cells of Martinotti and (iv) horizontal cells of Cajal. Of these, only pyramidal cells are projection cells while the other three are confined to the cortical layers.

Cytoarchitecturally, 6 layers are present in the cerebral cortex. These laminae, that are numbered I to VI outside in, are as follows. (I) **Molecular (plexiform) layer** consists of horizontal nerve fibers with interspersed horizontal *cells of Cajal*; (II) **Outer granular layer** contains *stellate cells* and small pyramidal neurons; (III) **Outer pyramidal layer** contains medium-sized pyramidal cells and a few stellate cells. (IV) **Inner granular layer** is densely packed with stellate neurons. The inner zone of this layer is traversed by the tangential fibers of the *external band of Baillarger* are derived from association fibers. (V) **Inner pyramidal (ganglionic) layer** contains large pyramidal cells. Some of the largest pyramidal cells are seen in the precentral gyrus where they are called the *giant pyramidal cells of Betz*. Tangential fibers of the *internal band of Baillarger* traverse this lamina. (VI) **Polymorphous (pleomorphic) layer** contains the *cells of Martinotti* and multipolar neurons which are probably modified pyramidal neurons.

### Name the different motor areas of the brain and explain their functions.

Motor (precentral) areas include the primary motor area (area 4), premotor area (areas 6 and 8) and supplementary motor area (Fig. 112.1). The supplementary motor area is located on the medial surface of the hemisphere in the posterior part of medial frontal gyrus as a continuation of area 6. The giant pyramidal cells of

Betz are confined to the posterior part of area 4 along the central sulcus and are more numerous in the paracentral lobule.

The **primary motor cortex** controls *movements of voluntary muscles* of the contralateral side of the body. Centers for movements are represented *somatotopically*, with head end below and leg end up (the **motor homunculus**) (Fig. 112.2). The extent of the cortical representation of a muscle depends on the precision requirements of its movements and not on its size. The **premotor area** is concerned with integrated movements and not for individual muscles.

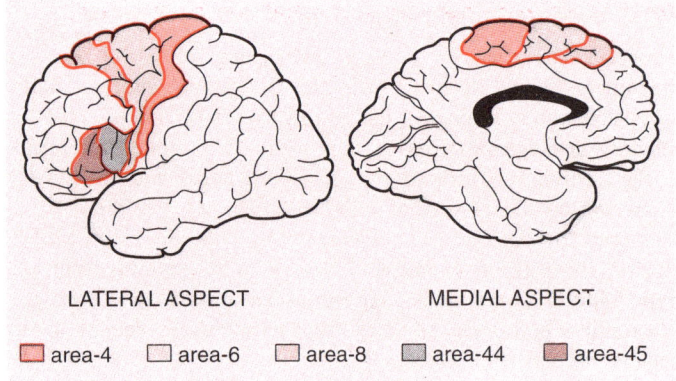

LATERAL ASPECT    MEDIAL ASPECT

☐ area-4    ☐ area-6    ☐ area-8    ☐ area-44    ☐ area-45

**Fig. 112.1**

A narrow strip of cortex between areas 4 and 6 is known as the **motor suppressor area** or *area 4-s*, stimulation of which produces suppression of voluntary movements. Areas 4 and 6 also have some sensory functions. Hence these areas may be designated as the **Ms-I** (motorsensory).

*Areas 6 and 8* are called the **premotor area**. The premotor area acts as cortical center for extrapyramidal system. The premotor area initiates *complex movements* by stimulating preset arrays of sites in area 4. *Area 8* is known as the **frontal eye field**, and regulates the voluntary conjugate movements of the eyes. Stimulation of this area produces conjugate deviation of eyes to the opposite side. *Upper part of area 6* has the **writing center of Exner**, which is concerned with the coordinated movements of writing. The **Broca's area** (*areas 44 and 45*) acts as the motor speech center and regulates the coordinated movements of the lips, tongue, palate, larynx and pharynx that are required for speech.

The **supplementary motor area** is located on the medial surface of the hemisphere in the posterior part of medial frontal gyrus as a continuation of area 6. It is designated as **Ms-II**. Lesion of this area alone does not produce permanent motor defect.

**Area 8** is the **frontal eye field**, which is important for conjugate

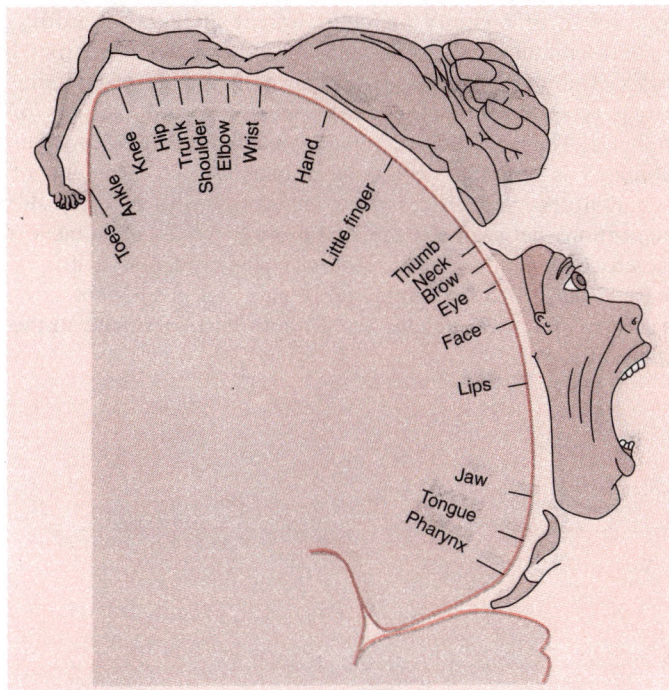

**Fig. 112.2**

and disjugate eye movements. The **perisylvian areas** (areas around the lateral sulcus) are concerned with speech. In includes the **area 22**, which is also known as the **Wernicke's area**.

### Name the different sensory areas of the brain and explain their functions.

The **primary somesthetic area** (*areas, 3, 1, 2*) is located in the postcentral gyrus and extends onto the medial surface in the posterior part of the *paracentral lobule* (Fig. 112.3). This area localizes, analyses and discriminates different modalities of cutaneous and proprioceptive senses.

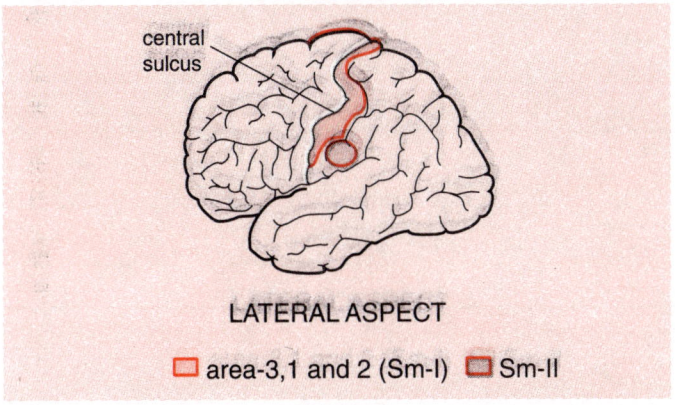

**Fig. 112.3**

Areas of sensation are somatotopically represented upside down with head below and leg up (**sensory homunculus**) (Fig. 112.4). Sensory area in the paracentral lobule receives the sense of distension from the *bladder and rectum*. The lower part of the postcentral gyrus acts as **taste receptive center**. Areas 3, 1, 2 also have some motor functions. Hence the area is designated as Sm-I.

Further processing of the somesthetic input takes place in the

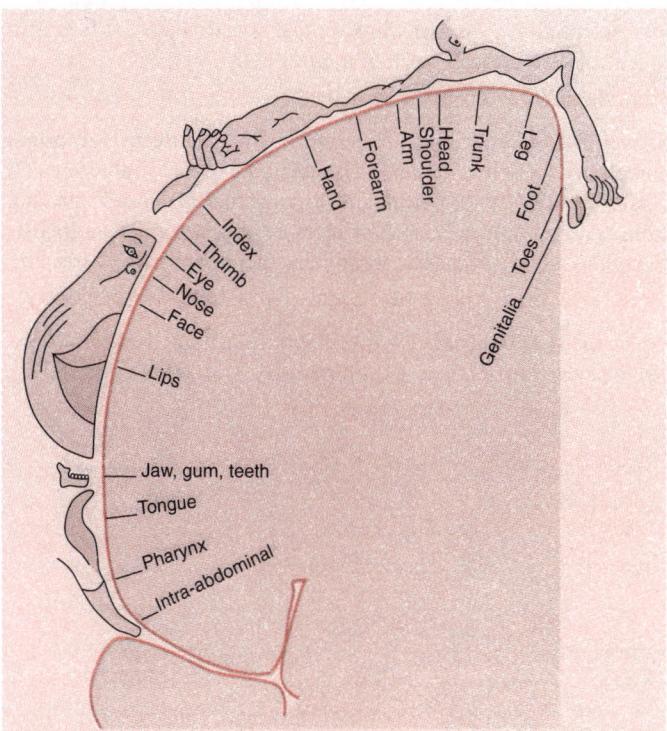

**Fig. 112.4**

sensory association areas. A lesion affecting *area-40* produces astereognosis. The auditory and visual areas include the **primary visual area** (visuostriate area, area 17 or visual area 1), **visual association area** (areas 18 and 19 and inferotemporal cortex), **primary auditory area** (*area 41, auditory area I*) and **auditory association area** (*area 42, auditory area II*).

### Name the different psychic areas of the brain and outline their functions.

Anatomically, the limbic areas are located in the border regions of the cerebral hemisphere. Functionally, the limbic areas are concerned with emotions and motivation. The limbic area includes: the **inferotemporal cortex** (area 21), which lends a logical and emotional insight to visceral perception. Ablation of this area causes psychic blindness: the animals are able to see but do not understand what they see. Monkeys with such ablations would attempt to grasp flames or play with snakes, which they normally abhor. The **anterolateral temporal area**, stimulation of which results in recall of complex visual and auditory images, an experience of déjà vu (*Fr:* already seen). The **uncinate area**, stimulation of which results in a dreamy state, olfactory and gustatory hallucinations and masticatory movements. The **parahippocampal gyrus**, bilateral ablation of which, when performed along with the hippocampus, causes severe loss of ability to learn or establish new memories (**Korsakoff's psychosis**). The **piriform cortex**, ablation of which produces hypersexuality. Cats and monkeys after the ablation would even approach animals of other species e.g. hen. The **amygdalar cortex**, destruction of which abolishes rage and induces docility, hyperphagia and oral tendencies.

The **prefrontal area** (areas 9 to 12) is the part of the frontal lobe rostral to the premotor area. The prefrontal area controls emotions.

It is essential for abstract thinking and social behavior. It is also called the 'silent area' of the brain.

### What is Kluver-Bucy syndrome?

Kluver-Bucy Syndrome occurs following **bilateral temporal lobectomy**, which removes a sizeable part of the limbic area. It results in docility, hyperphagia, hypersexuality, visual agnosia, increased oral tendency, loss of memory and hypermetamorphosis (failure to ignore peripheral stimuli and therefore easily distracted).

### What are the clinical features of prefrontal lobectomy?

**Prefrontal lobectomy** in monkeys result in hyperactivity, excessive expression of emotions, socially aggressive, impairment of memory and impairment of learning ability. Patients with tumors of frontal lobe or with atrophy of prefrontal cortex exhibit lack of a sense of responsibility in personal affairs, vulgarity in speech, clownish in behavior and feelings of euphoria. The operation of bilateral **prefrontal leucotomy** or **lobotomy** is sometimes practised in patients with symptoms of mental illness and distressing somatic pain, by severing the connections between the prefrontal area and the dorsomedial nucleus of thalamus. The resulting changes include a loss of anxiety and relief from intractable pain. Surgical lobotomies make the individual docile, and without much response to the surroundings.

# 113

# Autonomic Nervous System

## Define autonomic nervous system (ANS).

The ANS is essentially an **efferent visceral nervous system** that influences (excites or inhibits) the *contraction of cardiac and smooth muscles* as well as certain *secretory and metabolic processes*. Visceral afferents are sometimes called *autonomic afferents*. However, many disagree and consider the *autonomic system to be solely an efferent system.*

The autonomic system has two components: the **sympathetic** and the **parasympathetic**. Anatomically, the sympathetic fibers originate from the thoracic and lumbar segments of the spinal cord (the **thoracolumbar outflow**), while the parasympathetic fibers originate from the sacral segments of spinal cord and from the brainstem (the **craniosacral outflow**). Functionally, the sympathetic system is triggered during fight-or-flight situations and is associated with catabolic processes while the parasympathetic system is concerned with the vegetative aspects of day-to-day living and supports the anabolic processes of the body.

Most nerves have a few *autonomic nerve fibers* in them. The autonomic pathway from the spinal cord to the target organ is made of two neurons that synapse in an autonomic ganglion. The neuron originating from the spinal cord is the **preganglionic** neuron while the one that reaches the target organ is the **postganglionic neuron**.

## Which areas of the brain control the ANS?

The **hypothalamus** plays an important role in the regulation of autonomic activity and has been called the **head ganglion of the ANS**. However, the **limbic cortex** is equally important in the regulation of the ANS. It was earlier believed that the ANS is *not under voluntary control*. However, persons skilled in the arts of *yoga, meditation and relaxation* have demonstrated *voluntary control over their blood pressure and heart rate* that are normally regulated by the ANS.

## Briefly describe the anatomy of the sympathetic nervous system.

The *cell bodies of the preganglionic sympathetic fibers are located in the intermediolateral horn* of the thoracolumbar ($T_1$-$L_3$) spinal gray matter while the *cell body of the postganglionic sympathetic fiber is located in a ganglion*. The ganglia of the sympathetic fibers are most commonly located in the paravertebral sympathetic chain and less commonly, in a collateral ganglion close to the target organ, for example, the celiac ganglion, the otic ganglion etc. The ganglion may be present inside the organ itself.

The preganglionic fiber leaves the spinal cord through its ventral root along with the somatic nerves. However, it soon exits the ventral root through the **white rami communicantes** to enter the

ganglion on the sympathetic chain. The white ramus communicantes is white because it is formed entirely of preganglionic sympathetic fibers, which are *thinly myelinated B fibers*. The postganglionic fibers exit the ganglion through the **gray rami communicantes** and reenter the ventral root to enter the spinal nerve (Fig. 113.1-A). The gray ramus communicantes is gray in color because the postganglionic sympathetic fibers are *unmyelinated C fibers*.

Some fibers ascend or descend along the sympathetic trunk to a variable extent and make synapses with the cells of the upper or lower sympathetic ganglia (Fig. 113.1-B). A few fibers pass uninterrupted through the ganglia of the sympathetic chain and appear as the medial branches of the ganglia to form thoracic splanchnic and lumbar splanchnic nerves, and makes synapses in the collateral ganglia (e.g., celiac, mesenteric etc.) as shown in Fig. 113.1-C).

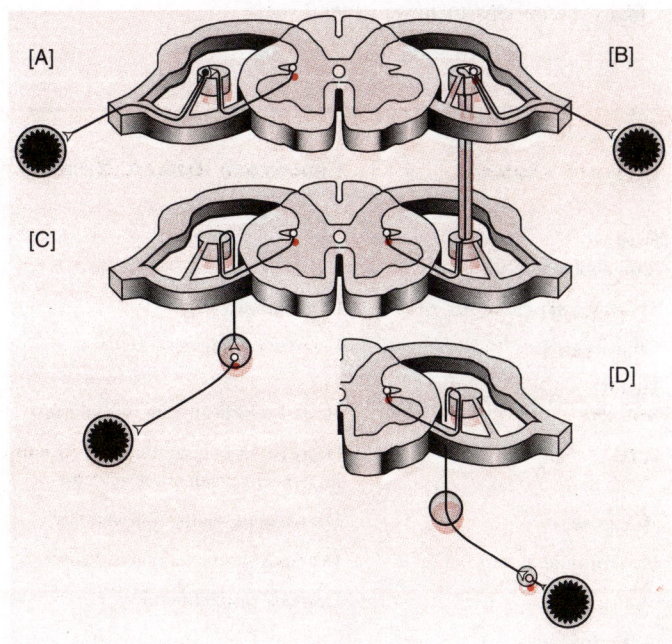

**Fig. 113.1**

Parts of the uterus and the male genital tract are innervated by the **short noradrenergic neurons** with cell bodies in ganglia in or near these organs, and the preganglionic fibers to these organs pass uninterrupted even through the collateral ganglion to synapse in ganglia in or near the organ (Fig. 113.1-D). (This type of arrangement is however typical of parasympathetic fibers.) Some of these also synapse with **terminal ganglia**, which are found only in the adrenal medulla as the chromaffin cells liberating adrenaline.

## Briefly describe the anatomy of the parasympathetic nervous system.

Parasympathetic fibers are present in the **craniosacral outflow** from the central nervous system. In the cranial nerves, the parasympathetic nerves are present in the *3rd, 7th, 9th and 10th cranial nerves* and originate in the nuclei of the corresponding cranial nerves. In the sacral part of the spinal cord, the parasympathetic fibers originate in the intermediolateral gray horn of $S_1$-$S_4$ and pass out through the ventral spinal root of the corresponding nerves. In either case, the *parasympathetic preganglionic fibers* travel all the way to the target organ and synapse with the *postganglionic neuron* in ganglia located near or in the organ.

## Name the main autonomic neurotransmitters and their receptors.

Postganglionic parasympathetic fibers release mostly **acetylcholine** as their neurotransmitter. Postganglionic sympathetic fibers release mostly **noradrenaline**. However in case of sympathetic vasodilator fibers and sympathetic fibers innervating sweat glands, the neurotransmitter is *acetylcholine*.

The adrenergic receptors are $\alpha$, $\beta_1$ and $\beta_2$. Noradrenaline acts mainly on $\alpha$ receptors and to a lesser extent, on $\beta$ receptors. In general, (i) $\alpha$ receptors mediate excitation of smooth muscles; (ii) $\beta_1$ receptors mediate excitation of cardiac muscle, and (iii) $\beta_2$ receptors mediate inhibition of smooth muscles. However, there are many exceptions to these general rules.

## Name the neurotransmitters and their receptors present in the autonomic ganglia.

At the synapse between the preganglionic and postganglionic neurons, the neurotransmitter is mostly **acetylcholine**, *which* acts on **nicotinic cholinergic receptors** located on the postsynaptic membrane. Although the receptors are nicotinic, they are not blocked by tubocurarine, the drug that blocks the nicotinic receptors in the motor end plate. Instead, they are blocked by a different set of nicotinic blockers that include the drug **hexamethonium**. Some cholinergic receptors in the ganglia are of the muscarinic type. Moreover, there are other types of ganglionic neurotransmitters too, like dopamine and GnRH. They act through **$D_2$ receptors** and **GnRH receptors** respectively.

Activation of the postsynaptic receptors in the ganglion mostly leads to the generation of EPSP in the postganglionic cell, and occasionally, produces an IPSP. The various neurotransmitters, the receptor they activate and the type of postsynaptic potentials they produce are summarized below.

| Neurotransmitter | Receptor | Postsynaptic potential and its duration |
|---|---|---|
| Acetylcholine | Nicotinic | Fast EPSP (30 milliseconds) |
| Acetylcholine | Muscarinic | Slow EPSP (30 seconds) |
| Dopamine | $D_2$ | Slow IPSP (2 seconds) |
| GnRH | GnRH receptor | Late slow EPSP (4 seconds) |

## What are the major differences in sympathetic and parasympathetic action in various tissues?

| EFFECTOR ORGANS | CHOLINERGIC IMPULSE RESPONSE | NORADRENERGIC IMPULSES RESPONSE | RECEPTOR TYPE |
|---|---|---|---|
| **Eyes**<br>Radial muscle of iris | | $\alpha$ | Contraction (mydriasis) |
| Sphincter muscle of iris | Contraction (meiosis) | | |
| Ciliary muscle | Contraction for near vision | $\beta$ | Relaxation for far vision |
| **Heart**<br>S-A node | Decrease in heart rate, vagal arrest | $\beta$ | Increase in heart rate |
| Atria | Decrease in contractility and (usually) increase in conduction velocity | $\beta$ | Increase in contractility and conduction velocity |
| A-V node | Decrease in conduction velocity | $\beta$ | Increase in conduction velocity |
| His-Purkinje system | Decrease in conduction velocity | $\beta$ | Increase in conduction velocity |
| Ventricles | Decrease in contractility | $\beta$ | Increase in contractility |
| **Arterioles**<br>Coronary | Constriction | $\alpha$<br>$\beta$ | Constriction<br>Dilation |
| Skin and mucosa | Dilation | $\alpha$ | Constriction |
| Skeletal muscle | Dilation | $\alpha$<br>$\beta$ | Constriction<br>Dilation |
| Cerebral | Dilation | $\alpha$ | Constriction |
| Pulmonary | Dilation | $\alpha$<br>$\alpha$ | Constriction<br>Dilation |
| Abdominal viscera | | $\alpha$<br>$\beta$ | Constriction<br>Dilation |

| | | | |
|---|---|---|---|
| Salivary glands | Dilation | α | Constriction |
| Renal | | α | Constriction |
| | | β | Dilation |
| **Systemic veins** | | α | Constriction |
| | | β | Dilation |
| **Lungs** | | | |
| Bronchial muscle | Contraction | β | Relaxation |
| Bronchial glands | Stimulation | α | Inhibition |
| | | β | Stimulation |
| **Stomach** | | | |
| Motility and tone | Increase | α, β | Decrease (usually) |
| Sphincters | Relaxation (usually) | α | Contraction (usually) |
| Secretion | Stimulation | α | Inhibition |
| Intestine Motility and tone | Increase | α, β | Decrease (usually) |
| Sphincters | Relaxation (usually) | α | Contraction (usually) |
| Secretion | Stimulation | α | Inhibition |
| **Gallbladder and ducts** | Contraction | β | Relaxation |
| **Urinary bladder** | | | |
| Detrusor | Contraction | β | Relaxation (usually) |
| Trigone and sphincter | Relaxation | α | Contraction |
| **Ureters** | | | |
| Motility and tone | Increase (?) | α | Increase (usually) |
| **Uterus** | Variable | α | Contraction (pregnant) |
| | | β | Relaxation (pregnant and non-pregnant) |
| **Male sex organs** | Erection | α | Ejaculation |
| **Skin** | | | |
| Pilomotor muscles | | α | Contraction |
| Sweat glands | Generalized secretion | α | Slight, localized secretion |
| **Spleen capsule** | | α | Contraction |
| | | | β Relaxation |
| **Adrenal medulla** | Secretion of epinephrine and norepinephrine | | |
| **Liver** | | α, β | Glycogenolysis |
| **Pancreas** | | | |
| Acini | Increased secretion | α | Decreased secretion |
| Islets | Increased insulin and glucagon secretion | α | Decreased insulin and glucagon secretion |
| | | β | Increased insulin and glucagon secretion |
| **Salivary glands** | Profuse, watery secretion | α | Thick, viscous secretion |
| | | β | Amylase secretion |
| **Lacrimal glands** | Secretion | α | Secretion |
| **Nasopharyngeal glands** | Secretion | | |
| **Adipose tissue** | | α, β | Lipolysis |
| **Juxtaglomerular cells** | | | Increased renin secretion |
| **Pineal gland** | | | Increased melatonin synthesis and secretion |

# 114

# Synaptic Transmission

### Define a synapse.
A synapse is a site where impulse travels from one neuron (the presynaptic neuron) to another (the postsynaptic neuron).

### What are the differences between electrical and chemical synapses?

| Chemical synapse | Electrical synapse |
|---|---|
| Synaptic transmission is mediated by release of neurotransmitters. | Synaptic transmission is ephaptic transmission of electrical impulses through gap junctions. |
| Can occur only in one direction: from the presynaptic terminal containing neurotransmitters to the postsynaptic membrane bearing receptors for the neurotransmitters. | Can occur in both directions. |
| Speed of synaptic transmission is much slower than the speed of nerve conduction, which results in a **synaptic delay** of about 0.5ms. | Speed of synaptic transmission equals the speed of nerve conduction. |
| Vulnerable to **synaptic fatigue** (fatigue on repeated stimulation) and to the effects of hypoxia and pH changes | Much less susceptible to fatigue. |

### Briefly outline the mechanism of synaptic transmission.
The pre- and postsynaptic elements are separated by a 20 to 30 nm wide cleft called the **synaptic cleft**. The synaptic cleft contains enzymes that destroy the neurotransmitters released into the cleft. Synaptic transmission occurs through the following steps: (1) The action potential arriving at the presynaptic nerve terminal depolarizes the presynaptic nerve terminal. (2) The depolarization stimulates the influx of free $Ca^{2+}$ into the nerve terminal by opening of voltage-gated $Ca^{2+}$ channels. (3) $Ca^{2+}$ stimulates the sliding of synaptic vesicles along the presynaptic grid towards the presynaptic membrane, presumably by triggering the cross-bridge movements. (4) The vesicles discharge their neurotransmitters into the synaptic cleft by exocytosis. (5) The neurotransmitter released from the presynaptic terminal do not persist in the synaptic cleft for long as it is removed from these in one of the following ways: (i) *reuptake by the presynaptic terminal*, which by far is the commonest mechanism. Exceptions are peptide neurotransmitter and acetylcholine; (ii) *rapid dissociation by enzymatic action* e.g. acetylcholine is dissociated by acetylcholinesterase into acetyl CoA and choline and only the choline is taken up; and (iii) *diffusion away from the synaptic cleft.*

### What is Dale's phenomenon?
Usually, only one type of neurotransmitter is released from all the terminals of a single neuron. This was first propounded by Dale, and is called Dale's phenomenon.

### How is an EPSP produced? What is the magnitude and duration of an EPSP?
The transmitter attaches to the receptors on the postsynaptic membrane. This triggers the opening of the ligand-gated $Na^+$ channels on the postsynaptic membrane. The resultant rise in the $Na^+$ conductance produces depolarizes the postsynaptic membrane. The depolarization thus produced is called the **excitatory postsynaptic potential** (**EPSP**). The magnitude of the EPSP is 8 mV. The depolarization starts with a latency of 0.5ms, rises to its peak in 2.0ms, and then declines with a half-life of 4.0ms (Fig. 114.1).

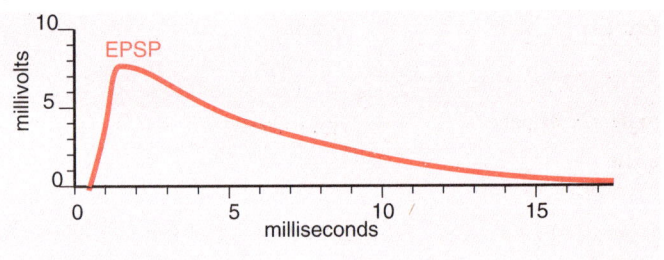

**Fig. 114.1**

### What is an initial spike?
The initial spike is the spike potential produced in the **initial segment** of an axon, which comprises the axon hillock and the proximal unmyelinated part of the nerve fibers. The initial segment has the lowest threshold of excitation (only 6 to 10 mV) as compared to the other parts of the nerve. The magnitude of the initial spike is 30 to 40 mV from the threshold level (Fig. 114.2).

### How is an IPSP produced? What is the magnitude and duration of an IPSP?
An inhibitory postsynaptic potential (IPSP) is produced when the neurotransmitter increases the permeability of the postsynaptic membrane to $K^+$ ions, producing hyperpolarization of the membrane. Its magnitude is -2 mV. The hyperpolarization has a latency of 2.0ms, attaining its maximum at 4ms and then returning towards the RMP with a half-life of 3 ms (Fig. 114.3).

### Compare and contrast EPSP and IPSP.

**SIMILARITIES**

Both are post-synaptic potentials.

Both undergo spatial and temporal summation.

**DIFFERENCES**

| EPSP | IPSP |
|---|---|
| Produced when excitatory neurotransmitters (like glutamate) are released | Produced when inhibitory neurotransmitters (like GABA and glycine) are released |
| Associated with the opening of ligand-gated Na⁺ channels | Associated with the opening of ligand-gated K⁺ channels |
| Has a potential of + 8 mV | Has a potential of - 2 mV |

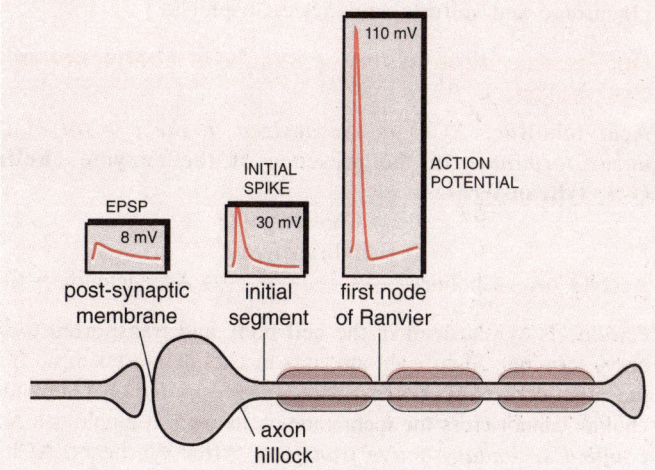

**Fig. 114.2**

## Explain the terms spatial and temporal summation.

The release of neurotransmitters in the synaptic cleft results in a number of small, subthreshold potential changes on the post-synaptic membrane. These post-synaptic potentials, which may be EPSP or IPSP, get added up or summated (Fig. 114.4). The summation of post-synaptic potentials may be temporal or spatial depending on whether the PSPs are separated in time or space. Temporal summation occurs when multiple PSPs are produced in same area of the postsynaptic membrane in quick succession. Spatial summation occurs when two PSPs are produced on adjacent areas of the postsynaptic membrane simultaneously. Summation of potentials is made easier by the membrane characteristics of the dendrites: the EPSP's and IPSP's produced on the dendrites *do not fade off quickly* – a property called the *holding capacity* of the dendrites.

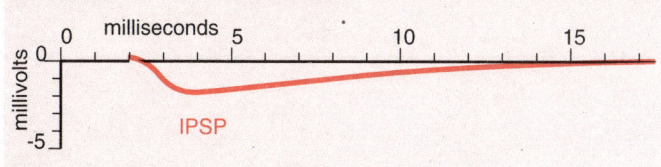

**Fig. 114.3**

## What is a soma-dendritic spike? What is its role?

The **action potential (AP)** spike triggered by the initial spike travels not only anterogradely along the axon but also gets conducted retrogradely over the soma and dendrites. This retrogradely conducted potential, although identical to the action potential, is called by a different name – the **soma-dendritic (SD) spike**. The SD spike *quickly restores the potential of the entire soma-dendritic*

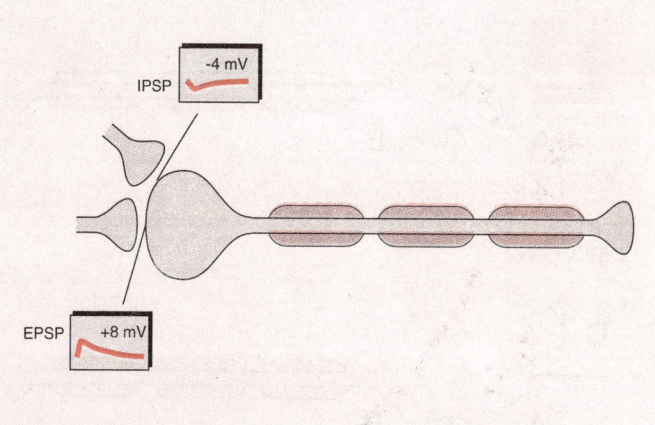

**Fig. 114.4**

*tree to the resting potential*. This allows a fresh set of postsynaptic potentials to be summated on the soma-dendritic membrane.

## What is presynaptic inhibition?

In presynaptic inhibition (Fig. 114.5), the inhibitory neuron (neuron C) does not make direct contact with the postsynaptic neuron (neuron B). Instead, it synapses on the presynaptic axon terminal (neuron A) and inhibits the release of the excitatory neurotransmitters from it. There are different mechanisms through which the release of excitatory neurotransmitter is decreased. (i) The inhibitory neuron (C) releases neurotransmitters that increase the permeability of the presynaptic membrane (A) to Cl⁻ or K⁺. As a result, the action potentials produced at the presynaptic membrane are smaller and there is lesser release of neurotransmitters. (ii) The inhibitory neuron (C) releases a neurotransmitter that closes $Ca^{2+}$ channels in the presynaptic membrane. Closure of the $Ca^{2+}$ channels results in reduced release of neurotransmitters from the presynaptic neuron. A neurotransmitter commonly released from the presynaptic inhibitory neuron is GABA.

## Compare and contrast presynaptic and postsynaptic inhibition.

**SIMILARITIES**

Both result in inhibition of synaptic transmission.

**DIFFERENCES**

| Presynaptic inhibits | Post-synaptic inhibits |
|---|---|
| Is heterosynaptic, i.e. involves a third neuron | Is homosynaptic, i.e. it does not involve a third neuron |
| Results in reduced neurotransmitter output from the presynaptic nerve terminal, leading to reduced EPSP formation | Results in IPSP formation |
| Occurs due to increased Cl⁻ or K⁺ permeability or reduced $Ca^{2+}$ permeability of the presynaptic nerve ending | Occurs due to increased K⁺ permeability of the postsynaptic neuron |

## What is subliminal fringe?

Neurons connected end-to-end rarely form a perfect chain. Rather, branches of neurons in the central chain synapse on other neurons

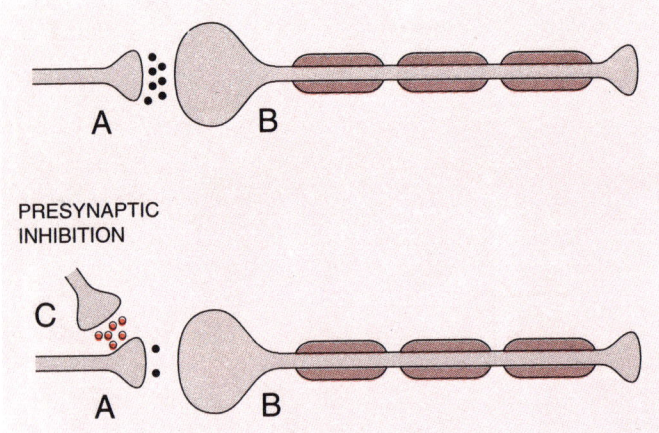

**PRESYNAPTIC INHIBITION**

**Fig. 114.5**

lateral to them. If the lateral neurons are facilitated, the neurons around the central chain remain in *state of subthreshold excitability* and constitute a zone called the **subliminal fringe**. A subliminal fringe would allow the passage of a weak neural signal that would normally fade out during its course through that zone (Fig. 114.6).

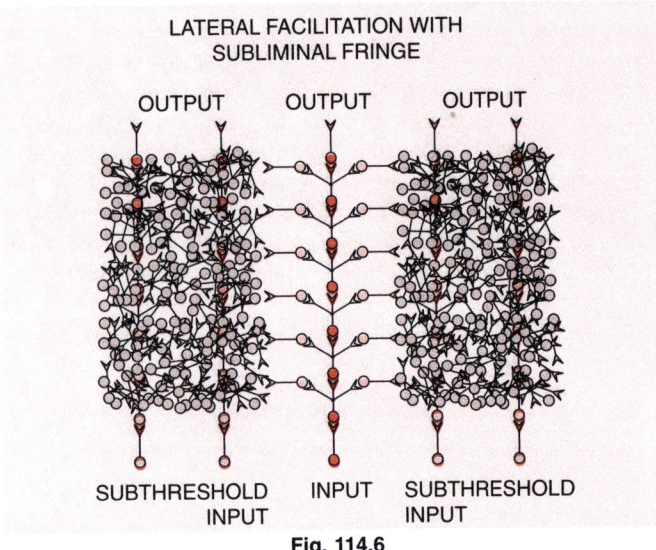

LATERAL FACILITATION WITH SUBLIMINAL FRINGE

OUTPUT        OUTPUT        OUTPUT

SUBTHRESHOLD    INPUT    SUBTHRESHOLD
INPUT                    INPUT

**Fig. 114.6**

### What is meant by the term occlusion?

In convergent circuits, multiple neurons synapse on a single neuron. Wherever there is convergence, the phenomenon of occlusion is observed. Conversely, if there is occlusion, there must be at least some amount of convergence. Occlusion is the phenomenon in which the *total output* of a neuronal network obtained by stimulating all the input neurons together *is less than the sum of outputs obtained by stimulating the input neurons individually*.

### Outline the steps in adrenaline synthesis in the neuron.

Noradrenaline (NA) and Dopamine (DA) are synthesized and stored in the vesicles in the axon terminals. The three catecholamines (NA, adrenaline and DA) are synthesized from the aminoacid phenylalanine.

Unlike ACh, NA released into the synaptic cleft is only partially destroyed and a part is taken up again by the sympathetic nerve endings. The end products of NA and Adr metabolism are excreted in urine in a free form and as conjugates of glucuronic and sulfuric acids (See Chapter 98).

### Outline the steps in the synthesis of acetylcholine in the neuron.

Acetylcholine (ACh) is *synthesized in the cytosol of the nerve terminals* in the presence of the enzyme **choline O-acetyltransferase**.

$$\text{Acetyl-CoA} + \text{Choline} \xrightarrow{\text{Choline O-acetyltransferase}} \text{Acetylcholine} + \text{CoA}$$

Choline is synthesized in the cell body and transported to the nerve terminal. Significant amounts of choline are taken up from the junctional cleft. Being a quaternary ammonium compound, choline cannot cross the membrane on its own: it employs a $Na^+$-*coupled secondary active transport*. After synthesis, ACh is incorporated into the synaptic vesicles. Some vesicles originate *in the soma* and are transported distally by axoplasmic flow. Some are formed *in the axon* while some are formed *in the terminal button* itself.

### Name some excitatory and inhibitory aminoacid neurotransmitter.

**Glutamate** is an excitatory aminoacid transmitters while **GABA** and **glycine** are inhibitory aminoacid neurotransmitters.

### What is the mechanism of action of tetanus toxin?

**Tetanus toxin** acts mainly by interfering with the release of **glycine**, which is an inhibitory neurotransmitter.

### What is the mechanism of action of strychnine?

**Strychnine** (an alkaloid obtained from the seeds of *strychnos nux vomica*) produces convulsions by acting as a competitive antagonist of **glycine** at the postsynaptic inhibitory site.

# 115

# Sensory Mechanisms

## What is difference between conscious and unconscious senses?

Sensations that can be discerned at the conscious level, i.e., the **conscious sensations** are touch, position sense (as sensed by the joint proprioceptors), temperature, pain, sense of gravity and acceleration (sensed by the labyrinth), vision, hearing, taste and smell. There are other senses that never reach conscious appraisal but nevertheless effect crucial reflex responses. These **unconscious senses** are mostly visceral (e.g. baroreception) but may be somatic (e.g. joint positions as sensed by the muscle spindles and the Golgi tendon organ).

## How are sensory receptors classified based on the type of energies they detect?

According to this classification, sensory receptors may be: (i) **photoreceptors** sensing light, e.g., the rods and cones. (ii) **chemoreceptors** sensing chemicals. These are used for the sensations of taste and smell as well for sensing the internal milieu, e.g., the glucoreceptors in the hypothalamus. (iii) **thermo-receptors** sensing temperature. Thermoreceptors present in the skin sense the external temperature while those present inside the body sense the body temperature. (iv) **mechanoreceptors** sensing mechanical changes. These include a wide variety of receptors that sense force and pressure in their various forms. For example, the inner hair cells of the ear senses *sound pressure*; the otolith organs sense the direction of *gravitational force*, pacinian corpuscles sense *pressure* applied on the skin; the muscle spindle respond to *stretching forces applied on muscle*; baroreceptors sense *blood pressure*. (v) **Nociceptors**, which respond to a variety of energies when applied at high intensity. They produce pain.

## How are sensory receptors classified based on the source of the stimulus?

According to this classification, sensory receptors may be exteroceptors, proprioceptors or interoceptors. (i) **Exteroceptors** provide information about the *external environment*, like touch, pressure, temperature, light, sound, taste, smell etc. Sometimes receptors sensing light, sound and smell, which provide information about the *distant environment*, have been called **telereceptors**. Exteroceptors are further subdivided into **general exteroceptors** that are present in the skin (**cutaneous** or the **tactile receptors**), and the **special exteroceptors** present in the head, represented by the receptors for vision, hearing, taste and smell. (ii) **Proprioceptors** provide information about the *position and posture of our body in space*. They sense stimuli from the muscles, tendons and the joints as well from the vestibular apparatus. Proprioceptors are sometimes further subdivided into **general proprioceptors** present in the locomotor system (muscle spindles, Golgi tendon organ and Pacinian corpuscle of the joints; and the

**special proprioceptors** present in the head (receptors of the vestibular apparatus). (iii) **Interoceptors** or **visceroceptors** provide information about the *events in the viscera*, e.g., receptors sensing blood pressure, plasma osmolarity, blood glucose concentration or the degree of stretching of the urinary bladder.

## What are the different types of cutaneous receptors?

General exteroceptors (**cutaneous receptors**) are involved with four types of sensations: touch-pressure-vibration, cold, warmth and pain. Accordingly, tactile receptors are divided into three broad groups: **tactile receptors**, **thermoreceptors** and **nociceptors**. Touch, pressure and vibration are considered to be different forms of the same sensation. Pressure is felt when the force applied on the skin is sufficient to reach the receptors located in the deeper layers of skin, whereas touch is felt when the force is insufficient to reach the deeper layers. Vibrations are felt when there is rhythmic variations in the force.

Whether a tactile receptor senses touch, pressure or vibration depends, among other factors, on whether they are rapidly-adapting or slowly-adapting receptors. **Slow adapting tactile receptors** are meant for signaling sustained pressure: they are useless for signaling vibrations. Conversely, **rapidly-adapting tactile receptors** are of no use in signaling sustained pressure: they are useful only when the pressure fluctuates rapidly, i.e., during vibration. *Higher the adaptation rate of the receptor, greater is the vibration frequency it can detect.*

| RAPIDLY ADAPTING TACTILE RECEPTORS | | | |
|---|---|---|---|
| **Name** | **Location** | **Receptor field** | **Effective stimulus** |
| Pacinian Corpuscle | Subcutaneous | 100 mm$^2$ | Vibration (40 – 600 Hz) |
| Krause end bulb | Dermis of | 2 mm$^2$ | Vibrations |
| Meissner corpuscle | glabrous skin | 12 mm$^2$ | (10 – 200 Hz |
| Hair follicle receptors | Dermis of glabrous skin | 1.5 cm$^2$ | Vibrations (5 – 200 Hz) |
| | Hair follicles | | Hair movement; Vibration (5 – 40 Hz) |

| SLOWLY ADAPTING TACTILE RECEPTORS | | | |
|---|---|---|---|
| **Name** | **Location** | **Receptor field** | **Receptive field** |
| Merkel receptor | Base of epidermis | 11 mm$^2$ | Pressure |
| Ruffini ending | Dermis | 60 mm$^2$ | Pressure |
| C-mechano-ceptor | Dermo-epidermal boundary | 2 mm$^2$ | Slow movement |

**THERMORECEPTORS**

| Name | Location | Receptor field | Receptive field |
|------|----------|----------------|-----------------|
| Cold | Base of epidermis | 1 mm$^2$ | Cold |
| Warmth | Base of epidermis | 1 mm$^2$ | Warmth and heat |

**NOCICEPTORS**

| Name | Location | Receptor field | Receptive field |
|------|----------|----------------|-----------------|
| Mechanical | skin | 3 mm$^2$ | Sharp, fast pain |
| Thermomechanical | Skin | 3 mm$^2$ | Dull, slow pain |

### What is a sensory unit? What is a receptor field?

Groups of sensory receptors are connected to the dendritic ends of a single neuron. Such a neuron, with all its peripheral terminals and their receptors is called a **sensory unit**. The total area encompassed by all the receptors of one sensory unit is called the **receptor field**.

### What is meant by the punctate character of sensations?

Sensations are not present uniformly all over an innervated surface but are present only in areas overlying sensory receptors. The small intervening areas between receptors are devoid of sensations. This is referred to as the **punctate character** of sensations.

### What are hot and cold spots?

Normally, receptor fields overlap considerably. Hence, a tactile stimulus at any one spot invariably falls within the confines of multiple receptor-fields, and therefore stimulates several neurons. However, the *receptor fields of thermoreceptors do not show any overlap*, probably because precise localization of thermal stimulus is rarely important to the body. Because of the lack of overlap, it is possible to delineate distinct 'hot' and 'cold' spots on the skin that respond respectively to warmth and cold.

### Define adequate stimulus.

A sensory receptor responds only to a particular stimulus, called the **adequate stimulus** and do not respond to the others.

### What is a generator potential?

On application of the adequate stimulus, a local potential proportional to stimulus intensity is generated within the receptor (the **generator potential**). A generator potential of about 10 mV is able to depolarize the adjacent areas of the membrane and trigger action potentials. The frequency of the action potentials generated is proportional to the magnitude of the generator potential and therefore, to the stimulus intensity.

### What is sensory adaptation? Which are the senses that show least adaptation?

Most sensations when present continually, tend to be perceived with decreasing intensity. This phenomenon is called **adaptation** and occurs due to the adaptation of the receptors themselves, which fire at progressively lesser frequency on sustained application of a stimulus. Some receptors notably *pain endings, vestibular receptors and muscle spindle do not show adaptation.*

### What is Bell-Magendie's law?

As the spinal nerve approaches the spinal cord, it divides into the dorsal (sensory) and ventral (motor) roots. All sensory fibers reach the spinal cord through dorsal nerve roots, and all motor nerves exit the spinal cord through the ventral nerve root. This is known as **Bell-Magendie's law**.

### What do you understand by the terms 1st, 2nd and 3rd order sensory neuron?

The dorsal root contains sensory fibers that are the first in *a chain of three neurons* that ultimately reach the cortex: The **1st order neuron** carries it from the sensory receptor to the spinal cord or the brain stem. The **2nd order neuron** carries the sensations from the spinal cord or brainstem to the specific relay nuclei of the thalamus. The **3rd order neuron** projects the sensations from the specific thalamic nuclei to the sensory cortex, mostly to its 4th layer.

### How do sensory physiologists classify sensory nerve fibers?

Sensory physiologists use the Lloyd and Hunt classification of sensory fibers. The 1st order neurons in the dorsal nerve root comprise Aα, Aβ, Aδ and C group fibers and are often referred to as group I, II, III and IV respectively by the sensory physiologists. *Fibers Aγ and B fibers are not present in sensory pathways.*

| Sensory group | Fiber type | Origin |
|---------------|------------|--------|
| Ia | Aα | Annulospiral endings on intrafusal muscle fibers |
| Ib | Aα | Golgi tendon organ |
| II | Aβ | Flower-spray endings on intrafusal muscle fibers Touch and pressure receptors |
| III | Aδ | Receptors for pain (fast), cold and crude touch |
| IV | C | Pain (slow) and temperature |

### What is sensory homunculus?

The sensory cortex receives general sensation from all parts of the body. However, the various parts of the body have a cortical representation proportionate, not to their extensiveness but to their sensory acuity. When the cortical areas are charted out for their peripheral connections and depicted figuratively, the distorted shape of a 'little man' emerges. This is called the **sensory homunculus** and is the diagrammatic representation of the peripheral connections of the sensory cortex (Fig. 112.4).

### What are the senses carried by the dorsal column sensory pathway and what is its course?

As shown in the table, the *Aα (Ia) and Aβ (II) fibers carry touch (fine-touch), pressure and proprioceptive information*. They run in the spinal cord through the *dorsal columns* to end on the *nucleus gracilis et cuneatus* in the medulla. The nucleus gracilis *et* cuneatus gives rise to the 2nd order sensory neurons which decussate in the medulla as the *internal arcuate fibers* and ascend in the brainstem as the *medial lemniscus*, terminating finally in the *ventroposterior-lateral* (VPL) nucleus of the thalamus. From the VPL nucleus of thalamus, sensory fibers ascend to the sensory cortex through the thalamic radiations (Fig. 115.1).

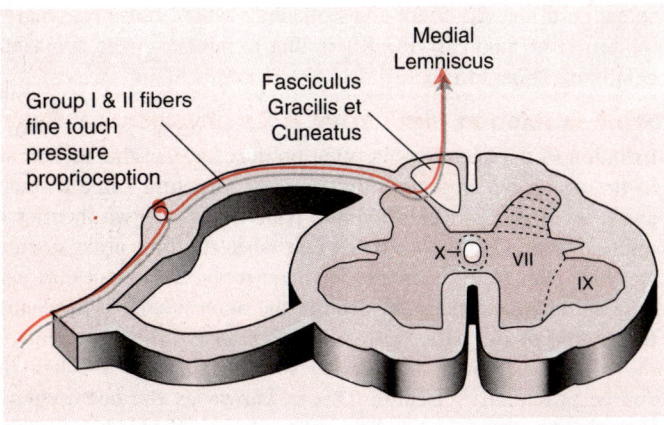

**Fig. 115.1**

## What are the senses carried by the anterolateral sensory pathway and what is its course?

After entering the spinal cord, the *Aδ (III) and C (IV) fibers carrying pain and temperature* fibers separate into short ascending and descending branches which constitute the *dorsolateral tract of Lissauer*. They finally terminate on the *nucleus proprius* of the spinal cord, one or two segments rostral and caudal to the point of entry of the dorsal root. Some sensory afferents end on the short interneurons in the *substantia gelatinosa*, which connect them to the nucleus proprius (Fig. 115.2).

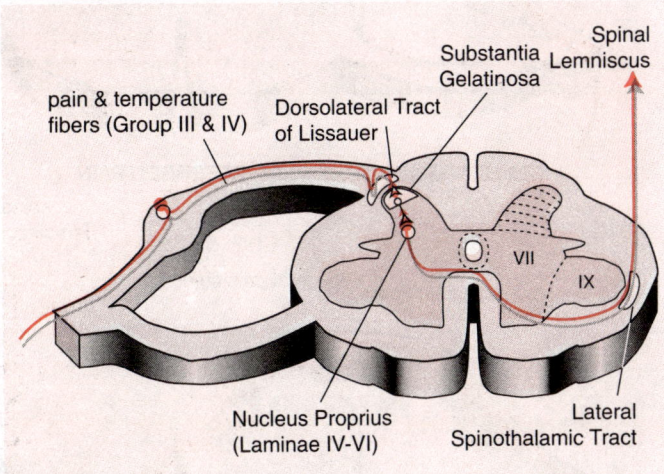

**Fig. 115.2**

The nucleus proprius gives rise to the 2$^{nd}$ order sensory neurons, which cross the middle line in front of the central canal in the anterior white commissure. After crossing, the fibers for *pain and temperature* ascend in the contralateral *lateral spinothalamic tract,* which higher up in the brainstem, is called the *spinal lemniscus.*

The fibers carrying sensation of *crude touch* ascend in the contralateral *anterior spinothalamic tract.* Higher up in the brainstem, the anterior spinothalamic tract joins the *medial lemniscus* (Fig. 115.3). The spinal and medial lemnisci terminate in the *ventroposterior-lateral* (VPL) nucleus of the thalamus. From the VPL nucleus of thalamus, sensory fibers ascend to the sensory cortex through the thalamic radiations.

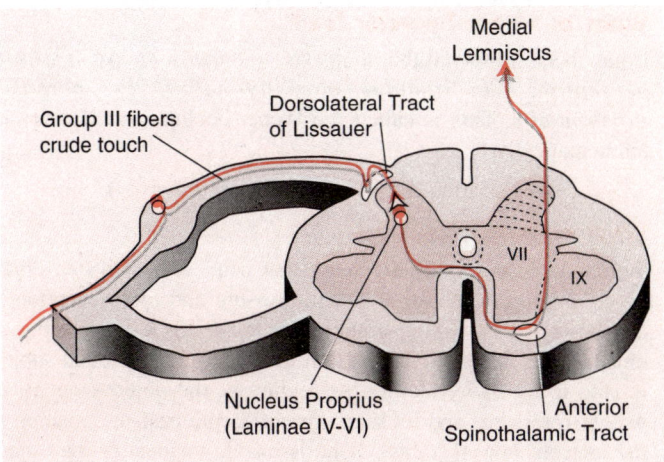

**Fig. 115.3**

## Why is the sensation of touch seldom lost in spinal cord lesions?

Touch is seldom completely lost in cord lesions because it has pathways through both the dorsal as well as the anterolateral columns of the spinal white matter. (i) The dorsal columns contain ipsilateral Aβ (group-II) fibers carrying fine touch; these run in the fasciculus gracilis and cuneatus. (ii) The anterior columns contain contralateral Aδ (group-III) fibers carrying crude touch; these run in the anterior spinothalamic tract.

## What is two-point discrimination and what does it indicate?

Two-point discrimination indicates the acuity of sensory perception. When a single receptor field is stimulated at multiple sites, it will be perceived as a single stimulus by the brain. For two stimuli to be perceived distinctly, they must impinge on two distinct receptor fields, stimulating two different sensory units. Hence, smaller the receptor field, the more acute is the power of two-point discrimination.

## What is the doctrine of specific nerve energies?

The type of sensation evoked depends on the class of sensory unit stimulated. A sensory unit connected to thermal receptors will always evoke thermal sensation, whether it is stimulated naturally through its receptors or whether the nerve is stimulated directly. Even if a sensory nerve is denuded of its receptors, it will still evoke the sensation characteristic of the severed receptors. The phenomenon is called the doctrine of specific nerve energies.

## What is the law of sensory projection? What is phantom limb?

The sensation evoked by a sensory unit will always be projected to (i.e., appears to originate from) the area innervated by its peripheral endings. This is known as the law of sensory projection, which remains true even if the peripheral end of the nerve is severed and the central stump is stimulated, or even though the area innervated by the nerve is ablated. Thus, in a person with an amputated leg, if a sensory nerve originally carrying pain from the toe is stimulated in the thigh region, pain will be felt in (referred to) the non-existent toe. The phenomenon is often referred to as the phantom limb (non-existent limb).

## What is Weber-Fechner law?

It has been observed that *to provide a linear increase in sensory perception, the stimulus intensity has to be increased exponentially*. This is called the Weber-Fechner law. Expressed mathematically,

$$\text{Sensation felt} = \text{Log (Stimulus intensity)}$$

## What is stereognosis?

Stereognosis is a **synthetic sense** that helps to identify an object by combining the sense of touch, pressure and proprioception. It can be tested by asking a subject to close his eyes, placing an object in his hand and asking him to identify it. A normal subject is able to do so by feeling the texture of the object (touch), its weight (pressure) and its shape (proprioception of the position of the interphalangeal joints). If he is unable to identify the object, he is suffering from astereognosis, probably due to a defect in the parietal cortex (sensory association area).

## What are the receptors for pain?

The receptors for pain are the naked nerve endings found in almost every tissue of the body.

## Which types of nerve fibers carry pain?

Pain is transmitted to the CNS by two types of fibers: the thinly myelinated Aδ, and the unmyelinated C fibers. Both conduct slowly but the Aδ fibers are relatively faster. Aδ fibers terminate in laminas I and V where as the C fibers terminate in laminas I and II.

## What are fast and slow pains?

An acute painful stimulus results in two 'waves' of pain. The first wave of pain is sharp and localized while the second wave of pain is dull and diffuse. Fast pain is carried by Aδ fibers while slow pain is carried by C fibers.

## What is the difference between hyperalgesia and allodynia?

In *allodynia*, pain is caused by innocuous stimuli. In *hyperalgesia*, stimuli that would normal cause minor pain produces intense pain.

## What is gating of pain?

Stimulation of touch fibers (Aβ) is known to reduce pain. This is called the gating of pain and occurs because after entering the

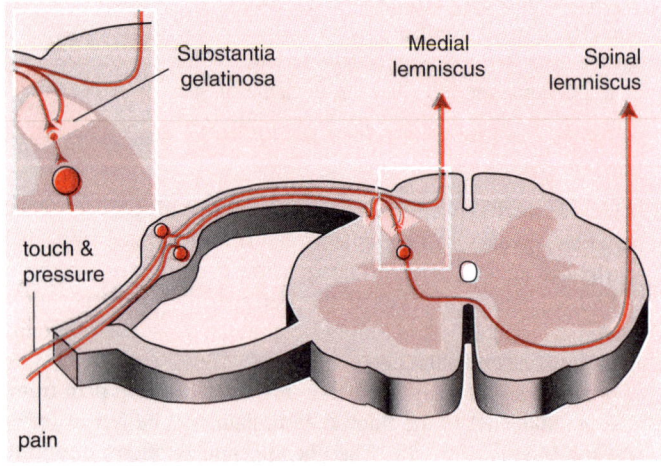

**Fig. 115.4**

spinal cord, the Aβ fibers give collaterals which cause presynaptic inhibition of pain-carrying fibers that terminate in the substantia gelatinosa (Fig. 115.4).

## What is referred pain? What is its physiological basis?

Irritation of a visceral organ often produces a pain that is felt, not in the organ but in some other somatic structure some distance away. Such pain is called referred pain. There are two theories of referred pain. One theory holds that when the first order neurons carrying pain from a somatic area and a visceral organ converge on a common second order neuron, the brain is unable to identify the source of the pain. *Since somatic pain is far more common, the brain interprets all pain as somatic pain* even when the source is actually visceral. This is known as the **convergence theory** of referred pain. The other theory holds that visceral irritation is inadequate for producing pain by itself. However, it facilitates pain fibers from somatic structures so that even minor somatic irritation produces perceptible pain. This is known as the **facilitation theory** of referred pain (Fig. 115.5).

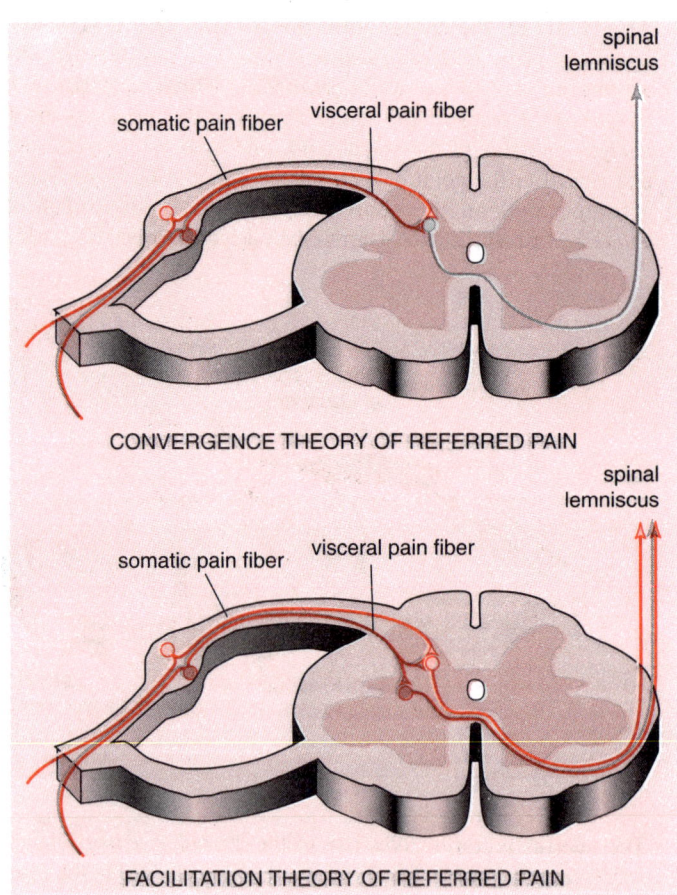

CONVERGENCE THEORY OF REFERRED PAIN

FACILITATION THEORY OF REFERRED PAIN

**Fig. 115.5**

## What are the surgical ways of abolition of pain?

Severe pain can be dissociated from its unpleasant feeling by cutting the deep connections between the frontal lobes and the rest of the brain (**prefrontal lobectomy**). Patients operated in this way feel the pain but are 'not bothered by it'. Another way of surgical abolition of pain is to cut the pain-carrying fibers in the anterolateral spinothalamic tract (**anterolateral cordotomy**).

### Briefly outline the supraspinal control of pain.

The synapse between the first order neuron (**primary nociceptive afferent**) and the second order neuron carrying pain is the site of inhibition by the neuron descending from **raphe nuclei** in the medulla (Fig. 115.6). The neuron descending from the **periaqueductal gray** in the midbrain also inhibits pain by stimulating the brainstem raphe nuclei. Both the brainstem centers of pain inhibition are stimulated by descending neurons from the **hypothalamus** and **frontal cortex**.

At all the sites of pain modulation, postsynaptic inhibition is mediated by a **serotonergic inhibitory interneuron** while stimulation is mediated by *inhibition of the inhibitory interneuron* by an **opioid-containing neuron**. In the spinal cord, pain is also inhibited through presynaptic inhibition of the primary nociceptive afferents.

### What are the various chemicals that produce pain?

Neurotransmitters producing pain are **bradykinin, prostaglandins, serotonin, histamine, leukotrines,** and **potassium ions**. These chemicals act on receptors located on nociceptive nerve endings, sensitizing them to pain. Many of these chemicals are released following cell death. All cells release $K^+$ after death. Dying cells also release proteolytic enzymes that react with circulating globulins to form bradykinin. Serotonin is released from platelets and histamine is released from mast cells.

Activation of a nociceptive nerve terminal stimulates the *axon reflex* and releases **substance P** and **calcitonin gene-related peptide (CGRP)** from the other terminals of the same nociceptive nerve fiber. These chemicals bring about the inflammatory changes that usually accompany pain.

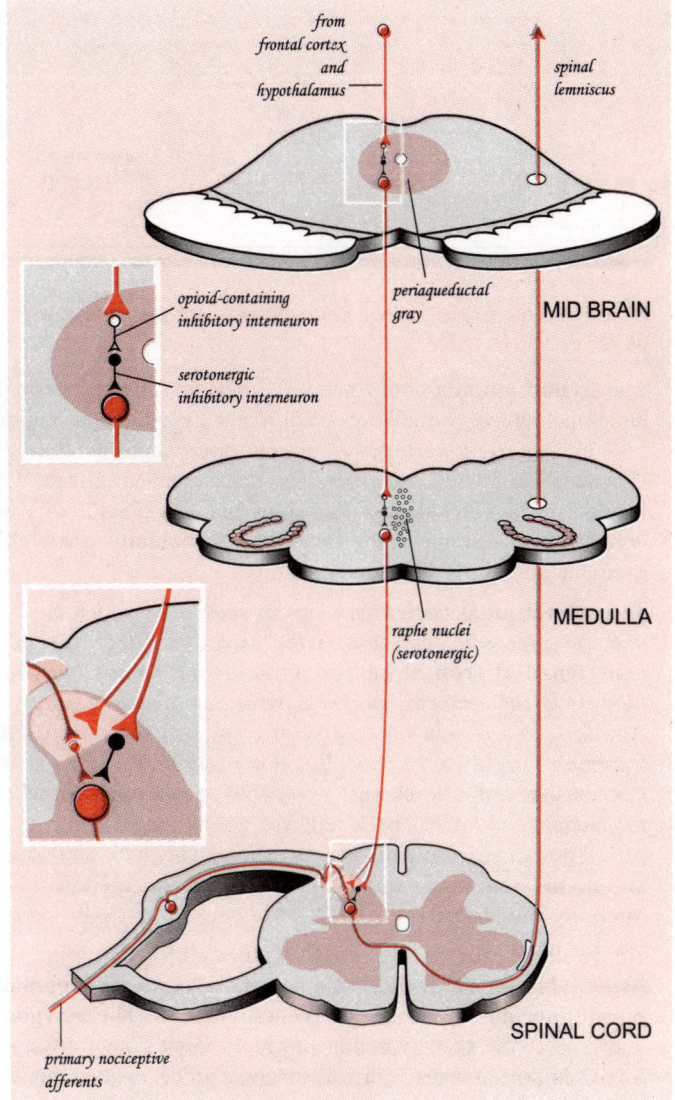

**Fig. 115.6**

# *Physiology of emotions*

## Name some brain areas associated with emotions and explain their role.

The **hypothalamus** coordinates the peripheral expression of emotional states. Stimulation of different hypothalamic regions evokes different patterns of autonomic reactions that are characteristic of different emotions. For example, animals with lesions in the **lateral hypothalamus** become placid, whereas animals with lesions of the **medial hypothalamus** are highly excitable and easily become aggressive.

The **orbitofrontal cortex** provides *the means by which memory and imagination too can evoke emotional feelings.* The **ventromedial frontal cortex** provides *the means by which conscious thought can suppress reflex emotional responses.* Another cortical area for control of emotional responses is the **anterior cingulate cortex.** Lesions of this area reduce the emotional response to chronic intractable pain. Patients in whom the cingulate gyrus has been removed are no longer bothered by pain. They experience pain as a sensation and exhibit appropriate autonomic reactions, but the sensation is not perceived as intensely unpleasant.

While the autonomic responses to emotion involve the **hypothalamus**, the feeling of emotions involves the **cingulate**, **parahippocampal** and the **prefrontal cortices**. The **amygdala** coordinates the two. A major amygdala input comes from the **inferotemporal cortex**, which is involved, in the explicit memory of facial identity, and hence, the amygdala can mediate emotional responses to facial expressions.

## What is sham rage?

Cats in which the whole cerebral cortex had been removed retain fully integrated emotional responses, termed **sham rage** because the responses appear to lack elements of conscious experience that are characteristic of genuine, naturally occurring rage (*sham* = false). Sham rage also differs from genuine rage because responses can be *triggered by very mild stimuli*, such as a weak touch, or can even occur spontaneously, without provocation. It is undirected, and the *animals sometimes even bite themselves.* No matter how it is elicited, sham rage *subsides very quickly* once the stimulus is removed. Sham rage largely *disappears when the hypothalamus is ablated.*

## What is the Papez circuit and what is its role in emotions?

In 1937 James Papez proposed that the neocortex influences the hypothalamus by means of connections to the cingulate gyrus and from the cingulate gyrus to the hippocampal formation. The hippocampal formation processes information from the cingulate gyrus and conveys it to the mamillary bodies of the hypothalamus by way of the fornix. In turn, the hypothalamus provides information to the cingulate gyrus by a pathway from the mamillary bodies to the anterior thalamic nuclei (the mamillothalamic tract) and from there to the cingulate gyrus. This circuit is known as the Papez circuit.

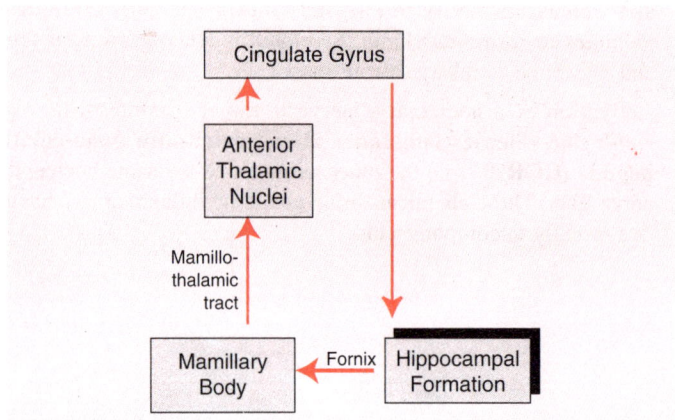

**Fig. 116.1**

The role of Papez circuit in emotions is now largely discarded. Parts of the circuit may be important to the hippocampus for its role in explicit (declarative) memory for facts and personal events that are associated with emotions.

# *Regulation of Muscle Length & Tension*

## Describe the muscle spindle. What is its function?

The muscle spindle is the sensory (proprioceptive) receptor sensing muscle stretch. It acts as a **length-detector** for the muscle. It is located within the muscle, intermingled with the muscle fibers. The ends of the muscle spindle are fixed to an adjacent muscle fiber. Within the spindle, a few specialized muscle fibers are present. They are called **intrafusal fibers** to distinguish them from the fibers of the muscle itself, which are called **extrafusal fibers**.

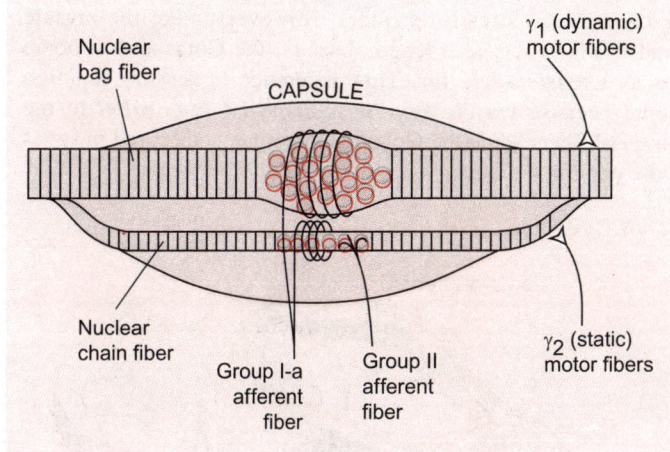

**Fig. 117.1**

Intrafusal fibers are of two subtypes: the nuclear bag fibers and the nuclear chain fibers. The **nuclear bag fibers** have a bulge in the equatorial region due to presence of an aggregation of nuclei. The **nuclear chain fibers** have no such bulge since the nuclei in its equatorial region are arranged in a single file. The peripheral parts of the intrafusal fibers contain contractile proteins, which show as cross striations in the periphery.

## Describe the sensory innervation of the muscle spindle.

Two types of sensory nerve fibers originate from the intrafusal fibers: the **annulospiral endings** are wound around the equatorial regions of intrafusal fibers. They are present on both nuclear bag and chain fibers. These fibers are of the Aα type and are called **type IA** by the sensory physiologists. The **flower-spray endings** are present predominantly in the nuclear chain fibers - innervating its peripheral parts. These fibers are of the Aβ type but are called **type II** by sensory physiologists (Fig. 117.1).

## What is the motor innervation of the muscle spindle and what is its function?

The peripheral parts are innervated by motor fibers which are of the Aγ type, and hence often called **γ-motoneurons** or **fusimotor**

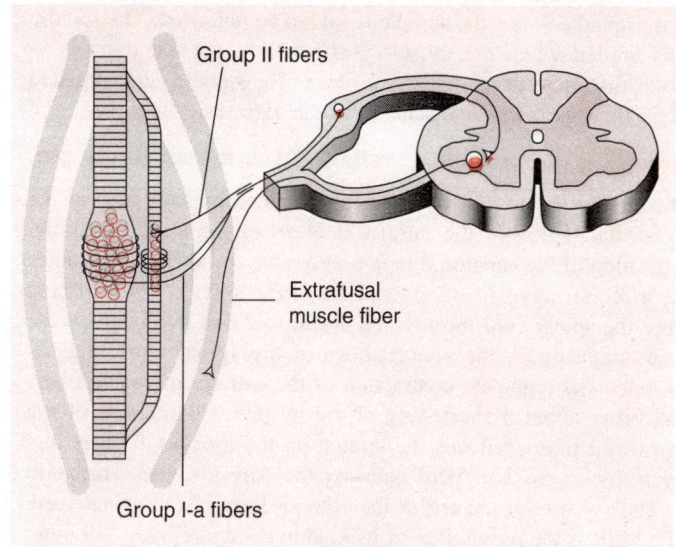

**Fig. 117.2**

**neurons**. These γ-motoneurons have their cell bodies in the anterior gray horn of the spinal cord, where they are interspersed among the cells of α-motoneurons (Aα), which supply the extrafusal fibers.

Motor innervation of the spindle is also of two types: the $\gamma_1$ and $\gamma_2$ fibers, which innervate the polar regions of the bag fibers and the chain fibers respectively. Aγ fibers alter spindle sensitivity to stretch. $\gamma_1$ *alter the dynamic sensitivity* while $\gamma_2$ *alters the static sensitivity* of the stretch reflex.

## How many spindles are there in a muscle?

The number of spindles in a muscle is proportionate to the proprioceptive acuity and the feedback control present in the muscle. Thus, the gastrocnemius muscles contain as few as 5 to 10 spindles per gram of muscle while the interossei muscles of the hand contain as many as 100 spindles per gram of muscle.

## What is the functional difference between the nuclear bag and nuclear chain fibers?

When the intrafusal fiber is stretched, the primary and secondary afferents respond differently. The secondary group II afferents discharge with a frequency that is proportional to the degree of stretch (**static response**). The primary group I afferents discharge with frequency that depends not only degree of stretch but also the rate at which the fiber is stretched (**dynamic response**). This is because bag fibers show dynamic response, while chain fibers show static response. Hence, group I afferents, which innervate both bag and chain fibers, show both static as well as dynamic response. Group II afferents innervate only chain fibers and therefore show only static response.

### How is the sensitivity of the receptors controlled?

The sensitivity of the receptors (bag and chain fibers) is increased by loading the spindle and decreased by unloading the spindle.

### What is meant by spindle loading? How is the spindle loaded and unloaded?

When the equatorial part of the intrafusal fibers is stretched, the spindle is said to be loaded. Conversely, when the equatorial part of the spindle is lax, the spindle is said to be unloaded. The spindle gets loaded when the muscle is stretched or when there is γ-motor discharge to the intrafusal fibers. The spindle gets unloaded when there is α-motor discharge to the extrafusal fibers.

### What is a monosynaptic reflex? Describe its reflex arc.

The monosynaptic reflex (MSR) is stimulated by stretching of the equatorial region of the intrafusal fibers of the muscle spindle. Stretching of the equatorial region of the intrafusal fiber stimulates the afferent nerve fibers (Ia and II) of the spindle. These fibers enter the spinal cord through the dorsal root and terminate on the α-motoneuron in the ventral horn of the spinal cord. The α-motoneurons stimulate contraction of the extrafusal muscle fibers and bring about a shortening of the muscle. Contraction of the extrafusal fibers reduces the stretch on the intrafusal fibers and the reflex stops. The MSR pathway has only a single synapse in it. The synapse is located in the anterior horn of the spinal cord. The MSR is the only reflex of its kind in the entire body. All other reflexes are either bisynaptic or polysynaptic (Fig. 117.2).

### What is the length servomechanism?

The **length servomechanism** is a hypothetical mechanism that seeks to explain how a muscle can be contracted to a desired length even when it faces unpredictable resistance to contraction. According to it, the brain makes the extrafusal fibers contract reflexly through the MSR instead of stimulating the Aα directly. *Contraction of intrafusal fibers is not affected by external load.* Hence, for making the intrafusal fibers contract to the desired length, the brain does not have to evaluate the external load. Hence, the *intrafusal fibers contract to the desired length regardless of the uncertainties of the external load.* The contracted intrafusal fibers trigger the MSR and results in the contraction of the extrafusal fiber. The MSR does not stop till the extrafusal fibers contract exactly the same amount as the intrafusal fiber, thereby unloading the spindle to its original level. The advantage of the length servomechanism is that it is *resistant to perturbations of external load.* Also, at the end of contraction, the *spindle sensitivity is retained.* However, it has been found that in reality, such reflex contractions are *too weak to move heavy loads.*

### What is α-γ coactivation?

According to another hypothesis called the **follow-up length servomechanism**, the motor cortex sends its *length-signal simultaneously to both extrafusal and intrafusal fibers* through α-motoneurons and γ-motoneurons respectively (α-γ coactivation). The α-mediated stimulation makes the muscle contract powerfully and quickly. If, due to unexpected changes in the external load, the extrafusal fibers fail to contract to the desired length, it results in a mismatch between the degree of extrafusal and intrafusal fiber shortening. This causes loading of the spindle and triggers off the MSR till the disparity is eliminated and the extrafusal fibers contract to the desired length. According to this hypothesis, the *MSR provides only a follow-up mechanism* to ensure that the extrafusal fibers contract to the desired length.

### What is the difference between stretch reflex and the monosynaptic reflex?

When the monosynaptic reflex is elicited by stretching of a muscle, it is called the stretch reflex. The monosynaptic reflex can be stimulated in other ways too, for example, by γ-motor discharge.

### Describe the inverse stretch reflex. What is its physiological significance?

The Golgi tendon reflex (also called negative or inverse stretch reflex) is a **bisynaptic reflex**, initiated by the **Golgi tendon organ** located in muscle tendons. Like muscle spindles, Golgi tendon organs are also stretch receptors. However unlike the muscle spindle, which acts as a length-detector, the Golgi tendon organ acts as a *tension-detector*. This difference in sensory function occurs because *muscle spindle is disposed in parallel* to the extrafusal fibers while the Golgi tendon organ is disposed in series to the extrafusal fibers.

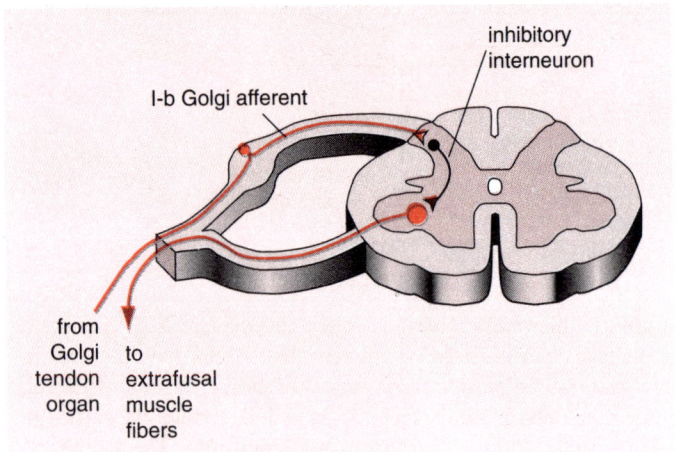

**Fig. 117.3**

The Golgi tendon organ is innervated by Aα sensory fibers, which are called I-b fibers by sensory physiologists. These afferent fibers terminate on **inhibitory interneurons** in the dorsal gray horn of the spinal cord. The interneurons terminate on the α-motoneurons in the ventral gray horn of the spinal cord. The Golgi tendon reflex is *a protective reflex that prevents excessive rise in muscle tension.* When the muscle contracts isometrically, the tendon gets stretched and the tension in the tendon rises markedly. This *rise in tension is sensed by the Golgi tendon organ*, which stimulates the **I-b afferents**. These afferents stimulate the inhibitory interneurons in the spinal cord and thereby, inhibit the α-motoneuron discharge to the muscle, which consequently relaxes. This reflex relaxation of the extrafusal muscle fibers in response to rise in muscle tension is called the **negative (inverse) stretch reflex** (Fig. 117.3).

## Define muscle tone and describe its supraspinal control.

All muscles in the living body are maintained at *a slightly contracted state*, which is called the **muscle tone**. This muscle tone is normally brought about through *reflex contraction* of the muscle fibers, caused by tonic discharge of γ-motor neurons.

Muscle tone is normally under elaborate supraspinal controls. The γ-motoneurons in the ventral horn of spinal cord are stimulated by descending fibers from the **facilitatory reticular formation** which extends from the upper medulla to the midbrain. They also receive descending inhibitory fibers from the **inhibitory reticular formation** in the pons and medulla. However, the facilitatory effect predominates, resulting in a tonic discharge of γ-motoneurons to the muscles.

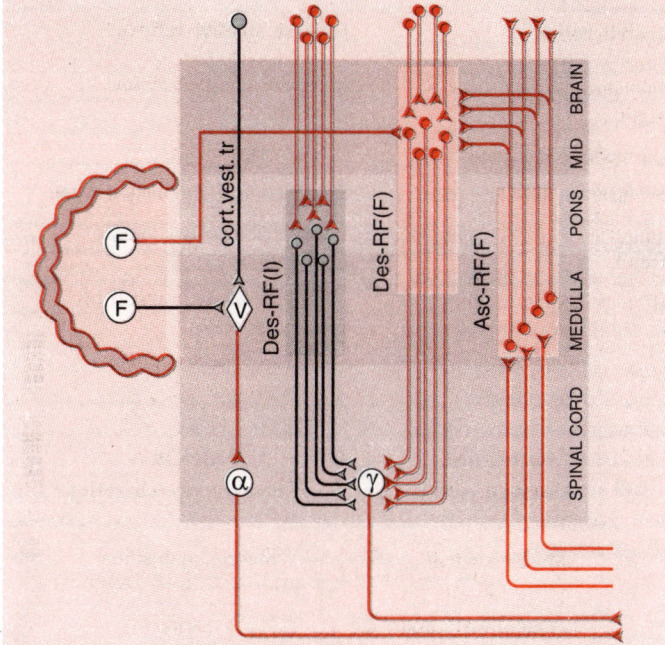

**Fig. 117.4**

Muscle tone is normally not under tonic control of α-motoneurons. *Tonic control of α-motoneurons is exerted almost entirely through vestibulospinal pathways.* However, the vestibular nucleus (esp., the Dieter's nucleus) is itself constantly inhibited by corticospinal fibers as well as fastigiovestibular fibers from the cerebellum. It is only under certain abnormal or experimental situations that the vestibular nucleus gets disinhibited, resulting in an exaggerated muscle tone that is α-led rather than γ-led (Fig. 117.4).

## How is muscle tone affected in cerebellar disorders?

Cerebellar disorders cause *hypotonia*. Cerebellar disorder is associated with a reduction of the inhibition of the vestibular nuclei. However, in the *continued presence of descending inhibition from the cortex*, the vestibular nuclei do not get disinhibited significantly and the α-motoneuron activity does not increase. On the other hand, a reduction of facilitatory impulses to the descending facilitatory reticular formation results in reduced γ-motor discharge and hypotonia.

## What is spinal shock? What is the cause of spinal shock?

*The net supraspinal influences descending on the γ-motor neuron is excitatory.* When this facilitatory supraspinal influence is suddenly removed, the γ-motor neurons become quiescent for a period of days to weeks. This is called the **spinal shock**. The duration of the spinal shock is much lesser in lower animals, possibly because the supraspinal facilitation is normally much lesser in them. Since the γ-motor discharge determines the gain of spinal reflex, *all spinal reflexes are abolished in the absence of γ-motor discharge.*

After a period of weeks, the γ-motor neurons start discharging excessively, due to denervation hypersensitivity and the sprouting of collaterals from interneurons that excite the γ-motor neurons. This recovery phase is associated with hyperactive muscle tone and reflexes (**spasticity**).

## What is decerebrate rigidity? What is the difference between classical and ischemic decerebration?

Decerebrate rigidity is produced experimentally, mostly in cats, by making a mid-collicular section of the midbrain (**classical decerebration**). The exaggerated muscle tone affects both flexors and extensors, but is *specially marked in the antigravity extensor muscles*. Antigravity muscles are those extensor muscles which keep the weight-bearing joints of the body extended, e.g., erector spinae muscles, the extensors of the hip and knee etc. Even under normal conditions, the antigravity muscles are endowed with a higher resting muscle tone. In decerebrate rigidity, the same pattern gets exaggerated (hypertonia), resulting in a *caricature exaggerated of the normal erect posture*. In classical decerebration, the muscle tone is increased due to exaggerated γ-motor discharge. The rigidity observed following classical decerebration is actually a form of **spasticity**.

Since classical decerebration was frequently associated with death of the experimental animal, a safer method was attempted. This was called **ischemic decerebration** in which the cerebral cortex was rendered ischemic and nonfunctional by tying off the basilar artery. Soon it was discovered that ischemic decerebration did not result in spasticity: it resulted in a different form of rigidity that was due to exaggerated α-motoneuron discharge (**α-rigidity**). The α-overdrive resulted in direct stimulation of extrafusal muscle fibers.

## How can α-rigidity be distinguished from γ-rigidity?

γ-rigidity is produced through the monosynaptic reflex and is therefore *abolished by deafferentation*, i.e., sectioning of the proprioceptive afferents from the muscle to the spinal cord, which interrupts the monosynaptic reflex arc. α-rigidity is not reflex in nature and therefore it is *not abolished by muscle deafferentation*.

## What is spasticity? What is clasp-knife rigidity?

A muscle with increased muscle tone due to excessive γ-motor discharge is called a **spastic** muscle. When a spastic muscle is stretched passively, there is an *intense initial resistance due to the exaggerated stretch reflex*. The resistance, which increases muscle tension, suddenly gives way due to the activation of the Golgi tendon reflex, producing the feel of a **clasp-knife**. This clinical sign is called spasticity. Spasticity will not be observed if the increase in muscle tone is due to α-overdrive.

## What is the mechanism of decerebrate rigidity?

The γ-drive to muscles is maintained by descending fibers from the descending reticular formation. The descending influences are both facilitatory (from facilitatory reticular formation) as well as inhibitory (from the inhibitory reticular formation). The facilitatory influence predominates.

The facilitatory and inhibitory descending reticular formations have no intrinsic activity of their own: they have to be kept energized by neurons from other sources. *The inhibitory reticular formation is kept activated by descending supraspinal fibers, mostly from the basal ganglia.* Hence, following decerebration, it gets totally orphaned and its inhibitory effect on γ-motoneurons vanishes. The *facilitatory reticular formation, in contrast, is also activated by ascending sensory stimuli that relay to it through the ascending reticular formation.* Hence even following decerebration, the facilitatory reticular formation remains reasonably active and continues to facilitate the γ-motoneurons. The balance of descending influence on γ-motoneurons therefore shifts heavily towards facilitation.

*Although cerebellar disorders cause hypotonia* (see above), *cerebellectomy in a decerebrate preparation accentuates the muscle tone.* This is because of the total disinhibition of the vestibular nuclei, which are now free from both – the descending cortical inhibition (due to midcollicular section) and cerebellar inhibition (because of cerebellectomy). Although cerebellectomy decreases the γ-motor output, in the presence of high α-motor discharge, the reduction in γ-motor discharge becomes immaterial.

The α-rigidity of ischemic decerebration occurs due to an entirely different reason. *Ischemic decerebration is unavoidably associated with ischemia and consequent necrosis of a large part of the cerebellum.* A reduction in cerebellar activity leads to a disinhibition of α-motoneurons and a reduction of γ-facilitation. This leads to α-rigidity.

## Compare and contrast classical and ischemic decerebrate rigidity.

### SIMILARITIES

In both, the brainstem reticular formation gets isolated from higher cortical influences.

Both are associated with hypertonia of antigravity extensor muscles.

### DIFFERENCES

| Classical decerebrate rigidity | Ischemic decerebrate rigidity |
|---|---|
| Produced by a midcollicular section | Produced by ligating the basilar artery |
| Isolates the brainstem RF from higher cortical influence | Isolates the brainstem RF from higher cortical influences and also causes necrosis of a large part of the cerebellum. |
| The hypertonia is abolished by deafferentation of the muscles | The hypertonia is not abolished by deafferentation of the muscle |
| Occurs due to excessive Aγ discharge to the muscles | Occurs due to excessive Aα discharge to the muscles |

## What is decorticate rigidity?

A decorticate preparation is made by *removing the whole cerebral cortex but leaving the basal ganglia and brainstem intact.* The decorticate animal does not have such intense hypertonia as a decerebrate preparation. This is because the basal ganglia, which is intact in the decorticate animal, activates the descending inhibitory reticular formation, and thereby prevents hypertonia.

## Compare and contrast stretch reflex and inverse stretch reflex.

### SIMILARITIES

Both are spinal reflexes.

Both influence the muscle tone.

### DIFFERENCES

| Stretch reflex | Inverse stretch reflexes |
|---|---|
| Maintains constant muscle length | Maintains constant muscle tension |
| Is a monosynaptic reflex | Is a bisynaptic reflex |
| Originates in muscle spindle | Originates in Golgi tendon organ |
| Stimulated by passive muscle stretch | Stimulated by active muscle contraction |
| Afferents belong to group I-a and II sensory fibres | Afferents belong to group I-b sensory fibres |
| Causes muscle contraction | Causes muscle relaxation |

| Reflex arc of stretch reflex | Reflex arc of inverse stretch reflex |
|---|---|
| Muscle stretch | Muscle contraction |
| ↓ | ↓ |
| ↑ length of extrafusal muscle fibres | ↑ tension in muscle tendon |
| ↓ | ↓ |
| Detected by the intrafusal (inside spindle) muscle fibers | Detected by Golgi tendon organ |
| ↓ | ↓ |
| ↑ discharge of group I-a and II fibres | ↑ discharge of groups I-b fibres |
| | ↓ |
| | Inhibitory interneuron in the dorsal gray horn of spinal cord |
| ↓ | ↓ |
| Motor neuron in the ventral gray horn of the spinal cord | Motor neuron in the ventral gray horn of the spinal cord |
| ↓ | ↓ |
| Stimulation of extrafusal muscle fibres | Inhibition of extrafusal muscle fibres |

# Motor Mechanisms & Regulation of Posture

### What is ideomotor apraxia?

When the **motor association** area is damaged, the patient will have defective motor plans resulting in **ideomotor apraxia**. The **motor plan** refers to the framing of right ideas for motor acts. An example of a motor plan would be to work out all the sequential steps for 'lighting a cigarette'. A patient with ideomotor apraxia, who was provided with a cigarette and a matchbox, tried to light the cigarette by striking it on the side of the matchbox. His ideas were wrong and therefore, his motor plan was faulty.

### What is final common pathway?

The neurons supplying skeletal muscles have their cell bodies located in the ventral horn of the spinal cord. The neurons which are of the Aα type (hence called the α-**motoneuron**) receive and integrate inputs from various parts of the brain as well from sensory receptors. Hence, they serve as the **final common pathway** to the muscle. In general, the final common pathway receives *two types of inputs*: (1) **Inputs through sensory nerves**. These come from receptors in the muscle (the muscle spindle), the tendon (Golgi tendon organ) and skin (nociceptors). As these sensory neurons relay on the α-motoneuron, they constitute a reflex arc and subserve important spinal reflexes like the stretch reflex, negative stretch reflex and the withdrawal reflex. (2) **Descending motor pathways from supraspinal centers**. These descend from various parts of the brain like the cerebral cortex, basal ganglia, cerebellum and descending reticular formation.

### What is reciprocal inhibition?

The α-motoneurons supplying **antagonistic muscles** are usually not stimulated simultaneously. When a muscle is stimulated, its antagonist muscle is inhibited. This is true for both descending supraspinal fibers as wells as sensory fibers of reflex arcs. This reciprocal inhibition is made possible by the interposition of an inhibitory neuron – called the **Golgi bottle neuron** – as shown in the Fig. 118.1.

### What is Renshaw cell inhibition?

Present in Rexed lamina VII of the spinal cord, the **Renshaw cell** is an inhibitory neuron which inhibits the α-motor neuron. It also inhibits the Golgi bottle neuron. The Renshaw cell is stimulated by the axonal branch of the α-motoneuron itself. Thus, every time the α-motoneuron discharges, there is a recurrent inhibition of its own discharge (Fig. 118.2). (1) Since the Renshaw cell inhibits the α-motor neuron supplying an agonist muscle and also inhibits the Golgi bottle neuron that inhibits the antagonist muscle, the Renshaw cell discharge is able to promote the simultaneous contraction of the agonist and antagonist muscles. Thus by

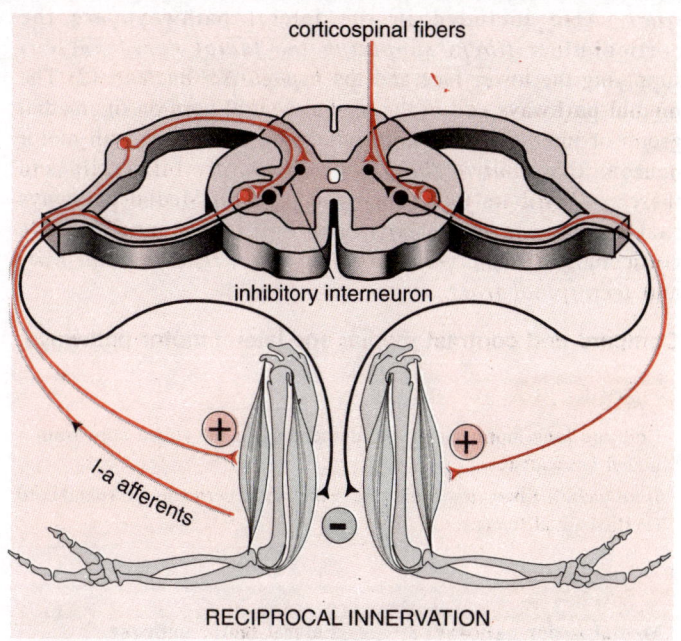

**RECIPROCAL INNERVATION**

**Fig. 118.1**

controlling the Renshaw cell excitability, the *cortex is able to choose between a selective control of the agonist alone, or the simultaneous control of an agonist-antagonist pair*. (2) Also, since the Renshaw cell inhibits the α-motoneuron but does not affect the discharge of the γ-motoneuron, Renshaw cell discharge can tilt the balance of α-γ coactivation towards a greater γ-motoneuron stimulation. Thus by controlling the Renshaw cell excitability, the *cortex is able to fine-tune the ratio of α-motoneuron versus γ-motoneuron stimulation*.

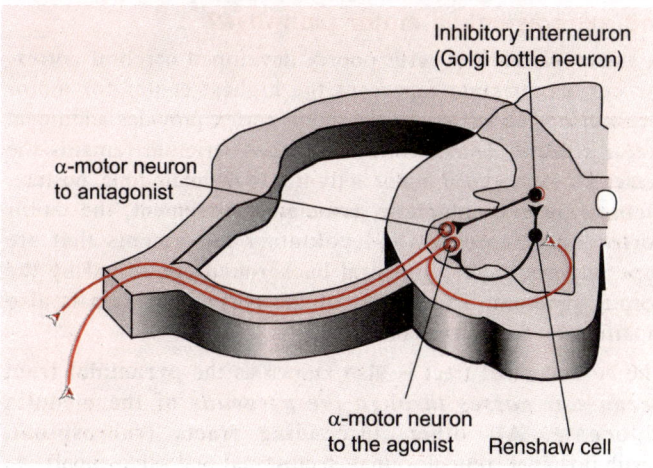

**Fig. 118.2**

## Name the medial and lateral motor pathways and mention their functional characteristics.

Functionally, the descending motor fibers can be categorized into two major type of pathways. (1) The **lateral pathways** are those that terminate directly on motor neurons or on the interneuronal groups in the lateral parts of the spinal cord gray matter. They excite motor neurons directly and influence reflex arcs that control the fine movements of the distal limbs as well as those that activate supporting musculature in the proximal limbs. It includes principally the *lateral corticospinal tract*. Also included in the lateral pathways are the corticobulbar *fibers supplying the facial nerve nucleus* supplying the lower face and the *hypoglossal nucleus*. (2) The **medial pathways** end in the medial ventral horn on the medial group of interneurons. These interneurons connect with motor neurons that *control the axial musculature* bilaterally and thereby contribute to balance and posture. Medial pathways include the *anterior corticospinal tract*, most of the corticobulbar tracts, *vestibulospinal tract*, *reticulospinal tract* and *tectospinal tract*.

## Compare and contrast medial and lateral motor pathways.

| SIMILARITIES |
| --- |
| Both are long motor pathways, descending to the spinal cord from higher brain areas. |
| Both include fibers descending from the motor cortex to the spinal cord (corticospinal tract). |

| DIFFERENCES | |
| --- | --- |
| **Medial motor pathway** | **Lateral motor pathway** |
| Controls axial musculature | Controls appendicular musculature |
| Important for regulation of posture | Important for fine, skilled movements |
| Includes the anterior corticospinal tract. Also includes the vestibulo- reticulo-and tecto-spinal tracts | Includes the lateral corticospinal tract. Also includes the cortico- bulbar tract supplying the VII and XII cranial nerve nuclei. |

## What are the functional differences between pyramidal and extrapyramidal motor pathways?

In lower vertebrates with poorly developed cerebral cortex, the corpus striatum represent the highest center for motor mechanisms. In mammals, the motor cortex provides additional motor control. Thus, while the corpus striatum remains the center for stereotyped motor activities to maintain tone, posture, locomotion and automatic associated movement, the motor cortex coordinates skilled voluntary movements that are superimposed on the postural background controlled by the corpus striatum. The output of the corpus striatum is also modified by the motor cortex.

The corticospinal tract is also known as the **pyramidal tract** *because it passes through the pyramids* of the medulla oblongata. All other descending tracts (rubrospinal, vestibulospinal, reticulospinal, tectospinal and olivospinal) are collectively called the **extrapyramidal motor fibers** and are largely under the control of the basal ganglia. However, the distinction between the pyramidal and extrapyramidal is now largely abandoned because pyramids *contain fibers other than those originating in the motor cortex. Conversely, the area 6 of the motor cortex, which gives rise to pyramidal fibers, actually represents the cortical center for the extrapyramidal system* because of the considerable control it exerts on the basal ganglia.

## Compare and contrast pyramidal and extrapyramidal pathways.

| SIMILARITIES |
| --- |
| Both are motor fibers descending to the spinal cord and brainstem from higher centers. |

| DIFFERENCES | |
| --- | --- |
| **Pyramidal pathway** | **Extrapyramidal pathway** |
| Descends through the medullary pyramids | Does not descend through the medullary pyramids |
| Originates mostly from area 4 and 6. Some fibres originate from the pyramidal cells of Betz | Originates from area 6 of cerebral cortex as well as subcortical structures like red nucleus, vestibular nucleus, tectal nucleus, olivary nucleus and reticular nuclei |
| Predominantly under cortical control | Predominantly under control of basal ganglia and cerebellum |
| Controls skilled movements of hands and fingers | Controls posture and axial movements |
| Lesion causes decrease in muscle tone | Lesion causes spasticity or rigidity |

## What is Bell-Magendie law?

When a sensory input relays on to the $\alpha$-motoneurons, it constitutes a **motor reflex arc**. The sensory fibers enter the spinal cord through the dorsal root, and ends on the motor fibers that leave the cord through its ventral horn. This basic rule of a reflex arc is called the **Bell-Magendie law**.

## Classify reflexes.

Depending upon the number of synapses in the reflex arc, the reflex may be monosynaptic, bisynaptic or polysynaptic. The $\alpha$-motoneurons are involved in three types of reflexes. Of these, *one is monosynaptic*, the *other is bisynaptic* and the *third is polysynaptic*. (1) The **stretch reflex**. This is a *monosynaptic* reflex, which is triggered by stretching of the muscle. Sensory receptors in the muscle – the **muscle spindles** – detect changes in muscle length and reflexly bring about $\alpha$-motoneuron discharge. (2) The **inverse stretch reflex**. This is a protective reflex, which is triggered by excessive rise in muscle tension. The tension-detecting receptors are located in the tendons and are called **Golgi tendon organ**. Stimulation of these receptors brings about a reflex inhibition of the α-motoneurons. The inhibition is possible by the interposition of an inhibitory Golgi bottle neuron in the reflex arc, which is *bisynaptic*. (3) The **withdrawal (flexor) reflex**. This also is a protective reflex, which is triggered by painful stimuli. It results in flexion of the affected limb. The reflex arc is *polysynaptic*. Withdrawal reflex is associated with a **crossed-extensor reflex**, the physiological significance of which is discussed in the context of regulation of posture (*see below*).

Clinicians classify reflexes as superficial and deep. **Superficial reflexes** are actually *polysynaptic withdrawal reflexes* while the **deep reflexes** are *monosynaptic stretch reflexes*.

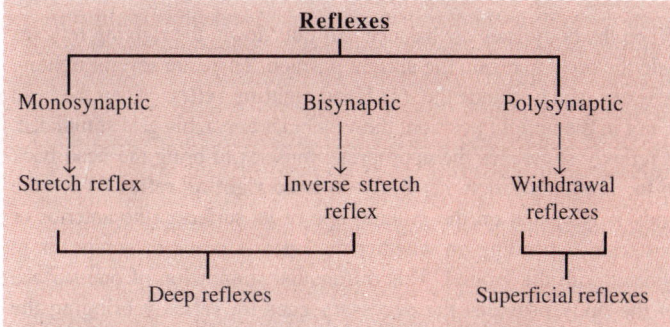

### Describe the reflex arc of the withdrawal reflex.

In the withdrawal reflex and especially, in the crossed extensor reflex, the tension in the contracting muscle rises slowly and also declines slowly. The slow rise in muscle tension is due to the phenomenon of motor recruitment. The slow decline in the muscle tension is due to the phenomenon of **after-discharge**. The after discharge occurs due to the presence of multiple parallel connections between the sensory afferent and the motor efferent fibers, constituting what are called the 'reverberating circuits' as shown in Fig. 118.3.

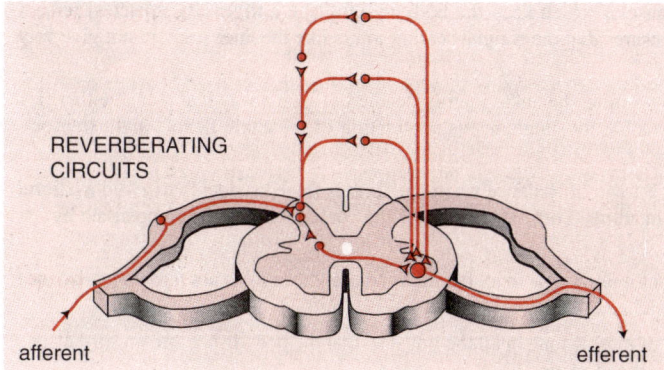

REVERBERATING CIRCUITS

afferent    efferent

**Fig. 118.3**

### What is the crossed extensor reflex? What is its functional significance?

This reflex and its importance in postural regulation are best understood in reference to quadrupeds. If a cat inadvertently places its right-front paw on a sharp object and gets hurt, it reflexly flexes the limb (withdrawal reflex). The flexion of the *right-front limb* will tend to destabilize its erect posture. The destabilization is prevented by other associated reflexes, i.e., hyperextension of the left-front limb, flexion of the left-hind limb and hyperextension of the right-hind limb (Fig. 118.4).

### Compare and contrast superficial and deep reflexes.

| SIMILARITIES | |
|---|---|
| Both are mostly spinal reflexes. | |

| DIFFERENCES | |
|---|---|
| **Deep reflexes** | **Superficial reflexes** |
| Elicited from deep structures like muscle and tendon, mostly by stretch | Elicited from superficial structures like skin and fascia, mostly by pain |
| Are monosynaptic or bisynaptic | Are polysynaptic |
| Are mostly postural reflexes | Are mostly protective reflexes |
| Involve a single muscle and move a single joint | Involve a group of muscles and often more than one joint |
| Are always centered in the spinal cord | Have reverberatory circuits passing through cerebral cortex |
| Are exaggerated in UMNL | Are abolished in UMNL |
| Examples are knee jerk, biceps jerk etc. | Examples are nociceptive withdrawal reflex, abdominal reflex etc. |

### What is central excitatory state?

The central excitatory state refers to the *level of activity of the facilitatory reticular activating system*. When one muscle is stretched, the proprioceptive afferents from the muscle not only result in the stimulation of its own α-motoneuron through the monosynaptic reflex but also places a large part of the facilitatory reticular activating system in the **subliminal fringe**. When the state of activity in the facilitatory reticular activating system (the **central excitatory state**) is high, the γ-motor discharge to all muscles are increased and all somatic motor reflexes are exaggerated.

### What is Jendrassik's maneuver?

When a clinician is unable to elicit a tendon jerk like the knee jerk, he employs **reinforcement** or the **Jendrassik's maneuver**. In this, the subject is asked to make a strong voluntary effort with his

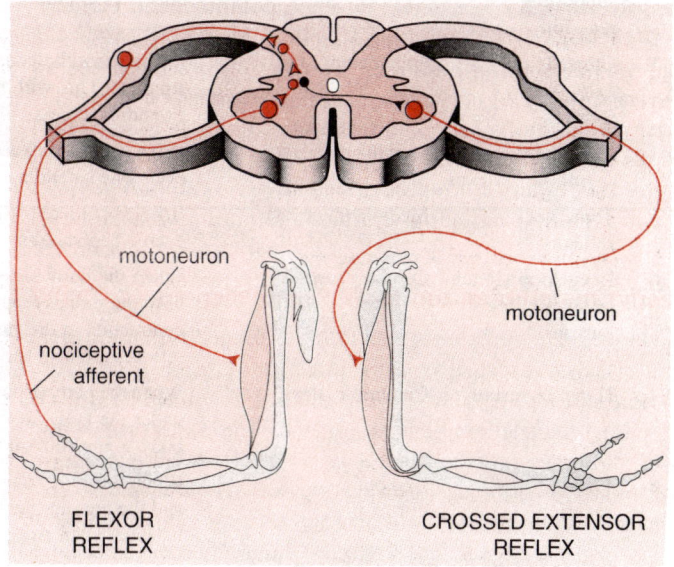

motoneuron

motoneuron

nociceptive afferent

FLEXOR REFLEX

CROSSED EXTENSOR REFLEX

**Fig. 118.4**

upper limbs; for example, to hook the fingers of the two hands together and then to pull them against one another as hard as possible. This increases the sensitivity of the monosynaptic reflex by increasing the central excitatory state and also diverts the attention of the subject from the muscle reflex being tested. The clinician is thus able to obtain a brisk knee jerk.

### What are antigravity muscles?

The antigravity muscles are those muscles which prevent flexion of the joints under the effect of gravity. The antigravity muscles of the body are endowed with a somewhat higher muscle tone than the other muscles of the body. In humans, the extensor muscles like erector spinae, erector capitis, glutei and quadriceps act as antigravity muscles and therefore have higher muscle tone. This higher muscle tone is provided by *supraspinal mechanisms*. In decerebrate preparations, the hypertonia occurs in the antigravity muscles, resulting in a caricature (i.e., exaggerated mimicry) of the normal posture. Interestingly, in bats, it is the flexor muscles that act as antigravity muscles. Accordingly in bats, the exaggerated muscle tone is present in the flexor and not the extensor muscles.

### Define posture and enumerate the postural reflexes, centers and functions.

Posture refers to the static position of any part of the body. Movements are the transition from one posture to another. The postural reflexes and their functions are summarized in the table given below.

### What is Romberg's sign?

The body behaves like an inverted pendulum hinged at the ankle joint. **Long-loop stretch reflexes** are continuously active in the erect posture and brings about a continuous correction of our 'sways' that occur from moment-to-moment during standing. There are *two*

*long-loop reflexes*: one is triggered by *proprioceptive afferents* from the muscles, and the other by *visual inputs*. Patients with lesions of the dorsal columns (as in tabes dorsalis) suffer from **sensory ataxia** due to loss of proprioceptive input. For maintaining the erect posture, they are entirely dependent on visually-triggered long loop postural reflex. The patient walks on a broad base with the legs apart, eyes are fixed to the ground for correcting the steps, associated with raising of the legs excessively high and slapping the feet on the ground. Closing of the eye accentuates the sensory ataxia (**Romberg's sign**). The *Romberg's sign is characteristic of sensory ataxia* and helps to distinguish it from cerebellar ataxia, in which the sign is absent.

### What are righting reflexes?

When the body goes off balance and falls down, the righting reflexes help the body to regain the upright position. There are several righting reflexes, which include the: (1) **Head righting reflex**. When the head is not in the upright position, the vestibular apparatus gets stimulated. It reflexly stimulates the appropriate muscles to bring the head back to the upright position. (2) **Body-on-head righting reflex**. When the body is lying flat on the ground, one of its surfaces (the anterior or posterior, depending on whether the body is prone or supine) is in contact with the ground. This differential stimulation of one surface of the body provides the necessary cues for reflexly bringing the head back to the upright position. (3) **Neck-on-body righting reflex**. Righting of the head (through head righting reflex) while the body continues to be in the horizontal position results in the stretching of the neck and activation of the neck righting reflexes. The neck righting reflex stimulates the appropriate postural muscles to bring the whole body back to the upright position. (4) **Body-on-body righting reflex**. When the body is lying flat on the ground, the differential stimulation of its anterior and posterior surfaces provides the necessary cues for bringing the body back to the erect position.

| | Postural reflex | Integrating center | Functional significance |
|---|---|---|---|
| 1. | Muscle tone | Spinal cord | Ensures that the extensor muscles which keep the body upright (the **antigravity muscles**) remain tonically contracted. This ensures that the weight-bearing joints like the knee joint do not give way under the effect of gravity. |
| 2. | Positive supporting reaction | Spinal cord | Ensures that in the standing position, the ankle joint is steadied in such a way that it can neither flex nor extend. This is made possible by simultaneous contraction of the ankle flexors and extensors. |
| 3. | Crossed extensor reflexes | Spinal cord | Ensures that the body is not thrown off-balance when one limb is flexed suddenly to avoid a painful stimulus. This will throw a quadruped off-balance unless the contralateral limbs compensate by extending excessively. |
| 4. | Tonic labyrhynthine reflexes | Medulla oblongata | Bring about a redistribution of muscle tone in all the limbs so that the body is not thrown off-balance even when standing on an inclined plane. |
| 5. | Tonic neck reflexes | Medulla oblongata | Bring about a redistribution of muscle tone in all the limbs so that the body is not thrown off-balance even when standing on an inclined plane. |
| 6. | Long loop stretch reflexes of leg muscles | Cerebral cortex | When the body sways forwards, there is *stretching of the gastrocnemius muscle*. This triggers not only the monosynaptic stretch reflex but also a long loop stretch reflex, which brings about reflex contraction in the gastrocnemius muscle with consequent correction of the sway. Long-loop postural reflexes are also triggered by visual inputs that suggest that the body is swaying. |
| 7. | Hopping reaction | Cerebral cortex | When the body is pushed forward, the leg hops in the direction of the displacement, bringing the foot under the body so that the center of gravity of the body is kept between the legs. Ensures that the body is not thrown off-balance when tipped over its center-of-gravity. |
| 8. | Placing reaction | Cerebral cortex | When the foot comes in contact with any firm surface, the foot is reflexly placed on the surface and the leg muscles are adjusted so as to support the body. Ensures that the body is not thrown off-balance when tipped over its center-of-gravity. |
| 9. | Righting reflexes | Midbrain | Ensure that the body regains its upright stance even after it is thrown off-balance. |

# Electroencephalogram

## What are different types of normal EEG waves and what are their characteristics?

The main types of EEG waves are alpha, beta, theta and delta waves. **Alpha waves** are the most prominent component of the EEG. They are *most marked in the parietooccipital area* of the scalp when the person is awake, quite and resting with eyes closed. They *disappear on opening the eyes* and *on attentive mind*. They *disappear entirely during deep sleep*. They are fairly regular pattern of waves at a frequency of 8 – 13 / sec and an amplitude of 50 – 100 μV. The mean peak alpha frequency is 10.2 Hz and *decreases in old age* due to decreased cerebral perfusion leading to decreased cerebral metabolic rate. Frequencies of alpha rhythm are also decreased in conditions like *low blood glucose level*, *low body temperature*, *low level of adrenal glucocorticoids* and *high arterial partial pressure of $CO_2$*. If there is a consistent difference of 1 Hz or more in alpha frequency between two cerebral hemispheres, the side of lower frequency is likely to be involved in pathological process.

**Beta waves** have frequency more than 13 cycles per second and may be as high as 25Hz. They have lower voltage than alpha waves. They are frequently recorded from the *parietal and frontal region*. They are seen during tension or CNS activation. When attentive to external stimulus or thinking hard about anything, the α wave is replaced by β rhythm. This transformation is known as EEG arousal. The seniles are found to have significantly less alpha or more beta activity that the young adult group. In infants, there is a fast beta like activity in EEG and occipital rhythm is slow 0.5-2/sec pattern. Barbiturates induce beta activity typically at a frequency of 18 – 24 Hz.

**Theta waves** have frequency between 4 – 8 Hz and have larger amplitude than alpha waves. They are seen in parietal and temporal region in children. They are seen in emotional stress in adults particularly during disappointment and frustration, and also occur in many brain disorders. The incidence of transient theta component is about 30% in an alert adult. Amplitude of theta component is greatest at 6 – 9 month (up to 150 μV when eyes are closed) of age. The theta component of EEG often accentuates during crying of children. Theta components persist into adult life in 10 – 15% of normal subject.

**Delta waves** have frequency of less than 3 Hz. They are seen in deep sleep (stage III and IV NREM) and in infancy. When they occur in awake state, they indicate serious organic brain disease.

| EEG wave | Frequency (Hz) | When seen |
|---|---|---|
| Alpha | 8-13 | When eyes are closed and mind is relaxed. Decreased in the aged, in hypoglycemia, hypothermia, hypercapnia and hypocortisolism. |
| Beta | 13-25 | Normally in children, during attention in adults. Induced by barbiturates. More in the aged. |
| Theta | 4-8 | Normal in infants. Present during emotional stress in adults. |
| Delta | < 3 | Normally in infants, during deep sleep in adults. Indicates brain disorder when present in awake state. |

## What is the functional significance of EEG?

Possible functions of EEG are: (1) The slowly repeating and highly synchronized discharges and inhibitory periods in thalamic and cortical cells actively induce **unconsciousness**. (2) The spontaneous spindles, initiated in the thalamus and imparted to the cortex, are essential for **memory and learning**. (3) During natural sleep, EEG waves may be involved in **suppression of sensorimotor activity** in spinal cord and brainstem.

## What are the clinical uses of recording an EEG?

Variations in EEG waves (frequency, morphology and seizure potentials) can be of diagnostic value in certain diseases. (1) **Epilepsy-seizure** potentials can be seen in different types of epilepsies. Epilepsy is associated with distinctive high amplitude (up to 1000 μV) wave patterns known as spikes or combination of spikes (polyspikes) or waves. In **grand mal (tonic-clonic) seizures**, there is fast EEG activity during the tonic phase. Slow waves, each preceded by a spike, occur at the time of each clonic jerk. In **petit mal (absence) seizures**, there is a characteristic spike and dome pattern of EEG with about 3 doublets occurring per second. (2) Other general changes such as slowing and irregularity accompany diffuse organic brain disease or follow cerebral **trauma** or **metabolic intoxication** (coma). (3) **Tumors** often produce local changes in EEG. (4) An area of electrical silence on the scalp could be due to an underlying subdural hematoma. (5) Many medications especially psychoactive drugs affect EEG. (6) An isoelectric or flat EEG indicates **brain death**.

# Sleep & Wakefulness

### Define sleep.

Sleep is a *reversible behavioral state* of *perceptual dissociation* from the environment and *unresponsiveness* to the environment. Sleep is usually (but not necessarily) accompanied by *postural recumbency, quiescence and closed eyes.*

### What is the normal duration of sleep?

Most young adults report sleeping approximately 7½ h a night on weekday nights and ~ 8½ h, on weekend nights. Sleep length depends upon genetic factors, volitional factors (staying up late, waking by alarm etc.) and circadian rhythms (i.e., the time of the day when one sleeps determines how long one sleeps).

### What are the differences between REM and NREM sleep?

Within sleep, there are two separate states: non-rapid eye movement (Non-REM) and rapid eye movement (REM). **Non-REM sleep** is also called **deep sleep**. It is subdivided into 4 stages based on the EEG. Sleep is lightest in stage 1 and deepest in stage 4 sleep. NREM sleep is usually associated with a lack of mental activity. A series of body movements usually signals a drift to the lighter NREM sleep stages.

**REM sleep** is characterized by: (1) **EEG activation**. The EEG shows the desynchronized or wakefulness pattern. Hence, REM sleep is also called **desynchronized sleep**. Yet, a person is usually more difficult to awake in REM than in non-REM sleep. Hence, REM sleep is also called **paradoxical sleep**. (2) **Dreaming**. Human REM sleep is associated with dreaming. There is vivid dream recall from approximately 80 per cent of arousals from REM sleep. (3) **Muscle atonia**. Inhibition of spinal motoneurons via brain-stem mechanisms mediates suppression of postural (antigravity) muscle tone in REM sleep. (4) **Rapid-eye movements**. During REM sleep, there are bursts of rapid eye movements, twitches in other phasic muscles and changes in respiratory pattern. (5) **Impaired thermoregulation**. Sweating or shivering during sleep in response to ambient temperature occurs in NREM sleep and ceases in REM sleep. (6) **PGO waves**. In cats, rapid eye movements are associated bursts of **ponto-geniculo-occipital waves**. PGO waves are not detectable in humans by scalp EEG but are *recordable by depth EEG recordings.*

### Why is REM sleep called paradoxical?

In REM sleep, the EEG shows the desynchronized or wakefulness pattern. Yet, a person is usually more difficult to awake in REM than in non-REM sleep. Hence, REM sleep is also called **paradoxical sleep**.

### Compare and contrast REM and NREM sleep.

**SIMILARITIES**

Both are stages of normal sleep.

**DIFFERENCES**

| NREM | REM |
| --- | --- |
| Is deeper than REM sleep | Is lighter than NREM sleep |
| EEG is synchronous with characteristic waveforms like sleep spindles, K-complexes, and high voltage slow waves | EEG is desynchronised, which is characteristic of wakefulness. PGO spikes are recorded in depth electrodes |
| Consists of 4 stages. Stages 3 and 4 are together called deep sleep | Not subdivided into stages |
| Not associated with dreaming etc. | Associated with dreaming, rapid eye movements, muscle atonia and impaired thermoregulation |
| Difficult to awake in deep sleep but not so in stages 1 and 2 | Difficult to awake |
| Sleep normally begins with NREM sleep | REM onset sleep occurs in infants, in jet lag, sleep deprivation, narcolepsy and withdrawal of REM-suppressing drugs. |
| Comprise 75% of total sleep | Comprise 25% of total sleep |

### Does sleep begin with REM or NREM sleep?

In infants, entry into sleep occurs via REM sleep. However, in normal adults, sleep *mostly begins with non-REM sleep*. In adults, REM-onset sleep occurs in jet lag, chronic sleep deprivation, narcolepsy, acute withdrawal of REM-suppressing drugs, endogenous depression, narcolepsy.

### What are sleep cycles? How many sleep cycles are there in a night's sleep?

NREM sleep and REM sleep alternate cyclically through the night. The average duration of a sleep cycle is 90 min. A typical sleep cycle progresses through stages 1 to 4 and then back through stages 3 to 1. The cycle ends in the REM sleep. A night's sleep usually progresses through 4 to 5 sleep cycles. Towards the end of the night, the cycles are often separated by brief intervals of awakening. These interruptions in sleep usually do not last long enough to be remembered in the morning. The transition from wakefulness to sleep is always through stage 1. The transition

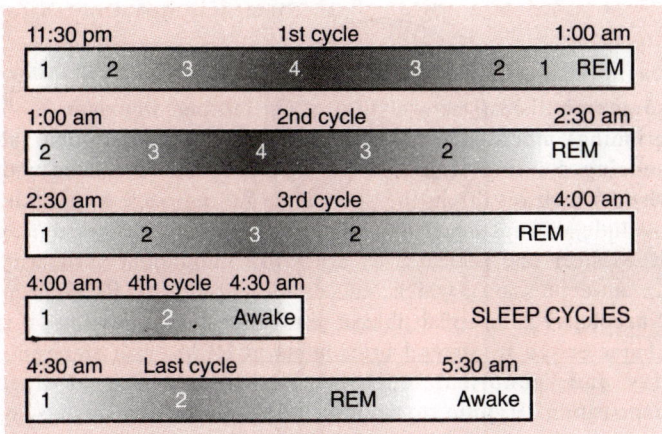

**Fig. 120.1**

from sleep to the awake state occurs either at the end of REM sleep or at the end of stage 2 (Fig. 120.1).

### How do the characteristics of the sleep cycles change through the sleep?

The $1^{st}$ cycle lasts 70 – 100 min. while the $2^{nd}$, $3^{rd}$ and $4^{th}$ cycles last for 90 – 120 min. each. Stages 3 and 4 (slow wave sleep) occupy less time in the second cycle and may disappear altogether from later cycles. The duration of stage 2 increases greatly and expands to occupy most of the NREM portion of the later cycles. REM sleep episodes become longer in the later cycles.

### Describe the EEG characteristics of the sleep stages.

The EEG pattern in NREM sleep is synchronous, with such characteristic waveforms as sleep spindles, K complexes, and high-voltage slow waves. In **stage 1 sleep**, the EEG changes from a rhythmic alpha (8 to 13 Hz) activity, particularly in the occipital region, to a relatively *low-voltage, mixed-frequency pattern*. Bursts of relatively high-voltage, very synchronous theta (3 to 7 cps) activity are common during the onset of stage 1 sleep in children and young adolescents (Fig. 120.2).

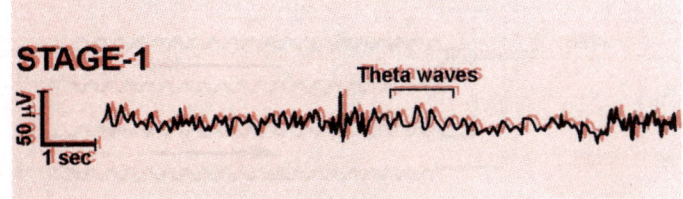

**Fig. 120.2**

There is still considerable sensitivity to sensory stimuli. However, the mild or moderate stimuli are often unable to produce a full arousal; instead, they produce a sharp electronegative wave at the vertex called the **vertex sharp wave** or **V-wave**. They can be regarded as the rudimentary form of the K-complexes that appear in stage-2. They look similar too, except that the V-waves are sharper and have shorter duration. Slow eye movements commonly precede the EEG transition from wakefulness to stage 1 sleep.

**Stage 2** is signaled by the appearance of **sleep spindles** in the EEG. These are up to 100μV in amplitude, and have a frequency of about 14 Hz. Each burst last about 0.5 to 1.5 sec. Auditory

stimuli during this phase readily evokes the **K complexes** in the EEG. They also occur spontaneously during this stage. The K-complex consists of one or two high voltage waves followed by a brief 14 Hz activity (Fig. 120.3). As stage 2 sleep progresses, there is a gradual appearance of high-voltage slow wave activity in the EEG till the onset of stage 3 sleep.

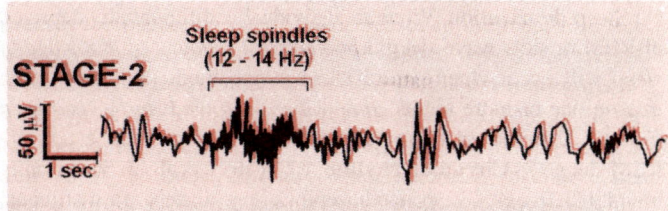

**Fig. 120.3**

**Stage 3 sleep** usually lasts only a few minutes in the first cycle. It is characterized by a high-voltage ($\geq 75$ μV) and slow ($\leq 2$ Hz) wave activity, the **delta waves** (Fig. 120.4), which *accounts for 20-50% of the EEG activity*. It lasts for about 20 to 40 min (or so) in the first cycle. It is characterized by *delta activity accounting for >50% of the EEG activity*. The *stage 3 and stage 4 sleep together* are referred to as **slow wave sleep**, **delta sleep**, or **deep sleep**.

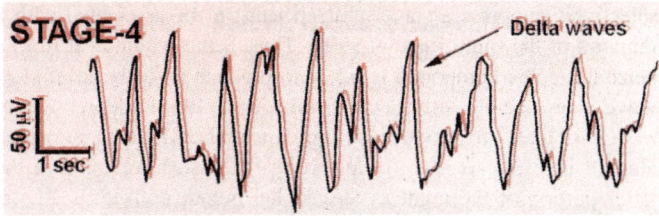

**Fig. 120.4**

### Give examples of discriminant responses during sleep.

During sleep, a person tends *to respond to only a few selected stimuli that are most meaningful* while ignoring the rest. This is called **discriminant response**. For example (1) a person tends to have a lower arousal threshold for his/her own name versus someone else's name; (2) a sleeping mother is more likely to hear her own baby's cry than the cry of an unrelated infant; (3) a captain wakes up to the cry of 'iceberg' in the midst of the din and bustle of a ship.

### Why are early morning dreams better recalled than midnight dreams?

The transition from wakefulness to sleep tends to produce a **retrograde amnesia**. This is because *sleep inactivates the consolidation of short-term* into long-term memory. If sleep persists for approximately 10 min, memory is lost for the few minutes before sleep. Midnight dreams are rarely followed by more than 10 minutes of wakefulness and therefore, are mostly forgotten.

### How does sleep change with age?

50% of the sleep in *neonates* is REM sleep. In preterm neonates, REM sleep is as high as 80%. The sleep cycles are shorter, about 60 min in the newborn. *Infants* have REM onset sleep. *Slow wave sleep is maximal in young children* and decreases markedly with age. It is nearly impossible to waken youngsters in the slow wave sleep of the night's first sleep cycle. *In adolescence*, slow wave sleep decreases by nearly 40%. *By age 60,* slow wave sleep may no longer be present, particularly in men. The age-related decline in nocturnal slow wave sleep parallels loss of cortical synaptic density.

### What are the factors affecting sleep-stage distribution?

(1) **Sleep deprivation**. When an individual is differentially deprived of REM or slow wave sleep, a *preferential rebound of that stage of sleep* will occur when natural sleep is resumed. *With total sleep loss* on one or more nights, *slow wave sleep tends to be recovered first.* (2) Extremes of **temperature** tend to disrupt sleep, especially REM sleep. (3) **Circadian rhythm**. REM sleep peaks in the morning hours. (4) **Drugs**, like benzodiazepines (e.g. diazepam), marijuana, tricyclic antidepressants, monoamine oxidase inhibitors (MAOIs) and alcohol.

### How do different drugs affect sleep?

Slow wave sleep is suppressed by **benzodiazepines** (e.g. diazepam) and by chronic ingestion of marijuana. REM sleep is suppressed by **tricyclic antidepressants** and **monoamine oxidase inhibitors** (MAOIs). **Alcohol** intake immediately before sleep produces REM suppression early in the night. *Withdrawal from drugs* that selectively suppress a stage of sleep tends to be associated with a rebound of the same stage of sleep. Thus, acute withdrawal from a benzodiazepine compound is likely to produce an increase of slow wave sleep; acute withdrawal from a tricyclic antidepressant or MAOI is likely to produce an increase of REM sleep; pre-sleep alcohol ingestion is often followed by REM sleep rebound in the latter portion of the night as the alcohol is metabolized.

### Give some examples of abnormal behavior during sleep.

Several abnormal behaviors can occur during sleep, e.g., **somnambulism** (sleepwalking), **sleep talking**, **bruxism** (tooth grinding), **nocturnal enuresis** (bedwetting), **sleep apnea** and **snoring**. Snoring occurs due to the hypotonia associated with sleep which results in the soft palate falling back to partially occlude the nasopharynx. Nocturnal enuresis occurs during REM sleep and is treated by drugs like imipramine (primarily, an antidepressant), which reduces the duration of REM sleep. **Narcolepsy** is an irresistible urge to sleep during daytime; it is characterized by several brief bouts of REM-onset sleep in a day. It is abnormal if it occurs in the absence of sleep deprivation. **Hypnic myoclonia** is the contraction of muscles associated with vivid visual imagery. It is a fairly common experience during sleep-onset. Normally REM sleep and dreaming are associated with inhibition of muscle tone. When REM sleep is not associated with inhibition of muscle tone, there may be motor responses to some of the dream-events, resulting in hypnic myoclonia.

### What is cerveau isole? What is its importance in relation to sleep?

Transections separating the cerebrum from the brainstem and spinal cord (the **cerveau isole**) produce a sleep-like state with cortical slow waves.

### How is sleep behavior studied in patients?

Sleep behavior is studied using **polysomnography**, i.e., simultaneous recording of EEG, EOG, EMG, ECG etc.

# 121

# Memory & Learning

## What are the four processes involved in memory?

Memory is the *acquisition, storage and retrieval* of sensory informations. It involves *four distinct processes.* (1) **Encoding** is the process by which newly learned information is attended to and processed when first encountered. (2) **Consolidation** is the process that alters the newly stored information so as to make it more stable for long-term storage. (3) **Storage** occurs at specific sites in the brain following which memory is retained for a long time. It involves the expression of genes and synthesis of new proteins. (4) **Retrieval** refers to the processes that permit the recall and use of stored information.

## What are the approximate durations of sensory, primary, secondary and tertiary memory?

Memory has different levels depending on the permanency of its storage : (1) **Sensory memory** lasts for less than 1 second; (2) **Primary (short-term) memory** lasts for several seconds; (3) **Secondary (intermediate-term) memory** lasts for minutes to years; (4) **Tertiary (long-term) memory** is permanent.

## What is the difference between implicit and explicit memory?

**Implicit memory** is also called **non-declarative** or **reflexive memory**. These are memories that one is never aware of like skills, habits and behavioral reflexes (habituation, sensitization, conditioning). For example as infants, we all have learnt and remembered how to stand. However we seldom realize that 'standing' is something we have learnt or memorized. **Explicit memory** is also called **declarative** or **recognition memory**. It is the memory – of facts and events – that we are aware of.

## What are the two types of explicit memory?

Explicit memory is of two types: episodic and semantic. **Episodic memory** is the memory of events. It is stored in the prefrontal cortex. Patients with frontal lobe damage have a tendency to forget events. For example, they may forget how a piece of information was acquired – a deficit called *source amnesia*. However, patients with loss of episodic memory still have the ability to recall vast stores of factual (semantic) knowledge. **Semantic memory** is the memory of objects, facts and concepts as well as words and their meaning. It is distributed at multiple sites in the brain. As a result, damage to a specific cortical area can lead to loss of specific information and therefore a *fragmentation of knowledge*.

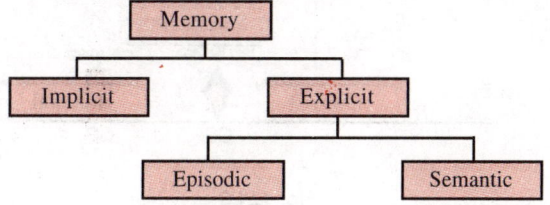

## What is retrograde amnesia?

A critical amount of time – about 5 to 10 minutes – is required for the transfer of short-term memory to a more stable intermediate-term memory through a process called **consolidation of memory**. If this time is not allowed for the consolidation to occur, the data in short-term memory is completely forgotten. This is seen in patients of concussion and electroconvulsive therapy who are unable to recall the events immediately preceding the concussion or convulsion. This phenomenon is called **retrograde amnesia**. A similar retrograde amnesia occurs before the onset of sleep – the reason why one is unable to remember the precise time of one's own sleep onset.

## Define learning.

Learning is a *modification of behavior* based on *individual experience*. It is *an enduring change* in behavior lasting at least a few seconds but mostly lasting a lifetime, which distinguishes it from transient reactions to sensory stimuli. Learning must have a teleonomic function i.e., *it must serve a purpose*. Not every experience results in learning. Similarly, not every instance of learning directly materializes into behavior: some types of learning result in the *potential to react, i.e., knowledge*.

## Classify the different types of learning.

Learning may be reflex or incidental. (1) In **reflex learning,** the learning is associated with an immediate behavioral change. Reflex learning may be of two types non-associative and associative: (i) In **non-associative learning**, the organism is **habituated** or **sensitized** to a stimulus. (ii) In **associative learning**, the organism learns relations among events in the world – either between stimuli, or between stimuli and actions. The two main categories of associative learning are **classical conditioning** and **instrumental conditioning**. (2) In **incidental learning**, the behavioral change is not immediately apparent. The individual acquires information about the world while attending 'incidentally' to sensory inputs, and thereby develops the potential to behave differently. Incidental learning occurs *in the absence of an identifiable instructive situation*. Incidental learning *results in knowledge*. However, its behavioral consequences are not apparent immediately but are manifested later in a number of ways. For example, it may alter the perceptual distinctiveness of sensory attributes (**perceptual learning**) or, it may contribute to the reorganization of internal representations, resulting in sudden solutions to previously unresolved problems (**insight**).

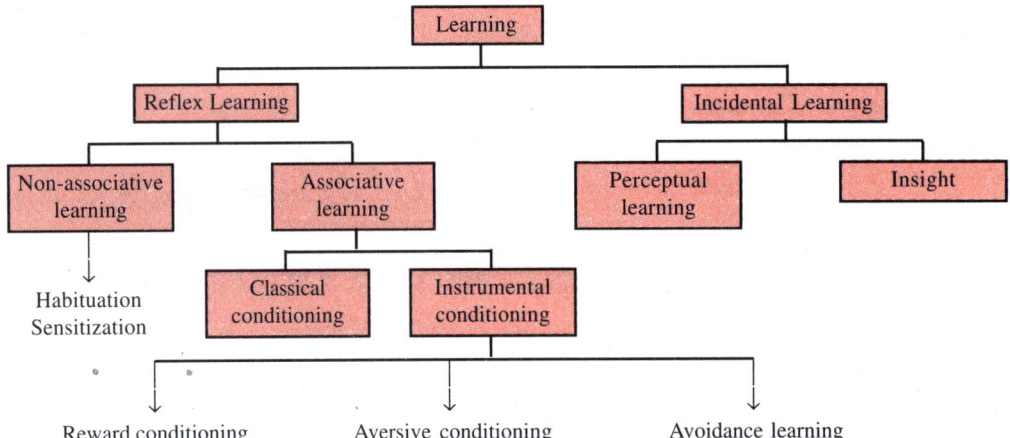

## What is the relation between learning the memory?

Learning follows memory. Implicit memory results in reflex learning. Explicit memory results in incidental learning.

## Name some parts of the brain that are important for memory.

Explicit memory is acquired through the polymodal association cortices (the **prefrontal**, **limbic** and **parietooccipital-temporal cortices**) that synthesize visual, auditory and somatic information, From there, the information is conveyed to the **parahippocampal** and **perirhinal cortices**, then the **entorhinal cortex**, the **dentate gyrus**, the **hippocampus**, the **subiculum**, and finally back to the entorhinal cortex, From the entorhinal cortex, the information is sent back to the polymodal association areas of the neocortex.

## What is classical conditioning? Explain giving examples.

In **classical conditioning**, the organism is presented with a stimulus that evokes a certain behavioral response. This stimulus is called the **unconditioned stimulus** (US). The response to the US is the **unconditioned response** (UR). Another stimulus, which is neutral with respect to the UR, is then presented in association with the US. This stimulus is called the **conditioned stimulus** (CS). The association between the CS and US alters the response to the CS, resulting in a **conditioned response** (CR), which is similar to the UR. Classical conditioning was first illustrated by Pavlov in 1927 with his experiments on dog. When the dog was presented with food (US), there was salivation (UR). After the dog had been repeated presented with food immediately after ringing a bell (CS), the dog started salivating on hearing the bell (CR) (Fig.121.1).

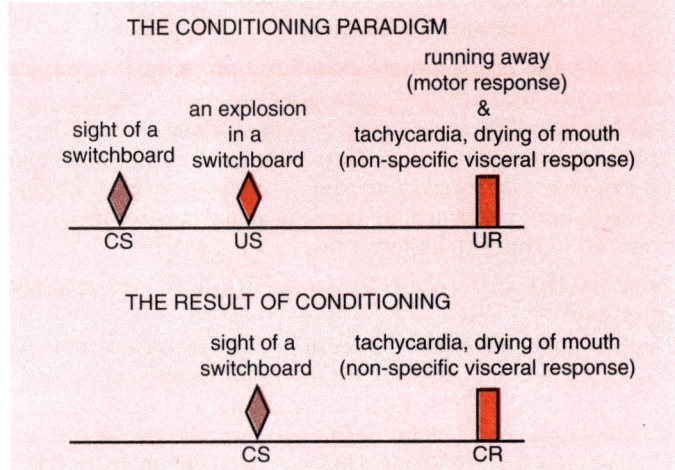

**Fig. 121.2**

When a CS is paired with an aversive US, specific motor CRs are accompanied with visceral reactions signifying arousal and fear e.g., altered heart rate, blood pressure, and respiration. These visceral reactions are called **conditioned emotional response** or

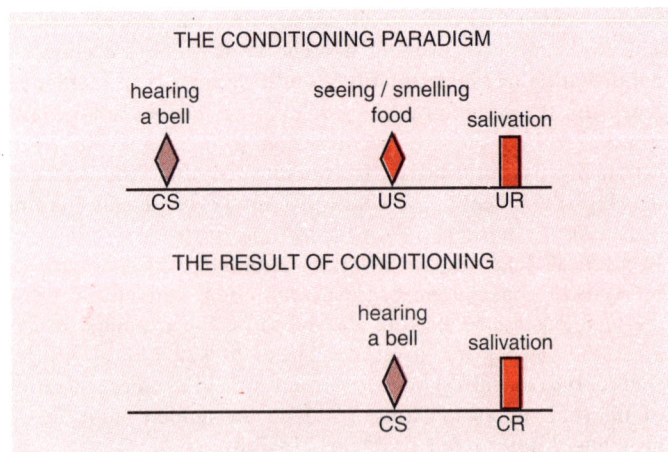

**Fig. 121.1**

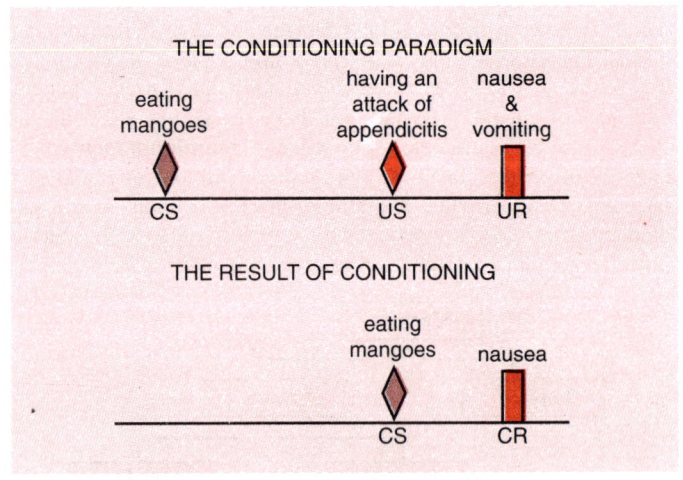

**Fig. 121.3**

**conditioned fear** and are important factors in the development of a psychiatric condition called **anxiety neuroses** (Fig. 121.2)

Conditioning is sometimes possible even when there is an extensive delay between the CS and the US. These cases involve gustatory reflexes, in which food is followed hours later by vomiting and cramps. This suggest that nature has evolved a mechanism to ensure that when survival is very much at stake, conditioning tolerates a long delay between cause and effect. For example, a person falling ill after consuming some food frequently develops an aversion for that particular food, even if the food was not responsible for his illness (Fig. 121.3)

The cellular mechanisms of classical conditioning have been studied in the gill-withdrawal reflex of *Aplysia*. Conditioning requires the activation of **NMDA receptors** for glutamate present on the soma of the motor cell, as opposed to the non-NMDA receptors that are activated during sensitization.

### What is instrumental conditioning? Explain giving examples.

Learning the impact of actions on the world is referred to as **instrumental conditioning** (also called **operant conditioning**). In this type of learning, the intensity of a spontaneous behavioral response is altered by a reinforcing stimulus. The term 'instrumental' denotes that the organism's behavior is *instrumental* (i.e., necessary or helpful) in the delivery of the US. In instrumental conditioning the organism learns *which of its own actions are responsible* for the occurrence of a reinforcer (US). There are three major categories of instrumental conditioning: (i) **reward conditioning**, in which an appetitive reinforcer (e.g. food) increases the intensity related of behaviors; (ii) **aversive conditioning**, in which an aversive reinforcer (e.g. electric shock) decreases the intensity of related behaviors; (iii) **avoidance learning**, in which an aversive reinforcer is delivered in the absence of a particular response, but is omitted, in the presence of that response. For example, a rat would learn to press a lever if this prevents a shock.

### What are the conditions that have to be satisfied for producing conditioned learning? How is it inhibited?

Successful conditioning is critically dependent on: the *duration* of the US and CS, their *rate,* the *interval* between them, and the *order of their presentation*. If the CS is presented repeatedly without the US, the conditioned reflex eventually dies out. This process is called **extinction** or **internal inhibition**. On the other hand, if the animal is disturbed by an external stimulus immediately after the CS is applied, the conditioned response may not occur (**external inhibition**).

### What is the role of corpus callosum in learning and memory?

If an experimental animal (cat or monkey) is conditioned to a visual stimulus presented only to the left eye, then the conditioned response can occur subsequently even if the visual stimulus is presented only to the other eye. The response occurs even after the optic chiasma has been sectioned in the middle so that the visual stimulus is transmitted only to the ipsilateral visual cortex. It suggests that the learning/memory got transferred to the contralateral cortex i.e., there has been an intercortical transfer of the learnt behavior. However, *if the training is imparted after sectioning the corpus callosum too* (in addition to the optic chiasma), the intercortical transfer fails to occur. Such failure of intercortical transfer of learning and memory is also seen in human subjects in whom the corpus callosum is congenitally absent or in those in whom the corpus callosum have been surgically sectioned in an effort to control epileptic seizures. Studies in subjects indicate that the *transfer of visual memory occurs in the posterior part of the corpus callosum* while *transfer of auditory and somesthetic memory occurs in the anterior part of the corpus callosum*.

### What is sensitization?

Sensitization is an *augmentation of a response to a stimulus*, following presentation of the same or another stimulus. In other words, it is *learning to intensify a response*. The sensitizing stimulus is usually strong or noxious. Sensitization is termed *non-associative* because it does not result from specific associations between particular stimuli, as opposed to associative learning. Rather, *a sensitizing stimulus increases the responsiveness to a wide variety of stimuli*. For example a man bitten by a snake might react sharply to a piece of rope. Repetitive exposure to noxious stimuli may lead to *long-term sensitization*, lasting weeks or even longer.

### What is the cellular mechanism of sensitization?

The cellular mechanisms of sensitization have been best studied in the *Aplysia* (snail). In the gill-withdrawal reflex, the snail withdraws its gill when its *siphon is touched* or when *a painful stimulus is applied to* its *tail* or its *mantle shelf*. The neurotransmitter released at the synapse between the sensory and motor neuron is glutamate. Glutamate acts on the non-NMDA receptors present on the motor neuron.

After *a painful stimulus is applied to the tail repeatedly*, the snail subsequently withdraws its gill much more vigorously in

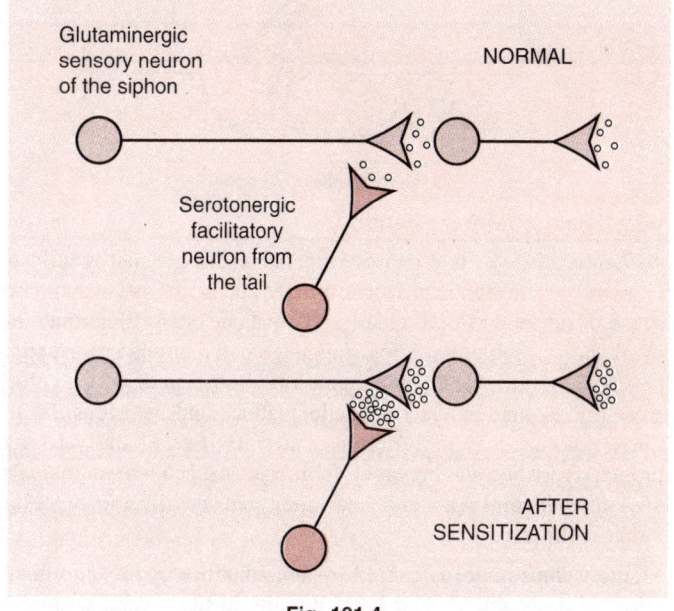

**Fig. 121.4**

response to an innocuous touch on the siphon. The sensitization is associated with increased release of neurotransmitters from the axonal ending of the sensory neuron. This is brought about by a third neuron called the **facilitator neuron** that synapses presynaptically on the sensory nerve terminal (Fig. 121.4). The facilitator neuron releases serotonin, which binds to serotonin receptors on the sensory nerve terminal. The binding leads to the phosphorylation of channel proteins through two different pathways: (i) The Gs-cAMP-phosphokinase-A pathway *phosphorylates and inactivates $K^+$ channels*. Inactivation of $K^+$ channels prolongs the duration of action potential, resulting in greater influx of $Ca^{2+}$ into the terminal. (ii) The $G_o$-phospholipase C-protein kinase C pathway *phosphorylates and activates L-type $Ca^{2+}$ channels*. Activation of $Ca^{2+}$ channels increases the $Ca^{2+}$ influx into the nerve terminal and increases the release of neurotransmitters.

### What is habituation?

**Habituation** is a *gradual diminution of response to a stimulus, following repeated presentation of the same stimulus*. The weaker the stimulus, and more rapid the frequency of stimulation, the more rapid and/or pronounced is habituation. Strong stimuli may fail to produce habituation. Presentation of another, usually noxious stimulus results in recovery of the habituated response i.e. **dishabituation**. Habituation of the gill-withdrawal reflex occurs when *the siphon of the snail is touched repeatedly*, and the snail does not withdraw its gill anymore. Habituation is associated with a decrease in neurotransmitter released at the synapses, which in turn is due to the inactivation of $Ca^{2+}$ influx at the axon endings (Fig. 121.5)

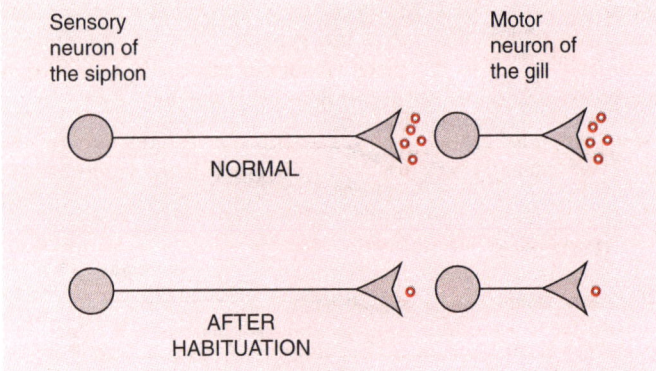

Sensory neuron of the siphon

Motor neuron of the gill

NORMAL

AFTER HABITUATION

**Fig. 121.5**

### What is Alzheimer disease?

Alzheimer disease is a neurodegenerative disease that manifests clinically in the seventh decade of life and is the most common cause of dementia in the elderly. The patients show abnormalities of memory, problem solving, language calculation, visuospatial perception, judgment, and behavior. Some patients develop psychotic symptoms, such as hallucinations and delusions. In all these patients mental functions and activities of daily living progressively become impaired. In the late stages these individuals are mute, incontinent, and bedridden and usually die of other medical illnesses.

Memory impairment is caused by abnormalities of the entorhinal cortex, hippocampus, and other circuits in the medial temporal cortex. Memory difficulties and attention deficits are due to abnormalities in the association areas of the neocortex that are due to alterations in the **basal forebrain cholinergic systems**. The behavioral and emotional disturbances occur due to involvement of the limbic cortex, amygdala, thalamus, and several **brain stem monoaminergic systems** that project to the hippocampal cortex.

Alzheimer disease is associated with cytoskeletal abnormalities in neurons. In affected nerve cells the cytoskeleton is often altered. The most common cytoskeletal alteration is **neurofibrillary tangles**. Another hallmark of Alzheimer disease are the **amyloid** (fibrillar peptides) deposits. The brain regions affected by Alzheimer disease also contain **neuritic** or **senile plaques** in which extracellular deposits of amyloid are surrounded by dystrophic axons as well as the processes of astrocytes and microglia (inflammatory cells).

Mutations in genes like the **APP** or **presenilin** promote the formation of more toxic forms of peptides (**Ap peptide**). It is likely that these forms of Ap peptide promote fibril formation and are central to the pathogenesis of Alzheimer disease.

### Compare and contrast habituation and sensitization.

| SIMILARITIES |
| --- |
| Both are forms of non-associative learning. |
| Both result from repeated stimuli. |

| DIFFERENCES | |
| --- | --- |
| **Habituation** | **Sensitization** |
| Occurs with weak stimuli | Occurs with strong, painful stimuli |
| Results in gradual decrease in response | Results in gradual increase in response |
| Helps in avoiding fatigue | Helps in survival |
| Associated with decreased neurotransmitter release | Associated with increased neuro-transmitter release |
| Occurs due to inactivation of $Ca^{2+}$ channels in presynaptic nerve ending (homosynaptic) | Occurs due to presynaptic facilitation by a third, serotonergic neuron (heterosynaptic) |

# 122

# Language & Speech

## What are the cortical areas of speech and what are the disorders caused by lesions in those areas?

(1) *Spoken words* are first perceived in the primary auditory area (areas 41, 42) and then recognized and understood in the **Wernicke area** (area 22). Thoughts and words also originate in the Wernicke's area. (2) *Written words* are perceived in area 17 and are subsequently processed at higher levels of visual association areas like Area 18 and 19, and in the **angular gyrus** (area 39). The written words are fully understood when the information passes to the Wernicke's area. (3) The *thought of words* generated in the Wernicke's area are transmitted to the Broca's area through a neuronal tract called the **arcuate fasciculus**. (4) It is in the Broca's area (area 44 and 45) that the *motor plans for the words* are formulated. The motor plan is forwarded to the primary motor cortex from where impulses are sent down to the muscles of articulation and the vocal cords, resulting in speech (Fig. 122.1)

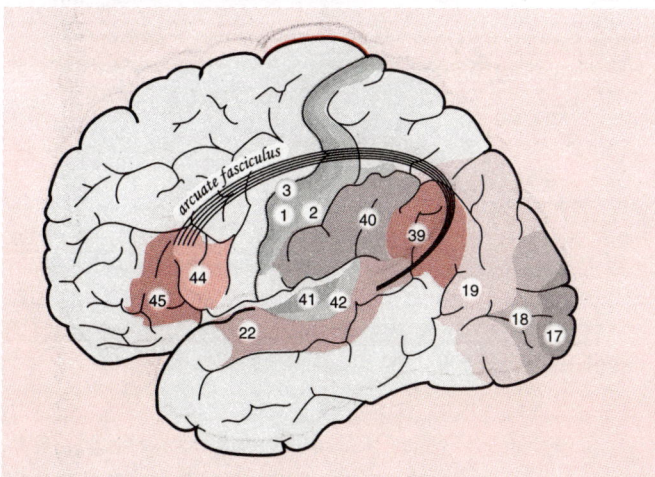

**Fig. 122.1**

The above model explains the various speech defects as follows. (1) A *lesion of speech center* of the dominant hemisphere results in aphasia, in which the affected individual is unable to appreciate or express written and spoken words. The aphasia may be sensory or motor. (2) A *lesion of area 22 or Wernicke's area* produces **word deafness (sensory aphasia)**. The patient is unable to interpret the spoken words, which he could appreciate under normal condition. He can speak fluently with occasional uses of incorrect and meaningless words. (3) A *lesion of area 39* results in **word blindness**, in which words are seen but not comprehended. Inability to read is known as **dyslexia** and inability to write is called **agraphia**. The patient can speak and understand spoken

language as long as the arcuate fasciculus between the Wernicke's and Broca's areas remains intact. (4) A *lesion of area 40* produces **astereognosis** in which an individual is unable to recognize a familiar object (without the help of vision) by touch and proprioception. Such tactile agnosia also interferes with speech function. (5) *Lesion of the Broca's area* results in **motor aphasia**. The patient cannot speak properly, although he knows what he intends to communicate. The speech is very slow, and certain grammatical words and phrases are dropped. Therefore, his spoken language is agrammatical and nonfluent. (6) *Lesion of the arcuate fasciculus* connecting the Broca's and Wernicke's areas results in **conduction aphasia** in which speech is fluent, comprehension is intact but repetition of spoken language is extremely difficult.

## Define aphasia.

**Aphasia** refers to *a disorder of language* apparent in speech, writing or reading. Aphasias must be distinguished from **dysarthria**, *a disorder of speech* in which articulation of word is impaired. Examples of aphasias include Wernicke's aphasia, transcortical aphasia, conduction aphasia, anomic aphasia, and Broca's aphasia.

## What is the difference between fluent and non-fluent aphasia?

Disorder of language and disorder of speech may coexist. Accordingly, aphasias are categorized into non-fluent (with difficulty in articulation) or fluent (with no difficulty in articulation). **Fluent aphasias,** in which there is fluent speech but *difficulties in the comprehension or repetition* of words, phrases, or sentences spoken by others. **Non-fluent aphasias,** in which there are *difficulties in articulating* but relatively good comprehension of spoken speech (auditory verbal comprehension).

## What is Broca's aphasia?

In Broca's aphasia (also called **motor, expressive,** or **nonfluent** aphasia), the individual has *difficulty in speaking but continues to understand speech.* The person *speaks in a very slow, deliberate manner using a simple syntax.* Only the keywords necessary for communication are used. Nouns are most apt to be expressed only in the singular, and *conjunctions, adjectives, adverbs, and articles are very uncommon.* The deficit in Broca's aphasia is not one of making sounds, but rather one of switching from one sound to another.

## What is Wernicke's aphasia?

Wernicke's aphasia, or **sensory aphasia,** is the inability to comprehend words or to arrange sounds into coherent speech. There is no dysarthria and the *speech is fluent.* It has three characteristics: (1) **Deficit in the categorization of sounds.** The inability to isolate the significant phonemic characteristics of speech and to classify sounds into known phonemic systems. An example will illustrate. In the Japanese language, the sounds "l" and "r" are not distinguished; a *Japanese-speaking person hearing English cannot distinguish the sounds "l" and "r"* because the necessary template is not in the brain. Thus, although this distinction is perfectly clear to English-speaking persons, it is not so to a native Japanese. This is precisely the problem that a person with Wernicke's aphasia has in his or her own language. (2) **Defect in speech**. The affected person can speak a great deal, but the speech is often associated with: (i) **anomia** i.e., difficulty in finding an appropriate word to express a thought; (ii) **neologism** i.e., using or creating new words or new meanings for established words; (iii) **paraphasias** i.e., the production of *unintended* syllables, words, or phrases during the effort to speak. Paraphasia differs from difficulties in articulation in that sounds are correctly articulated, but they are the wrong sounds; people with paraphasia either distort the intended word (for example, "pike" instead of "pipe") or produce a completely unintended word (for example, "my mother" instead of "my wife"). Confusions associated with phonetic characteristics while speaking is often called a **word salad**. (3) **Impairment in writing**. A person who cannot discern phonemic characteristics cannot be expected to write, because he or she does not know the **graphemes** (pictorial or written representations of a phoneme) that combine to form a word.

## Compare and contrast Broca's aphasia and Wernicke's aphasia.

**SIMILARITIES**

Both are associated with a disorder of language that is apparent in speech.

**DIFFERENCES**

| Broca's aphasia | Wernicke's aphasia |
| --- | --- |
| It is a form of motor aphasia | It is a form of sensory aphasia |
| There is difficulty in speaking and is therefore called non-fluent aphasia | Speech is fluent (fluent aphasia) though often associated with incorrect or meaningless words |
| Has no difficulty in understanding speech | Has difficulty in understanding spoken words |
| Writing is not affected | Has difficulty in expressing through writing |
| Associated with lesion of Broca's area (areas 44 and 45) | Associated with lesion of Wernicke's area (area 22) |

# 123

# Regulation of Food Intake

## What is the difference between hunger and appetite? What is satiety?

**Hunger** is a bodily need to fulfil the caloric requirements of the body while **appetite** is a psychic or emotional desire to eat, and may or may not be associated with the need for food. Appetite is acquired, and is dependent upon pleasurable past experiences associated with eating. An individual when *hungry* will eat almost any wholesome food so long as it is reasonably palatable. After he has reached a state of satiety, he may still have the *appetite* to eat some dessert, which is entirely unnecessary so far as caloric requirements are concerned. Cessation of eating is a voluntary act, and is induced by a conscious sensation called satiety when sufficient food has been eaten.

## What is the role of hypothalamus in regulation of food intake?

Injury to the **ventromedial hypothalamic nucleus** causes obesity. If this area is destroyed, instead of being satisfied with an amount of food appropriate to its caloric requirements, the animal continues to eat as long as it is able to swallow food or as long as food is available, with the result that it becomes excessively obese. Injuries to the **lateral hypothalamic nuclei** cause the animal to stop eating altogether. Animals with such injuries absolutely refuse food even though they starved to death. Electrical stimulation of the lateral hypothalamic nuclei by means of implanted electrodes produces **hyperphagia** in animals. During the period of stimulation, the animals exhibit a compulsive desire to eat. It was concluded from these observations that the nuclei in the lateral area of the hypothalamus contain a **feeding center**, and that the medial hypothalamic nuclei contain a **satiety center**. Since injury to the satiety center was effective only if the feeding center was intact, it was concluded that the *medial satiety center acted by inhibiting the lateral feeding center*. B. K. Anand is credited with the discovery of the feeding center.

## What are the other brain areas involved in the regulation of food intake?

The *mechanics* of feeding are controlled by centers in the *brain stem*. The **area postrema** and the caudal medial **nucleus of the solitary tract** affect the degree of eating. The **amygdala** and the **prefrontal cortex**, which are closely coupled with the hypothalamus play important role in the control of feeding, particularly in the control of **discriminative appetite**. Destruction of the amygdala causes **psychic blindness** in the choice of foods, i.e., the animal becomes indifferent to the type and quality of food that it eats. The **neocortex** can modify feeding behavior as a result of habits and conditioning.

## What are two types of peripheral regulation of food intake?

Peripheral regulation of quantity of food is of two types. The **short term regulatory system** is based on *gastrointestinal feedback* and serves to limit the size of each meal. Smaller quantities of food passes through gastrointestinal tract at a steadier pace and digestive and absorptive mechanisms work out at optimal rates. Large amounts of food at each meal would be too much for storage systems once food has all been absorbed. The **long term regulatory system** for feeding is based on *metabolic feedback* and helps to maintain constant stores of nutrients in tissues preventing them from becoming too low or too high.

## What is leptin and what is its role in obesity?

**Leptin** is a circulating protein produced primarily in fat cells. It mediates a feedback loop by which the size of the body's fat depots regulates food intake. Leptin acts on the hypothalamus to decrease food intake and increase energy consumption. Leptin receptors are found in various peripheral tissues as well as the brain.

In humans, inactivating mutations of the leptin gene and the leptin receptor gene cause obesity that starts early in life. Plasma leptin levels are higher in women than in men, and this difference is partly due to the fact that women have more body fat. Leptin levels are increased in obese humans with normal leptin genes in direct proportion to the percent of body fat, and there is a similar positive correlation between the leptin mRNA concentration in adipose tissue and percent body fat. In many cases of human obesity, there is a defective leptin receptor gene, a defect in the mechanisms activated by the human gene, or a defect in the transport of leptin into the brain.

## Which are the other hormones involved in regulation of food intake?

Gastrointestinal hormones that inhibit food intake include GRP, glucagon and glucagon-like polypeptide (GLP), somatostatin, cholecystokinin (CCK). Food entering the gastrointestinal tract triggers the release of substances, which act on the brain to produce satiety by short-term, meal-to-meal control of food. **Neuropeptide-Y** is a polypeptide hormone that increases food intake when injected into the hypothalamus. **Orexins** are polypeptides that increase food intake. They are synthesized in neurons located in the lateral hypothalamus. **Pro-opiomelanocortin** (**POMC**) derivatives decrease food intake. Food intake is also increased by **melanin-concentrating hormone**, a polypeptide found in the lateral hypothalamus and the zona incerta. Neuropeptides that inhibits food intake include **cocaine and**

**amphetamine-regulated transcript** or **CART** found in the hypothalamus, and **corticotropin releasing hormone (CRH)**. **Catecholamines** depress appetite and food intake. **Amphetamine** and related drugs are used clinically to suppress appetite by releasing norepinephrine in the brain.

### Name the feedback mechanisms from the GIT that are involved in the regulation of food intake.

**Hunger contractions** contribute to hunger state but are not solely responsible for the hunger sensation. Cutting the splanchnic nerve and vagus nerve abolishes the hunger contractions but does not abolish the hunger sensation. The effect of **gastric distention** on hunger and appetite is due to the presence in the stomach of stretch receptors situated in the muscular walls and connected to afferent fibers of the vagus nerves. Section of the vagi abolishes the effects of gastric distention on appetite. **Oral metering** of food intake is performed by the various oral receptors related to feeding such as chewing, salivation, swallowing and tasting meter the food as it passes through the mouth. As a result, after a certain amount of food has passed through the mouth, the hypothalamic feeding center becomes inhibited. This can be demonstrated in an experimental animal prepared with an esophagostomy so that food, which is eaten, passes through the mouth and pharynx and upper esophagus but does not enter the stomach (**sham feeding**). Although no food enters the stomach, feeding still stops after sometime.

### Enumerate the metabolic feedback mechanisms involved in the regulation of food intake.

The **glucostatic hypothesis** proposes that there are glucoreceptors sensitive to blood glucose present in hypothalamic areas as well as in the periphery. When the tissues are utilizing glucose rapidly, thus establishing a high *arteriovenous glucose difference*, the glucoreceptors are stimulated, and through their central connection produces satiety. On the other hand, when glucose is not available for tissue utilization, and the arteriovenous glucose difference tends towards zero. This is sensed by the hypothalamic centers, which then facilitate the feeding reflexes.

*Hypoglycemia is an appetite stimulant*, and it decreases glucose utilization by reducing the amount of glucose reaching the cells. **Polyphagia** or *increased food intake occurs in diabetes mellitus despite hyperglycemia because cellular utilization of glucose by the satiety center is low* due to insulin deficiency. There may also be a direct stimulation of appetite by insulin. The **lipostatic hypothesis** holds that adipose tissue produces a humoral signal that is proportionate to the amount of fat and acts on the hypothalamus to decrease food intake and increase energy output. This hypothesis is now borne out by the discovery of leptin. The **thermostatic hypothesis** holds that a fall in body temperature below a given set point stimulates appetite and a rise above the set point inhibits appetite.

### Briefly describe the causes and clinical types of obesity.

Obesity is caused by excess energy input over energy output. For each 9.3 Calories of excess energy that enters the body, 1 gram of fat is stored. *Muscular activity* is by far the most important means by which energy is expended in the body. Hence, obesity results from a high ratio of food intake to daily exercise. The common clinical types of obesity are: (1) **Psychogenic obesity**. (i) The most common psychogenic factor contributing to obesity is the prevalent idea that healthy eating habits require three meals a day the children continue to practice it throughout life as forced into this habit by parents. (ii) During or after stressful situations people are known to gain large amounts of weight. Eating seems to be a means of release from tension. (2) **Neurogenic Abnormalities**. Lesions in the ventromedial nuclei of the hypothalamus cause an animal to eat excessively and become obese. **Frolich syndrome** is a condition in which persons have a tendency to become obese due to tumors of the hypophysis. (3) **Genetic obesity**. Obesity definitely runs in families. Genetic abnormalities in fat storage also cause obesity. Deficiency of *hormone sensitive lipase* leads to storage of fat. (4) **Childhood overnutrition**. In first few years of life, the rate of formation of new fat cells is rapid. The number of fat cells is three times more in obese children. Overnutrition of children in infancy can lead to lifetime obesity.

# 124

# Regulation of Body Temperature

## What is the normal body temperature and what are its normal variations?

In humans, the normal value for the oral temperature is traditionally considered to be *37 °C, but it can be as low as 36°C*. The extremities are generally cooler than the rest of the body. The temperature of the *scrotum is maintained at 32 °C*. Factors causing variations in body temperature are as follows: (1) **Diurnal variations**. The normal human core temperature undergoes a regular circadian fluctuation of 0.5-0.7 °C. In individuals who sleep at night and are awake during the day it is lowest at about 6 AM and highest in the evenings. (2) **Sex**. In women, there is a monthly cycle of temperature variation characterized by a rise in basal temperature at the time of ovulation. (3) **Age**. Temperature regulation is less precise in young children, and their body temperature is 0.5 °C higher than that of adults. The aged have subnormal temperature and are intolerant to extremes of ambient temperature. (4) **Metabolic rate**. Body temperature is lowest during sleep, is slightly higher in the awake but relaxed state, and rises with activity. During exercise, the rectal temperature normally rises as high as 40 °C. Body temperature also rises slightly during emotional excitement, probably owing to unconscious tensing of the muscles. (5) Some normal adults chronically have a temperature above the normal range (**constitutional hyperthermia**).

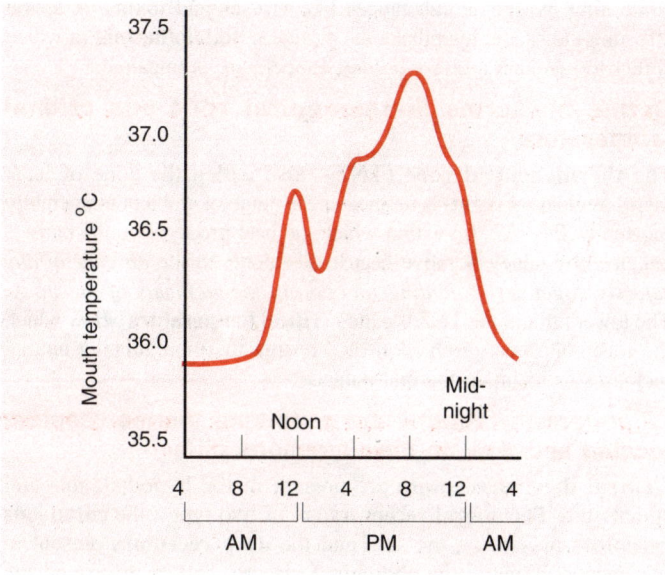

**Fig. 124.1**

## What is the difference between core and shell temperature? Where are they measured from?

Shell temperature is the **skin temperature** where as core temperature is the **visceral temperature**. The core temperature of

the body is easily measurable by the **rectal temperature**, which varies least with changes in environmental temperature. The **oral temperature** is normally 0.5 °C lower than the rectal temperature, but it is affected by many factors, including ingestion of hot or cold fluids, gum chewing, smoking, and mouth breathing. The core temperature is best represented by the **aortic blood temperature**. The intracranial temperature is also important considering that the central thermoreceptors located in the hypothalamus sense the intracranial temperature rather than the general core temperature. The **tympanic membrane temperature** best reflects the intracranial temperature.

## Enumerate the body mechanisms activated by heat and cold.

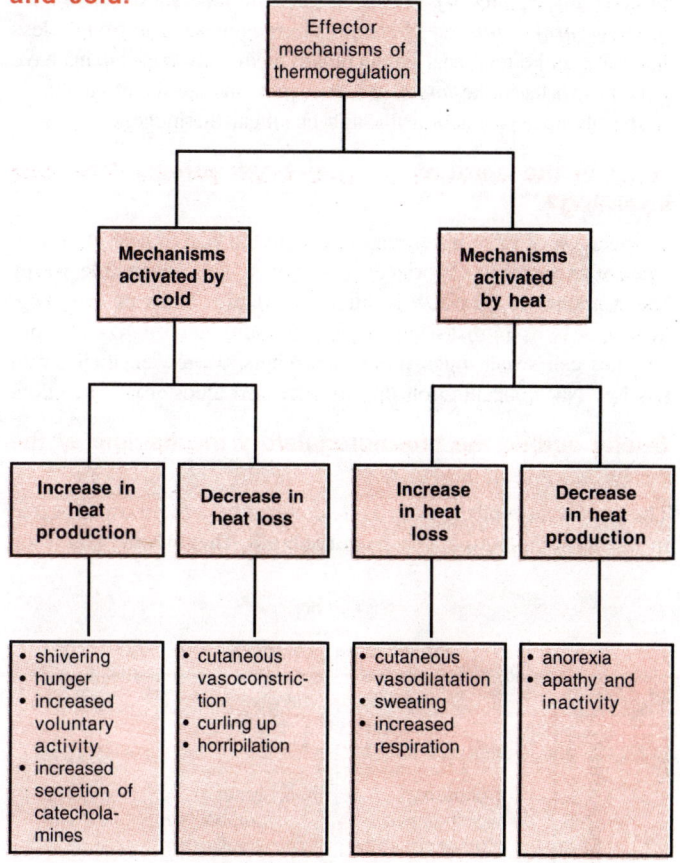

## What is the mechanism of shivering?

Shivering is a *cortical reflex* in which stimulation of cold-receptors in the skin reflexly increase the muscle tone of the body. The efferent arc of the reflex is mediated by the *lateral motor pathways*

– *tectospinal and rubrospinal*. When the muscle tone increases a certain threshold, it results in a muscle clonus, which is commonly known as shivering. Shivering, or even the increase of muscle tone denotes greater metabolic activity and greater heat generation. A **primary motor center for shivering** is located in the *posterior hypothalamus*. During maximum shivering, body heat production can rise to four to five times normal.

### What is chemical (nonshivering) thermogenesis and what is the role of brown fat in it?

Sympathetic stimulation and increased plasma levels of catecholamines cause an immediate increase in the rate of cellular metabolism. It results from *uncoupling of oxidative phosphorylation*, i.e., the oxidation of foodstuffs is associated with release of heat rather than generation of ATPs. This is known as **chemical thermogenesis**. Chemical thermogenesis is also promoted by *thyroxine*. Cold temperature stimulates hypothalamic release of TRH, which in turn stimulates the secretion of TSH and thyroxine. However, several weeks of cold-exposure are required before the thyroid gland secretes more thyroxine.

The amount of chemical thermogenesis is proportional to the amount of **brown fat** in the tissues. Brown fat contains large numbers of *special mitochondria where the uncoupled oxidation occurs*. Brown fat cells are supplied by strong sympathetic innervation. *Adults do not have brown fat* and chemical thermogenesis contributes less than 15% to the total heat production in them. However, infants have some brown fat in the *interscapular region*, and are therefore able to double its heat production through chemical thermogenesis.

### What is the amount of insensible perspiration and sweating?

Evaporation of 1g of water removes about 0.6 kcal of heat. A certain amount of water is vaporized at all times. This **insensible water loss** amounts to 50 mL/h in humans. At high rates of sweating, heat loss is as high as 900 kcal/h. Persons acclimatized to hot climates can sweat much more than others. Moreover, their sweat has low $Na^+$ concentration due to increased aldosterone secretion.

### Briefly outline the thermoregulatory mechanism of the body.

The temperature of the body is determined by a thermostat located in the hypothalamus. The **hypothalamic thermostat** has a set point, which is normally set at 37°C but can be reset. When the body temperature rises above or falls below the set point, the thermostat activates appropriate effector mechanisms for restoration of the body temperature.

The various effector mechanisms activated by the hypothalamus (*see flow chart* above) broadly fall in three categories: the **sympathetically mediated mechanisms** (vasoconstriction / vasodilatation, sweating, chemical thermogenesis), the **somatic mechanism** (shivering) and **behavioral mechanisms**. The threshold temperature is 37 °C for sweating and vasodilatation, 36.8°C for vasoconstriction. 36°C for chemical thermogenesis and 35.5 °C for shivering.

The hypothalamus has *two thermoregulatory mechanisms* built into it: one for raising the body temperature and another for cooling the body temperature. *Both the systems have their own cut-off temperatures* at which the heating or cooling mechanisms are activated or deactivated. The **anterior or rostral hypothalamus** contains catecholaminergic neurons and acts as heat-loss center (heat-dissipating or **anti-rise center**) and tends to prevent rise of body temperature. Stimulation of this region, specially the **preoptic area**, produces heat loss by cutaneous vasodilatation, sweating, panting and by lessening heat production. Information reaches the heat-loss center from the peripheral heat receptors by neural pathways, and through blood stream from warmer areas. Destruction of rostral hypothalamus produces heat production of hyperthermia (**neurogenic fever**).

The **posterior or caudal hypothalamus** (near the mamillary body) contains serotonergic neurons and is concerned with heat production (**anti-drop center**). Stimulation of this region activates heat production by cutaneous vasoconstriction, shivering and increasing the metabolic rate through the release of the thyroid-stimulating hormone (TSH). Afferent signals reach the heat-production region from the peripheral cold receptors, and by blood from cooler areas and blood containing pyrogenic substances like viruses and toxins. A lesion affecting the caudal hypothalamus produces **poikilothermia** in which ability to maintain a uniform body temperature is impaired.

### Define the terms thermoneutral zone and critical temperature.

The **thermoneutral zone (TNZ)** (also called the zone of least thermoregulatory effort) is defined as the range of ambient temperature (normally 25° - 27° C) within which the heat produced in the body is balanced by nonevaporative heat losses alone, in the *absence of any reflexly-engendered heating or cooling mechanisms of the body*. The lower limit of the TNZ is called **critical temperature** below which the metabolic heat production of a resting thermoregulating animal increases to maintain thermal balance.

### Where are the central and peripheral thermoreceptors located and how do their functions differ?

**Central thermoreceptors** are present in the hypothalamus and spinal cord. **Peripheral receptors** are of two types: the **cutaneous receptors** present on the skin and the **deep receptors** present in the deeper tissues – the abdominal viscera, and in or around the great veins in the upper abdomen and thorax.

The *central thermoreceptor* sense temperature of the blood flowing through them. The *cutaneous thermoreceptors* sense the ambient temperature: Most of them are cold-detecting receptors. The *deep receptors* share features of both the central and

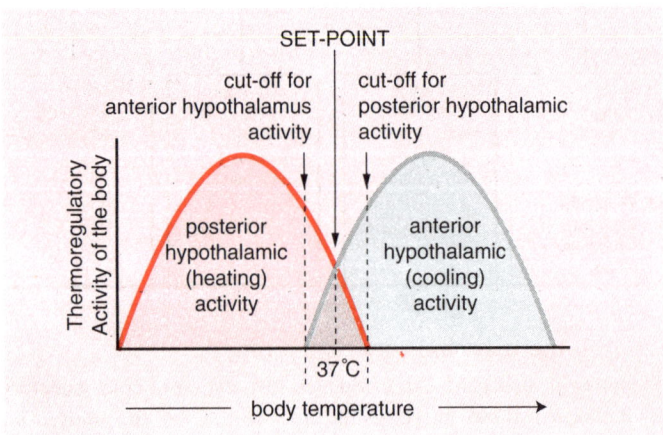

**Fig. 124.2**

cutaneous receptors: they are exposed to the body core temperature rather than the body surface temperature. Yet, like the skin temperature receptors, they mainly detect cold rather than warmth. Both cutaneous receptors and the deep body receptors are concerned with preventing hypothermia.

The central and peripheral thermoreceptors often provide *conflicting information* about body temperature. The posterior hypothalamus therefore calculates an **integrated temperature** from the informations obtained from both the central and peripheral thermoreceptors. Thus, if the hand is exposed to heat, the peripheral thermoreceptors evoke local vasodilatation through segmental spinal reflex. However, if the core temperature, as sensed by the central thermoreceptors, is less than 37°C, the hypothalamus inhibits the spinal vasodilatory reflex.

### Briefly outline the pathophysiology of fever.

An elevation of the body temperature above the normal range is called fever or **pyrexia**. Fever is presumably beneficial because many microorganisms grow best within a relatively narrow temperature range, and a rise in temperature inhibits their growth. In addition, antibody production increases when body temperature is elevated. Before the advent of antibiotics, *fevers were artificially induced* for the treatment of neurosyphilis and proved to be beneficial. Hyperthermia benefits individuals infected with anthrax, pneumococcal pneumonia, leprosy, and various fungal, rickettsial, and viral diseases. Hyperthermia also slows the growth of some tumors.

Very high temperatures are however harmful. Body temperatures above 41°C (**hyperpyrexia**) are accompanied by tachycardia, raised respiratory rate, weakness, headache, mental confusion, abnormal behavior and finally brain damage with loss of consciousness. A *persistent temperature of over 43°C is not compatible with life.*

Fever is produced if heat is generated in the body at greater rates than can be balanced by heat loss. This can happen in *hard exercise* and *hyperthyroidism*. However, fever most commonly occurs when the *hypothalamic setpoint is reset to a higher temperature*, resulting in the activation of heat-generating and heat-conserving mechanisms of the body till the body temperature equals the hypothalamic set point. The onset of fever is signaled by the 'chills' and its offset, by the 'crisis'. **Chills** are felt in fever when the heat generating and heat conserving mechanisms of the body are active. These mechanisms continue to be active until the body temperature remains below the elevated hypothalamic set point of fever. **Crisis** is characterized by sudden sweating. It occurs when the hypothalamic setpoint suddenly lowers to normal and the heat losing mechanisms are activated.

The hypothalamic set point is elevated by fever-producing substances called **pyrogens**. Pyrogens like *lipopolysaccharide endotoxins* derived from bacterial cell membrane are called **exogenous pyrogens**. Pyrogens that are formed in the body are called **endogenous (leucocytic) pyrogen**. They are actually **cytokines** (1L-IB, IL-6, β-IFN. γ-IFN, and TNF-α) that are released from monocytes and macrophages that phagocytose bacteria. These cytokines act on the organ vasculosum of lamina terminalis (OVLT) lying outside the blood-brain barrier. This in turn activates the *preoptic area of the hypothalamus.* Cytokines are also produced by cells in the CNS when these are stimulated by infection, and these may act directly on the thermoregulatory centers. Cytokines induce the synthesis and release of **prostaglandin E$_2$**, which in turn act on the hypothalamus to increase the setpoint. **Antipyretics** like aspirin prevent the formation of prostaglandin E$_2$ from arachidonic acid. Fever is also caused by *brain tumors* pressing on the hypothalamus and by surgery in its proximity.

In **malignant hyperthermia**, a defective ryanodine receptor leads to excess $Ca^{2+}$ release during muscle contraction triggered by stress. This in turn leads to contractures of the muscles, increased muscle metabolism, and a great increase in heat production in muscle leading to hyperthermia which is fatal if not treated.

### What is the difference between heat exhaustion and heatstroke?

**Heat exhaustion** occurs due to excessive sweating leading to circulatory failure. **Heat stroke** occurs at very high ambient temperatures that upset the normal heat balance of the body, leading to a rise in body temperature. The rise in body temperature impairs the thermoregulatory capability of the hypothalamus, leading to a further rise in body temperature. A vicious cycle is thus set off which culminates in loss of consciousness.

### What is hypothermia and what are its effects?

Thermo regulatory mechanisms fail if the body temperature falls below 32°C. Shivering is replaced by muscular rigidity, consciousness is impaired and reflexes are sluggish. Death usually occurs below about 25°C though some patients have survived core temperatures as low as 18°C.

### What is artificially induced hypothermia?

Hypothermia is sometimes induced artificially in surgery so that the O$_2$ needs of the tissues are greatly reduced and circulation can be stopped for relatively long periods. The induction of hypothermia during surgery is made easier with the use of anesthesia and muscle relaxants, both of which abolish shivering.

A temperature of 27 °C can be easily induced for surgical purposes. At this temperature, metabolism is reduced by 30 – 40%, the heart rate, blood pressure and respiratory rate decrease, and the patient passes into a state of *suspended animation* from which he can completely recover if he is allowed to warm up slowly. In such a state the circulation can be interrupted for 10 to 15 minutes so that surgical operations on the heart and large blood vessels become practicable. *At temperatures below 27° C ventricular fibrillation occurs* fairly often but normal rhythm can be restored on rewarming by injecting potassium citrate or by applying an electric shock to the ventricle.

### What is poikilothermia?

Poikilothermia occurs when thermoregulation is impaired. It occurs in hypothalamic lesions and in lesions interrupt descending hypothalamic fibers to the thoracolumbar sympathetic outflow of the spinal cord. Some local vasodilatation and sweating is still possible through spinal reflexes, but are too weak for effective control of body temperature. The *body temperature becomes labile, rising and falling easily.* Such patients have to depend largely on conscious behavioral thermoregulatory mechanisms. If he is covered with blankets and surrounded by hot-water bottles his body temperature quickly rises and may reach a dangerous level.

# 125

# Structure & Functions of the Eye

## What is aqueous humor? How does it form and circulate?

Aqueous humor is a clear optically transparent fluid, filling the anterior and posterior chambers of the eye. It provides nutrition and oxygen to the lens and the cornea, and also serves as a vehicle for elimination of metabolic waste products. It is formed by the **ciliary body**, mostly through active secretion of the **ciliary epithelium**.

## Describe the pathway for aqueous circulation in the eye.

The ciliary epithelium secretes aquous humor into the posterior chamber of the eye. The aqueous humor then flows from the posterior to the anterior chamber through the pupil. It then flows out into the **canal of Schlemm**, a venous channel at the limbus (junction between the iris and the cornea). As it drains out through the canal of Schlemm, it passes through the **trabecular mesh** (Fig. 125.1).

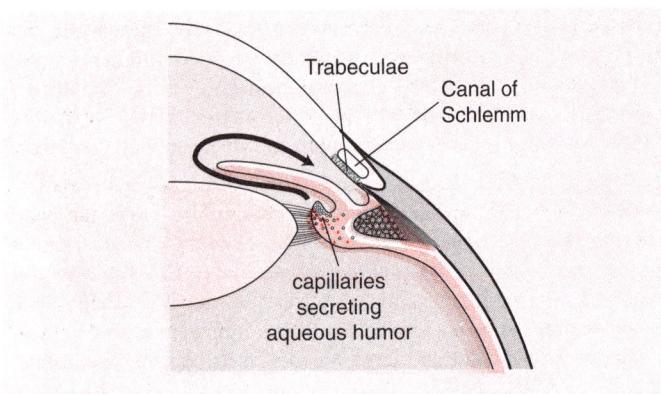

**Fig. 125.1**

## What is the normal intraocular pressure? What are the factors affecting it?

The average intraocular pressure (IOP) is between 10 – 21 mm Hg. The factors affecting IOP are: (i) **Age**. After 40 years, the mean IOP increases due to reduced aqueous outflow. (ii) **Heredity**. Individuals with family history of glaucoma tend to have a higher level of IOP. (iii) **Axial length of the globe**. Myopes tend to have higher intraocular pressure. (iv) **Diurnal variation**. Diurnal changes in IOP occur due to the cyclical variations in the serum levels of adrenocortical steroids. (v) **Postural changes**. IOP rises by 0.3 – 6 mm Hg when reclining from a sitting to supine position. (vi) **Exercise**. Physical exertion lowers IOP. (vii) **Irritation**. Corneal or conjunctival irritation alters

aqueous humor formation through axon reflex. (viii) **Hormones**. IOP pressure rises in response to administration of ACTH, glucocorticoids and GH and drops in response to progesterone, estradiol, chorionic gonadotropin and relaxin. (ix) **Drugs**. Trichlorethylene (an anesthetic drug) tends to lower IOP while depolarizing muscle relaxants like succinylcholine and suxamethonium cause a sudden increase in IOP. Oral ethyl alcohol, heroine, and marijuana lower IOP while tobacco smoking, caffeine and LSD elevate IOP.

## Define glaucoma. What are the two main types of glaucoma?

Glaucoma is an elevation of IOP with *characteristic degenerative changes in the optic nerve head*. There are two distinct types of glaucoma: the angle-closure glaucoma and open-angle glaucoma. The differentiation is based, as the names suggest, on the *magnitude of the sclerocorneal angle*, (Fig. 125.2) which can be assessed with an instrument called the **gonioscope**.

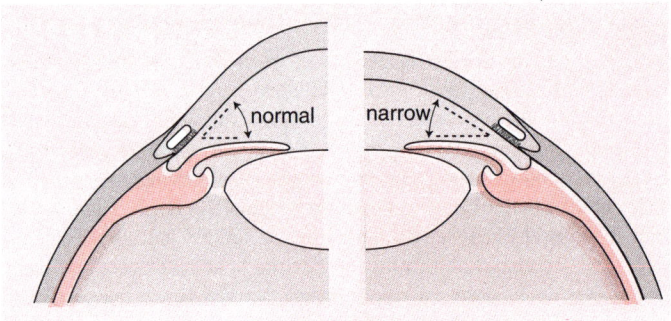

**Fig. 125.2**

## Explain the pathophysiology of angle closure glaucoma.

In angle closure glaucoma, the sclerocorneal angle (which is also called the angle of anterior chamber) is narrow and therefore easily occludable by the peripheral part of the iris as shown in Fig. 125.3. The occlusion, which may be slight initially, causes pooling of aqueous in the posterior chamber, further accentuating the occlusion. This is called the **appositional closure** of the angle and results in a sudden rise in intraocular pressure. Repeated attacks of appositional closure may be followed by an irreversible closure of the angle due to adhesions (**synechiae**). The rise in IOP in this type of glaucoma is sudden: it is extremely painful and associated with red congested eye and corneal edema, thus accounting for its previous name of **acute congestive glaucoma**.

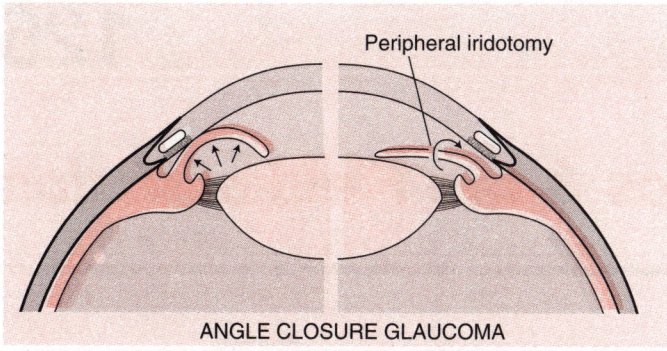

ANGLE CLOSURE GLAUCOMA

**Fig. 125.3**

## Explain the pathophysiology of open angle glaucoma.

In this type of glaucoma, the *anterior chamber angle is not reduced*. One of the commonly identifiable causes of the increased IOP is the *increased resistance of the trabeculae to aqueous outflow* (Fig. 125.4).

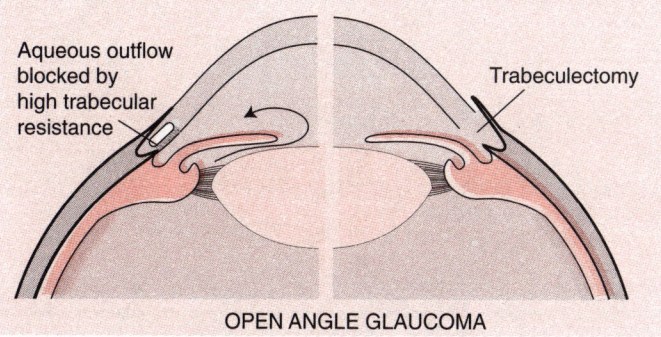

OPEN ANGLE GLAUCOMA

**Fig. 125.4**

Increased trabecular resistance is often due to deposition in the trabecular meshwork of pigments and mucopolysaccharides. What causes such deposition is not known; however, some predisposing factors include myopes above 50 years of age, patients with diabetes and thyroid disorders and patients with family history of glaucoma. Such cases are diagnosed as having **primary open angle glaucoma**. Cases where the cause can be discerned are diagnosed as **secondary open angle glaucoma**. This can be due to either an *increase in the episcleral venous pressure* or due to *deposition of pigment and exfoliative materials from the iris and lens capsule.*

## How is glaucoma treated?

Medical treatment is common to both types of glaucoma and comprises an immediate reduction in the intraocular pressure with the help of *hyperosmotic agents* like mannitol, glycerol, sorbitrate or urea which causes shrinkage of the vitreous, hence reducing the IOP, and *intravenous acetazolamide* which reduces aqueous formation. Subsequent reduction in pressure can be maintained with drugs that reduce aqueous formation like β-*adrenergic blockers* and *cholinergic agonist*. Recent drugs include $PGF_2\alpha$ agonist and $\alpha_2$ blockers.

Miotics (drugs causing constriction of the pupil) are useful in both types of glaucoma. In angle-closure glaucoma, pupillary constriction *flattens the iris and draws it away from the cornea*, thus increasing the outflow of aqueous. In open angle glaucoma, the ciliary muscle contraction induced by miotics *exerts traction on the scleral spur*, thus *opening out the sclerosed trabecular meshwork*, improving the outflow (Fig. 125.5).

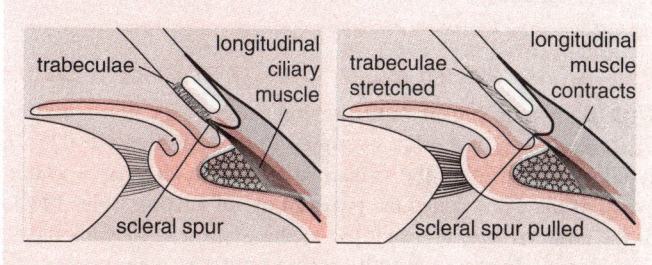

**Fig. 125.5**

Surgical treatment is different for the two types of glaucoma. Appositional closure is often relieved by **peripheral iridectomy**, i.e., punching a small hole in the iris. The hole allows aqueous flow from the posterior to the anterior chamber and thereby relieves the IOP (Fig. 125.4). Surgical treatment of open angle glaucoma involves **trabeculectomy**, i.e., the formation of a fistula between the anterior chamber and the subconjunctival space (Fig. 125.4).

# 126

# Visual Optics & the Field of Vision

## Where in the eye does the maximum refraction of light take place?

The passage of light through the eye involves refraction at multiple interfaces. Thus, there is bending of light when it passes from the air to cornea, cornea to aqueous humor and aqueous humor to vitreous. The degree of bending at an interface is proportional to the ratio of the refractive indices (μ) of the two media it separates. The *maximum bending of light occurs at the air-cornea interface* (for air, μ=1).

## What is the reduced eye of Listing? Describe it briefly.

With light bending at multiple interfaces, any mathematical treatment of visuooptics becomes very complicated. This is avoided by confining the mathematical approach to a simplified model of the eye – called the **reduced eye of Listing**. (Fig. 126.1). In the reduced eye, the multiple media – cornea, aqueous humor and vitreous humor – are all replaced with a single media of a refractive index of 1.336. The edge of this hypothetical medium (air-medium interphase) is located 1.4 cm behind the corneal surface. The edge is spherical, with its radius of curvature being 5.6 mm. The nodal point or optical center of the medium is therefore located 5.6 mm behind the air-medium interphase. Rays of light passing through the nodal point do not undergo any refraction.

## What is the diopteric power of the eye?

Although the refraction of light first takes at the air-medium interphase, for all practical purposes, the entire refraction is assumed to occur at the plane of the nodal point as shown in the Fig. 126.2. In an eye with normal dimensions and refractive power, all parallel rays come to focus on the retina. Thus, the focal length of the eye equals the distance between the nodal plane and the retina, which is equal to 17 mm. The relation between focal length and diopteric power is given by the formula:

$$\text{Power in diopters} = \frac{1}{\text{Focal length in meters}}$$

*Substituting:*

$$\text{Power in diopters} = \frac{1}{0.017}$$

$$= 59\,D$$

Although calculated on the basis of the schematic eye, the diopteric power of the real eye too is 59 D. This power represents the *combined refractory power* of the cornea, aqueous humor, lens and the vitreous humor. The *contribution of the lens in it is 16 D.*

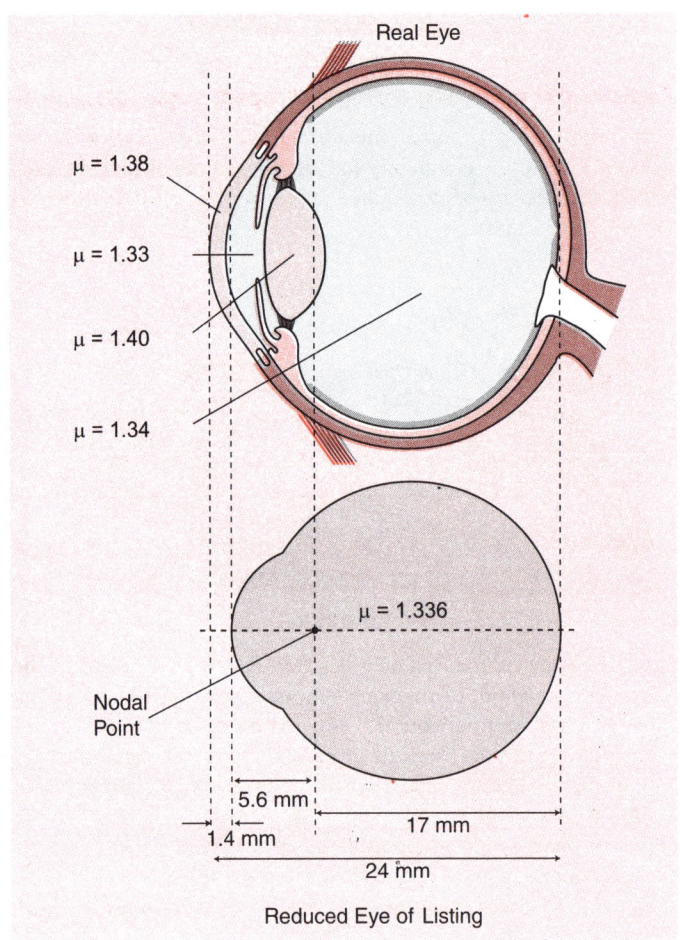

Real Eye

μ = 1.38

μ = 1.33

μ = 1.40

μ = 1.34

μ = 1.336

Nodal Point

5.6 mm

1.4 mm

17 mm

24 mm

Reduced Eye of Listing

**Fig. 126.1**

## What is accommodation?

The normal optics of the eye is designed for focusing on the retina parallel rays from infinity. Hence, anything nearer than infinity should produce a blurred retinal image. That however does not happen because the *lens of the eye increases its refractive power* and brings to focus on the retina divergent rays originating from near objects. This increase in the diopteric power of the eye is called **accommodation** and is brought about by the contraction of the *ciliary muscles*.

Accommodation is the *ability of the eye to focus on objects at varying distances*. This is made possible by changes in the curvature of the *anterior surface of the lens*. The radius of curvature of the anterior surface of the lens is 12 mm when the eye is adapted for distant vision (resting position) and 6 mm when the eye is accommodating maximally for near vision. The posterior surface of the lens hardly alters its radius of curvature, remaining nearly unchanged at 6 mm.

### What is range of accommodation?

The diopteric power of the eye can increase by up to 10 diopters increase (from 59 D to 69 D) when looking at near objects. This increase in power, which is the maximum possible increase in power of the eye, is called the **range of accommodation**. In an emmetropic eye, the range of accommodation can be calculated by the formula:

$$\text{Range of accommodation} = \frac{1}{\text{Distance of near point (in meter)}}$$

### Define far point and near point.

**Far point** is the most distant point that can be clearly focused on the retina. The **far point** of an emmetropic eye is infinity ($\alpha$). **Near point** is the point nearest to the eye that can be clearly focused on the retina by using maximum accommodation. In a normal eye, it is about 10cm.

### What is an emmetropic eye?

An eye whose *far and near points are normal* is called an emmetropic eye. In an emmetropic eye, parallel rays coming from infinity get focussed on the retina.

### Name the common refractory errors and explain their cause.

There are three common errors of refraction (Fig. 126.2). In **myopia** or shortsightedness, parallel rays incident on a myopic eye come to focus in front of the retina, resulting in a blurred retinal image. Use of accommodation increases the blurring further. Only divergent rays originating from a close distance come to focus on the retina. Myopia occurs either because the diopteric power of the eye is greater than normal or *more commonly, because the anteroposterior diameter of the eye is greater*. In **hypermetropia**, parallel rays incident on a hypermetropic eye come to focus behind the retina. This occurs either because the diopteric power of the eye is lesser than normal or *more commonly, because the anteroposterior diameter of the eye is smaller*. The problem can be overcome by employing accommodation and increasing the diopteric power of the eye. However, continuous use of accommodation for overcoming hypermetropia can, in the long run, result in a particular type of cortical blindness called *amblyopia ex anopsia*. **Presbyopia** is an inadequacy of the accommodative power of the eye that occurs with aging, usually after the age of 40 years. **Astigmatism** occurs when the eye shows two different powers in two different axes.

### How do the refractory errors affect the far and near points?

| | Far point | Near point |
|---|---|---|
| Emmetropia | $= \alpha$ | = 10 cm |
| Myopia | $< \alpha$ | < 10 cm |
| Hypermetropia | $> \alpha$ (behind the eye) | > 10 cm |
| Presbyopia | $= \alpha$ | > 10 cm |

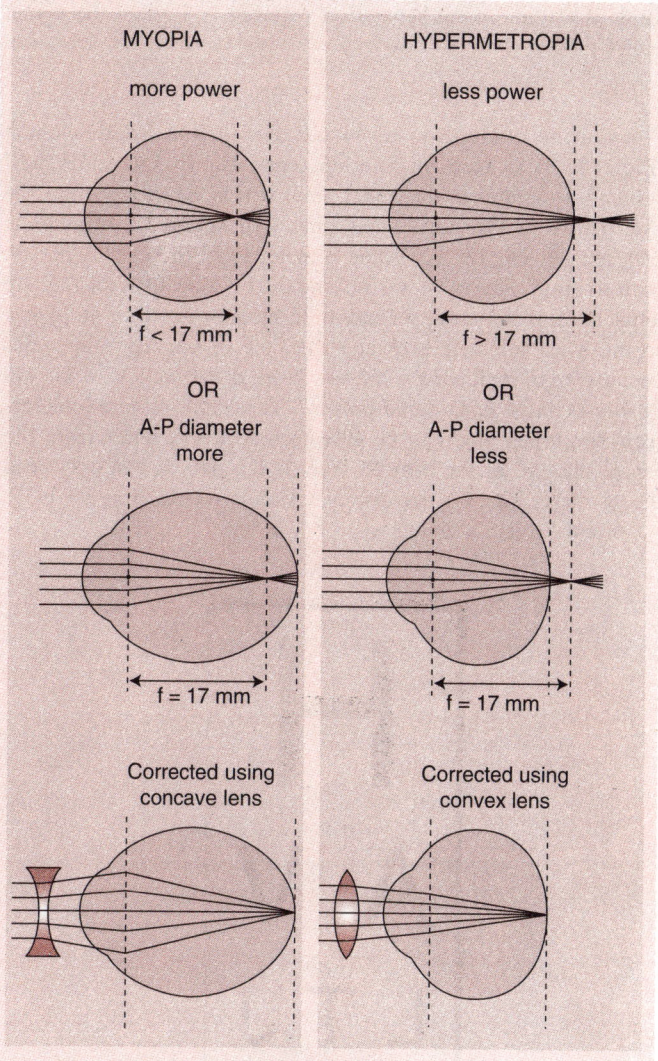

**Fig. 126.2**

### How are the refractory errors corrected?

Myopia is corrected by wearing **concave lenses**. Hypermetropia is corrected by wearing **convex lenses**. Presbyopia is corrected by wearing convex lenses for near vision only. Astigmatism is corrected with lenses that have two different powers in two different planes i.e., **cylindrical lenses**.

### Define visual acuity.

When two point-objects are brought very close together, they are no longer seen as separate. To be seen as discrete points, they must be so separated that between them, they subtend an angle of at least 1 minute (1') at the eye. The angle subtended at the eye by two point objects is called the **visual angle**. It can be calculated that a 1' visual angle corresponds to a 4.5 μm separation of the images on the retina. Since an average cone is about 3 μm wide, at least one unstimulated cone must be interposed between two stimulated cones if the images falling on them are to be perceived as discrete.

If the vision is impaired, a greater separation is required. The *reciprocal of the minimum visual angle required for two point objects to be recognized as discrete* is called the **visual acuity**.

Thus, if the minimum separation required is 2', then the visual acuity is ½.

### Describe the method for determining visual acuity.

For routine evaluation of visual acuity, the Snellen chart (Fig. 126.3) is used. In Snellen types, the largest letter will subtend 5 minutes at the nodal point if it is 60 meters from the eye. Those in the subsequent lines will subtend 5 minutes if they are 36, 24, 18, 12, 9 and 6 meter from the eye. A person with average acuity of vision should be able to read the top letter at 60 meters, the second at 36 meters, the third at 24 and so on. The patient is kept at a distance of 6m from the types because *rays incident on the eye from a distance of 6 meters or more can be considered parallel.* A normal subject 6 meters from the types ought to be able to read every letter from the top to the end of the 6-meter line. If the patient can only read the 18 meter line, his/her distant vision is recorded as V= 6/18. A normal subject's vision will be V = 6/6.

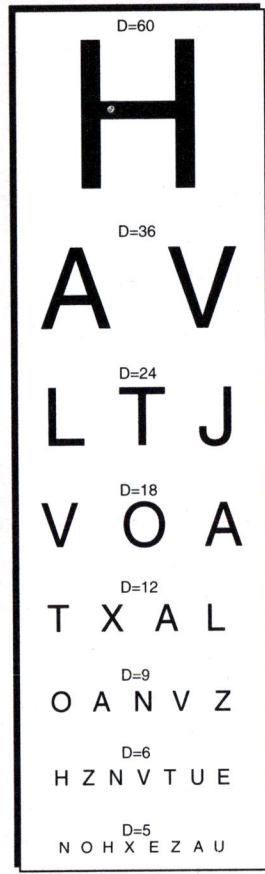

**Fig. 126.3**

### Define visual field and describe a normal visual field.

The eye can see clearly only an extremely small area at a time. This point-sized area – which the eye focuses and looks directly at – is called the **fixation point**. The total area of the external world that is visible to the eye that is fixated straight ahead is called the **field of vision** (Fig. 126.4). The measure of the visual field is given by the angle it subtends with the visual axis at the center of the cornea.

Using an instrument called the **perimeter**, the entire field of vision can be charted out, and the technique is called **perimetry**. The visual field is divided into the nasal and temporal halves by a vertical line passing through the fixation point in the visual field. The field is further charted out by meridians and isopters as shown in the Fig. 126.4 The normal field of vision is *50° superiorly* (restricted by eyebrow), *60° nasally* (restricted by nose), *70° inferiorly* (restricted by zygoma) and *90° temporally* (unrestricted).

### What is the location of the blind spot in the visual field?

The part of the field that gets focused on the optic disc remains invisible to the eye. It is called the **blind spot**. Normally, the blind spot is located between the 12° and 18° isopters, a little below the 180° meridian (i.e., on the temporal side). There are no photoreceptors in the blind spot.

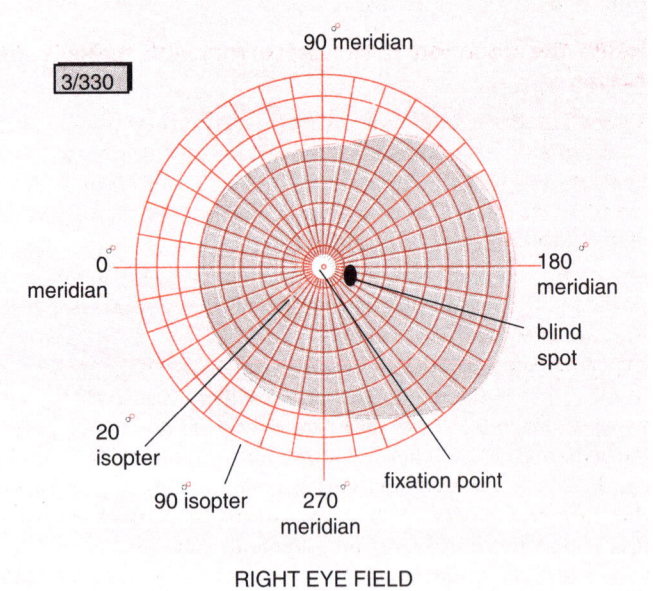

RIGHT EYE FIELD

**Fig. 126.4**

# 127

# The Retina & Phototransduction

## Enumerate the retinal layers and the cells present in them.

The retina consists of 10 layers. Outside in, they are as follows: (i) **Pigment layer**, which lies adjacent to the choroid and sometimes, is considered being a part of it. (ii) **Layer of rods and cones**, which consists of the outer segments of the photoreceptor cells. (iii) **Outer limiting membrane**, which is not a real membrane but the row of zona adherentes between the photoreceptors and the neuroglial **Müller's cells**. (iv) **Outer nuclear layer**, which is the row of nuclei of the **photoreceptors cells**. (v) **Outer plexiform layer**, which is the layer of synapses between photoreceptors, bipolar cells and the **horizontal cells**. (vi) **Inner nuclear layer**, which is the layer of nuclei of **bipolar cells**; (vii) **Inner plexiform layer**, which is the layer of synapses between bipolar cells, ganglion cells and the **amacrine cells**. (viii) **Ganglion cell layer**, which contains **ganglion cells**. (ix) **Optic nerve layer**, which contains the axons of the ganglion cells; (x) **Inner limiting membrane**, **which** lies next to the vitreous.

## Compare and contrast rods and cones.

### SIMILARITIES

Each photoreceptor (rod or cone) has an outer segment, an inner segment and an innermost segment.

The **outer segment** contains stacks of *disks* and $Na^+$ *channels* on the outer membrane.

The double-membrane discs are formed by invagination of the cell membrane.

The disk membrane contains photopigment molecules stitched into it.

The outer segments grow in length and their tips are shed and phagocytosed by the pigment epithelial cells.

The **inner segment** contains the *nucleus, mitochondria* and $Na^+$-$K^+$ *pumps*. The outer and inner segments are connected by an eccentrically placed modified cilium.

The **innermost segment** is the synaptic zone. In darkness, it releases transmitters continuously.

### DIFFERENCES

| Rods | Cones |
|---|---|
| The outer segment of a rod is a slender cylindrical structure. | The outer segment of the cone is a long conical structure. |
| In rods, the invaginated cell membrane gets separated from the cell surface. | In cones, the invaginated cell membrane retains continuity with the cell surface. |

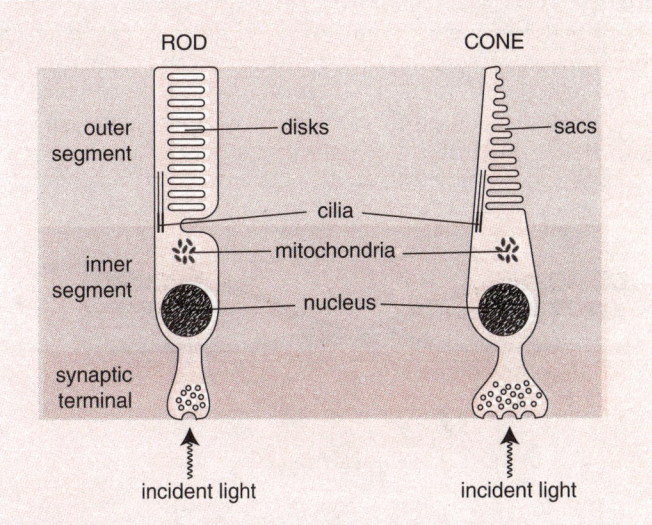

**Fig. 127.1**

| | |
|---|---|
| The photopigment is **rhodopsin**, which mediates **scotopic vision** (vision in dim light). Can detect even a single photon of light. | The photopigment is **photopsin**, which mediates **photopic vision** (vision in bright light) and **color vision**. |
| Membrane proteins synthesized in the inner segments are assembled into new disks at the inner end of the outer segment. The newly formed discs slowly move toward the tip of the rod as additional discs are formed behind them. | Membrane proteins synthesized in the inner segment are inserted into the disc membranes throughout the outer segment. Discs do not move toward the pigment epithelium continuously as in rods. |
| The nucleus of the rod is smaller and its chromatin is more condensed. | The nucleus is larger and relatively pale staining. |
| The synaptic terminal is narrower than that of cones. | The synaptic terminal is expanded into a triangular **cone-pedicle**. |

## The axons of which nerve cells constitute the optic nerve?

The photoreceptor synapses with the bipolar cell, which in its turn synapses with the ganglion cell. The *axons of the ganglion cells form the optic nerve*, which leaves the eye to reach the lateral geniculate body.

## What is the fovea centralis? What are the causes of the high visual acuity at the fovea?

About 2.5 mm lateral to the border of the optic disk, the inner surface of the retina shows a shallow round depression, the **fovea**, which contains *a dense and orderly aggregation of cones* (Fig. 127.2). The fovea and its immediate vicinity contain yellow pigment and are called the **macula lutea**. Vision at the fovea is unusually clear (high visual acuity) for several reasons. (i) There is a *high concentration* of foveal photoreceptors. The foveal photoreceptors are *all cones*; there are no rods in the fovea. (ii) The *inner retinal layers are thinned out at the fovea* exposing the cones better to light. In other areas of the retina, light has to pass through all the layers before it can strike the photoreceptors. (iii) The fovea contains only fine arteries, veins, and capillaries. The larger blood vessels pass above and below the central fovea. *In the very center of the fovea, even the capillaries are absent*, greatly increasing its transparency. (iv) There is *no convergence* of the efferents of the foveal cones. Each foveal cone relays to a single ganglion cell. Hence, there is a disproportionately *large representation of the fovea in the visual cortex.*

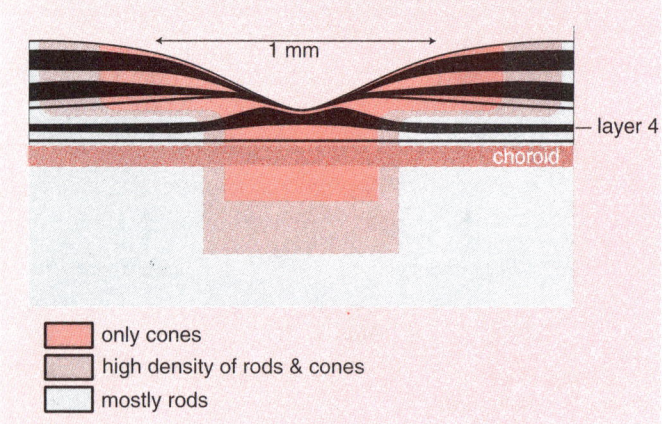

only cones
high density of rods & cones
mostly rods

**Fig. 127.2**

## What are the functions of the pigment epithelium of the retina?

The functions of the pigment epithelium are as follows. (i) The tight junctions between adjoining pigment epithelial cells *protect the retina from toxic metabolites* that may be present in the stroma of the choroid. (ii) The pigment granules *absorb light* after it has traversed the photoreceptor layer, thus preventing its reflection from the external ocular tunics. (iii) The pigment epithelium is involved in the continuous renewal of the underlying photoreceptors. Membranous discs are continuously exfoliated from the tips of the outer segment of the rods, which are surrounded by processes of the pigment epithelium. These *discs are phagocytosed by the pigment epithelium.* (iv) The pigment epithelium participates in the visual cycle by *reducing all-trans-retinal to all-trans-retinol*, i.e., vitamin A, followed by isomerization of the vitamin and regeneration of 11-*cis*-retinal. During the visual cycle, the vitamin-A derivatives move to the pigment epithelium in the course of light adaptation and return to the photoreceptors during dark adaptation. In the pigment epithelial cells, vitamin A is stored in the membranes of the smooth endoplasmic reticulum.

## Enumerate the steps of phototransduction.

The photoreceptor cell has a membrane potential of –40 mV. It is

attributable largely to a greater outward diffusion of $K^+$ than the inner diffusion of $Na^+$. The $K^+$ channels are located in the inner segment of the photoreceptors while the $Na^+$ channels are located in the outer segments. The $Na^+$ - $K^+$ pump is located in the inner segment (Fig. 127.3).

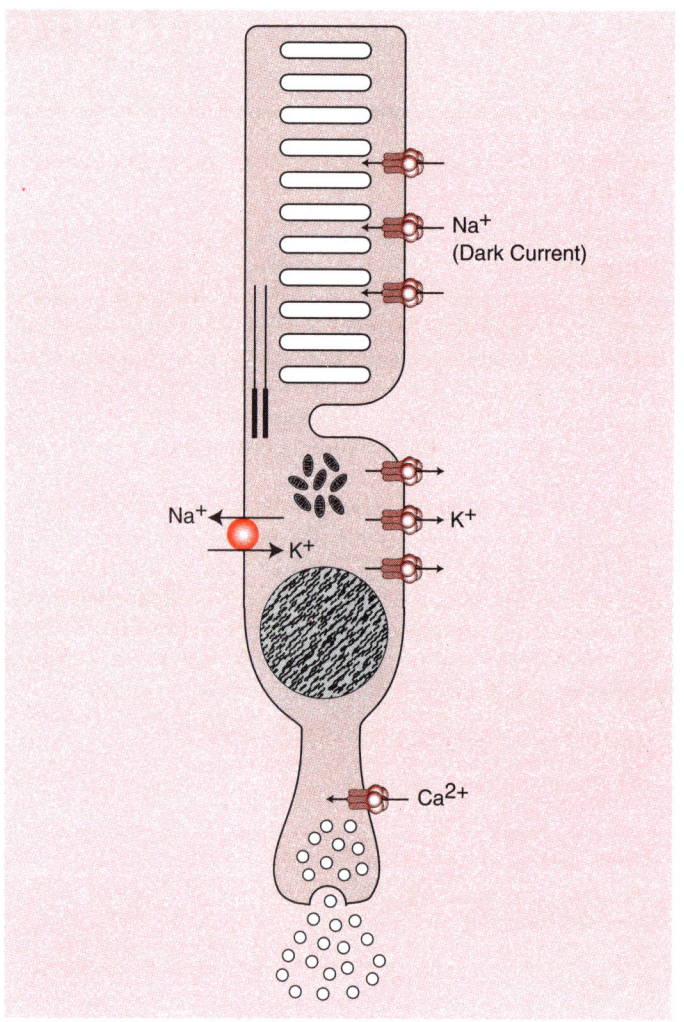

$Na^+$ (Dark Current)

$Na^+$

$K^+$

$K^+$

$Ca^{2+}$

**Fig. 127.3**

The $Na^+$ channels are open when no light falls on the photoreceptor. Hence in darkness, $Na^+$ continuously flows into the outer segment of the photoreceptor. This is called the **dark current**. Due to the dark current, the photoreceptor remains depolarized in dark and *a steady stream of neurotransmitter is released* from its terminal. The neurotransmitter release is mediated by $Ca^{2+}$ influx into the synaptic terminal through voltage-gated $Ca^{2+}$ channels. The neurotransmitter is **glutamate**.

When light falls on the retina, the light energy is trapped in the photosensitive pigments present in the photoreceptors and through *a series of steps* – called the **visual cycle** – results in the closure of the $Na^+$ channels with consequent reduction in the dark current. Reduction in $Na^+$ current hyperpolarizes the photoreceptor to –70mV and reduces its neurotransmitter output. Phototransduction is thus *a unique example of sensory transduction* that is associated with hyperpolarization and a reduction in the signal output from the sensory receptor.

## Describe the visual cycle.

The disks contain photosensitive pigments (rhodopsin and iodopsin) stitched into the membranes of the disks. Both these pigments are composed of *a protein moiety called opsin* (**scotopsin** in rods, **photopsin** in cones), and *11 cis-retinal* (retinal is also called retinene), an aldehyde of Vitamin A.

When light falls on the receptors, the *11 cis-retinal in the photopigment gets converted into all-trans-retinal,* forming **prelumirhodopsin**. This *cis-trans transformation* triggers a chain reaction (proceeding through *lumirhodopsin, meta-rhodopsin-I, meta-rhodopsin-II*) that culminates in the *separation of retinal from metarhodopsin-II*, leaving behind opsin.

*Metarhodopsin II closes the Na⁺ channels* in the outer segments, thereby hyperpolarizing the membrane and *reducing the neurotransmitter output* from the synaptic zone of the receptor. The action of metarhodopsin II is mediated by a G-protein called **transducin**. When transducin is activated by the formation of metarhodopsin-II, the GDP on transducin gets replaced by GTP and the α subunit separates. The α-subunit activates the enzyme phosphodiesterase which converts cGMP to 5'-GMP. The Na⁺

channels are kept open in darkness by the action of cGMP. In the presence of light, the lowering of cGMP due to its conversion to 5'GMP results in the closure of Na⁺ channels.

The *11 cis-retinal gets regenerated* from *all*-trans retinal by the enzyme *retinal isomerase*. Some of the 11-all-trans retinal gets converted into all-trans retinol (vitamin A) by alcohol dehydrogenase in the presence of NADH. The all-trans retinol thus produced, as well as that obtained as vitamin A from the diet is converted to 11 *cis* retinal required for refurbishing the rhodopsin stock of the retina (Fig. 127.4).

## What is the effect of vitamin A deficiency on vision?

Since vitamin A is important for replenishing the retinal stores in photoreceptors, a dietary deficiency of vitamin A produces visual abnormalities. The earliest to appear is **night blindness (nyctalopia)** due to impaired functions of rods. Impairment of cone function occurs later. Chronic avitaminosis A is associated with structural abnormalities in rods and cones followed by degeneration of other layers of the retina. Treatment with vitamin A restores retinal function if administered before the receptors are destroyed.

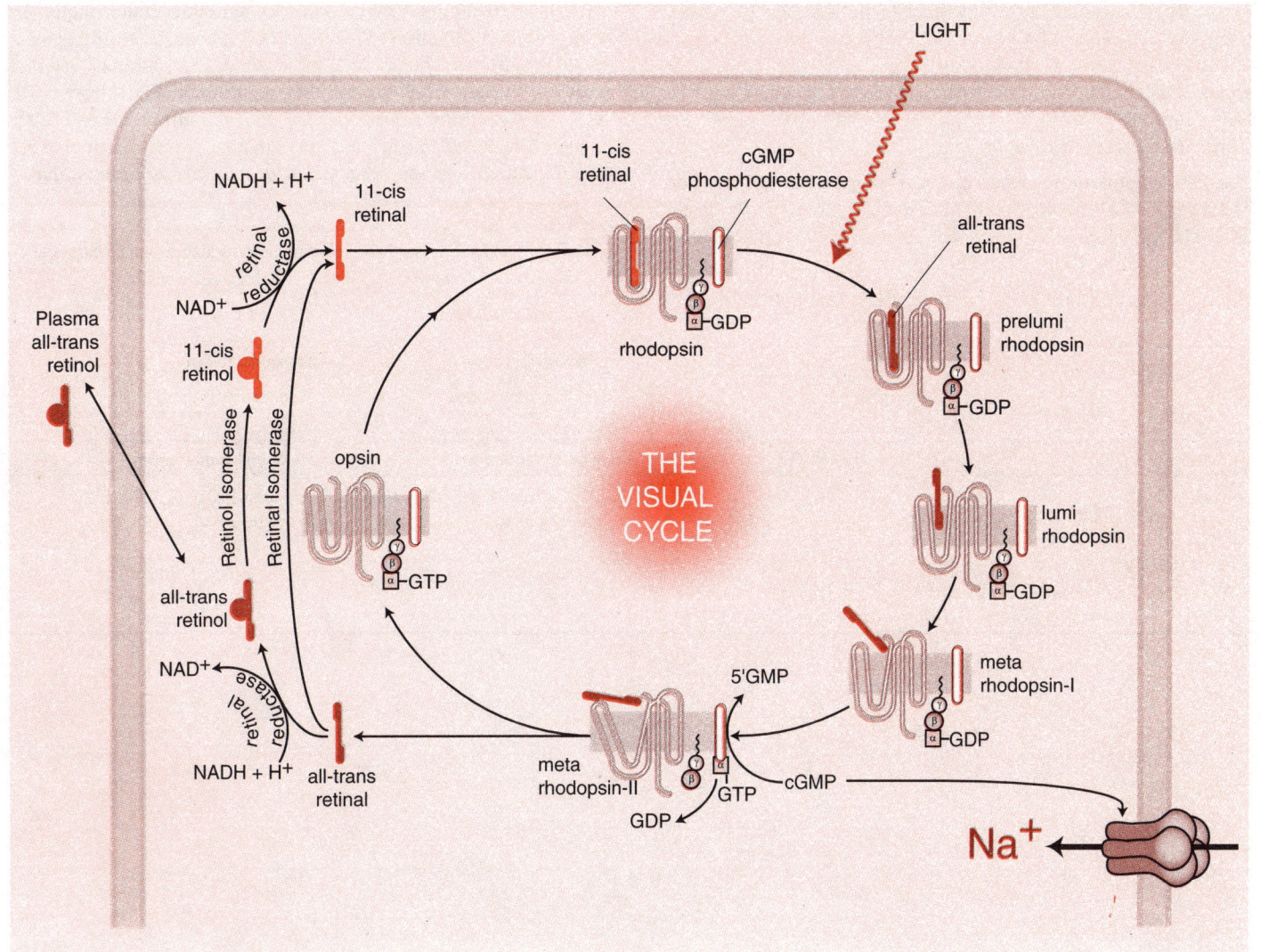

**Fig. 127.4**

## What is the difference between scotopic and photopic vision?

The human eye responds to a remarkable range of luminance. A white surface lit by moonless night sky has a luminance of $10^{-6}$ milliamberts whereas in bright sunlight, the same surface has a luminance of $10^4$ milliamberts. Neither rods nor cones have the ability to provide effective vision over such a wide range of luminance. Rods function effectively in the range of *$10^{-7}$ to $10^{-3}$ milliamberts*. Vision in this range of luminance is called **scotopic vision**. The spectral sensitivity of scotopic vision is maximum at *500 nm (i.e., the blue-green wavelength)*. Cones function effectively in the range of 1 to $10^8$ milliamberts. Vision in this range of luminance is called **photopic vision**. Prolonged exposure to higher luminance damages the retina. Comfortable reading requires 10 milliamberts. The spectral sensitivity of photopic vision is maximum at *560 nm (i.e., the green-yellow wavelength)*.

## What is the mechanism of dark adaptation? What are the two phases of dark adaptation?

If a person spends a considerable length of time in brightly lighted surroundings and then moves to a dimly lighted environment, the retina slowly become more sensitive to light as the individual becomes accustomed to the dark. This increase in visual sensitivity is known as **dark adaptation**. It becomes maximal in about 20 minutes. The time required for dark adaptation is the time required to build up the photopigment stores, which are constantly depleted in bright light.

The dark adaptation response has two components (Fig. 127.5). The *initial rapid but small rise* in visual sensitivity is due to the *dark adaptation of cones*. A *late but large rise* in visual sensitivity occurs due to the *dark adaptation of rods*. It occurs only in the

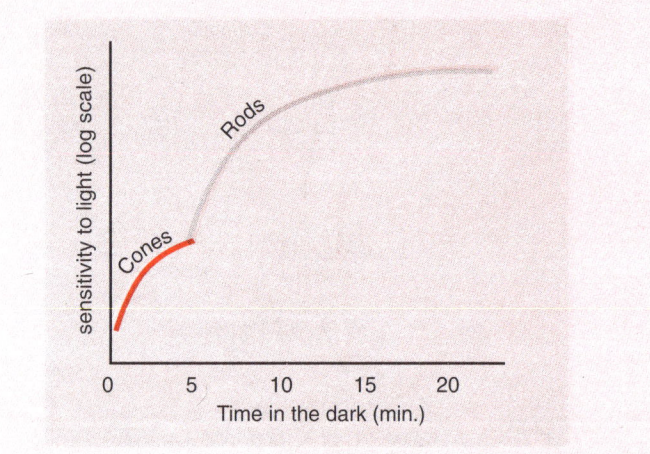

**Fig. 127.5**

peripheral portions of the retina and not in the fovea, which contains only cones.

## Why do aircraft pilots wear red goggles when on ground in bright light?

Aircraft pilots taking off into the night sky cannot afford to wait for 20 minutes after take-off for dark adaptation to occur. Hence they wear red goggles when on ground in bright light. Red light ($\lambda=650$ nm) is a poor stimulator of rods which have peak spectral sensitivity at $\lambda=500$ nm. However, red light causes reasonably good stimulation of S-cones, which have peak spectral sensitivity at $\lambda=560$ nm. Therefore, pilots wearing red glasses can see in bright light and yet their rods remain dark-adapted.

## What is light adaptation?

When one passes suddenly from a dim to a brightly lighted environment, the light seems intense until the eyes adapt to the increased illumination. This adaptation occurs over a period of about 5 minutes and is called **light adaptation**.

The mechanism of light adaptation is as follows. When light falls on a photoreceptor, there is closure of $Na^+$ channels leading to its hyperpolarization and reduction of its reurotransmitter output. In cones, light also causes *closure of $Ca^{2+}$ channels*, resulting in a reduction in intracellular $Ca^{2+}$. Intracellular $Ca^{2+}$ normally inhibits guanylyl cyclase - the enzyme that synthesizes cGMP from GTP. *A low intracellular $Ca^{2+}$ therefore elevates intracellular cGMP levels*. The cGMP keeps the $Na^+$ channels open leading to its depolarization and the *resumption of neurotransmitter output*.

**SIMILARITIES**

Both have indentical mechanisms of phototransduction and visual cycle.

**DIFFERENCES**

| Photopic vision | Scotopic vision |
|---|---|
| Mediated by cones | Mediated by rods |
| Effective luminance range is 1 to $10^{-3}$ milliamberts | Effective luminance range is $10^{-7} - 10^{-3}$ milliamberts |
| Peak sensitivity is at 560 nm (green yellow) | Peak sensitivity is 502 nm (blue-green) |

# 128

# Visual Pathway & Image Processing Cells

### Name the four neural pathways originating from the retina.

The fibers from the nasal halves of the retina cross over at the optic chiasma while those from the temporal halves continue ipsilaterally. Thereafter, they reach *four different destinations*. *(i)* 90% of them reach the striate cortex via the lateral geniculate body, forming the **retinogeniculostriate pathway**. (ii) The second strongest retinal projection is to the *superior colliculus of midbrain*. From there, fibers project to the *pulvinar of thalamus*, which in turn projects to the *extrastriate cortex*. When the geniculocalcarine pathway is damaged, this **colliculo-pulvino-extrastriate pathway** is responsible for the persistence of some very limited stimulus detection and eye movement toward objects in the visual field. This residual vision is called **blindsight**. (iii) A third **retinotectal pathway** is a much weaker retinal projection that terminates in the pretectum and accessory optic nuclei. It controls **visuomotor mechanisms**. (iv) Finally, a very small number of axons terminate immediately above the optic chiasma in the suprachiasmatic nucleus of the hypothalamus. These form a part of the **retinohypothalamic** pathway that mediates **circadian rhythms**.

### Describe the retinal pathway reaching the visual cortex.

The axons of retinal ganglion cells (which are equivalent to the 2nd order sensory neurons) relay in the **lateral geniculate nucleus (LGN)**, which is a part of the thalamus. Fibers from the LGN fan out as the optic radiation to terminate in the **primary visual cortex**, which is also known as area 17, striate cortex or visual area 1(V1). Fibers from the nasal half of the retina decussate in the **optic chiasma** before relaying in the contralateral LGN. Fibers from the temporal half of the retina do not decussate but relay in the ipsilateral LGN. Fibers from the LGN terminate in the ipsilateral primary visual cortex. Fibers from the inferior half of the retina take a detour of the temporal lobe as the **Meyer's fibers** before terminating in the cortex.

### Describe the effect of lesions in the visual pathway.

All lesions of geniculostriate pathway other than those in the optic nerve tend to cause hemianopia – i.e., blindness in only one half of the visual field. The term **homonymous** is used when the hemianopia affects only the left or right halves of the visual field, while the term **heteronymous** is used when the hemianopia affects only the temporal halves (**bitemporal**) or nasal halves (**binasal**) of vision. *Lesions of the striate cortex are rarely large enough to abolish macular (foveal) vision completely*. Hence, hemianopia with **macular sparing** is characteristically seen in lesions of the striate cortex. The effect of lesions at different sites is shown in Fig. 128.1.

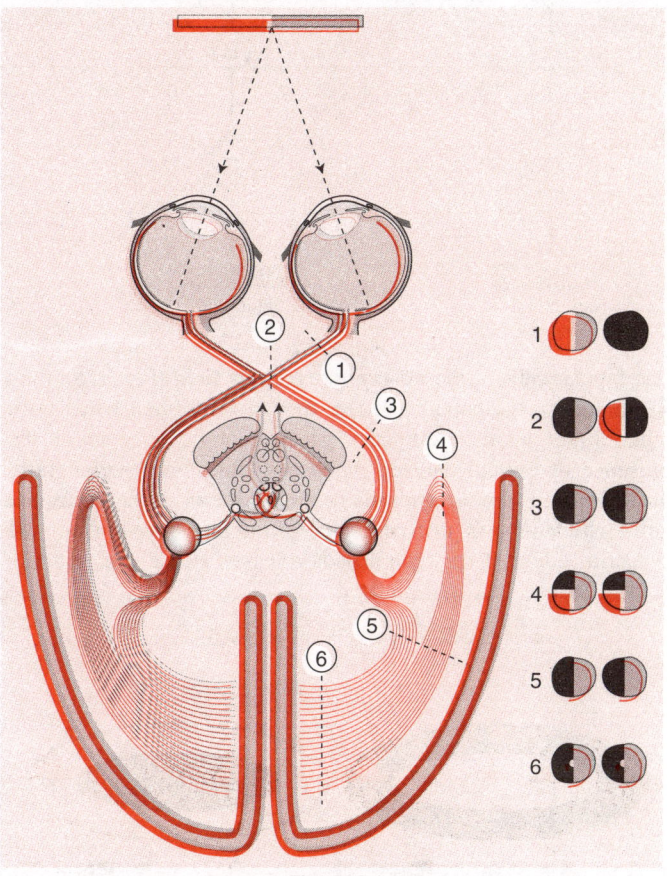

**Fig. 128.1**

### What do you understand by the terms on-center and off-center responses?

The bipolar, ganglion and LGN cells have **concentric-antagonistic receptor fields**. Depending on the characteristics of their receptor fields, the ganglion cells are called on-center or off-center cells. An **on-center cell** is stimulated by a light stimulus at the center of its receptor field and inhibited by light in the periphery of the field. Conversely, an **off-center cell** is stimulated by light in the periphery of the field and inhibited by light in its center.

The bipolar cells of the **on-center receptor field** (Fig. 128.2) are inhibited by glutamate. Hence, they are disinhibited (stimulated) when the glutamate output of photoreceptors decreases, as occurs in the presence of light. However, when light falls on a peripherally located photoreceptor, it results in the disinhibition (stimulation) of the horizontal cell, which in turn increases the glutamate output from the synaptic ending of the central photoreceptor. Hence, the centrally located bipolar cell is inhibited.

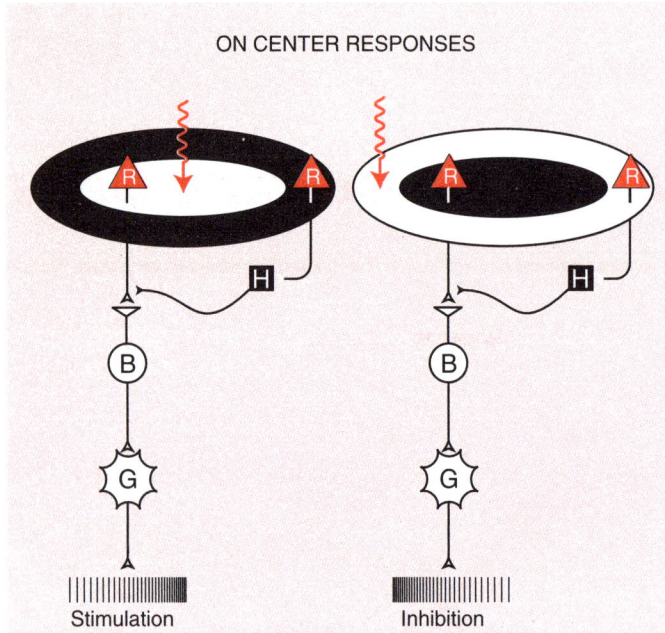

**Fig. 128.2**

The bipolar cells of the **off-center receptor field** (Fig. 128.3) are stimulated by glutamate. Hence, they are inhibited when light reduces the glutamate output of photoreceptors, as occurs in the presence of light. However, when light falls on a peripherally located photoreceptor, it results in the inhibition of the horizontal cell, which in turn decreases the glutamate output from the synaptic ending of the central photoreceptor. Hence, the centrally located bipolar cell is stimulated.

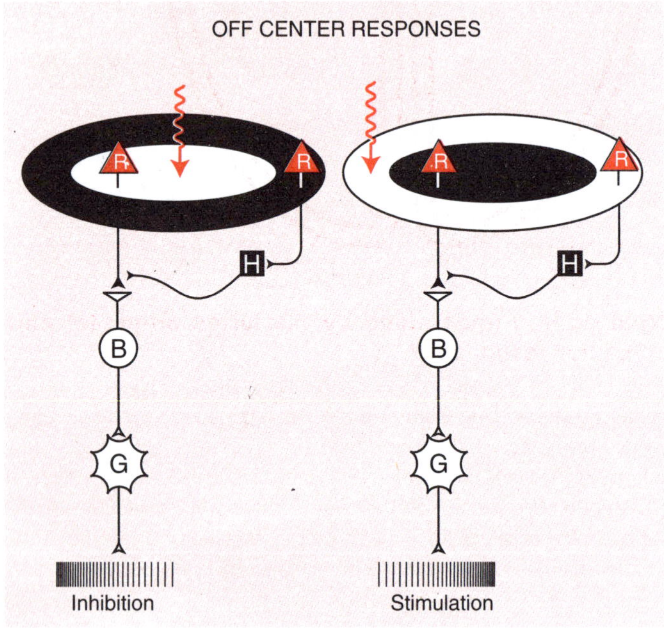

**OFF CENTER RESPONSES**

**Fig. 128.3**

### What are ocular dominance columns?

**Ocular dominance** columns (Fig. 128.4) are important for **stereopsis** (binocular vision). Cells of these columns receive input from corresponding points of both retinas. However, the inputs from two eyes, in most cases, are not equal, and the stimulus from *one of the eyes usually dominates. Cells that are located directly*

*above or below one another are dominated by the same eye* forming **ocular dominance columns**. Adjacent columns show differences in ocular dominance.

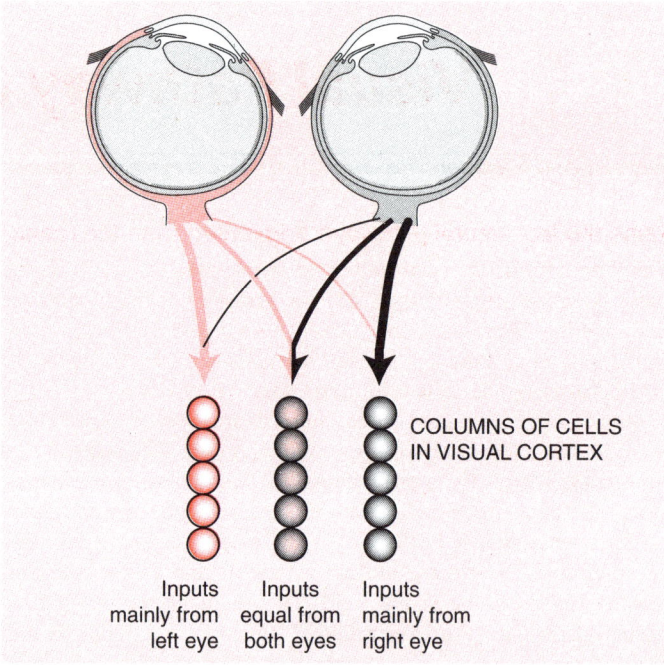

**Fig. 128.4**

### What are orientation columns?

The simple cells of the striate cortex, which respond to a particular orientation, are aligned in columns, disposed perpendicular to the cortical surface. These columns (Fig. 128.5) are referred to as **orientation columns**. The optimal stimulus-orientation of successively adjacent columns is progressively tilted, and within a width of 1 mm, all the orientations are represented.

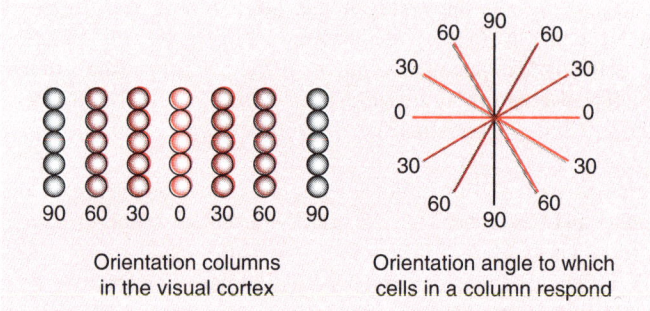

**Fig. 128.5**

### Name the cortical visual areas and briefly outline their functions.

**Visual area-1 (V1)** is variously known as the primary visual cortex (visual area-*one*), *Brodmann area 17* and the *striate cortex* (because the myelinated fibers of LGN that terminate there are visible as prominent stripes on a cross section of cortex). V1 is situated along the lips and walls of the posterior part of calcarine sulcus (Fig. 128.6). The peripheral part of the retina is represented in the anterior part of the area 17. The upper quadrants of the retina project on the upper wall of the calcarine sulcus and lower quadrants project on the lower wall of the sulcus. Macular part of retina projects mainly to the posterior part of area 17 and anteriorly, to a thin strip along the calcarine sulcus. The macular area occupies nearly one-third of area 17.

In V1, most cells respond optimally only to stimuli that have linear properties, such as a line or bar, and do not respond to small spots of light. These cells belong to two major groups, the **simple cells** and the **complex cells**.

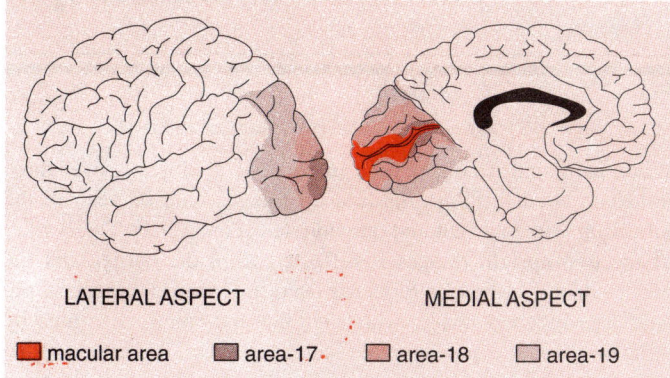

LATERAL ASPECT          MEDIAL ASPECT

■ macular area   ■ area-17·   ■ area-18   □ area-19

**Fig. 128.6**

**Visual area 2 (V2)** is also called the secondary visual cortex. It occupies much of area 18. Staining with cytochrome oxidase gives a striped appearance to the V2 cortex. The stripes are of two types: the **thick stripes** and the **thin stripes**. The interstripe regions are sometimes called **pale stripes**. Cells in V2 are sensitive to the orientation stimuli, to their color, and to their binocular disparity. V2 carries out more complex analysis of contours than V1, and *can respond even to illusory contours.*

**Visual area 3 (V3)** is a narrow strip adjoining the anterior margin of V2, still within Brodmann area 18. The functions of this area are not well defined.

**Visual area 4 (V4)** lies within area 19 anterior to V3. The V4 cells are responsive to both color and form. V4 cells are also responsible for **color constancy** – the ability of the visual system to identify different colors under different illumination conditions.

The **inferior temporal cortex** area is located in inferior temporal gyrus, the temporal pole and the lateral and medial occipitotemporal gyri. The cells of this area have the ability to recognize the same object regardless of its location in the visual field (**position invariance**). Some inferotemporal cells respond only to specific types of complex stimuli, such as the hand or face. Lesions of this region lead to specific deficits in face recognition (**prosopagnosia**).

**Visual area 5 (V5)** is the cortical area dedicated to detection of motion across the visual field. The area corresponds to the *junction of the parietal, temporal, and occipital cortices*, lying in Brodmann Area 19. The V5 cells respond to moving objects and forms and are therefore called *pattern direction-sensitive*. This is in contrast to V1 cells, which respond only to moving lines and edges and are therefore called *component direction-selective*.

### What are the theories of color vision?

The two main theories of color vision are trichromatic coding and opponent color-coding. According to the **trichromatic coding**, there are 3 types of cones: the S cone for yellow ($\lambda$=560nm) color, M cone for green ($\lambda$=530nm) color and L cone for blue ($\lambda$=440nm) color. The spectrum of S-cones is wide enough to sense red light. The letters S, M and L denotes the short, middle and long

wavelength of light that the cones absorb. All colors are coded at the receptor by differential stimulation of these 3 types of cones.

According to the **opponent color-coding theory**, there are three distinct opponent mechanisms. One captures *red-green* variation in the image: it is excited by red light and inhibited by green light. Another captures *blue-green* variation in the image: it is excited by blue light and inhibited by yellow light. A third opponent mechanism captures the *achromatic* (light-dark) variations in the image: it is excited by light and inhibited by dark. All the three opponent mechanisms are formed by summation or subtraction of signals from the three types of cones. Summation occurs when the photoreceptors facilitate each other. Subtraction of signals occurs when one photoreceptor inhibits the other.

### What are the different types of color blindness?

Colorblind people may be monochromats, dichromats or anomalous trichromats. **Monochromats** are unable to distinguish colors at all: they are of two kinds. *Rod monochromats* lack normally functioning cones. They see very poorly in bright light. *Cone monochromats* lack rods. They see very badly in dim light. Monochromats, especially cone monochromats are rarely seen. **Dichromats**, who can see two colors, are of three kinds. The *protanopes* (red-blind) and *deuteranopes* (green-blind) are often grouped together as 'red-green' blind. They confuse red and green objects, though they can usually distinguish yellow objects. **Tritanopes**, sometimes called 'blue-blind', are rare. They have little ability to distinguish blue from green. **Anomalous trichromats** can see all the colors but still have defective color vision due to the presence of abnormal pigments.

### How is color blindness inherited?

Color blindness is common in men (~8%) but much less common in women (~0.4%). It is inherited as a X-linked recessive character. Though hereditary color-blindness is very much commoner, defects of color vision can also be acquired as a result of diabetes mellitus or diseases of the retina, optic nerve or visual cortex (Fig. 128.7).

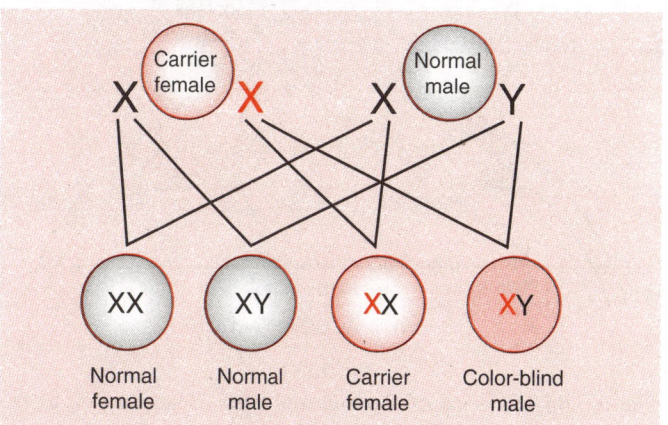

**Fig. 128.7**

### How is color blindness diagnosed?

The detection of color-blindness is important in selecting people for jobs in which it is necessary to be able to distinguish colored markings or colored light signals. A convenient quick test consists of a set of pseudoisochromatic plates, like the **Ishihara's Chart**.

# 129

# Motor Mechanisms of the Eye

### What is the ocular mechanism of accommodation?

The intraocular muscles are smooth muscles. They include the **ciliary muscle**, which is responsible for the process of accommodation, and the **iris muscles** (the sphincter pupillae and the dilator pupillae), which control the pupillary diameter.

Accommodation is the *ability of the eye to focus on objects at varying distances*. This is made possible by changes in the curvature of the *anterior surface of the lens* (Fig. 129.1). The radius of curvature of the anterior surface of the lens is 12 mm when the eye is adapted for distant vision (resting position) and 6 mm when the eye is accommodating maximally for near vision. The posterior surface of the lens hardly alters its radius of curvature, remaining nearly unchanged at 6 mm.

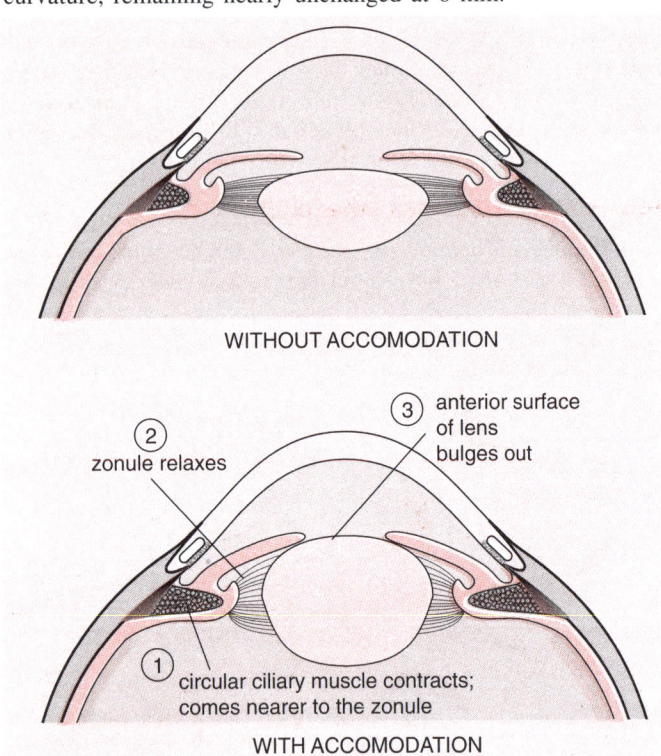

WITHOUT ACCOMODATION

② zonule relaxes

③ anterior surface of lens bulges out

① circular ciliary muscle contracts; comes nearer to the zonule

WITH ACCOMODATION

**Fig. 129.1**

The bulging forward of the anterior lens surface is due to the relaxation of tension in the lens capsule, which permits the elastic lens to assume a more spherical form. When the ciliary muscle contracts, it pulls the ciliary body forwards and inwards towards the lens: correspondingly, the tension exerted by the zonula on the lens capsule is reduced. As a result, the elastic lens bulges forwards. Paralysis of accommodation is called **cycloplegia** and can be induced by atropine and homatropine (cycloplegics).

### What are Purkinje Sanson images?

When a lighted candle is held in front of a subject's eye, three images, called the Purkinje Sanson images, can be seen in the reflection – two upright and one inverted (Fig. 129.2). The smaller of the two upright images is reflected from the cornea and the other, which is larger, is reflected from the anterior surface of the lens. The inverted image, which is faint and small, is formed by reflection from the posterior surface of the lens. The image formed at the anterior surface of the lens becomes smaller as the subject accommodates. The other two images do not show any change with accommodation. This shows that during accommodation, only the anterior curvature of the lens increases.

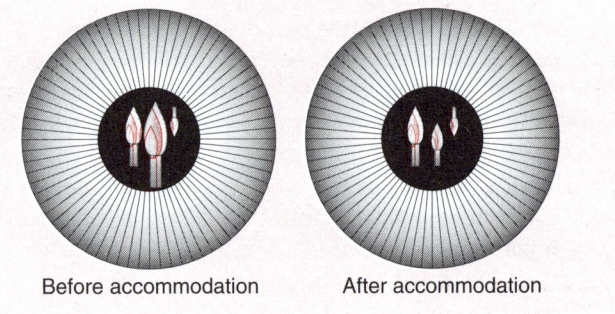

Before accommodation     After accommodation

**Fig. 129.2**

### What is the normal diameter of the pupil? How is it controlled?

The iris contains two sets of smooth muscles: the **sphincter pupillae**, a circular bundle running round the pupillary margin, and the **dilator pupillae**, arranged radially near the root of the iris. These two muscles regulate the size of the pupillary aperture. The normal diameter of the pupil varies between 2 to 4 mm.

### Describe the pathway of the light reflex.

When light is shone in one eye, there is an ipsilateral constriction of the pupil (**direct light reflex**) and simultaneously a constriction of the contralateral pupil (**consensual light reflex**). The reflex pathway is as follows (Fig. 129.3).

The afferent neurons from the retinal ganglion cells run in the optic nerve and partially decussate to enter the optic tract. The fibers pass through the lateral geniculate body uninterrupted, and enter the superior colliculus to relay in the **pretectal nucleus**. Fibers originating in the pretectal nucleus partly decussate in the midbrain and enter the **Edinger-Westphal (EW) nucleus** on both sides. (EW nucleus is one of the several cell groups in the 3rd nerve nucleus; it gives rise to parasympathetic fibers to the eye.) Parasympathetic fibers originating in the EW nucleus leaves the midbrain through the 3rd cranial nerve and relays in the ciliary

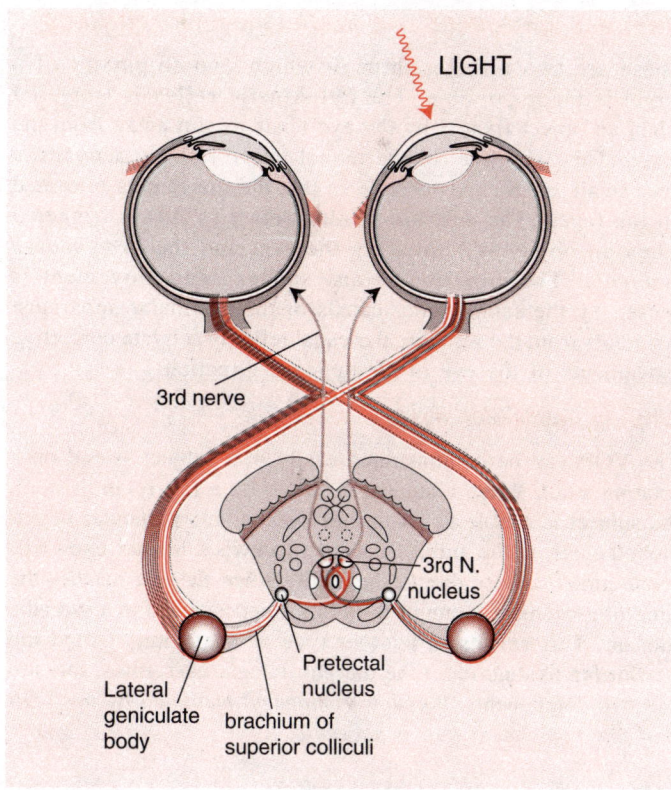

**Fig. 129.3**

ganglion. Postganglionic parasympathetic fibers leave the ciliary ganglion through short ciliary nerves to innervate the pupillary sphincter. Consensual reflex occurs because *light from each eye reaches the pretectal nuclei of both sides.* Also, the *pretectal nucleus of each side innervates the EW nuclei bilaterally.*

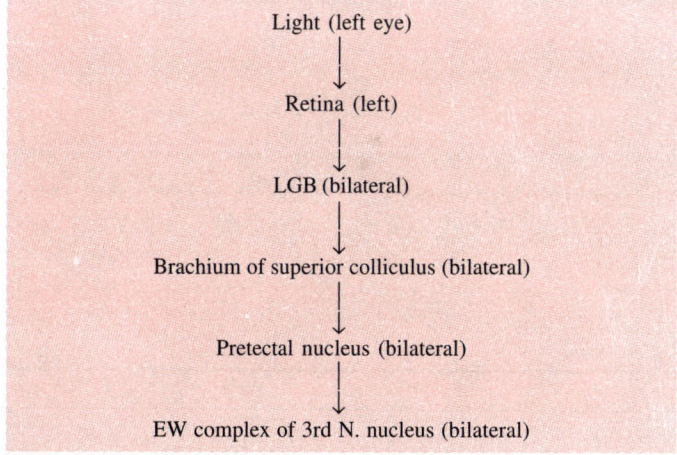

### What is near reflex? Describe the pathway of the near reflex.

The near reflex (or the accommodation reflex) occurs when an object on which the eye is fixed and focused is suddenly moved nearer to the eye. This is a synkinesis characterized by the triad of **convergence**, **accommodation** and **pupillary constriction**. The reflex is triggered by any of the several monocular and binocular visual cues of depth perception that suggest that the object is moving closer to the eye.

The afferent pathway of the reflex (Fig. 129.4) is the same as the visual pathway as it travels from the retina to the **cortical visual areas** (the striate, parastriate and the peristriate cortex). The fibers then travel through the *long associations fibers* to the **frontal eye field** (area 8). Projection fibers from the frontal eye field descend through the internal capsule and terminate on the oculomotor nuclear complex where they stimulate the **nucleus of medial rectus** and the **Edinger-Westphal nucleus**.

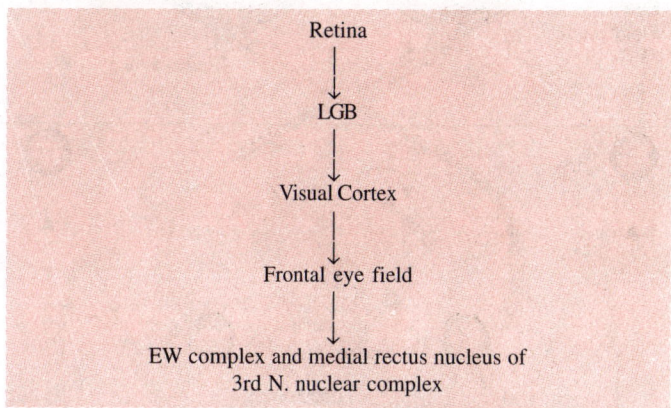

### What is an Argyll Robertson pupil (ARP)?

In *lesions of the pretectal nucleus* (which are almost always due to syphilis), the pupillary light reflex is abolished. However, the visual pathway to the cortex is unaffected. Also not affected is the pathway for accommodation reflex. Thus, there is pupillary constriction in response to the accommodation reflex but not in response to light reflex. (ARP=*A*ccommodation *R*eflex *P*resent).

### What are the different types of conjugate ocular movements?

Conjugate movements are of two types: saccadic and smooth pursuit. **Saccades** are rapid, involuntary jumps made by the eyes from one fixed point to another, as in reading. Visual perception is momentarily suppressed between saccades. This prevents blurring of vision during the interval in which the eye jumps from one target to fixate another. Saccades are seen not only when searching for new visual targets but also while gazing at a fixed target. The slight saccadic movements associated with a fixed gaze are probably beneficial in that they prevent adaptation of the photoreceptors. **Smooth-pursuit movements** occur when the eyes follow a target moving sideways (left-to-right or right-to-left). The movement of the target is relative. Thus, smooth-pursuit movements are also seen in a person looking out of the window of a moving vehicle.

### What is physiologic nystagmus?

A person seated in a moving vehicle tends to fixate any object of interest outside the window and follow it all the way as it moves back, with the eyes moving in *smooth pursuit*. Just after it passes by, the eyes fixate a new object, moving in a *saccade*, and again follows it all the way back. This type of rhythmic eye movements (nystagmus) comprising a slow smooth pursuit and a fast saccadic component is called **physiological nystagmus**. *The direction of the nystagmus* refers to the *direction of its fast component.*

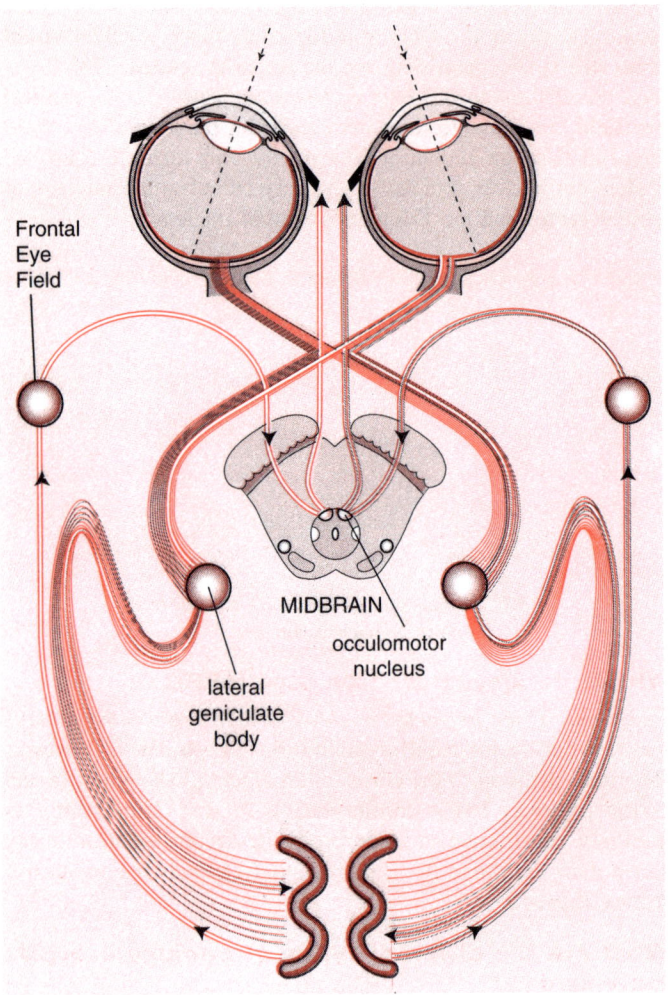

Frontal
Eye
Field

MIDBRAIN

occulomotor
nucleus

lateral
geniculate
body

**Fig. 129.4**

## What are optokinetic and vestibuloocular reflexes?

These are two reflexes through which smooth-pursuit of a target is made possible. The **optokinetic reflex** is triggered when an object fixated by the eye tends to slip away from the fovea. This 'slippage' of the retinal image reflexly activates a very small, *corrective saccade* so that the image gets relocated on the fovea. The **vestibuloocular reflex** (VOR) is triggered when an object is fixated by the eye, and the *head moves suddenly*. The direction of any sudden head movement is sensed by the semicircular canals of the vestibular apparatus. Afferents from the semicircular canal reflexly activate corrective movements of the eye in the opposite direction.

## What is vestibular nystagmus?

The VOR can be demonstrated easily in a subject seated on a rotating stool. When a subject is seated on a fast-rotating stool, the subject is unable to fix his/her eyes on any particular target. Nonetheless, if the subject rotates clockwise, his/her eyes will rotate anticlockwise due to the VOR. When the eye reaches the limit of movement, it jumps back to the opposite end in a saccadic motion. This results in another type of nystagmus called the **vestibular nystagmus**. Like the physiologic nystagmus, this too has two components: the *slow component mediated by the VOR and fast component that is saccadic.*

# 130

# Auditory Mechanisms

## Which characteristics of the sound waves determine the pitch, loudness and quality of the sound?

The **pitch** or **tone** of the sound is what is perceived by the human ear as higher or lower musical notes. It is directly related to its frequency: the greater the frequency, higher the tone. The **intensity** or **loudness** of a sound is related to the amplitude of the sound waves. The **quality** or **timber** of sound is related to frequency and amplitude of its component harmonics.

## What is the unit of frequency? What is the range of frequency response of the human ear?

The frequency, or the number of waves per unit of time is measured in Hertz (Hz) or cycle per second (cps). The normal human ear is sensitive to pure tone with frequencies in the range of *20 – 20,000 Hz*, with the *greatest sensitivity in the 1000 – 4000 Hz* range.

## What is the unit of loudness?

Loudness is measured in decibels (dB), which is a logarithmic scale. 1 Bel is defined as the number of times a sound is louder than a standard sound.

$$1 \text{ Bel } \frac{\text{Intensity of sound}}{\text{Intensity of standard sound}}$$

Sound intensity is proportionate to the square of sound pressure. Therefore:

$$1 \text{ Bel} = 2 \log \frac{\text{Pressure of sound}}{\text{Pressure of standard sound}}$$

One Bel is equal to 10 decibels. The pressure of standard sound is *0.000204 dynes/cm²*. *A sound that is barely audible at the threshold of hearing - has an intensity of zero decibels.* Since decibel scale is a log scale, every 10 decibels indicates a tenfold increase in sound intensity. The *usual loudness of speech is 65 dB*. A 100dB sound damages the peripheral auditory apparatus while 120dB causes pain. 150dB causes permanent damage to hearing apparatus.

## What is the function of the Eustachian tube?

The auditory (Eustachian) tube connects the middle ear to the nasopharynx. It serves to equalize the pressure on both side of the tympanic membrane. The auditory tube is usually collapsed so that debris and infectious agents are prevented from traveling from the oral cavity to the middle ear. In order to open the auditory tube, the tensor tympani muscle attaching to the auditory tube and the malleus must contract. This occurs during *swallowing, yawning and sneezing*. People sense a popping sensation in their ears as they swallow when driving up a mountain because the opening of the auditory canal permits air to move from the region of higher pressure in the middle ear to the lower pressure in the nasopharynx. *In children the direction of Eustachian tube is nearly horizontal,* hence they suffer from middle ear infections more often then the adults.

## What are the functions of the middle ear?

The tympanic membrane and the chain of ossicles serve as an **impedance matching** device. For hearing, the pressure waves in air must be converted into pressure waves in fluid. The acoustic impedance of water is much higher then that of air. Therefore without a special device for impedance matching, most sound reaching the ear would simply be reflected. Impedance matching in the ear depends on: (i) the *ratio of the surface area of tympanic membrane and that of oval window.* Since force is equal to pressure multiplied by the area, the pressure collected over the tympanic membrane is applied to the much smaller area of the stapes footplate and *a 17 fold net pressure gain is achieved.* (ii) The *mechanical advantage of the lever system* (1:1.3) formed by the ossicle chain.

## What is the acoustic reflex?

Two muscles are found in the middle ear: the tensor tympani and the stapedius. These muscles attach respectively to the malleus and stapes. (i) Contraction of **tensor tympani** pulls the manubrium of the malleus medially and decreases the vibrations of the tympanic membrane. (ii) Contraction of the **stapedius** pulls the footplate of the stapes out of the oval window. Loud sounds initiate a reflex contraction of these muscles, called the **tympanic reflex** or **acoustic reflex**. Thus they dampen the movements of the ossicular chain and so decrease the sensitivity of the acoustic apparatus. This action can *protect the acoustic apparatus against damaging sounds that can be anticipated.* However, *a sudden explosion can still damage the acoustic apparatus* because the reflex contraction of the middle ear muscles does not occur quickly enough.

## Describe the structure of the cochlea.

The part of the inner ear that is concerned with hearing is the cochlea. The **membranous cochlea**, the coiled portion of the inner ear is encased in the **osseous cochlea**. It takes approximately $2\frac{2}{3}$ turns from base to apex and is about 35 mm long in humans. It consists of three spiraling chambers: **scala vestibuli**, **scala media** (or the **cochlear duct**) and the **scala tympani**. The **vestibular** or **Reissner's membrane** separates the scala vestibuli from scala media while the **basilar membrane** separates the scala media from scala tympani. The basilar membrane is attached internally to the **spiral lamina**, which arises from the **modiolus**. Externally, the basilar membrane is anchored to the wall of the cochlea by the **spiral ligament**. Contained within the spiral ligament is a vascular structure – the **stria vascularis**. The scala vestibuli and scala tympani are continuous at apex of the cochlea because the cochlear duct ends blindly, leaving a small space called the **helicotrema** between the end of the cochlear duct and the wall of the cochlea.

### Describe the structure of the organ of Corti.

The organ of Corti (or the spiral organ) is the *functional unit of hearing*. It is made of the tunnel of Corti, hair cells, the tectorial membrane, and the nerve fibers innervating the hair cells (Fig. 130.1).

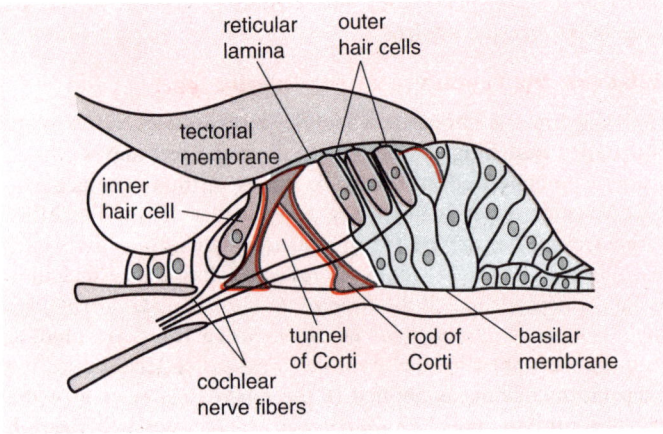

**Fig. 130.1**

The sensory **hair cells** are located on the basilar membrane, with their 'hair' or **stereocilia** projecting into the endolymph of the cochlear duct. These hair cells are arranged in a single row on inner cells and three rows of outer hair cells. The **tunnel of Corti** is formed by the inverted Y-shaped **rods of Corti** that support the hair cells. The stereocilia of the outer hair cells are embedded within a gelatinous **tectorial membrane** that overhangs the hair cells within the cochlear duct.

The cell bodies of the afferent neurons innervating the bases of the hair cells are located in the **spiral ganglion** within the modiolus, the bony core around which the cochlea is wound. 95% of these afferent neurons innervate the *inner hair cells, which are the actual auditory receptors*. Only 5 % innervate the outer hair cells, with each neuron innervating several of these outer cells. *Efferent fibers in the auditory nerve terminate on the outer hair cells.*

### What is endolymphatic potential?

The scala media is electrically positive (+80mV) relative to the scala vestibuli and scala tympani. This positive **endolymphatic potential** occurs due to the selective secretion and absorption of ions by the stria vascularis.

### What are the different types of fluids in the cochlea?

The scala media contains endolymph while the scala tympani are filled with perilymph. The composition of **perilymph** resembles that of plasma (high Na$^+$ and low K$^+$) while the composition of the endolymph resembles that of the intracellular fluid (low Na$^+$ and high K$^+$). The tunnel of corti is filled with perilymph.

### Describe the auditory pathway.

The cochlear nerve terminates tonotopically (i.e., in an orderly sequence representing the various frequencies) in the **cochlear nucleus** in the medulla. The fibers of the cochlear nuclei pass to the **olivary nucleus**, which is the first part of the auditory system to receive inputs from both ears. From each olivary nucleus, fibers project to the ipsilateral **inferior colliculus** via the lateral lemniscus and thence, to **medial geniculate body** of the thalamus. From the medial geniculate body, auditory fibers project to the **primary auditory cortex**. At all levels above the cochlear nuclei, there is strong bilateral representation of auditory information. Hence, *unilateral lesions of auditory pathway usually do not produce significant impairment of hearing.*

### Name the auditory areas in the cortex and outline their functions.

The **primary auditory cortex** lies principally in **area 41** in the *anterior transverse temporal* (Heschl's) *gyrus*. It projects to the **auditory association area (area 42)** which lies immediately behind area 41, and is formed by the posterior transverse temporal gyrus. The superior temporal gyrus behind the areas 41 and 42 forms the **higher auditory association area** (area 22). This area, which is better known as the **Wernicke's area**, is concerned with the interpretation of sounds and *comprehension of spoken language* (Fig. 122.1).

### Explain the mechanism of auditory transduction.

At the top of each hair cell, the stereocilia occur in several rows of increasing length. The tips of stereocilia are connected to the sides of the next tallest stereocilium by longer filaments known as **tip links**. These links control the opening of specific ion channels in the stereocilia, known as **transduction channels**, which are *very permeable to potassium*.

When the cochlear duct is displaced by pressure waves of perilymph (in the scala vestibuli), *a shearing force is created* between the basilar membrane and the tectorial membrane. This *causes the stereocilia to bend*.

Deflection of the stereocilia *towards the tallest stereocilium* causes K$^+$ channels in the apical portions of the stereocilia to open. The large potential difference between the endolymph (+80mV) and the hair cell interior (-70mV) creates a force of 150 mV that drives K$^+$ into the cell, depolarizing the cell. This depolarization in turn causes voltage gated Ca$^{2+}$ channels at the base of the hair cells to open, allowing Ca$^{2+}$ to enter the cell. The influx of Ca$^{2+}$ causes synaptic vesicles to release their transmitter (*aspartate or glutamate*) into the synaptic clefts, and the afferent fibers respond by undergoing depolarization and increasing their rate of firing. When the stimulus subsides, the stereocilia return to their resting position, allowing most Ca$^{2+}$ channels to close and voltage gated K$^+$ channels at the base of the cell to open. K$^+$ efflux returns the hair cell membrane to its resting potential. Conversely when the stereocilia are bent away from the tallest stereocilium, the tension in the links is reduced and more of the transduction channels become closed leading to hyperpolarization.

## What are cochlear microphonics?

Cochlear microphonics develop in the hair cells of cochlea before the development of action potential in auditory nerve fibers. It is called 'microphonics' because when these potentials are fed into a speaker through an amplifier, the sounds that elicited these potentials are accurately reproduced. This proves that the waveform of *cochlear microphonic potential is an exact replica of the sound wave that produces it.*

Cochlear microphonics is produced in the hair cell through **piezoelectric effect** – a property exhibited mostly by certain crystals of generating electricity when subjected to mechanical stresses. The following observations indicate that *cochlear microphonics are not biological in origin.* (i) It does not have a latent period. (ii) It does not have a refractory period. (iii) It does not show fatigue and is resistant to ischemia and hypoxia. (iv) Its frequency can be unusually high for any biological signal. (v) It persists several hours after death! Cochlear microphonics *do not have any major physiological role in hearing mechanism.* At best, it might have a role in boosting receptor excitation. Cochlear microphonics have been put to clinical use for testing the integrity of cochlea, since they *disappear when the hair cells are damaged.*

## What are the theories of pitch discrimination?

There are several theories of pitch discrimination like the resonance theory, traveling wave theory, standing wave theory, and telephone theory etc. that differ only in their finer points. Broadly speaking, there are only two theories of pitch discrimination – the place theory and the volley theory. A third theory – the duplex theory – combines both. According to the **place theory**, the brain infers the pitch of a sound from *the place along the basilar membrane,* which responds with the maximum displacement, stimulating the organ of Corti located on it. The basal end of the cochlea is sensitive to high frequencies and the apical end of the cochlea is stimulated by low frequencies. A particular variant of the place theory is the **traveling wave theory**, which says that sound is propagated in the cochlea in the form of a traveling wave in the basilar membrane. This wave travels from the base to the apex of the cochlea. The maximum amplitude of the wave occurs at a point along the basilar membrane that corresponds to the frequency of the stimulus. According to the **frequency theory** (also called **volley theory**), the frequency of action potentials set up in an auditory nerve fiber equals the frequency of the impinging sound (*volley = simultaneous burst*). Thus, a sound stimulus of frequency of 500 Hz would cause fibers within the auditory nerve to discharge at the rate of 500 times per second. However, since the maximum possible frequency of discharge in a nerve fiber is much lower than the highest frequency of audible sound (20,000 cps), the discrimination of high pitches cannot be explained on the basis of a frequency theory. The **duplex theory** combines the place and frequency theories. It holds that perception of pitch for frequencies up to 5000 Hz are due to nerve impulses firing in volleys, and that higher frequencies are perceived through the place of maximal excitation along the basilar membrane.

## What is the function of the olivocochlear fibers?

Although the cochlea is essentially a sensory organ, it is under some degree of motor control exerted through the **olivocochlear fibers**. These fibers innervate the outer hair cells, which seem to have a role in controlling the sensitivity of the inner hair cells to particular frequencies. It is a common experience that in a noisy radio channel, we are able to selectively hear the song or speech of our interest and ignore the rest. To some extent, this is made possible by *'tuning' our inner hair cells to selected frequencies.* Such *'tuning' is mediated by the olivocochlear fibers.*

# 131

# Deafness & Tests for Hearing

## What is conductive deafness? What are its causes?

Conductive deafness is a hearing loss that results from a failure of the outer and middle ear to transmit sound efficiently to the inner ear. It can result from various causes like: (i) wax or foreign body in external ear; (ii) middle ear infection (which can lead to a condition known as **glue ear**); (iii) **otitis media** (in which fluid accumulates in the middle ear) and (iv) **otosclerosis** in which the movement of the foot plate the stapes is impeded by the growth of bone around the oval window.

## What is sensorineural deafness? What are its causes?

Sensorineural deafness results when some part of cochlea or auditory nerve is damaged. It is quite commonly the result of: (i) **Traumatic damage** to the cochlea by very loud sound. A special variant of traumatic damage is the **boiler makers' disease** in which there is damage to only those hair cells of the cochlea that respond to the *high intensity sounds of the particular frequency* caused by industrial processes. (ii) **Presbycusis,** which is an age-related sensorineural deafness that specifically affects the high frequencies. (iii) Loss of hair cells can be caused by **ototoxic drugs** (e.g. streptomycin and neomycin). The ototoxic effect of some aminoglycoside antibiotics e.g. streptomycin and gentamycin may be due to direct reduction of the transduction currents of hair cells.

## What is tinnitus?

*Tinnitus* is the sensation of sound generated within the ear itself. It masks the natural sound reaching the ear, and thereby impairs hearing.

## What is masking?

The presence of one sound decreases an individual's ability to hear other sounds. This phenomenon is known as **masking**. In conductive deafness, there is less masking of air conduction by external noise. Hence, *hearing through bone conduction is better in conductive deafness than in normal individuals.*

## What are the bedside tests for hearing?

The common bedside tests for hearing are the voice test and tuning fork tests, viz., the Rinne's test, Weber's test and the Schwabach test. In the **voice test**, the distance at which the patient can hear a forced whispered voice with the opposite ear occluded in a quiet room is measured and the result recorded of each ear. A person with normal hearing should be able to hear words at about 5.5 m. The tuning fork tests are performed with a stainless steel tuning fork of *frequency 512Hz.* In **Rinne's** test, the base of a vibrating tuning fork is placed on mastoid process until subject no longer hears it, and then its prongs are held in air next to ear. A normal subject is still able to hear the sound, suggesting that his air conduction is better than bone conduction. A patient with conductive deafness however has better bone conduction than air conduction and the *Rinne's test is said to be negative in conductive deafness* and *positive in normal subjects.* In sensorineural deafness, air conduction remains better than bone conduction and Rinne's test remains negative. In **Weber's** test, the base of vibrating tuning fork placed on vertex of skull, allowing the sound to be conducted through bone to both ears. A normal subject hears equally on both sides. If hearing is deficient in one ear, it indicates either a sensorineural deafness in that ear or a conductive deafness in the opposite ear. *Bone-conducted sound is better heard in the ear with conductive deafness* because of reduced background noises conducted though air. The sound is poorly heard in the normal ear due to the *masking* effect of background noise.

In **Schwabach** or **absolute bone conduction** test, the examiner compares the bone conduction of patient with his own, assuming that he himself has a perfect hearing. The base of the vibrating tuning fork is placed first on the mastoid of the patient till he stops hearing the sound. The examiner then places the tuning fork on his own mastoid. If he still can hear the sound, it indicates that the patient's bone conduction is impaired, presumably due to sensorimotor deafness.

## When is Rinne's test false negative?

Rinne's test is usually positive in sensorineural deafness. However, in severe unilateral sensorineural deafness, Rinne's test is negative. Air conduction is absent, but bone conduction may be good because the sound is transmitted to the opposite cochlea through the skull bones. This result may mislead the examiner

|  | Normal | Conductive deafness | Nerve deafness |
|---|---|---|---|
| Rinne | Positive, i.e., air conduction is better. | Negative, i.e., bone conduction is better. | Positive, i.e., air conduction is better than bone conduction. |
| Weber | Hearing equal in both ears. | Hearing is better in (i.e., lateralized to) the affected ear. | Hearing is better in (i.e., lateralized to) the normal ear. |
| Schwabach | Bone conduction of subject and examiner are equal | Bone conduction of the subject is better than that in the examiner . | Bone conduction of the subject is poorer than that in the examiner . |

into making a wrong diagnosis of conductive deafness. In this situation Weber's test helps in avoiding a wrong diagnosis.

## Compare and contrast conductive and sensorineural deafness.

| SIMILARITIES |
|---|
| Both are associated with a rise in hearing threshold. |

| DIFFERENCES | |
|---|---|
| **Conductive deafness** | **Sensorineural deafness** |
| Defect lies in the external or middle ear | Defeat lies in the internal ear |
| Rinne's test negative | Rinne's test positive |
| Weber's test lateralized to the affected side | Weber's test lateralized to the normal side |
| Sehwabach test shows better bone conduction than examiner's | Schwabach test shows poorer bone conduction than examiner's |
| Can be corrected by hearing aids | Cannot be corrected by hearing aids |

## Describe pure-tone audiometry.

In pure tone audiometry, a pure tone audiometer delivers tones of variable frequency and intensity to the ear through earphones. The frequencies tested are at octave steps i.e. 125, 250, 500, 1000, 2000, 4000 and 8000 Hz. Each frequency is tested in the intensity range of 10 dB – 120 dB. Both the air conduction and bone conduction are measured. For each frequency, a series of tone pips are delivered at intensities above the patient's presumed threshold and the patient is instructed to signal every time he hears a sound. The intensity is reduced until no sound is heard and then increased in 5dB steps until half of the tone pips are consistently heard. This is the patient's threshold for that frequency. The threshold for the remaining frequencies measured in the same way. Thereafter, bone conduction is measured by putting a receiver onto the mastoid bone and repeating the test protocol. The results are charted as **audiograms** (Fig. 131.1 to 131.3).

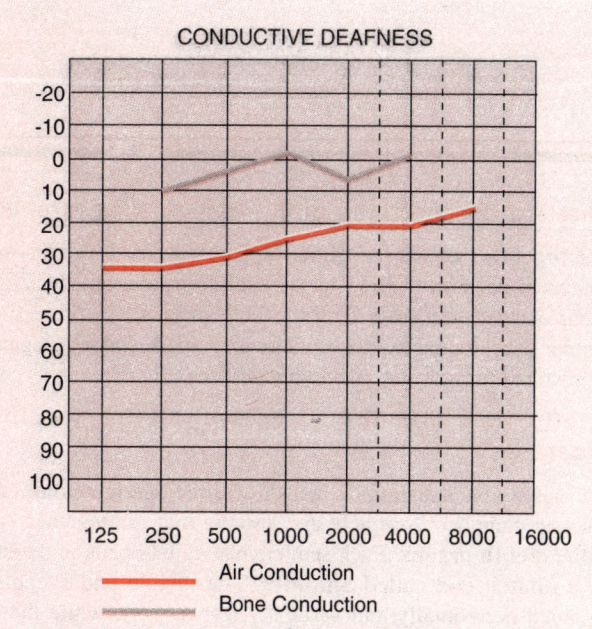

**Fig. 131.2 Conductive deafness. Bone conduction better than air conduction.**

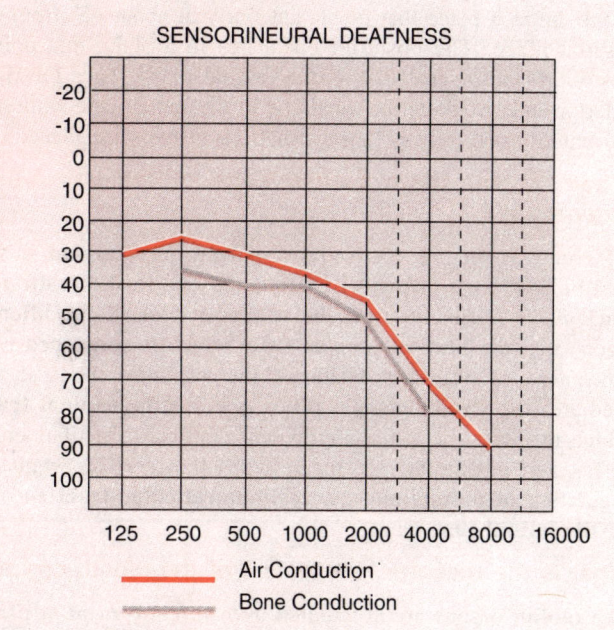

**Fig. 131. 3. Sensorineural deafness. Deafness is specially marked for higher frequencies as happens in presbycusis.**

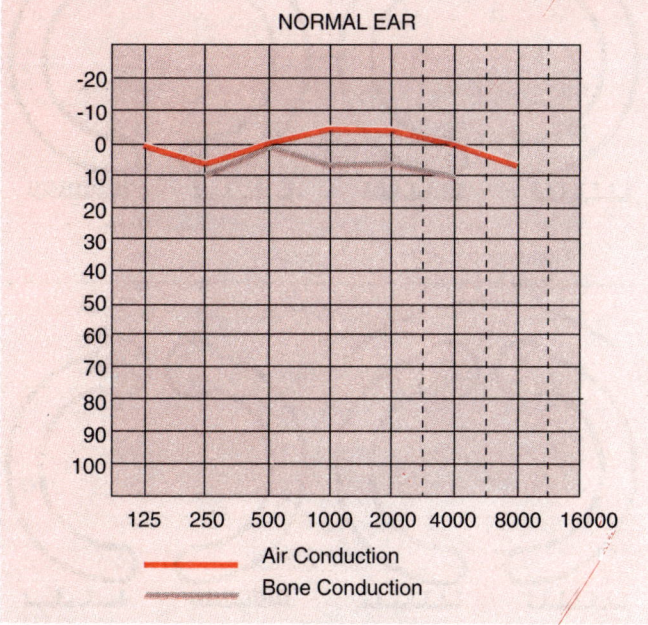

**Fig. 131.1. Pure-tone audiogram of the normal ear. Air conduction is better than bone conduction.**

# 132

# *Vestibular Senses*

## What are the functions of the vestibular apparatus?

The functions of the vestibular apparatus are: (i) detection of change in position of head by the otolith organs; (ii) detection of linear acceleration, also by the otolith organs; (iii) detection of angular acceleration by the semicircular canals, and (iv) regulation of posture through the vestibular reflexes.

## Briefly describe the structure of the vestibular apparatus?

The vestibular apparatus consists of three **semicircular canals** and two chambers – **utricle** and **saccule** that are together known as the **otolith organs**. Each semicircular canal opens in the utricle by a dilated end called **ampulla**. The utricle and saccule are arranged horizontally and vertically respectively, while the three semicircular canals (lateral or horizontal, anterior and posterior) are arranged at right angle to each other, with the lateral canal inclined at an angle of about 30° from the horizontal. The anterior canals lie in a plane that points anteriorly at about 45° from the sagittal plane. The posterior canal lies in a plane that points posteriorly at about 45° from the sagittal plane. Thus the right anterior and left posterior canals lie in the same plane while the left anterior and right posterior canals lie in the same plane.

## What are the main connections of the vestibular apparatus?

Afferents from the vestibular apparatus are carried in the vestibular branch of the VIII nerve and end in the **vestibular nucleus**. The efferents from the vestibular nuclei form different tracts, i.e., the **vestibuloocular tract** which is concerned with movements of eyeballs in relation to the position of the head, and mediates the vestibuloocular reflex, the **vestibulospinal tract**, which mediates the tonic labyrhynthine reflexes, vestibulocollic reflex and vestibular righting reflexes that are important for regulation of posture and the **vestibuloreticular tract** and the **vestibulocerebellar tract**.

## What is the receptor mechanism of the otolith organs?

The otolith organs are stimulated by *change of head position*. The sensory receptors are the hair cells, which are covered by a gelatinous membrane (the **otolith membrane**) containing small crystals of $CaCO_3$ called **otoliths**. The otoliths increase the specific gravity of otolith membrane as compared to endolymph. Hence, a change in the direction of gravitational pull exerted on otolith membrane bends the cilia of hair cells. This change in direction of gravitational pull occurs whenever head is tilted from its normal position. The force of gravity bends the cilia of hair cells more than the tilt of hair cell itself, thus changing the activity of hair cells.

The otolith organs are also stimulated by *linear acceleration*. As the head accelerates in linear direction, the otolith membrane having more specific gravity lags behind due to inertia. This causes the bending of cilia embedded in otolith membrane and excitation of vestibular afferents.

## What is the receptor mechanism of the semicircular canals?

The sensory portion of semicircular canal is located in the ampulla. The sensory epithelium in the ampulla is called a **crista ampullaris,** which consists of a ridge on which are located vestibular hair cells. These are innervated by primary afferent fibers of the vestibular nerve. The cilia projecting from the hair cells are embedded in a large gelatinous mass called the **cupula**, which is in loose contact with the wall of ampulla at its free end. As a result, it closes the lumen of the canal, preventing free circulation of endolymph. Movements of endolymph produced by angular acceleration of head deflect the cupula and consequently bend the cilia on the hair cells. The cupula has same specific gravity as

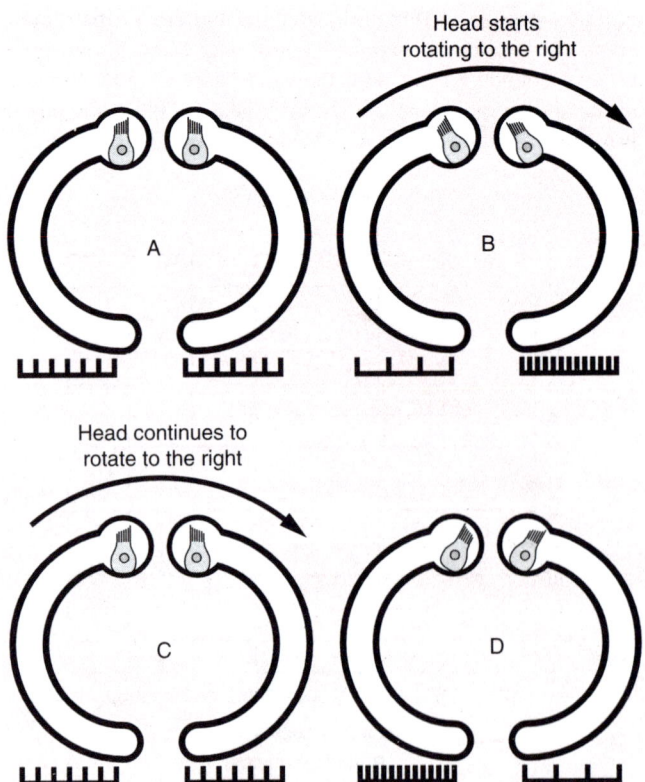

**Fig. 132.1**

the endolymph and so it is unaffected by linear acceleration force, such as that exerted by gravity.

### What is the vestibuloocular reflex?

The vestibuloocular reflex helps to maintain a stable image on retina during rapid head rotation. This reflex produce conjugate movements of the eyes in the direction opposite to and in an amount equal to the head movement so that the retinal image does not move. The reflex is triggered by angular acceleration of head.

### What is motion sickness?

It is a syndrome of physiological response during movement (travel) to which the person is not adapted. It is due to excessive and repeated stimulation of vestibular apparatus, which occurs due to rapid and repeated change in rate of motion while traveling. The psychological factor like anxiety about the unfamiliar modes of travel may be added up. The person feels nausea, vomiting, sweating, headache and disorientation. It can be prevented by avoiding greasy and bulky food before travel and by taking antiemetic drugs.

### What is caloric test?

The head is tilted backwards by 60° so that the horizontal canal is in the vertical plane. Then the auditory canal is rinsed with warm water. The heat from the auditory canal is conducted to the horizontal semicircular canal and this elicits convective currents that cause deflection of the cupula resulting in **vestibular nystagmus**. This test is performed to determine whether the canal is defective. This test is also one of several that are used to establish whether a comatose patient is brain dead.

### What is Meniere's disease?

Normally the balance between the ionic contents of endolymph and perilymph is maintained by specialized secretary cells in the membranous labyrinth and the endolymphatic sac. In Meniere's disease, there is disruption of normal endolymph volume resulting in **endolymphatic hydrops** (an abnormal distension of membranous labyrinth). There is loss of sensitivity to low frequency sounds accompanied by attacks of dizziness or vertigo that may be so severe that the patient is unable to stand. These attacks are frequently accompanied by nausea, vomiting and vestibular nystagmus.

# 133

# Olfactory & Gustatory Senses

## Briefly describe the olfactory receptors.

Olfactory stimuli are detected by specialized receptors located on the free nerve endings of the olfactory nerve fibers. The olfactory receptors are located within the olfactory mucosa is innervated by the olfactory nerve and some branches of the trigeminal nerve. The irritative character of some odors like ammonia results from stimulation of the free nerve endings of the trigeminal nerve. The olfactory mucosa contains three types of cells: (i) The **receptor cells** are bipolar neurons. Their dendrites terminate in a knob. Cilia project from the knob into the mucous layer of the olfactory mucosa. Their axons form the olfactory nerve. (ii) The **supporting cells** have a columnar shape. Microvilli extend from the surface of these cells into the mucous layer covering the nasal mucosa. (iii) The **basal cells** are stem cells from which new receptor cells are formed. There is a continuous replacement of receptor cells by mitosis of basal cells.

## Briefly describe the gustatory receptors.

Taste receptors (taste cells) are modified epithelial cells that communicate with gustatory nerve endings by synaptic transmission. They are located within **taste buds**, which, in turn, are located within **papillae.** Taste buds are located on the tongue papillae, hard and soft palate, epiglottis, and in the pharynx. Each taste bud is a cluster of 40-60 **taste cells** and numerous supporting and basal cells. Each taste bud contains a **taste pore** that allows substances to reach the interior of the taste bud. The taste receptors are located on microvilli, which project from the taste cells into the taste pores. Taste cells are innervated by branches of the VII, IX, and X, cranial nerves. The tactile and temperature receptors of the mouth, tongue, and pharynx are innervated by the V cranial nerve. The taste buds in the **anterior two-thirds** of the tongue are innervated by lingual branches of the **facial nerve;** the lingual nerve, which branches from the chorda tympani, is part of the facial nerve. The cell bodies are located in the geniculate ganglion, and the nerve terminals end in the **nucleus solitarius** of the medulla. The taste buds in the **posterior third** of the tongue are innervated by the **glossopharyngeal nerve.** The cell bodies lie in the superior and inferior ganglia of this nerve. The fibers relating to taste sensation terminate in the nucleus solitarius. Taste receptors in the **pharyngeal aspect** of the tongue and on the hard palate, soft palate, and epiglottis are innervated by fibers of the **vagus nerve.** The cell bodies are located in the superior and inferior ganglia of the vagus nerve and terminate in the nucleus solitarius.